OPIOIDS IN MENTAL ILLNESS:
Theories, Clinical Observations,
and Treatment Possibilities

ANNALS OF THE NEW YORK ACADEMY OF SCIENCES

VOLUME 398

OPIOIDS IN MENTAL ILLNESS:
Theories, Clinical Observations, and Treatment Possibilities

Edited by Karl Verebey

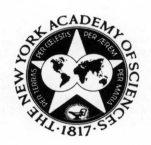

The New York Academy of Sciences
New York, New York
1982

Library of Congress Cataloging in Publication Data

Main entry under title:
Opioids in mental illness.

(Annals of the New York Academy of Sciences; v. 398)
Results of a conference held by the New York Academy of Sciences, Oct. 28–30, 1981.
Bibliography: p.
Includes index.
1. Opioids—Therapeutic use—Congresses. 2. Psychopharmacology—Congresses. I. Verebey, Karl, 1938–   . II. New York Academy of Sciences. III. Series. [DNLM: 1. Behavior—Drug effects—Congresses. 2. Endorphins—Pharmacodynamics—Congresses.   3. Mental   disorders—Drug therapy—Congresses.   4.   Narcotics—Pharmacodynamics—Congresses. W1 AN626YL v. 398/WL 104 061 1981]
Q11.N5 vol. 398 [RC483.5.064]   500s   82–19072
ISBN 0–89766–186–9   [616.89′18]
ISBN 0–89766–187–7 (pbk.)

PCP
Printed in the United States of America
ISBN 0–89766–186–9 (cloth)
ISBN 0–89766–187–7 (paper)

ANNALS OF THE NEW YORK ACADEMY OF SCIENCES

VOLUME 398

December 20, 1982

OPIOIDS IN MENTAL ILLNESS: THEORIES, CLINICAL OBSERVATIONS, AND TREATMENT POSSIBILITIES *

Editor and Conference Chairman
Karl Verebey

CONTENTS

---

* This series of papers is the result of a conference entitled Opioids in Mental Illness: Theories, Clinical Observations, and Treatment Possibilities, held by the New York Academy of Sciences on October 28–30, 1981.

Financial assistance was received from:

- BURROUGHS WELLCOME COMPANY
- CIBA–GEIGY
- E. I. DU PONT DE NEMOURS & COMPANY
- ENDO LABORATORIES, INC.
- HOFFMANN–LA ROCHE, INC.
- ICI AMERICAS, INC.
- McNEIL PHARMACEUTICALS
- MERCK SHARP & DOHME RESEARCH LABORATORIES
- NARCOTIC AND DRUG RESEARCH, INC.
- NEW ENGLAND NUCLEAR
- SCHERING CORPORATION
- THE UPJOHN COMPANY

INTRODUCTORY REMARKS

Karl Verebey

New York State Division of Substance Abuse Services
Testing and Research Laboratory
Brooklyn, New York 11217
and
State University of New York
Downstate Medical Center
Brooklyn, New York 11203

The scientific papers at this conference provide the first concentrated information on the influence on behavior of both internal and external opioids. The experimental observations of endorphins in animal and human subjects and the clinical experience with exogenous opiates suggest a relationship between behavior and the functional state of the endorphin system. These observations imply that some psychological disorders may result from or may be aggravated by an impaired endorphin-opiate receptor system.

On the basis of the similarities in the pharmacology of naturally occurring opioid peptides in the brain and exogenous opioids, it appears that normal human subjects are constantly under the influence of morphine-like substances. Thus exogenous molecules with opiate activity are not entirely foreign to the human organism. An acceptance of these facts by professionals and the public may free opiates from the social stigma and medico-legal restrictions that currently identify opiates entirely with addiction. Future research needs a prejudice-free environment to allow planning and performance of well-controlled clinical evaluation of opioids in the treatment of various psychiatric conditions.

The clinically observed antipsychotic effects of opiates seem very reasonable based on the anatomical distribution of opiate receptors and endorphins and on the biochemical and neurophysiological similarity between the effects of opiates and neuroleptic drugs. Confirmation of these findings are needed along with an attempt to identify diagnostic categories of mental disorders that respond to opiate treatment. The timeliness and need for new effective medication is demonstrated by the numerous reports describing tardive dyskinesia and other serious complications from the chronic use of antipsychotic drugs. Patients having such complications have to discontinue conventional antipsychotic medication and would be left without any psychopharmacological treatment. Effective psychoactive medication without the extrapyramidal side effects are needed. The effectiveness of opioid peptides in treating mental illness would suffer from the same difficulty as would the short-acting narcotic agonists such as heroin and morphine: they would have to be administered systemically at short intervals. For chronic treatment, the orally effective long-lasting opiates such as methadone and *l*-α-acetylmethadol would provide more suitable characteristics. With these thoughts I open this volume of the *Annals* hoping that it will provide the scientific foundation of a new and successful therapeutic approach for the treatment of mental illness.

PART I. HISTORICAL PERSPECTIVES

OPIATE USE IN ENGLAND, 1800–1926 *

Virginia Berridge

Institute of Historical Research
University of London
London, England

In 1857, when a Select Committee of the House of Lords dealing with the sale of poisons was taking evidence, it recorded the following exchange:

Q. Is much laudanum or opium sold by the druggists?
A. A very large quantity.
Q. By grocers?
A. By grocers in country towns.
Q. Do you know what it is used for principally? Who are the parties that purchase it?
A. I tried to discover that as far as I could, and was unable to do so; the druggists merely told me 'Anybody that asks for a pennyworth of laudanum I give it to them.'
Q. What quantity of laudanum or preparation of opium have you found sold in any case?
A. It is laudanum chiefly; and it is sold in pennyworths or twopennyworths. . . .[1]

Just over a century ago, opium was as easily available and acceptable as this in England. The more familiar historical images of Thomas De Quincey's *Confessions of an English Opium Eater*, or the mid-nineteenth-century Chinese opium wars are hardly a preparation for the prosaic reality of the everyday use of opium in English society at that time.

Yet what are now called "dangerous drugs" are severely restricted in contemporary English society. Public attitudes towards their use are distinctly harsher than those towards alcohol and tobacco. The first half of this paper will analyze how opium came to be seen in this way. The definition of opium as a "problem drug" was never simply a drug-centered matter of opium's own dangers. The natural corollary of this process of defining a problem is the evolution of a policy to deal with it. The second part of the paper will therefore examine why and how Britain developed the drug control policy she did in the first three decades of the twentieth century. We shall see how, in the 1920s, there were consistent attempts to establish a penal drug policy in England on the American model; but the 1926 Rolleston Report established an apparently liberal system of medically based control. This was the much-vaunted "British system" which operated until 1968.

THE NINETEENTH CENTURY:
THE OPEN SALE OF OPIUM

Turning to the nineteenth century, it perhaps needs to be stressed that opium was indeed, until 1868, freely available. The drug was imported, not from India, despite the flourishing Indo-Chinese opium trade, but from Turkey and

* The research on which this paper is based was originally funded by the Drug Abuse Council, Washington, and the United Kingdom Social Science Research Council.

1

to a lesser extent from Persia. It was bought and sold openly on the London drug market, either to organizations such as the Apothecaries' Company or to less august bodies. After grinding, and wholesaling, it ended up in any type of retail shop. There was no need for the vendor to have any sort of qualification. At this stage, indeed, even the pharmacists themselves were only just beginning to emerge as a profession. Opium was the aspirin of the time. Contemporaries, with few exceptions, accepted that it was just like any other commodity. Looking at the day book of a "chemist and grocer," for instance, one sees entries for ginger beer and half-grain morphia pills, or paint, turpentine, and laudanum; the drug was simply part of the everyday stock in trade of a general store.[2]

So much has been made of the dangers of such a situation (which undoubtedly existed) that it is important, too, to emphasize that in some respects, given the particular social and economic conditions that sustained it, this informal arrangement operated reasonably well. The poisoning death rate was relatively stable, between 5 or 6 per million population; home consumption had risen from 2–3 pounds per thousand population.[3] There was too, a general tolerance of the habit; it was not at this period categorized as a problem. Isaac Milner told the reformer of the slave trade, William Wilberforce, who was dependent on opium, which he took because of the pain of ulcerative colitis, "Do not be afraid of the *habit* of such medicines, the habit of growling guts is infinitely worse." [4] The drug had a central place both in orthodox medical practice and in self-medication. Even the medical profession, first involved in the question at the time of a life insurance case involving the Earl of Mar, tended to discuss only opium eating and longevity, not the nature of a separate condition defined as addiction.[5,6] That definition was yet to emerge.

The Development of an Opium "Problem": Public Health Questions

This relaxed attitude to opium use underwent considerable change in the course of the century. What can be called the public health reasons were a major cause of the shift in perceptions. The large number of deaths from opium poisoning, many of them accidental, the drug's use as an agent for would-be suicides, and its criminal usage (reflected in the inclusion of laudanum in the 1861 Offences against the Person Act) were increasingly publicized. Certainly the system of open sales could lead to horrifying mistakes—the selling of opium in mistake for other drugs, by ignorant and often semiliterate small shopkeepers, for instance.[7] The drug was heavily adulterated, too, so even orthodox medical preparations could vary wildly in the amount of effective opium they contained.[8]

The prime concern among reformers of the time was the dosing of children with opiate-based soothing syrups—Godfrey's Cordial, home-made infants' quietness, Mrs. Winslow's Soothing Syrup, and Dalby's Carminative among them. This is an issue that has always attracted the lion's share of the attention, both at the time and by historians subsequently.[9] But the reformers who criticized working class child-rearing practices were confusing cause and effect. Opiates did cause infant deaths—but many more babies died from malnutrition, general poor health, and living conditions. Opium was an effective palliative for the gastrointestinal disorders which in fact killed most young babies. The reformers were ignorant of working class living conditions and ignored popular belief in the positive power of the drug, that it was good for children, and "strengthening." Godfrey's and laudanum were given to children on the day they were born, and were even prepared in readiness for the event.[10]

This misunderstanding of the popular culture of opiate use arose out of the class tensions of the period. The dependence of middle class respectable people was much more acceptable than the spread of the habit within the working class. In the nineteenth century, the publication of De Quincey's *Confessions* was a matter for interested comment; but urban popular opium usage was seen as threatening. It was more worrying even than the undoubtedly widespread dependence within the rural population in the Fens of Eastern England.[11] There arose in relation to the urban working class the myth of "stimulant" or "recreational" working class use of opium. This was a belief, which owed much to De Quincey's endorsement of it in the *Confessions* (1821), that working people in the industrial towns were turning to opiates as a cheaper alternative to beer.[12]

In reality, much of this appears to have been founded on misconceptions of popular patterns of opiate use. The drug was very widely used in self-medication for all the small complaints for which no medical aid was available. Many people were undoubtedly dependent on it, but unconscious of the fact until supplies were cut off. Opium and alcohol were indeed linked. In orthodox medical practice, opium was used in the treatment of delirium tremens; and in popular usage, opium was well known as an antidote to over-indulgence in alcohol. In Liverpool, laudanum was on sale in the pubs; in the Fens, it was added directly to the beer. A basic misunderstanding of popular culture was displayed in the propagation of the "stimulant" myth.

PROFESSIONAL RIVALRIES AND CONSOLIDATION

The belief that an epidemic of working class recreational use threatened was a useful argument for the professional interests involved with opium, for it gave new force to their campaign for control of the drug. The theme of professionalization runs right through the history of opiate use in this and the succeeding period. The emergence and consolidation of professional groupings in the medical world had considerable impact on the way narcotic use was viewed and on the establishment of a problem of opiate use. The most practical impact this had was on the availability of opium. The restrictions eventually imposed on the sale of opium in the 1868 Pharmacy Act were in part the outcome of the public health campaign against the drug. They were also testimony to interprofessional rivalry.

Both doctors and pharmacists had designs to control the sale of drugs. The pharmacists won; the lax controls imposed on opium in 1868 owed much to the fact that pharmacists wanted the drug under their own professional control— but not too strictly controlled so that their trade in it would suffer.[13] This question of the conflict between professionalization and availability continued in other ways through the century, primarily in medical (and pharmaceutical) attempts to end self-medication with opiate-based patent medicines, chlorodyne in particular. There were also discussions at the end of the century on the question of the limitation of prescriptions (usually morphine ones), which marked an attempt to alter the balance of the doctor/patient relationship in favor of the former.

HYPODERMIC MORPHINE AND THE DISEASE THEORY OF ADDICTION

The allied questions of the use of hypodermic morphine and the disease theory of narcotic addiction were also connected with this professional impetus. Certainly hypodermic usage *was* a turning point in attitudes towards opium, and advocacy of the drug's use was in many ways over-free (although not every textbook suggestion was in fact taken up). But increasing medical concern about morphine addiction in the last quarter of the nineteenth century arose as much from the involvement of the profession itself as from the objective reality of an "epidemic." The epidemiological statistics are piecemeal, but suggest that numbers of addicts were small. Whereas morphine production was expanding, much of this was for export, not home consumption. Much opiate consumption and dependence had always been outside the medical ambit of control. But morphine by contrast had always been primarily a medically administered drug. Its users (and addicts) were reasonably well-to-do and likely, too, to have started on their habit by medical prescription. Many of them were, in fact, doctors themselves; a study of 580 cases admitted over 25 years to branches of the Norwood Sanatorium (in the period 1907–1932) found 250 male doctors and numerous chemists and dispensers.[14] There was some degree of hypodermic morphine addiction; that it became defined as a problem owed much to medical intervention and the professional perspective.

A similar process was at work in the elaboration of a disease theory of narcotic addiction. This was paralleled by the development of disease views of other conditions: insanity, alcoholism, and homosexuality most notably. It took place also at a time when physical disease entities—typhoid and tuberculosis— were also under discussion. The post-Darwinian revolution in scientific thinking encouraged the reclassification of conditions with a large social element in them on strictly biological lines. Addiction was part of medical expansion into new areas of specialism in the last quarter of the nineteenth century.[15, 16] The pioneers were mostly French or German—the work of Levinstein and Erlenmeyer was known in English medical circles soon after its publication. There were connections with American developments, too; and T. D. Crother's *Morphinism and Narcomanias from other Drugs* (1902) and J. B. Mattison's *The Mattison Method in Morphinism. A Modern and Humane Treatment of the Morphin Disease* (1902) joined Dr. H. H. Kane's earlier work for attention by English medical specialists.

English medical men began to develop their own version of disease theories. Most notable was the work of Dr. Norman Kerr. Kerr, chairman of the British Medical Association's (B.M.A.) Inebriates Legislation Committee, was closely involved in moves to secure the compulsory detention of alcoholic inebriates. His interest in narcotic addiction was an offshoot of his prime concern for alcoholic inebriety. Through his *Inebriety, its Etiology, Pathology, Treatment and Jurisprudence* (1889) and his establishment of the Society for the Study and Cure of Inebriety in 1884 (the "cure" part of the title was later dropped), he helped form the English version of disease theories. Soon no medical text was complete without a section dealing with this newly defined disease (often still defined as a form of "chronic poisoning") and medical-specialist texts, seminars, and debating papers were produced in increasing profusion. This was indeed a medical "growth area" by the turn of the century.

But the dimensions of disease theories owed much to moral emphases. In many respects the apparent scientific "progress" represented by their elaboration marked only the reformation of moral reactions to opiate use in a changed setting. Moral views were given scientific respectability through their propagation by medical specialists. Disease theories themselves were individualist and drug centered. Symptoms were described in terms of personal responsibility. Addiction was both disease *and* vice; it was, in the commonly-used term, a "disease of the will." According to Dr. Thomas Clouston, morphine addiction and alcoholism were the product of "diseased cravings and paralysed control." [17]

THE ANTI-OPIUM MOVEMENT

Doctors were reformulating and presenting old moral concepts in an area where, as examination of treatment methods very clearly shows, they really had little to offer. The moral emphasis within disease theory had its connections with temperance and anti-opium ideology. Many of the doctors most active in formulating concepts of addiction were also active in the anti-opium agitation. The Society for the Suppression of the Opium Trade (SSOT), founded in 1874, campaigned specifically against Britain's involvement in the Indian opium trade with China. It was a classic nineteenth century pressure group campaign involving meetings, pamphlets, and parliamentary pressure.[18] Its practical nineteenth century successes were limited. In domestic terms, the importance of the anti-opium agitation lay precisely in its connection with addiction theory. Many medical specialists involved in the establishment of disease theories were also workers in the anti-opium agitation. Norman Kerr himself, a temperance advocate, was active in the SSOT.[19]

There were striking parallels between medical opinion and moral propaganda on the subject. Both adopted the fundamental distinction between medical and nonmedical use of opium, which was to inform international control agreements and subsequent domestic narcotic policy. Storrs Turner, secretary of the SSOT, saw opium as "the physician's invaluable ally in his struggle against disease and death." But, he continued, "opium has been perverted from its rightful use into a means of vicious, because highly injurious, sensual pleasure." [20] The anti-opiumists, together with the medical specialists, saw moderate opiate use as impossible, dosages ever-increasing, and addiction inevitable. Doctors like Kerr and Benjamin Ward Richardson, a Vice President of the SSOT, and a leading English specialist on morphine addiction, strongly denied that moderation in opiate use could exist. Both disease theories of addiction and the propaganda of the anti-opium movement served to single out the addict as a distinct abnormal "deviant" personality, and addiction itself as a separately defined condition.

OPIUM "DENS"

The anti-opium campaign was linked also with the propagation of hostility to opium through racial feeling. The moral imperialism of the desire to save the "heathen Chinese" for Christianity and, at the same time, save them from smoking opium, was paralleled by increased domestic emphasis on the dangers of the opium den. Other factors lay behind this, too. Racial hostility at a time of increased immigration and economic decline was primarily reflected in turn-of-the-century anti-Semitic feeling, but also spilled over into anti-Chinese feeling, through competition for jobs and housing. In the last quarter of the nineteenth century, the popular image of the opium den appeared in fictional works like Dickens' *Edwin Drood* (1870), in Wilde's *Dorian Grey* (1891), in the numerous social surveys, and in exposes of low life which characterized this period. Clearly the stereotype had little foundation in reality.[21] All the evidence points to small numbers of opium dens, to the den not as a haunt of evil and mystery, but simply as a type of social club, a place where Chinese seamen enjoyed customary relaxation while on shore. An old Englishman, interviewed in Limehouse in East London, who as a boy had run errands for the Chinese seamen and had watched them smoke opium, put it thus:

> . . . you'd push a door open and you'd see them smoking. . . . I used to be in number 11, and in that house there on the second floor we had one bed, but on the ground floor, we had two, three beds. . . . It was quite natural for the people who lived in that house . . . they're ordinary working people that come in here and have their pipe, because they're paid off from the shipping and they have their pleasure time in the Causeway as long as their money lasts. . . .

Opium smoking, and the Chinese community, was never as extensive in London or Cardiff as it was, for instance, in San Francisco. But the association of opiate use with an alien minority fulfilled similar functions in both societies. When addiction did become a matter of social policy, attitudes towards opium smoking were initially much harsher.

By the end of the nineteenth century, opium was no longer freely available as it once had been. Medical practice was changing and the drug's effectiveness as a palliative was under challenge. Its use in insanity was declining; cannabis was much publicized as a more effective alternative. The bromides and chloral were replacing it in the treatment of pain and sleeplessness where it had long been the only standby. The 1908 Pharmacy Act placed opium and all preparations of opium and of poppies containing more than 1% morphine in the more restrictive part of the poisons schedule. Many patent medicines, as the B.M.A.'s investigations in the 1900s discovered, no longer contained opium, or included it in minute amounts.[22] The overall mortality rate for opium was in permanent decline. Restrictions on sale, together with the general improvement in living standards and in medical care that accompanied the "Great Depression" of the last quarter of the century, appeared to have achieved a considerable decrease both in levels of use and possibly levels of addiction to opiates too.

THE TWENTIETH CENTURY

But in the twentieth century controls were in fact increased. Legislation was no longer simply a matter of limitation of sale, but control of the user of the drug as well. For the first time the state became directly involved in the direction and implementation of policy—whereas the Pharmaceutical Society had "policed" the 1868 and 1908 Acts, under the lax control of the Privy Council Office. The second part of this paper will analyze how addiction became, not simply a "problem," but also a matter of public policy.

THE INTERNATIONAL CONTROL MOVEMENT

Certainly the restrictive attitudes developed in the course of the last quarter of the nineteenth century had much to do with the development of control policy. Few doctors would have argued against the notion that addicts should be patients, under medical control. The "problem" framework was at this professional level already established. The formation of control policy was affected primarily by the development of an international narcotics control movement and by particular emergency conditions during the First World War. The international narcotics control movement, which originated in the Shanghai Opium Commission of 1909 and culminated in the three Hague Conferences of 1911 to 1914 and the Hague Convention of 1912, have been presented as an example of American humanitarianism.[23] Humanity was not lacking, but the American decision to attempt to deal with the opium problem in the Far East (the original limited aim at Shanghai) also owed much to the imperatives of American power politics in that area. The "Open Door" policy, which the country hoped to use to gain economic advantage in China, America's recent acquisition of a Pacific power base in the Philippines, and a desire to mitigate the effects of an economic boycott of American goods in China, which had resulted from American anti-Chinese immigration legislation, were also involved. In short, the origins of international narcotics control were essentially self-interested; the desire of Bishop Brent in the Philippines to see some control of Far Eastern opiate use was in itself insufficient without the demands of strategic advantage.

Nor was America solely responsible for the institution of a world-wide movement of control. It was Britain who insisted on the inclusion of morphine and cocaine at the Hague Conferences. The Indian and Colonial Offices, at whose bidding the Foreign Office had acted, were indeed genuinely concerned about the spread of addiction to the two alkaloids. There is also little doubt that they hoped to use this issue to delay matters and divert attention from the Indo-Chinese opium trade.[24] It was Germany who insisted, largely to protect the interests of her own cocaine industry, that the Hague Convention must be of world-wide application. This ensured both a novel ratification procedure and a system of world-wide, not just Far Eastern, control. Domestic British narcotics policy was naturally thereby included.

THE WAR-TIME "EMERGENCY"

The Hague Convention had not come into force in Britain by the time war broke out in 1914. Desultory interdepartmental discussions about the likely form domestic legislation would take had envisaged little more than an extension of existing systems of professional control. Certainly no government department was keen to take on the responsibility. The pre-war discussions had been marked by much departmental "passing the parcel." At the outbreak of war, the Privy Council Office looked as if it was to be left holding it; the new system based on the Hague Convention could have been much like the old.

THE WAR-TIME EMERGENCY AND DORA 40B

Dramatic change occurred in 1916. An apparent "emergency"—the spread of drug use beyond the limited professional circle and the likely effect of this on the war effort—brought restrictive regulation. There was concern about the leakage of morphine, much of it smuggled on British ships, via Japan to the

Far East. But the main focus was the supposed spread of "recreational" cocaine use among soldiers on leave and mixing with prostitutes in the West End of London. Action under the Pharmacy Act was abortive. An Army Council order forbidding troops to possess the drug (and a wide range of others including cannabis and morphine) was introduced. This was followed, after intense police and army pressure, in July 1916, by Regulation 40B under the Defence of the Realm Act (DORA 40B). Cocaine and raw and smoking opium (but not morphine) were severely restricted, and possession and use as well as sale were controlled.[25]

DORA 40B was important in several ways. It marked the ascendancy of the penal over the professional approach. Doctors and pharmacists were consulted on several points and given some long-cherished aims, such as the limitation of prescriptions, but were largely left on the sidelines. The main driving forces were the police and the army. For the first time, too, a government department was directly involved. This was the Home Office, previously responsible for defending Privy Council Office decisions in the Commons. Sir Malcolm Delevingne, Assistant Under Secretary there, had taken charge in the weeks of hurried activity prior to the promulgation of DORA 40B.[26] He had been involved with drug matters in the Home Office since 1913, in particular in the operation of the inebriates acts, under which addicts could also be confined.

THE PENAL POLICY, 1916–26

The whole cocaine "epidemic" seems to have been blown up out of proportion. Professional dentists had hoped to use DORA 40B to withdraw the use of cocaine, a very effective dental anaesthetic, from nonprofessional dentists who mostly served working class areas. The investigations of a Commons Select Committee into the use of cocaine in dentistry, which extended its remit to cover the passing of the regulation itself, discovered that recreational use was very limited, confined to a few "broken down medical men." [27] The report was quietly shelved. Delevingne's own aim was to ensure that the regulations of 1916 set the tone of post-war government policy. Over the next decade, he had some success in laying the foundations of a policy towards narcotics that emphasized a penal and prohibitive approach, nonprofessional in its orientation, with considerable similarities to American practice at the same time. The 1920 Dangerous Drugs Act extended to morphine and made permanent the war-time regulations (Article 295 of the Treaty of Versailles had given control over the Hague Convention to the League of Nations and the implementation of that agreement formed part of the peace settlement). Regulations made under the Act in 1921 and 1922 severely restricted medical and pharmaceutical control of narcotics. The 1923 Dangerous Drugs (Amendment) Act imposed harsher penalties and more extensive police powers of search. This was the era of the "dope fiend" and the "alien trafficker." The Billie Carleton case of 1919 and the Freda Kempton affair in 1923, the conviction of Edgar Manning, a black drug trafficker, formed the backdrop to a hard-line policy.

The Home Office was attempting to defeat the medical profession's own conception of addiction. The regulations forbade doctors to prescribe narcotics for themselves; doctors not in actual practice were prohibited from prescribing. There were reports of addict doctors on the run from the police; Delevingne suggested that the police circulate a blacklist of addicts and doctors. There was disapproval of medical maintenance doses for addicts and of methods of gradual withdrawal. But the profession fought back. Intense grass-roots opposition forced the modification, or withdrawal, of the more restrictive regulations.[28] The dilemma for treatment and maintenance imposed by a penal policy was best expressed in an addict's own words. Thomas Henderson, addicted to morphia for nearly 40 years, called at the Home Office in 1922 to put the maintenance case:

> I claim to be a useful life to the state, teaching others to earn their living and only asking to be permitted to earn my own, and I appeal to you . . . to see with unbiased eyes, and I implore you . . . not to crush me out under this new law . . . morphia has not corrupted me . . . it has never tempted me to do wrong in any respect. . . . I only ask to be left in the hands of my doctor. . . .[29]

It was the usurpation of the profession's function that caused intense disquiet, both among ordinary general practitioners (GPs) and among addiction specialists in particular, who were concerned to defend the whole disease structure of addiction built up over the previous half century. Dr. W.E. Dixon, Reader in Pharmacology at Cambridge, put this forcefully in a letter to the *Times* in 1923.

> We do not seem to have learnt anything from the experience of our American brethren. . . . Cannot our legislators understand that our only hope of stamping out the drug addict is through the doctors, that legislation above the doctors' heads is likely to prove our undoing and that we can no more stamp out addiction by prohibition than we can stamp out insanity? [30]

The case for medical control and the maintenance of disease theory could hardly have been more clearly put.

The questions of treatment and maintenance led in 1924 to the appointment of a Departmental Committee on Morphine and Heroin Addiction under the Chairmanship of Sir Humphrey Rolleston, President of the Royal College of Physicians (with W.E. Dixon among its members). Its 1926 report reasserted medical control and established what became known as the "British system" of control. Addiction was seen within a medical model, as a doctor's proper concern. Regular maintenance doses were allowed, compulsory notification to the Home Office was abandoned, and a medical tribunal, not the courts, was to deal with "rogue" doctors and the doctor addict.[31]

The system certainly operated smoothly enough until the late 1960s. The drug explosion of that decade brought a tightening of control, the removal of addicts to treatment clinics, compulsory notification, the licensing of doctors able to prescribe heroin, and later methadone—the rest is current affairs. But the Report of 1926 is worth looking at in more depth. The Report did not mark the establishment of a liberal medically based system in the way it is often represented. Medical and penal approaches were not mutually exclusive. The Home Office remained in overall control, even if its guiding hand was muted for the next 40 years. Doctors themselves were no longer in any case professionally autonomous. They were involved in the machinery of state. In the case of narcotics, the role of the Ministry of Health, established in 1919 and a poor second to the Home Office in the departmental in-fighting for responsibility for dangerous drugs in 1920, was crucial. It was through that Ministry that the Home Office set up Rolleston as a medical committee on addiction; and important members of the committee were on the staff of the Ministry. The "British system" was in fact, a compromise, absolutism in a velvet glove. The medical profession was allowed the appearance of total professional self-regulation so long as addicts were, as they were in the 1920s, mainly middle class and primarily medical or iatrogenic in origin.

The official language of the Rolleston report seems far removed from open sale over a grocer's shop counter. What can one then conclude about the establishment of narcotic use as a social problem and eventually as social policy? Perhaps the most obvious answer is that reactions and later policies towards narcotics have always been much more than the result of a simple humanitarian desire to reduce their dangers. Ideals and self-interest have been closely linked, narcotics being the scapegoat for a complicated interaction of professional strategies, class tensions, and international power politics. Public opinion, and politicians in Britain at least, have historically had little influence to bear; and policies were evolved through the strategies and collaboration of elite groups of doctors and administrators. Even the analysis of the roots of this involvement is unlikely to change that.

ACKNOWLEDGMENTS

I am grateful to members of staff of the Addiction Research Unit of the Institute of Psychiatry, University of London for advice and assistance and especially to the Honorary Director, Professor Griffith Edwards. My thanks are also due to Lynda Bush for typing this paper.

REFERENCES

1. PARLIAMENTARY PAPERS. 1857. Report from the Select Committee of the House of Lords on the Sale of Poisons etc. Bill, XII: qs 1047–1054.
2. WELLCOME MANUSCRIPT COLLECTION. 1847–1899. Ms 978. W. Armitage's prescription book. London.
3. BERRIDGE, V. & N. RAWSON. 1979. Opiate use and legislative control: A nineteenth century case study. Soc. Sci. Med. 13A: 351–363.
4. POLLOCK, J. 1977. Wilberforce. Constable, London.
5. CHRISTISON, R. 1832. On the effects of opium eating on health and longevity. Lancet (1): 614–617.
6. BERRIDGE, V. 1977. Opium eating and Life Insurance, British J. Addiction 72: 371–377.
7. ANON. 1858. Poison Shops. Lancet (1): 486.
8. ANON. 1853. The Analytical Sanitary Commission. Lancet (1): 64, 116–117, 251–253.
9. ANON. 1894. Labour and the Poor. The Manufacturing Districts. Manchester. Morning Chronicle. Letter IX: 5.
10. PARLIAMENTARY PAPERS. 1843. Childrens Employment Commission: Appendix to the Second Report of the Commissioners (Trades & Manufactures): Report by R.D. Grainger on the Employment of Children and Young Persons in the Manufactures and Trades of Nottingham, Derby, Leicester, Birmingham and London and on the State, Condition and Treatment of Such Children and Young Persons. XIV, part 1: f.61–62.
11. BERRIDGE, V. 1979. Opium in the Fens in nineteenth century England. J. Hist. Med. All. Sci. 34(3): 293–313.
12. DE QUINCEY, T. 1822. Confessions of an English Opium Eater. Taylor and Hessey, London.

13. ANON. 1868. Report of the Pharmacy Bill Committee to the General Medical Council. Br. Med. J. (2): 39.
14. NORWOOD SANATORIUM LIMITED. 1932. Survey of a quarter of a century of the treatment of Alcoholism and other Drug Habits. Being the 25th Report of the Rendlesham and Beckenham Branches of the Norwood Sanatorium Limited.
15. PARSSINEN, T. & K. KERNER. 1980. Development of the disease model of drug addiction in Britain, 1870–1926. Med. History 24: 275–296.
16. BERRIDGE, V. 1979. Morality & medical science: Concepts of narcotic addiction in Britain, 1820–1926. Ann. Sci. 36: 67–85.
17. CLOUSTON, T. S. 1890. Diseased cravings and paralysed control. Edinburgh Med. J. 35: 508–521, 689–705, 793–809, 985–996.
18. JOHNSON, B. 1975. Righteousness Before Revenue: The Forgotten Crusade Against the Indo-Chinese Opium Trade. J. Drug Issues 5: 304–336.
19. ANON. 1892. The medical aspects of the opium question. Friend of China 13 (supplement to main issue).
20. TURNER, F. S. 1876. British Opium Policy and its Results to India and China. Sampson Low, London.
21. BERRIDGE, V. 1978. East End opium dens and narcotic use in Britain. London J. 4(1): 3–28.
22. BRITISH MEDICAL ASSOCIATION. 1909. Secret Remedies, What They Cost and What They Contain. British Medical Association, London.
23. TAYLOR, A. H. 1969. American Diplomacy & the Narcotics Traffic 1900–1939. University Press, Durham, NC.
24. FOREIGN OFFICE (F.O.) PAPERS, 1910–1911. Files dealing with negotiations leading to the Hague Conference of 1911: F.O. 371/1330, 1331, 1332, 1334, F.O. 415/5, 6.
25. BERRIDGE, V. 1978. War Conditions and Narcotics Control: The passing of Defence of the Realm Act regulation 40B. J. Social Policy 7: 285–304.
26. PRIVY COUNCIL OFFICE (PCO) PAPERS. 1916. Home Office memorandum to inter-departmental conference, June 1916: PCO8/803.
27. PARLIAMENTARY PAPERS 1917–1918. Report of the Committee on the use of Cocaine in Dentistry, VIII: 151–157.
28. BERRIDGE, V. 1980. The Making of the Rolleston Report 1908–1926. J. Drug Issues 10(1): 7–28.
29. HOME OFFICE (H.O.) PAPERS 1922–1923. Cases under the Dangerous Drugs Act: H.O. 45/432, 886.
30. THE TIMES, 1923. Letter from W. E. Dixon, 21 March.
31. ROLLESTON REPORT, 1926. Report of the Departmental Committee on Morphine & Heroin Addiction: His Majesty's Stationery Office, London.

HISTORY OF OPIATE USE IN
THE ORIENT AND THE UNITED STATES

E. Leong Way

Department of Pharmacology
School of Medicine
University of California, San Francisco
San Francisco, California 94143

This is a very different type of a meeting on opioids from ones that I have had the opportunity to attend and participate in. In the past, the conferences had rather narrow limits and were restricted either to the medical application of opiates for the treatment of pain or more often to various aspects of their misuse or abuse. With the recent discovery of peptides with morphine-like properties in the brain and other organs, a new door has been opened. We now find methionine- and leucine-enkephalin, β-endorphin, and dynorphin, to name but a few, present in neurons that were hitherto unrecognized and undoubtedly have important roles. Aberrations in the disposition, synthesis, and degradation of these peptides in the brain could lead to increased or decreased neuronal activity and ultimately to pathologic states. This possibility gives credence to the belief which many of us have held and which has been most eloquently expressed by Dole and Nyswander, that compulsive heroin use may be a manifestation of a metabolic disorder.

In the next few days we are going to examine some of the potential applications of opioids in mental illness. That we are going to hear about these possibilities does not, of course, mean that such applications have been established. However, in the light of the discovery of the endorphins, it would be conservatism to the extreme not to consider new avenues for the use of opioids. I hasten to add that such approaches must be made with well-designed studies to yield as much objective evidence as possible.

In recent years, the restrictions placed on narcotic usage by the so-called Moral Majority, which in actuality is a vocal activist minority, have greatly hampered thinking about the therapeutic applications of narcotics, other than for pain, and even this use has been subjected to rigid regulation. Now that we know that there are substances in our own body with opioid-like activity and much greater potency than heroin, it is time to readdress our thinking and educate those who attempt to impose their attitudes on the medical applications of opioids.

This should not be too difficult because history has shown repeatedly that medical and social attitudes towards narcotic use and misuse do change with time. All that is needed is more activism, and if this can be supported by hard data, a more healthy climate for rational narcotic usage can be established. The evanescent nature of social attitudes can be exemplified by an examination of the history of opioid use.

The assignment to discuss the history of opiate use only in the Orient and the United States seemed inappropriate if not incongruous to me. A more apt topic might have been opiate use in Great Britain and the United States because the two countries have much more in common with respect to ethnicity, culture,

0077-8923/82/0398-0012 $1.75/0 © 1982, NYAS

and the time-frame of opiate use and misuse. Despite the wide diversity in Oriental and Western culture, I shall try to justify the arbitrariness of the conference chairman, Dr. Verebey, and meet the challenge of the task. To do this, I shall narrow the focus on the Orient mostly to China and utilize my dual ethnicity to point out that some interesting parallelisms can be drawn with respect to social attitudes on opiate misuse in two diverse cultures. I hasten to state at the outset, since I am neither a historian nor a social scientist, that I am speaking only as a pharmacologist with a long and abiding interest in narcotic use and misuse. For this reason, I have leaned heavily on the experts in the field and have not checked on the primary sources. The secondary citations, in the main, relate to those not directly concerned with opiate use, but with dates and events in Chinese history [1-3] and to discussions concerning social attitudes with respect to opiate misuse.[4-7] In defense of myself I have heard "plagiarism" defined as when you steal from one and "research" when you steal from a dozen.

The parallels with respect to social attitudes related to narcotic use and misuse between China and the United States might well apply to many other countries. The story is often the same even though the chronology may be different. In the beginning, the use of the drug is well-accepted with many strong advocates. As the liabilities of chronic narcotic usage become increasingly apparent, tolerance to misuse changes to disfavor and then intolerance as reformers and moralists gradually impose their opinions and ways on a diffident majority.

Although the history of opium dates back several millenia, its use in China is of relatively recent origin, being for little more than a thousand years. Before and after this time, China enjoyed many periods of great cultural advances. While I would hardly venture that opium caused the fall of the Chinese empire, it ultimately provided the economic and political fuel to accelerate the decay of a great civilization that occurred a little over a thousand years after its advent.

Most writers [5, 6, 8] ascribed the introduction of opium into China by Arab traders during the Tang Dynasty (618–907 A.D.), a glorious period in Chinese history. It was a time of great prosperity and cultural progress. Historians write of the Tang Dynasty as the golden period of literature and art. Block printing and porcelain were invented. There were many famous poets and all forms of religion were greatly honored. The freedom of thought and study attracted many scholars to study in China. The Arabs, who brought the opium, also introduced Islam. Large numbers of the Muslims settled in the country, and some occupied high positions in the Tang court, but in time they were gradually assimilated.

Prior to the Tang Dynasty, China had been united as an empire 800 years earlier by Chin Shih Huang, who established the Chin Dynasty (221–206 B.C.), built highways and the Great Wall, standardized the written language, currency, weights, and measures, but also imposed thought control and burned books. His magnificent tomb has only recently been discovered in Xian and is still undergoing excavation. Chin's brief reign was followed by the Han Dynasty (206 B.C.–221 A.D.). Education flourished and civil service examinations were introduced. Trade routes were opened to the West and Chinese goods and culture spread across Asia. Paper was invented in 105 A.D. Corruption and chaos led to the disintegration of the Han Dynasty and although there were short periods of reunification, turmoil and frequent wars occurred until the establishment of the Tang Dynasty.

After the fall of the Tang dynasty, there were again brief periods of anarchy until reunification in the Sung dynasties (960–1284 A.D.). Printing from movable type was introduced. The period was renowned for its great painters and elegant simple porcelain. The reign then fell to Jenghis Khan and his invading Mongols; and under his son, Kublai Khan, the Mongols established the most extensive empire in world history. During this period (Yuan Dynasty 1280–1368), Marco Polo visited China and called the attention of the world to the riches in the Far East. This, of course, led ultimately to the discovery of America in 1492 by Columbus and begins the entwining threads of our story. By this time, however, Emperor Chu had disposed of the oppressive Mongols, and established the famed Ming Dynasty (1368–1644).

Great advances were made in sciences and literature in the Ming dynasty. Explorations were encouraged and there were seafaring expeditions throughout southeast Asia and to Africa. Near the end of the period, Jesuit missionaries came and brought with them the sciences of the European Renaissance. In this interim, the colonization of the Americas had started at Jamestown in 1607.

Between the intervening years of the Tang and Ming dynasties, which amounted to less than a millenium, there is little mention of the addicting liabilities of opium although its medicinal virtues were immediately and widely recognized. Mention is made of the use of opium for the treatment of pain and diarrhea, but not its addiction liability, in Pen Tsao Kang Mu, a voluminous materia medica treatise published in 1590 which has been republished and expanded many times with commentaries. It was originally written by Li Shin-Chen (1518–1593) who spent a lifetime studying and compiling the pharmacology of native plant and animal products. The social problems with opium appear to have arisen only after opium smoking began at some time toward the end of the Ming and the beginning of the Ching dynasty.

The Ching dynasty (1644–1911) was established after the Manchus, under the pretext of helping the Ming emperor exterminate bandits, occupied Peking and seized the government. The Manchus assimilated China's superior culture and encouraged arts and literature. During the initial 150 years much progress was made under three great successive rulers (Kang Hsi, 1662–1723); Yung Cheng, 1723–1736, and Chien-Lung, 1736–1797), but problems with opium smoking were already in evidence. At the same time we find the spawning of a revolution and the founding of the United States. Insofar as opium misuse was concerned, the gaps in time between the two countries were narrowing rapidly, but let us first get back to opium smoking.

The practice of smoking opium appears to have originated in the Dutch East Indies whence it spread to Formosa and then to China. In China, it followed the introduction of tobacco smoking by the Portuguese late in the 16th century.[9] In time, the Chinese smoked tobacco in combination with opium and later the smoking of opium alone prevailed. In subsequent years it became a problem peculiar to the Chinese, and it was carried to other countries by Chinese immigrants.

It is interesting to contrast the use of opium in India with that in China during these early times. According to Blum citing Chopra,[5] opium use in India probably developed in the 14th century and it was cultivated in the 16th century. The drug was popular among all classes. It was taken as a pill or as a liquid, the nobility drinking a mixture of wine, opium, and hemp. It was and continued to be used over the centuries as a folk medicine. It was used to soothe the crying of infants who were ill or when the mother had to abandon the child temporarily. Opium smoking was uncommon, but in time small sectors adopted the habit. However, in spite of the fact that the drug was readily accessible and its use was widespread, at no time has India been considered to have had a major opium problem. A puzzling mystery remains, why the Chinese became plagued by the narcotic and the Indians did not. Blum speculates on some possible explanations, but does not arrive at a definite conclusion.[5]

Whether opium use was considered to be dangerous, corrupting, and degenerating or relatively innocuous depended often on the eyes of the beholder.[5, 9] Missionaries, including physician missionaries, mostly condemned the practice as a vice. As Kramer writes,[9] "The missionary saw opium as a hindrance to the propagation of the Christian faith in China, or conversely, that the absence of Christianity deprived the Chinese of protection from the vice." On the other hand, other physicians, more often those employed by British companies favoring opium trade with the Chinese, while conceding some excessive use, emphasized the predominance of moderate use without deleterious effects. The British Inspector General of the Imperial Maritime Customs in his 1881 report [10] expressed puzzlement as to why the Chinese were opposed to the traffic when it was such a rich source of revenue to the Chinese government and only two-thirds of one percent of the population could be damaged by the habit. Based on an estimated population between 300 to 400 million at the time, "only" about 2,000,000 people were suffering.

By the 18th century the social problems engendered by increasing opium use, coupled with the drain on the treasury, compelled the Emperor Yung Cheng to issue an edict in 1729 prohibiting the sale of opium and decreeing punishments ranging from imprisonment to death by strangulation for the sellers of opium. The user was exempted. But, as the practice multiplied, punishment for the user was also decreed, still to no avail. Like prohibition laws in this country, the manifestos were largely ignored and opium consumption and importation in China continued to increase. Eventually, the bans became obsolete when the opium trade was legalized after the Opium Wars.

Reliable estimates of the extent of narcotic addiction are always difficult to obtain, and this was and still is particularly true in the Orient. The complexities were pointed out by Lindesmith.[4] Regardless of the system of control, smuggling has been rife throughout the Far East for centuries wherever there is opium smoking. Official connivance and police complicity in the traffic have been widely reported and, hence, figures are sometimes doctored to put officials in a good light. During the era of government monopolies, statistical data pertained only to registered smokers and ignored those who relied upon smuggled supplies. The sporadic attempts to reduce consumption by progressively reducing rations or raising opium prices resulted in the use of morphine or heroin as substitutes by hypodermic injection. This trend has been greatly accelerated throughout the Far East by the adoption of prohibitive measures.

Some rough approximations on the extent of opium use in China can be gleaned from a 1881 report by the British Maritime Customs, at which time the import of opium amounted to 6 million kilograms annually.[10] If allowance be made for losses incurred in preparing the opium for smoking, a 30 percent loss would still provide about 4.2 million kilograms that could be utilized. It was estimated that this amount would provide enough opium for one million smokers using 12 grams of opium daily. This amount represents a high estimate of average use. It would not be too difficult to increase the estimated number of opium users by two- or threefold if the esitmated daily dosage is lowered to 4 grams and allowance is made that opium ash still containing roughly one-half the original opium was repeatedly resmoked. Since opium is generally considered to contain 10 percent morphine (it often is less), 4 grams of opium would translate into 400 milligrams of morphine. However, the utilization of morphine in opium by smoking probably does not exceed 15 percent, so this would mean at most a 60 milligram morphine habit, a relatively mild one, for about 4 million smokers out of our estimated population of 400,000,000 people. Comparing this ratio of opium smokers of 1:100 to estimates of alcoholism in this country of about 1:15, the statistics on opium smoking do not support a severe degree of drug dependence by current standards in the United States, but it still represents a lot of silver being exchanged for the opium.

To the Europeans, trade with China was frustrating. Prior to the Opium Wars, all ports were closed to them except Canton and negotiations had to be conducted through a monopoly, the CoHong.[11] The main items of trade were cotton goods, raw cotton, ivory, and opium, the last being illegal since the 1729 anti-opium edict. As trade increased between China and the West, there was a gradual shift in the favorable balance of trade from China to the foreign traders. As the imperial treasury diminished, Emperor Chia Ching banned all importation of opium in 1800 and domestic growing of opium as well. However, English traders fronting for the East India Company in connivance with greedy local merchants continued to smuggle opium into China. The emperor sent an official, Lin Tse-Hsu, to Canton in 1839 to suppress the trade. Lin detained the merchants, and seized and destroyed over 20,000 chests of opium in possession of the British. Under the pretext of promoting free trade, England declared war against China. The disastrous Opium War (1839–42) followed, and with their overwhelming firepower the British won easily. The second Opium War in 1858 was a follow-up to insure the opium trade, which was being resisted. The defeat of the Manchus marked the beginning of their downfall, and China was placed at the mercy of Western imperialism for the next hundred years. Through the Treaty of Nanking in 1842 the English gained trade concessions and Hong Kong, which became the center of trade for opium. Following the Treaty of Tientsin in 1858, there were more territorial concessions to England and legalization of the opium traffic.[11]

The gains of England bothered the Western Powers, including the United States. For growing opium in India and shipping it into China for profit, Britain was roundly criticized on moral grounds and for less than altruistic reasons. American missionaries in China voiced their indignation concerning the ruination of the Chinese people, and American traders saw this as an instrument for obtaining for American products some of the silver that was being siphoned off for opium. After the Spanish–American War in 1898, the United States acquired the Philippine Islands and inherited their opium problem, and, to meet all these concerns, the United States State Department pushed for an international opium conference with the stated aim to help solve the opium problem in China. A conference was held in Shanghai in 1906 and another at the Hague in 1911, which resulted in the first international opium agreement, The Hague Convention of 1912. The treaty did little to help China with the opium problem, but it provided the incentive to initiate anti-narcotic measures in the United States shortly thereafter. While all this was going on there was much discontent and unrest in China.

The Manchu government was overthrown in 1911 by the Kuomintang (Nationalist Party) led by Dr. Sun Yat-sen. With the fall of the Ching dynasty, a Republic was established, but it took a few years to consolidate the country. Sun became President, but only briefly. He died in 1925 and was succeeded by Chiang Kai-shek who remained titular head of China until the Nationalists were driven out of the country to Taiwan in 1949. While Chiang was in power on the China mainland, he tried vainly to suppress opium smoking while attempting to modernize the country. In his efforts he was mainly thwarted by the Japanese who seized Manchuria in 1931, invaded China in 1937, and used opium to subjugate the country while deriving profits.

However, if one looks at the record in Taiwan, there is evidence that Chiang might have succeeded in China if given the time. The incidence of heroin addiction is extremely low in Taiwan due in great part to the death penalty for the narcotic traffickers and repeated users.[12]

Under the rule of the Communist party and Mao Tse-tung, narcotic addiction in China was for all practical purposes also abolished. This could be accomplished only by decreasing the availability of the drug through closing the coastal ports in China to the West, having an effective policing system, and having intensive moral educational and persuasive programs. I have no reason to doubt that the Government has been successful in controlling any substantial narcotic addiction. In 1962–63 I spent a year in Hong Kong where at the time there were an estimated 150,000 narcotic addicts.[13] Many of these individuals originated from China and were allowed to visit their relatives in China, but they returned to their home villages and cities with great reluctance and only when there was an important family event (funeral or weddings) because they stated that narcotics were not available. They were allowed to carry about a week's supply of an opium wine to fend off withdrawal signs, and they were happy to return to Hong Kong. Now that China is opening her doors for more trade with the capitalistic and democratic West, it would not be surprising to expect some resurgence of the opium problem, but for the time being anyhow, the two Chinas have more or less solved the opium problem.

While the opium problem in the Peoples' Republic of China and the Republic of China appears to have been substantially controlled, this does not appear to be the case in many other Asiatic countries. Opium smoking is still prevalent in the Middle East and Southeast Asia, and heroin use has become serious in Hong Kong and Thailand [7] due in large measure to the consequence of restrictive legislation on opium smoking.

The founding of the British Crown Colony of Hong Kong had its roots in opium, and since it was the base for furthering the opium trade, it is no surprise that narcotic addiction became a major social problem on the island and adjacent territories. After the Japanese drove the British out in 1940, they continued to condone opium use and profited from it. When the British reoccupied Hong Kong after World War II, in the atmosphere of enlightened colonialism they put a ban on opium smoking. This succeeded only in exacerbating the narcotic problem because heroin use became increasingly prevalent. During the initial phase of the opium ban, it was not that difficult for the police to limit its use because opium had a characteristic odor and it was not easy for the user to conceal a pipe about two feet long. To satisfy their needs, therefore, it was only natural for the addict to graduate to heroin, which is far easier to smuggle, use, and dispose of.[13]

During the early transition from opium to heroin use, heroin was seldom used by intravenous injection. The conditioning imposed by learning to smoke opium carried over into taking heroin by inhalation. One habit described as "ack ack" or "anti-aircraft gunning" involved placing heroin powder in a cigarette and smoking it with the head tilted backward to minimize loss of the heroin powder. The other mode of inhalation was known as "chasing the dragon" whereby the curling fumes emanated by heating a mixture of barbital and heroin are inhaled. Anti-aircraft gunning is a milder habit than dragon chasing because there is greater utilization of heroin by the latter method. We found that the high temperature (750° C) generated by a smoking cigarette destroys most of the heroin, whereas mixing it with barbital not only allows volatilization of heroin at a relatively low temperature (200° C) but also reduces greatly its decomposition.[14] At the time I was in Hong Kong, nearly 20 years ago, this was the tradition with nearly pure heroin, but I learned on my recent trip to Hong Kong in July that the drug has become increasingly adulterated, and with the decrease in potency the intravenous mode of administration has become more popular.

It would seem that one country should profit from another's mistake, but, as history has repeatedly shown, those who govern our daily lives always learn the hard way and awfully slowly. In America, from early colonial times up into the twentieth century, opium was indispensable. For the physician in the middle nineteenth and well into the twentieth century, one essential, if not the most important, drug to have in the black bag was morphine. There was no drug so universally useful, even though it afforded only symptomatic relief. It could be counted upon to be promptly effective in a variety of conditions. Its sphere of usefulness extended beyond its central application for relief of pain and sedation. It was widely employed also for disorders of the respiratory tract, digestive tract, endocrine glands, and the blood. Before antibiotics, morphine was used to lower body temperature and alleviate the coughing in respiratory infections as well as the diarrhea of intestinal infections. Before insulin, morphine was used to diminish the thirst, hunger, and itching of diabetes.

Even for central application, morphine was considered also to be a near panacea. It was used as a tranquilizer and sedative before the barbiturates, meprobamates, and benzodiazepines. It was used in mood disorders before the bromides, phenothiazines, monoamino-oxidase inhibitors, and the tricyclic antidepressants, until such applications were discouraged by enforcement.

During the nineteenth century, opium was easily available throughout the United States and at a price within reach of nearly everyone. In the latter part of this period and early into the twentieth, the same held true, to some extent, for morphine and heroin. Although most of the opium was imported for the manufacture of morphine and heroin, the opium poppy was also legally grown in New England and Southern states. Physicians freely dispensed opiates and the substances were sold over the counter not only in pharmacies but in grocery and general stores as well. In fact, they could be purchased from mail-order houses, and, in addition, many patent remedies contained opiates. They were extensively advertised not only for the treatment of pain and coughing, but also as cures for consumption and women's ailments.[4–6, 15–18] Congress did not ban the growth of the poppy until 1942, although some states enacted prohibitory legislation earlier.

Morphine was generally considered to be, and correctly so, substantially less inimical to health than alcohol. Even Kane, a severe critic of the opium habit, believed opiates to be less harmful than alcohol, and opined that in general the Chinese were better off as opium smokers than as drunkards.[9] As a matter of fact, many physicians used opium or morphine to treat chronic alcoholism.

This practice continued well into the twentieth century until pressure by regulatory officials discouraged such application.

The details of these practices were chronicled by the late John Donnell, whom many of us knew.[19] In his study, he reported that among the addicts living in Kentucky who were admitted to the Lexington Hospital for treatment of narcotic addiction between 1935 and 1959, at least 152 had a record of excessive alcohol drinking before becoming opiate dependent, and of those who shifted from alcohol to opiate dependence, in most instances it was a physician who gave the alcoholic his first injection of morphine.

Morphine has also been used to cure other types of drug habits. The most celebrated case is its use to overcome addiction to cocaine by the eminent physician, William Halsted (1852–1922), who is considered to be the father of modern surgery. He was a skilled surgeon who pioneered many surgical innovations. He introduced nerve block anesthesia and breast surgery, the concept of asepsis, and techniques for reducing bleeding, and he trained a school of distinguished surgeons. While carrying out research on cocaine, early in his career, he became addicted by self-administration. He tried many times to break the cocaine habit but succeeded only when he became a morphine addict. He joined the Johns Hopkins faculty at the age of 34 when an addict, and while dependent on 180 mg morphine daily, he earned himself international renown for his skill and ingenuity. At the age of 46 he reduced his daily morphine dose to 90 mg daily and remained active until his death at the age of 70.[20]

The attitude of the United States toward opiate use began to turn slowly in the nineteenth century. Although the Chinese government had sought by decree to control opium 100 years earlier, this was regarded as only a Chinese problem, and in all likelihood, the colonists were not even aware of the edict. Although there had been earlier warnings about the potential for opium to promote misuse, there was no general concern. The trials and tribulations of the famed poet, Samuel Coleridge, (*Kubla Khan* and *The Rime of the Ancient Mariner*) with opium and the writings of Thomas De Quincy (*Confessions of an English Opium Eater*) increased awareness in the West concerning opium misuse. The Opium War caused widespread attention to opium and raised cries of moral indignation, but mostly against England rather than against the drug, which was still largely believed to be not overly detrimental to health. Towards the latter half of the century the potential destructiveness of opiate misuse was brought into sharper focus during the Civil War when morphine was given to wounded soldiers by hypodermic injection, although it has been argued that addiction among the troops did not have a major impact on the incidence of addiction immediately after the war.[9] In any event, pharmacists and physicians began to notice that increasing numbers of their clients and patients were becoming dependent on opiates.

A survey of opiate use was conducted in 1888 in Boston. Of 10,000 prescriptions dispensed by 35 pharmacies, nearly 15 percent contained opium, and of the prescriptions refilled three times or more, 78 percent contained opiates.[6] Other surveys yielded similar results. Still, at the time opposition to alcohol was much greater than to opiates. Powerful organizations for the prohibition of alcohol existed in 1881 but there were no similar anti-opiate organizations because opium and morphine were not considered to be a serious menace to society. At the turn into the twentieth century, oral ingestion of opium or liquid preparations of morphine was the principal mode of opiate misuse and women outnumbered men among this population. There was little agitation at the time to regulate opiate use other than opium smoking and the roots of the latter ordinances had racial overtones at the local level.

There are those who have faulted the heathen Chinese for causing enslavement to narcotics in the United States. If blame is to be bandied about for innovating vices, however, Asiatics might well argue that addiction to narcotics was a relatively harmless practice when confined to opium smoking and really did not become serious until the West improved on the *status quo* by isolating morphine, introducing the hypodermic syringe, and synthesizing heroin. Forgetting the polemics, in actuality, narcotic addiction was well-established in this country long before the arrival of the Chinese in California during the 1849 Gold Rush. The Chinese might have exacerbated the problem to some extent in the Far West, but as I shall bring out later, they could not have been the primary causative factor for promoting opiate addiction in this country.

Many of the Chinese immigrants smoked opium recreationally, and although some became compulsive users the vast majority did not. As a boy, I recall living in a small town in California, and frequently visiting a bunkhouse where about 40 workers lived. In the evening, a large number of them smoked opium, but during the lunch hour only one of them extended the habit. The men were employed at an apple drying and packing house and worked from six in the morning to six at night. I do not recall any malingerers among the lot. For recreation, my father, with his cronies, visited places where opium was smoked, perhaps two or three times a year but did not particularly miss these ventures when we moved to San Francisco where the houses had died out because enforcement was more rigid. He did learn to sublimate occasionally with a nip of bourbon instead. My 90-year-old mother tells me that she tried it herself once, and that virtually every man in our home village had smoked opium but relatively few became dependent. I had one uncle who was heavily addicted and did not function effectively. I had also another uncle in this country who smoked opium daily for more than three decades. He was quite successful financially and so had no problems purchasing the drug. He died only recently, an octogenarian, of causes unrelated to opium.

Some of the non-Chinese residents in the larger cities of California, especially San Francisco, did pick up opium smoking and became frequenters of opium "dens" but there are no reliable statistics to indicate a serious epidemic of opium smoking had developed among the non-Chinese. However, instances of such practices were used by the labor agitator, Dennis Kearney, to foment racial tension. As is often the case, the real issue was economic; the Chinese could do more for less, the prime example being the building of the first transcontinental railway. As a consequence of labor activism, however, legislation was enacted to ban opium smoking, but more or less concurrently there were also immigration laws passed to discriminate against Chinese immigration; and such exclusion acts remained in effect for several decades until President Roosevelt rescinded them in 1943.

The bans against opium smoking proved to be unsuccessful. The first statute originated in San Francisco in 1875 and the second, a year later in Virginia City, Nevada. Not long afterwards other states and cities in succession followed suit. When the local regulations failed to control opium smoking, Congress began passing a series of laws. The first enactment, in 1883, raised the tariff on the opium used for smoking, the second, in 1887, limited its importation by Chinese, and the third, in 1890, restricted its manufacture only to American citizens. As opium smoking continued despite these regulations, Congress became less discriminatory and passed a law in 1909 prohibiting all persons from importing smoking opium. Such enactments did not stop opium smoking but were highly successful in stimulating the emergence of illicit enterprises. However, cities and states continued to pass laws prohibiting opium smoking and by 1914 there were 27 such laws, but the amount of smoking opium legally imported still continued to rise steadily.[4–6] We should have learned from these lessons, but instead Congress passed even more comprehensive restrictive narcotic legislation.

After the Hague Convention of 1912, the Secretary of State, William Jennings Bryan, a zealous prohibitionist with missionary convictions, urged that laws be passed to fulfill the United States obligation under the new international treaty for narcotic control. In a climate of growing fear among the public and among some physicians, misguided legislation was enacted that eventually resulted in the victimization of narcotic users and physicians.

The Harrison Narcotic Act was enacted in 1914 but its rigid enforcement did not begin until after World War I. On the face, the Act was not a prohibitory law against narcotics but an act to raise revenue. It placed a tax on those involved commercially in the distribution and preparation of opium and coca leaves and, in essence, appeared to be a law for the orderly marketing of these substances by importers, manufacturers, physicians, dentists, and pharmacists. However, law enforcement officers interpreted the law differently. Although the physician was allowed to prescribe narcotics in the course of his professional practice, according to enforcement this did not pertain to maintaining the habit of the addict because addiction was not a disease. Some physicians who dared to prescribe opiates to allay withdrawal stress were arrested under this interpretation, and this, needless to say, not only discouraged the dispensing of narcotics for the addict but also made the physicians overly cautious in providing narcotics for patients with severe pain, especially if the condition was chronic.

The Harrison Act did limit to some degree the illicit supply of opium and morphine, but it was an abysmal failure in controlling severe opiate addiction and it tended to promote a far more severe form of drug misuse, which created far graver social problems.

Although heroin had been synthesized by the Germans late in the nineteenth century and its addiction liabilities recognized early in the twentieth century, it had not become a major drug problem in the United States. At the time the Harrison Act was enacted, there was not much heroin available and its pharmacologic properties were still not widely known among the laity. However, within a few years after its application to "cure" opiate addiction, coupled with the passage of the Harrison Act, the demography of addiction began gradually to change. Instead of housewives inbibing opium wines, and writers and artists smoking opium, increasing numbers began to inject heroin, and among these there were many juvenile male delinquents.

The pleasure and relaxation heroin afforded by intravenous injection coupled with the aches and pain that resulted when it was not taken, motivated the desire to obtain heroin at the expense of family, home, job, and social position. Those who could not support the habit stole to acquire the ready cash. Neither punishment nor high costs deterred the heavily dependent addict from his drug-seeking behavior, and even as the penalties became more severe, the habit continued to flourish. The ban succeeded only in driving up the purchase price, proliferating a highly profitable black market for the drug. The willingness of the addict to pay any price for heroin enticed greedy entrepreneurs to capitalize on such misfortune. Smuggling could not be effectively controlled, and, in instances of successful apprehension, this only seemed to drive the price of heroin higher and forced the addict to steal even more.

The narcotic addict became a victim of relentless persecution by enforcement officials of the Bureau of Narcotics for over 50 years.[4-6] Additional legislation was tacked on existing ones to increase the penalties for narcotic use, which escalated from imprisonment for five years, to ten years, to life imprisonment. The consequence of this unfortunate situation has been described and can be summed up from a paragraph published in a volume by a consumer's group: [4]

It is important to note that opiate use was not subject to the moral sanctions current today. Employees were not fired for addiction. Wives did not divorce their addicted husbands or husbands their addicted wives. Children were not taken from their homes and lodged in foster homes or institutions because one or both parents were addicted. Addicts continued to participate fully in the life of the community. Addicted children and young people continued to go to school, Sunday school, and college. Thus, the nineteenth century avoided one of the most disastrous effects of current narcotic laws and attitudes—the rise of a deviant subculture, put off from respectable society and without a "road back" to respectability.

In summation then, while repressive legislation against narcotic usage may not have been a complete failure, the policy could hardly be called a success. Looking at the record, it appears that considerably more harm than good was engendered by punitive measures. It became increasingly paramount in the 1960s that changes were needed when other drug problems began to surface.

When the price of heroin rose too high, some compulsive drug users found it necessary to resort to other drugs for relief, and so, there were not only the "junkies," but also the "goofballers" opting for barbiturates and meprobamates, and "speed freaks" for the amphetamines. On top of this there were a new class of drug users spawned from united opposition to the Vietnam War. There were "acid heads" for LSD and the "potheads" for marijuana. Temporizing legislation was enacted to control each crisis until finally the comprehensive Controlled Substances Act of 1970 was passed by Congress.

The 1970 Act is certainly a marked improvement over the Harrison Act and the ones enacted in the sixties for stimulant and depressant drugs. The 1970 Act controls all substances with the potential for abuse and provides for five categorizations based on their established risk. A drug may be scheduled upwards or downwards as more becomes known about its effects. Significantly, first-time possession of controlled substances in Schedule I, including heroin, for example, constitutes a misdemeanor instead of a felony. I have been an ardent believer in the decriminalization of drug use, and while the 1970 Act does not fully appease me, it certainly makes a stride in the right direction. In any event, we need a little more time to assess the consequences of this new measure.

It is not the mission of the present conference to fight the cause for the "junkies" nor for heroin or methadone maintenance programs. However, we cannot ignore the social problems engendered by chronic heroin misuse, misguided legislation, and overzealous enforcement, particularly since they can be potential roadblocks for future rational research on opioid peptides and their synthetic surrogates. Over a span of 200 years we have seen narcotic usage in this country widely extolled, strongly advocated, fiercely rejected, excessively regulated, and reasonably tolerated. Although these attitudinal changes have been greatly colored by subjectivity, emotionality, and overreactivity, they resulted in the main from the steady accumulation of more knowledge. It remains for us to further the understanding of narcotics with objectivity and dispassionate well-designed studies for the medical benefit of the general public, including the junkie.

REFERENCES

1. HOBSON, R. L.   1976.   Chinese Pottery and Porcelain. Dover, New York.
2. CHUBB, O. E.   1964.   Twentieth Century China. Columbia Press, New York.
3. CHINN, T., H. M. LAI & P. P. CHOY, Eds. 1969. A History of the Chinese in California. Chinese Historical Society of America, San Francisco.
4. LINDESMITH, A. R.   1965.   The Addict and the Law. Indiana University Press. Bloomington, IN.
5. BLUM, R. H. AND ASSOCIATES.   1969.   Society and Drugs. pp. 45–58. Jossey-Bass, Inc. San Francisco.
6. BRECHER, E. M.   1972.   Licit and Illicit Drugs. Little Brown & Co. Boston, Ma.
7. EDWARDS, G. & A. ARIFLEDS.   1980.   Drug Problems in the Sociocultural Context: A Basis for Policies and Programme Planning. WHO, Geneva.
8. ADAMS, E. W.   1937.   Drug Addiction. Oxford University Press. London.
9. KRAMER, JOHN C.   1979.   Speculations on the nature and pattern of opium smoking. 6 J. Drug Issues (Spring): 247–256.
10. HART, ROBERT.   1881.   Opium. And 1887. Native Opium. Imperial Maritime Customs II Special Series No. 4 and 18 and Special Series No. 9, Shanghai Department of the Inspectorate General of Customs, Shanghai.
11. WHISSON, M. G.   1965.   Under the Rug: the Drug Problem in Hong Kong. South China Morning Post, Hong Kong.
12. SOLOMON, R., T. BARLOW & R. KOSTAL.   1981.   The opiate trade of Taiwan and Japan: An historical note. J. Psychoactive Drugs.
13. WAY, E. LEONG.   1965.   Control and treatment of drug addiction in Hong Kong. In Narcotics. D.M. Wilner & G.G. Kasselbaum, Eds. Chap. 17, pp. 274–289. McGraw Hill Book Co. New York.
14. MO, B. P. N. & E. LEONG WAY.   1966.   An assessment of inhalation as a mode of administration of heroin by addicts. J. Pharmacol. Exp. Ther. 154: 142–151.
15. KRAMER, J. C.   1979.   Speculation on the nature and pattern of opium smoking. J. Drug Issues: 247–256.
16. KRAMER, J. C.   1979.   Opium rampart. Medical use, misuse and abuse in Britain and the West in the 17th and 18th centuries. Brit. J. Addict. 74: 377–89.
17. KRAMER, J. C.   1980.   The opiates: Two centuries of scientific study. J. Psychodelic Drugs 12: 89–103.
18. KRAMER, J. C.   1981.   The metapsychology of opium. J. Psychoactive Drugs 13: 71–79.
19. O'DONNELL, JOHN A.   1969.   Narcotic Addicts in Kentucky. Publication No. 1881. U.S. Public Health Service. Washington, D.C.
20. PENFIELD, WILBUR.   1969.   Halsted of Johns Hopkins, the Man and His Problem. From the secret records of William Osler. J. Am. Med. Assoc. 210: 2214–18.

PSYCHOLOGICAL (STRUCTURAL) VULNERABILITIES AND THE SPECIFIC APPEAL OF NARCOTICS

Edward J. Khantzian

*Harvard Medical School and
The Cambridge Hospital Department
of Psychiatry
Cambridge, Massachusetts 02139*

The study of human dependence on opiates offers an opportunity to understand important, if not basic, aspects of mental life, emotional pain, and mental illness. The addictions are a place where the biology and psychology of the mind meet. It is a place that promises to resolve some of the mysterious manners in which the body and the mind affect each other, and to unravel better the "mysterious leap from the mind to the body," [1] with which psychoanalysts and clinicians have concerned themselves for a long time. Recent discoveries of the opiate receptors and endogenous opioid peptides have prompted us to consider how the brain and the mind produce their own analgesia for biochemical modulation of physical pain and to consider as well how such processes might also be involved in the modulation and regulation of emotional distress and human psychological suffering.

My presentation today will be based on my understanding of opiate dependence as a clinician and as a psychoanalyst.* However, before embarking on such a tack, I experience a certain sense of uneasiness and trepidation in my approach, given that the promising discoveries of opiate receptors and peptides have been based on very sophisticated methods of investigation. These discoveries have been the result of a fast-growing, complex technology that has allowed researchers a more concrete, precise means to examine microscopically, molecularly, and quantitatively how the brain and mind function. In contrast, the approach of a clinician and psychoanalyst involves less precise, more abstract techniques and methods of investigation that attempt to understand and explain the problems of opiate dependence in its human, experiental contexts, usually by studying single individuals in great detail and in depth, one-at-a-time. Such an approach utilizes macroscopic constructs concerned with structures, functions, and qualities of the mind and mental life. The two approaches need not compete, and more likely they are complementary, albeit the focus of their respective interests and observations at times seem far apart.

Having expressed a concern at the outset that sounds apologetic, I set it aside and proceed by assuring myself, and hopefully my audience, that my approach is a valid and useful one. It is an approach that needs no apology any more than the pathologist apologizes for the validity and usefulness of autopsies, instead of the electron microscope, in understanding pathology and dysfunction.

Considered from a psychoanalytic perspective, opiate dependence may be approached and considered in terms of human processes involving affects,

---

* Psychoanalysis is a method of treatment for emotional problems as well as a method of understanding and explaining mental life and human behavior. Unless otherwise specified, it is applied here in the latter sense as a method of investigation.

0077–8923/82/0398–0024 $1.75/0 © 1982, NYAS

drives, and behaviors, and the mental apparatus or structures responsible for the regulation of these processes. Addicts become dependent on drugs because they have had general and specific difficulties in regulating their affects, drives, and behaviors. There are different reasons why people use drugs and why a certain individual chooses or prefers a particular drug. Based on a representative clinical example, I would like to consider in this presentation, generally and specifically, the nature of the psychological/structural vulnerabilities that make opiates so appealing to narcotic addicts.

ARNOLD—A CASE HISTORY

Arnold is a 29-year-old white heroin addict from a wealthy family background. He sought psychotherapy after starting on an outpatient methadone maintenance program. At the time of his evaluation he appeared to be subdued, friendly, and compliant, and he related to the therapist in a strikingly reticent and apologetic manner. In reviewing his history he characterized his parents in idealistic terms and stressed his own culpability in relation to them and the troubles that had emanated from his drug use. His presenting qualities and manner contrasted sharply with a history of violent, sadistic behavior that dated back to his teenage years. As an adolescent he was in many provoked and unprovoked fights. Some of these occurred while under the influence of sedatives and amphetamines. He prided himself on his fearlessness and capacity for brutality.

He indicated that the initial effects of amphetamines appealed to him when he was a teenager because they helped him overcome feelings of vulnerability and weakness in social situations and in contact sports (despite a very hefty muscular physique). With continued use, however, he found himself repeatedly involved in brutally damaging fights, both for himself and his victims. In some instances the fights were provoked and premeditated, but in other instances, they erupted unpredictably and precipitously with little or no provocation. Initially he rationalized and glorified these episodes in a manner consistent with his need to maintain a sense of omnipotence and invulnerability. Later, with more sober reflection, he admitted to enormous terror and dysphoria as a result of his uncontrollable impulses while under the influence of stimulants.

As Arnold approached his early twenties, he found that his often uncontrollable rage and violence was interfering with his friendships and his work. During this period of his life he discovered the calming, subduing influence of heroin, to which he subsequently became heavily addicted.

He stressed how tranquil and relaxed he felt with heroin in contrast to amphetamines and sedatives, and, how at first, it helped him to feel organized, more energetic, and able to work.

During the initial phases of psychotherapy he continued to present himself in a subdued and deferential way, speaking politely and thoughtfully about his life, his parents, with whom he remained very involved, and his estranged wife. This was during a period of stabilization with methadone maintenance and at a time when he was on good terms with his family and was working regularly in his father's business. After approximately three months of treatment he decided to detoxify from the methadone. As he approached the end of the detoxification, a dramatic shift in his manner, attitudes, speech, and behavior occurred. He was visibly more restless and uneasy during his interviews, he began to falter at work, and he became involved in a barroom fight, sustaining a deep gash in his leg. Repeated fights ensued with his parents during which he was enraged, verbally assaultive, and intimidating. In his therapy he poured out vitriolic hatred and obscenities toward them, revealing for the first time impulses to kill his father; obscenities and paranoid feelings of jealousy were also directed toward his wife. Within two months of discontinuing the methadone, he dropped out of treatment.

Arnold's case reveals remarkable contrasts and shifts over time in his manifest behavior, attitudes, and feelings states. His history reveals he needed drugs both to regulate/overcome feelings of weakness and vulnerability as well as to help in expressing his aggressiveness and to behave more assertively. We also observe that his newly discovered self-assertiveness as a teenager was elusive, short lived, and devastatingly out of control. To combat his feelings of adolescent turmoil and amphetamine-induced rage and aggression, he then began to take advantage of the calming and comforting effects of opiates.

Sedatives and stimulants had initially helped to overcome a sense of inhibition, inertia, and powerlessness in his adolescence. As he approached some of the new challenges in his young adult life, he discovered that the muting and subduing effects of opiates now allowed him to feel more together, integrated, and effective in his personal relationships and work involvements that were otherwise eruptive, chaotic, and overwhelming. However, what was common to both phases of life was his general inability to face some of the specific emotions, affect states, and developmental challenges without relying on a drug to regulate himself and to cope with reality. In the course of therapy, it also became clear how opiate use represented a specific, if not necessary, means to counter the disorganizing effects of his rage and aggression.

Although Arnold is different in a number of respects from some addicts, in many more ways he shares qualities with the narcotic addicts whom I have evaluated and treated in a public narcotic treatment program, as well as with the opiate-dependent patients I have seen in my private practice. The common features are related generally to lifelong problems in regulating one's emotions and behavior, and, specifically, to enormous difficulties in modulating, regulating, and expressing feelings (affects) and drives associated with anger, rage, and aggression.

Some psychoanalysts, particularly those from an earlier generation, might focus and elaborate on Arnold's problems in terms of drive theory, fixations, and disturbances linked to certain phases of psycho-sexual development. Considered from such a perspective, Arnold's drug use might be interpreted to be the result of unresolved needs to seek regressive, pleasurable states, or caused by explosive impulses and tensions related to early problems around bowel control, or still further, his reliance on drugs might be viewed as a symptomatic expression of anxiety and inhibitions over sexual and aggressive impulses dating back to unresolved oedipal conflicts. This earlier psychoanalytic point-of-view would place emphasis on the discharge of drives, keeping them at a minimum and how drugs serve such an end.

In more recent years (i.e., the past 25 to 50 years) psychoanalysts have concerned themselves less exclusively with the influences of drives and conflicts emanating out of various phases of psychosexual development. Instead they have focused more on structures and mechanisms of the mind that help to regulate human drives, affects, and behaviors. Considered from this more contemporary psychoanalytic perspective, Arnold's problems might be seen more in terms of how unevenly he expressed and managed his feeling. At times he suffered from inertia and states of immobilization; at other times he seemed to be totally out of touch with his feelings, and on many other occasions he was overwhelmed with violent, aggressive, and uncontrollable impulses. In short, this more recent psychoanalytic perspective would focus on developmental impairments and deficiencies in psychological structures that otherwise not impaired are responsible for regulating feelings, behavior, inner states of well-being and satisfactory self–other relationships. This more recent perspective would place greater emphasis on maintaining optimal (as apposed to minimal) levels of feelings (e.g., anxiety and depression) as guides for regulating one's internal life, behavior, and relationships with other people. Viewed in this context, opiate dependence might then be interpreted as a way of shoring up one's impaired capacities to deal with one's feelings and as a means to regulate behavior and interpersonal relations.

VULNERABILITIES IN AFFECT REGULATION AND DEFENSE

With the benefit of a contemporary psychoanalytic perspective, I would like to review briefly some more recent explanations of why narcotic addicts generally become involved with drugs and find the action of opiates welcome, and to consider in more detail, then, how one of the principal actions of opiates, namely, its anti-aggression action, provides a specific appeal for narcotic addicts.

Wurmser has recently referred to drug use as a "protective system." [2] His term captures the essence of a recent psychoanalytic perspective of addictions that has better appreciated addicts' structural vulnerabilities and defects in coping with their internal emotions and external reality. In one of our early reports on clinical aspects of heroin use we reviewed some of the causes and consequences of heroin use and how it was used to overcome a range of emotions including pain, stress, and dysphoria.[3] Weider and Kaplan referred to the prosthetic function of drugs and their capacity to relieve tension and distress as major motivating influences for dependence on drugs.[4] Milkman and Frosch were able to present empirical findings suggesting that addicts used drugs either to shore up shaky defenses or to enhance limited ego capacities to engage one's environment.[5] Wurmser delineated how drugs are used to compensate for defects in affect defense, and, in the case of heroin dependency more specifically, how opiates offered protection against painful affects of rage, hurt, shame, and loneliness.[6] Along similar lines, some of my early work emphasized how the anti-rage and anti-aggression action of opiates were used to help addicts cope with defective or nonexistent defenses against these powerful feelings.[7, 8] Krystal's work in this context was important in explaining how addicts are developmentally disturbed in recognizing and experiencing their feelings because of the damaging trauma in their backgrounds, and how such individuals used drugs to overcome feeling states that, as a result, were only vaguely perceived, undifferentiated, somatized, and thus overwhelming.[9]

VULNERABILITIES IN SELF-CARE AND NEED SATISFACTION

More recently in my own work I have been impressed with two other general influences that predispose individuals to substance dependence. These have to do with addicts' structural vulnerabilities in taking care of themselves, and, special problems in accepting and pursuing their dependency needs and wants in more simple and ordinary ways.

Beyond the compulsive and driven aspects of drug dependence, I have been impressed that certain aspects of addicts' dangerous involvements, including the dangers of the drug use and its attendant practices, are results of failures in ego functioning responsible for self-care and self-protection. These functions are related to structures or ego capacities that are acquired in early phases of development and are derived from the caring and protective functions originally provided by the parents. They serve to protect against and anticipate harm and danger. Addicts give repeated evidence in their lives, prior to and while addicted, of being impaired in this capacity. Whereas most people would be fearful, apprehensive, or avoid the many aspects and elements of drug involvement that are dangerous, addicts fail to show worry, caution, or fear, or if present at all, lapse all too readily under the influence of psychological states of disorganization, stress, and/or other regressive influences.[10, 11]

In addition to vulnerabilities in self-care, addicts give much evidence of being very uneven, self-defeating, and conflicted in satisfying themselves around the dependency and needful aspects of life. Although they lack for a sense of self-worth, comfort, and nurturance from within and thus remain dependent on others and the environment to maintain a sense of well being, they are just as often counterdependent and disavow their needs. As a result, they alternate between seductive and manipulative attitudes to extract satisfaction from the environment, and disdainful, aloof postures of independence and self-sufficiency that dismiss the need for others. I have described in more detail elsewhere how these counterdependent and self-sufficient attitudes against ordinary forms of dependency leave addicts susceptible to adopting more extraordinary chemical dependencies to meet their needs and wants.[10, 11]

In brief, then, beyond having troubles (i.e., structural vulnerabilities) in regulating a range of painful feelings, addicts also suffer from an inability to take care of and protect themselves, and to satisfy their needs and wants.

THE SPECIFIC APPEAL OF NARCOTICS

In the previous sections I have tried to review the general psychological vulnerabilities that predispose an individual to become involved with drugs. In what follows I would like to describe and develop a little more what the specific appeal of opiates is and how this specific appeal malignantly combines with addicts general psychological vulnerabilities to make opiates so devastatingly compelling in their lives.

I believe that one of the major specific appeals of opiates resides in the anti-aggression action of these drugs. This action of opiates interacts with general and specific structural vulnerabilities to make opiates very appealing for individuals who suffer such vulnerabilities. In my early work with narcotic addicts I became impressed quickly with addicts' lifelong experiences and problems with rage and aggression, most often dating back to family and environmental influences where they were subject to and victims of physical abuse, brutality, violence, and sadism. I began to suspect that there was a connection between addicts' rageful/aggressive feelings and impulses, their own backgrounds of exposure to violence, and their attraction to opiates. After interviewing many addicts I began to suspect they craved less for euphoria, but that they craved more for a relief from dysphoria associated with anger, rage, and related restlessness, which, in the short term, narcotics seem to provide. This was evident in patients' descriptions of how narcotics helped them to feel normal, calm, relaxed, and soothed, and was even more apparent in observing addicts in treatment as they stabilized on methadone and their aggressiveness and restlessness subsided. I subsequently hypothesized that problems with aggression predisposed certain individuals to opiate dependence, and that the appeal of narcotics was related to the anti-aggression action of the drug. I proposed that opiates counteracted regressed, disorganized, and dysphoric ego states associated with overwhelming feelings of rage, anger, and related depression. This effect was particularly appealing and welcome given that the ego capacities in such individuals were shaky or absent, especially against aggressive drives. Opiates reversed regressed ego states by counteracting the disorganizing influences of aggression on the ego, helping addicts to feel and become more organized, and thus, better able to cope with life's demands and challenges. It was also this sustained, longer action of methadone that accounted for the "success" and better adaptation of individuals receiving this form of treatment.[7, 8, 11]

COMMENTS AND CONCLUSIONS

I would now like to reconsider briefly here this early formulation of the appeal of opiates as an anti-aggression agent with the benefit of an added ten-year perspective, and in the context of more recent psychoanalytic formulations and the discovery of naturally occurring endogenous opioid peptides and receptors.

Addicts' survival problems are formidable. They derive from lifelong developmental problems in coping both with their feelings and with external reality. These problems are further compounded by the artificial drives and painful affect states associated with the addictive intoxication-withdrawal cycles, and by the dangerous world of violence and threat in which addicts operate. Internal states of comfort, tranquility, and satisfaction have all too often been elusive or absent. In addition, although they fail to recognize their self-care problems and the related tendency for hazardous involvements, they nevertheless experience a vague sense of vulnerability in their existence because of their inability to take care of themselves, and as a result, they are even more unstable. Whatever equilibrium they attain is usually precarious. Given their unstable ego and self-structures for containing feelings and behavior, painful affects of any kind tend to compound further an all-too-ready tendency for psychological fragmentation and disorganization. In my experience, the affects and drives associated with rage and aggression are particularly devastating in this regard. I believe the dysphoria with which addicts suffer is intimately associated with the disorganizing influences of these affects and drives. A vicious cycle is set in motion in which shaky or brittle defenses for coping with internal emotions and external reality are further weakened by the uncontrolled aggression, and, given the subjective and objective threatening nature of these feelings in particular, one's very survival/existence seems more and more at stake. That is, uncontrolled aggression disorganizes from within by eroding ego structures, and threatens from without by jeopardizing needed relationships and by provoking counter-violence from others. The appeal of opiates resides then in the dramatic capacity of these drugs to reverse this state of affairs by muting, containing, and eliminating the rage and aggression that disorganizes and disrupts such individuals.

In closing, I cannot resist speculating how the concept of exogenous opiates as an anti-aggression agent might have implications for and be related to the exciting discovery of endogenous opiates, and the role endorphins might play in regulating human aggression. Could it be that under more ordinary circumstances, and in the course of development, the brain and mind elaborate endorphins not only to keep physical discomfort and pain at bay, but that differential elaboration of these substances play a crucial role in maintaining *optimal*, and I emphasize "optimal," feeling and comfort states. Endogenous opiates might be especially critical in regulating human aggression, given that it is such a necessary part of human existence in its controlled forms, but can be equally devastating in its uncontrolled forms. As we study further the role and function of endorphins in the workings of the mind, we might better understand how they fuel productivity by maintaining aggression at optimal levels, and how aberration and dysfunction of endorphin activity might be related to the destructive vicissitudes of human aggression. Perhaps, it is not too far fetched to suggest that we might some day bridge and better control the "mysterious leap from the mind to the body" by understanding how ego and self-structures function as endorphin regulators.

REFERENCES

1. DEUTSCH, F., Ed. 1959. On the Mysterious Leap from the Mind to the Body. International Universities Press, New York.
2. WURMSER, L. 1980. Drug Use as a Protective System. *In* Theories of Addiction. D. J. Lettieri, M. Sayers & H. W. Wallenstein, Eds. NIDA Monograph 30: 71–74. National Institute on Drug Abuse, Rockville, MD.
3. KHANTZIAN, E. J., J. E. MACK & A. F. SCHATZBERG. 1974. Heroin use as an attempt to cope: Clinical observations. Am. J. Psychiatry 131: 160–164.
4. WEIDER, H. & E. KAPLAN. 1969. Drug Use in Adolescents. Psychoanal. Study Child 24: 399.
5. MILKMAN, H. & W. A. FROSCH. 1973. On the preferential abuse of heroin and amphetamine. J. Nerv. Ment. Dis. 156: 242–248.
6. WURMSER, L. 1974. Psychoanalytic considerations of the etiology of compulsive drug use. J. Am. Psychoanal. Assoc. 22: 820–843.
7. KHANTZIAN, E. J. 1972. A preliminary dynamic formulation of the psychopharmacologic action of methadone. Proc. Fourth National Methadone Conference, San Francisco, CA.
8. KHANTZIAN, E. J. 1974. Opiate addiction: A critique of theory and some implications for treatment. Am. J. Psychother. 28: 59–70.
9. KRYSTAL, H. & H. A. RASKIN. 1970. Drug Dependence. Aspects of Ego Functions. Wayne State Univ. Press, Detroit, MI.
10. KHANTZIAN, E. J. 1978. The ego, the self and opiate addiction: Theoretical and treatment considerations. Int. Rev. Psychoanal. 5: 189–198. *Also in* 1977. Psychodynamics of Drug Dependence. J. D. Blaine & J. A. Demetrios, Eds. Research Monograph 12: 101–107. National Institute on Drug Abuse, Rockville, MD.
11. KHANTZIAN, E. J. 1980. An ego–self theory of substance dependence. *In* Theories of Addiction. D. J. Lettieri, M. Sayers & H. W. Wallenstein, Eds. NIDA Monograph 30: 29–33. National Institute on Drug Abuse, Rockville, MD.

DISCUSSION OF THE PAPER

H. D. KLEBER: (*Yale Medical School, New Haven, CT*): That was a very nice presentation, but I wonder how you reconcile your hypothesis with the findings of Mirin and Meyers who stated that chronic opiate administration is not normalizing, but is the exact opposite; it leads to dysphoria and anger.

E. J. KHANTZIAN (*Harvard Medical School, Cambridge, MA*): I am glad you asked that question. In other places I have tried to distinguish the effects of short-acting opiates like heroin from those of long-acting ones like methadone. The acute calming effects of short-acting opiates are counteracted by the regressive influences of the addiction-withdrawal cycle, which has a powerful disorganizing influence on mental functions.

When you ask addicts what they feel when they take heroin acutely, they say that they become calm and subdued. However, as the drug wears off and as they repeatedly go through the addictive cycles, they become more regressed. I think Leon Wurmser will agree with me that by definition in regressed states there is more aggression evident. So there is a vicious cycle. They never catch up with their dysphoria using the short-acting opiates. I think it is for this reason that methadone works better; that is, it is more effective because it has a longer sustained action. Individuals, I think, do begin to cope better and, in fact, this is evident in what we record in descriptive terms. They go to work, behave less impulsively, they do better with their families. In psychological/structural terms it means they are less regressed and better organized.

I also happen to believe that if you overshoot the mark with methadone with certain patients, they do become more regressed, because you dampen things down too much intrapsychically.

A. CORBASCIO, (*Oakland, CA*): The trouble with opiates stems from their improper classification as "narcotic analgesics" rather than "major tranquilizers." It has always been known that opiates exert their action only on certain components of pain such as anxiety, fear, tension, etc., rather than the perception of the pain itself, which is not abolished even by large doses of opiates. In this respect opiates differ radically from anesthetics, which block all perception of pain indiscriminately. The discovery of endogenous ligands of CNS opiate receptors that mimic the analgesic actions of opiates makes this revision all the more necessary. The inclusion of opiates under the heading of "major tranquilizers" would clarify some of the misconceptions that still plague this field and hinder their proper use. It would discourage further useless efforts aimed at dissociating analgesia from euphoria and place opiates under a more benign perspective. It may permit their use in the treatment of some psychiatric conditions such as endogenous depression that are resistant to current drugs. It would soften the rigid and uncomprehending attitudes of the medical profession toward opiates since these drugs mimic a physiological mechanism that is constantly operating in nature.

KHANTZIAN: Your comments are well received. Again, there is some literature on this with borderline syndromes. One of the features of patients with the borderline syndrome is that they do very poorly on phenothiazines, and it appears to be related to the fact that they are on very poor terms with their bodies. They are always feeling dysphoric, uncomfortable feelings in their body. As they experience the extrapyramidal side effects, it aggravates their condition. Opiates are marvelous drugs in that they lack the extra-pyramidal effects. One of the major actions of phenothiazines, for example, is their antiaggression effect. One might hypothesize that opiate addicts would therefore welcome the effect of these drugs, but I also believe that there is the attendant problem of these side effects and, maybe that is one of the reasons why they do not benefit by that particular action. Perhaps Dr. Jaffe may comment on this.

J. H. JAFFE (*University of Connecticut School of Medicine, Farmington*): I am not going to respond to the issue that dopamine blockers are anti-aggression agents. I do think that you made some very useful comments, but I think they need to be put into context. The exogenous opiates have multiple actions. Antiaggression effects are only one.

You warned us that you are seeing people one at a time and there may be some selective factors in the people who choose to interact in a psycho-therapeutic situation. You may be seeing a selective sample. I do not question what you see, but in epidemic situations there are people who have multiple difficulties, some of which are not related to aggression. Some of their problem may be much more related to other effects or, perhaps, to nothing at all other than a desire to achieve some kind of peer approval by opiate use. The final common pathway, as I am sure others will be discussing later, is that the repeated reinforcement of drug use by reduction of abstinence phenomena produces what Abe Wickler has called a disease *sui generis*. It is a disorder in and of itself, and that long after the users have resolved whatever problem may have given rise to the drug use, for some the addictive process remains even when their emotions are within the range that most of us would consider normal. I think we need to be alert to those users who suffer from dis-regulation of aggression, but we also need to recognize that there may be people whose problems lie in other spheres, or in no sphere other than the historical one: that they once decided to use opioids for recreational purposes and are now saddled with a new, somewhat autonomous disorder.

KHANTZIAN: I will only comment briefly. Before I started the paper this morning I wondered whether I ought to quickly retitle it, "a specific" appeal rather than "the specific" appeal of narcotics because I realize I am putting myself out on a limb. I decided to keep it that way primarily for heuristic purposes. I realize from my perspective as a clinician, doing it one patient at a time, that I might have a biased sample. However, a clinical perspective leads me to believe that this specific antiaggression effect of opiates is very important and we ought to study it more. For that reason I kept it as "the specific" appeal. I also agree with Dr. McKenna that opiates are great anti-depressants and great antianxiety agents.

JAFFE: May I make one last comment? We have to recognize that the people you are seeing in this culture, meaning the American culture, have suffered from a situation in which heroin is our most disapproved drug. Therefore, in order to use it you must be a deviate, and you have to be quite angry at the external world with which you interact to even sample it. So, the American heroin addict may be somebody who has a kind of angry reaction to most social interactions, an anger that facilitates breaking the rules and getting into this rather deviant behavior.

We have to keep in mind that in other cultures where opioid use does not evoke such an extreme form of disapproval, we might see different kinds of users. Your comments may apply to most American heroin users.

THE QUESTION OF SPECIFIC PSYCHOPATHOLOGY IN COMPULSIVE DRUG USE

Leon Wurmser

Department of Psychiatry
University of Maryland
Baltimore, Maryland 21201

INTRODUCTION

If there is any truth to the view that compulsive substance abuse is not simply an event of happenstance, a kind of gratuitous get-together of "innocence abroad" and ugly forces of temptation, or, in another formulation, of curious exploring and peer pressure matched by the sinister power of some addictive drugs, and if in the contrary we presume that there must be some eminent readiness in the individual to succumb to such ever present dangers, then we are immediately faced with the question: What prepares specifically the personality to acquire this illness and not any other?

Intensive as well as extensive work, informed by the psychoanalytic way of ordering experience, allows one to single out certain regularities of lower, middle, and high specificity that I am going to present. Before I do that though, two preliminary remarks are in order.

(1) So often in science it is not one perspective, one method of access, one model of understanding, that gives true insight, but the *complementarity* of opposite ways of looking at, and inquiring into, the phenomena.[1] One version of this dialectic germane to substance abuse is the primary versus the secondary view. In the *primary* view the focus is strictly on the phenomenon of compulsive use of some mind-altering substance and its medical and psychological sequels. The focus on the specific concrete abuse dictates the treatment philosophy: "Drug Abuse or Alcoholism is *the* disease. Our main task is to remove the misuse of this noxious agent: everything else is diversion." The *secondary* view sees substance abuse of any kind only as a symptom, an expression of a hidden agenda of great complexity, usually involving not just the abuser, but his immediate environment as well, and reflecting not only conscious cognition and feeling, but the intricate layers of deeper strata as well. The trickiness lies in that one of these views alone does not suffice. If one explores the unconscious depths, but fails to see and to treat the surface phenomena, one is bound not even to get started in effective treatment. In turn, if one just focuses on the dependency, he may obtain striking first success, but inevitably, if he wants to be more effective, he has to go beyond the immediately visible problem of substance abuse and study the underlying psychopathology. The difference between these two is a matter of method, not one of more or less truth (i.e., both are "true").

(2) The second preliminary statement is this: Psychoanalysis is the consistently applied model of understanding centered on *conflict* of motives— external and internal (mostly internal), conscious and unconscious. This one perspective as a method of understanding cannot exhaustively explain mental life, but, if consistently applied, still proves to be of astonishing richness and

33

0077–8923/82/0398–0033 $1.75/0 © 1982, NYAS

depth, of heuristic fertility and clinical applicability—far beyond the confines of its use as a method of treatment.[2]

The two large groupings of inner forces in conflict are the basic urges for union with the other, and for power for the self. Derived from these are sexual and aggressive wishes opposed first by limitations in outer reality, then, in addition, by those from within as well, i.e., the varied, highly complex defenses, and eventually by the entire inner system of the superego.

I turn now to the three levels of specificity in the individual's pathology, as gauged both by quantitative correlation and, more importantly, by psychodynamic ("meaningful") correspondence.[3]

MAJOR DYNAMIC FEATURES

This is the lowest level of specificity, really a summary of the main dynamic features as relatively easily visible.

(1) Drugs uniformly are used as an artificial *affect defense*, i.e., they are compulsively taken to bring about relief from overwhelming feelings. Very specifically, drug use is lastly only a pharmacologically reinforced denial—an attempt to get rid of feelings and thus of undesirable inner and outer reality. This presupposes not solely a particular proneness for this particular defense, but also an inclination for what has been described as affect regression [4]—the global, undifferentiated nature of emotions, that can often only scantily be put into words and other symbolic forms, but is instead partly converted into somatic sensations (many drug addicts are today's version of conversion hysterics!). The choice of drugs shows some fairly typical correlations with such otherwise unmanageable and deeply terrifying affects: Narcotics and hypnotics are deployed against rage, shame, jealousy, stimulants against depression, and weakness, psychedelics against boredom and disillusionment, alcohol against guilt, loneliness, and related anxiety.[5]

(2) More and more I see, at least in most addicts, a *phobic* core as the infantile neurosis underlying the later pathology, typically the fears (and wishes) around being closed in, captured, entrapped by structures, limitations, commitments, physical and emotional closeness, and bonds.[6]

It strikes us at once how the compulsive *search* of the addict is almost a mirror image of the compulsive *avoidance* of the phobic. Whereas the latter condenses all his dangers into one object or one situation, thus directing all his anxieties upon this one threat and arranging all of his life around its avoidance, the addict does exactly the reverse: his life's entire content and pursuit, that what he seeks above everything else and that he depends on, has also become condensed in one object or one situation. I shall come back to this important correlation at the end of my presentation.

(3) Where there are phobias, there are *protective fantasies*—fantasies of personal protective figures or of impersonal protective systems, specifically counter-poised to the threats. This search for a protector against the phobic object and the anxiety situation almost inevitably leads to a compelling dependency once such a factor is found—be it a love partner, a fetish, a drug, a system of actions, or the analyst. Most typically drug addiction enacts the protective fantasy that most potently defends the phobic core. Protectors are highly *overvalued*; i.e., they are "narcissistic objects" (self-objects),[7] expected

to be all powerful, all absolving, all giving, yet also feared to be all destructive, all condemning, all depriving.

(4) The helplessness of the state of primary phobia especially and the pain of repeated feelings of having been uncontrollably overwhelmed, traumatized, is defended against by a thick crust of *narcissism*. Grandiosity and haughty arrogance, more or less extensive and deep withdrawal of feelings from the painful environment (decathexis), and, hence, coldness and ruthlessness are typical features of such a narcissistic defense. It is often papered over by a superficial amiability, friendly compliance, and flirtatious charm—the hallmarks of the "sociopath."

(5) Torn between the fears of the condemning and humiliating powers on the outside and these narcissistic needs of a defensive nature from within, the personality assumes a strikingly unstable, unreliable quality. Periods of high integrity and honesty suddenly give way to episodes of ruthless coldness and criminality. The discrepancy may go so far that we actually encounter *split or multiple personalities*.

There is correspondingly a remarkable discontinuity of the sense of self, a global lability with no mediation and no perspective. It is an unreliability that is infuriating for others, humiliating and depressing for themselves. These *"ego splits" or "ego discontinuities"* are not a defense, but a functional disparity and contradictoriness derived from denial above all.

(6) *Acute narcissistic crises* (feared or real disappointments in others and the self) usually trigger the overwhelming affects described and launch the patients into compulsive drug use.

As a foil to the theoretical presentation, a patient will repeatedly—in brief illustrative vignettes—be quoted.

Jason had entered intensive treatment because of the severe anxiety underlying his massive, recurrently addictive abuse of narcotics, sedatives and cocaine. He was an only child. His parents' marriage had fallen apart when he was less than 5. His anxiety attacks and ensuing use of heroin increased very much after separation from his wife. The attack was described as resembling acute withdrawal: "a rush, chills, restless tossing and turning." He could not sleep and banged his hand against the bed in anger and frustration. He traced the terror back to similar fits of extreme, nearly murderous rage when he felt betrayed and rejected: "I am almost swollen inside, so full of steam, flushed. My heart would beat faster, I get 'stary' eyed, a look of danger around me, like another force taking over, the strangest feeling . . ." He was reminded of the many instances when he was left alone at home by his mother to whom he was excessively close, but whose presence was fickle and unreliable: "It was furious rage, feeling choked—and utter helplessness, when I kept screaming out of the window for her—deep into the night." When recounting it he was puzzled: "What do I do with these bits and fragments of information?" He felt—in his rage turned into panic—a dissolution of inner continuity and cohesion, a repetition of the traumatic state. The sedative drug assuaged the affect storm and almost instantaneously kept reconstituting this inner continuity.

As to the claustrophobia: There was a pervasive dread of being trapped by any closeness or limitation. In dreams he was smothered, pulled into a hole or under water by some monster, his screaming going unheard; he enjoyed sex, as long as it was not bound and confined by marriage. He had to break all limitations by transgressing whatever rule there was—thus inviting mortal danger and social ostracism (including imprisonment). He was engaged in motorcycle jumping, gambling, climbing along façades or jumping from roof to roof—and in illegal trafficking with drugs.

His fear of shame, his provocation of humiliation, and his seeking forgiveness through contrite self-debasement, were compulsively repeated time and again. With each drug-taking episode he expected to hear: "Now—you have had your chance. You should be ashamed for having abused my patience. Get the hell out of here!"

The next level of specificity is that already of a higher level of abstraction: the nature of the predominantly used defenses. I single out three of particular prominence.

DEFENSE ANALYSIS

Denial

Drug use is lastly only a pharmacologically reinforced denial, an attempt to get rid of feelings and thus of undesirable inner and outer reality. Denial can be defined as "a failure to fully appreciate the significance or implications of what is perceived" [8]; it is a defense making the emotional significance of a perception (including that of a memory) unconscious. Its content means: "I don't want to feel that way as I do and I resort to external means to shut out any inner perception of such feelings."

Not only are the painful feelings denied, but so is the awareness of inner conflict: "There is really nothing wrong with me. I take drugs only to have some fun, to feel relaxed and to enjoy the company of my friends," is a frequently encountered statement. Yet, such a disclaimer is only momentarily successful and quickly followed by the admission: "You are right, I do not feel well. There is something wrong with me." [3] The feelings denied are perceived, repudiated, and yet again acknowledged. This denial is inherently accompanied by a *split in the ego.* In Freud's words: "The disavowal is always supplemented by an acknowledgement; two contrary and independent attitudes always arise and result in the situation of there being a splitting of the ego." [9]

As far as we can ascertain now in compulsive drug users, this split has the following nature: What is both perceived and not perceived—in wild back-and-forth vacillation—is *not* presence or absence of the penis as in fetishism, but the presence of a more or less extensive province of emotions and impulses, that reminds the drug user often consciously of a severe trauma. More specifically this province can be determined as referring to affects that are in various ways related to the superego, i.e., to aspects of authority, responsibility, time, and limitation. More directly, they are affects expressing either a condemnation by the superego (shame and guilt), or the loss of approval by this inner agency (reduced self-esteem, sadness or vague dysphoria, emptiness, and loneliness), or the loss of ideals (disappointment, disillusionment, meaninglessness), or the upsurge of such feelings and striving that would evoke censure by the superego, especially aggressive affects and aggressive wishes.

This denial or disavowal pertains therefore specifically to the refusal to perceive and to take seriously (1) the superego as a relevant part of inner life; (2) the representatives of the superego in outer reality, be they now in personalized or abstract form (values, ideals, laws, limits of possibility, and considerations of time restraints, like delay); (3) the affects expressing condemnation by the superego; (4) the affects accompanying the loss of ideals; and (5) the affects and drives that would lead to condemnation by the superego. At the same token all these disavowed, superego-related parts of inner and outer life are time and again acknowledged. One knows "that" of course, but one acts as if that reality did not exist—again this doubleness.

Our patient: "I let my bills pile up. I let things go. I just deny their existence. I am shutting my eyes. It's the same like when I was driving around with several pounds of pot in my car. I was sure I would not be caught. All along I never faced up even to the possibility that I ever would have to go to jail: 'Somehow I'll be bailed out.' " When he is rejected or just mildly rebuked, it feels: "as if I had been hit with a knife." He feels crushed by shame and loneliness and then finds refuge in a system of fantasies that have to be made real—by lies and drug taking.

Reversal

A number of drive reversals are generally of much greater significance as defenses than the literature indicates: turning active into passive, turning passive into active, the turning against the self. It appears to me more and more persuasive to see in the defense of *turning passive into active* a cardinal type of defenses in severe psychopathology—especially against aggression—much as repression is in the more typical neurotics and particularly against libido.

Just as it is a main theme of the patient's life that he suffers and fears disappointment and helplessness, he does everything in his power first to enlist help, but then to turn the tables and to prove the therapist helpless and defeated. Thus he wants to inflict the same helplessness, defeatedness, and humiliation on others—his family, the therapist, the treatment or penal system—that he has suffered himself. He wants to defeat *them*, because he feels defeated; he wants to make *them* feel helpless, weak, and ashamed, because so does he; he tries to scare *them*, because he is so scared. He tries to corner them and box them in, because he feels so confined, limited, and wishes to break out. For example, in our case: "Everybody I get close to will betray me—so I must betray her (or him) first." This preemptive betrayal, deceiving, lying, and his anticipatory disappointing and disillusioning the other are a thorough-going attempt to turn passive into active: to be the one who inflicts it on the other instead of suffering it passively and helplessly: "Instead of my being passively fooled and feeling humiliated for it, I am fooling everyone else." In his life's experience: "I trusted my mother—yet how much has she cheated on me and has made me feel an absolute fool, a ridiculous imp. . . ."

Externalization

With this defense "the whole internal battle ground is changed into an "external one" [10]; put the same in different words: externalization is the defensive effort *to resort to external action in order to support the denial of inner conflict.* For example, ridicule, rejection, and punishment are provoked (not just suspected) from the outside world—a very frequent form, by no means restricted to compulsive drug users. Or: Limit-setting is invited and demanded from the therapist, but then fought against. Or: Oral and narcissistic "supplies" are quite concretely requested and sought from spouses and friends; their limitation is responded to with envy and rage. Much of the "acting out," the "impulsiveness" is such a defensive use of action, an action with the aim of taking magical, omnipotent control over the uncontrollable, of risking the ultimate threats (separation, humiliation, castration, dismemberment), yet—counterphobically—proving that these terrors are unfounded, that fate can be propitiated and forced to protect. It may be action by gambling, motorcycle jumping, and racing; it may be by lying, manipulating, cheating; it may be by violence and revenge; it may be just by any exciting action. Or it may be by drugs: "I have the power, with the help of this magical substance, to master the unbearable."

I have already postulated that the main defenses are directed not against the drives, but against the superego and considerable aspects of external reality. This postulate has important psychodynamic and systematic implications.

Let us look at some of the consequences of the defenses just described:

Instead of internal danger, instead of anxiety about drives, superego sanctions, and unconscious archaic castration anxiety, he encounters real, tangible anxiety about something "out there." He overcomes the other, inner dangers, by triumphing over the dangers in external reality. The denial consists in this: "There are no limits that I have to respect. I prove that the threats from out there are ineffectual and the laws and barriers invalid. Therewith I prove also that what I observed *then* as something so terrifying is not true."

In Jason's words: "Included in the denial was actively acting out the fantasies that were contrary to what I tried to deny."

This brings us now to what I believe to be the highest level of specificity and to a final passage. Though even more abstract, it may allow us that specificity in the deeper understanding that has eluded researchers so far.

THE STRUCTURAL SPECIFICITY OF CONFLICT SOLUTION

The following synopsis is derived from a schema that Freud used to distinguish neurosis and psychosis; [11] it was taken up by Waelder [12] and enlarged by Rangell.[13, 14]

In neurosis the ego stands on the side of the superego and outer reality and directs its main defense against the id. In schizophrenic psychosis it allies itself with archaic drives and equally regressive superego demands and directs its defensive efforts in form of denial and withdrawal of investment ("decathexis") mostly against outer reality. In severe depressions the ego almost completely submerges in the archaic superego. Its mirror image is "sociopathy" (and Rangell's "syndrome of the compromise of integrity") where the ego mainly battles against the superego and is allied with the id; while it certainly also makes "inoperative" crucial elements of outer reality, the latter is largely enlisted against the main enemy.

It appears that this defensive endeavor shifts when we come to toxicomania: In this syndrome the ego certainly also deploys such defensive action against the superego, but hardly less against external reality. Not only is the latter attacked insofar as it is bearer of limits, authority, responsibility, and commitment (that is perhaps to some extent also true in sociopathy), but much more generally, even where it has to do with self-preservation, with anticipation of consequences, with delay and later gratification, with basic contradictions and logical impossibilities. In other words: in compulsive drug use the ego eventually tries to invalidate not only values, authority, and responsibility (superego), but also the lines drawn between objects, the boundaries between the times, between inside and outside the borders, between social entities, the limits between concepts.[3] It is an attack on the syllogistic basis of rationality, very akin to the same event in psychoses. When drug use is compared with psychoses, I believe the difference is merely quantitative (apart of course from the different position of the superego).

Commonly these conflict solutions are transient and easily shift. Kubie used to say: "No one is 24 hours a day psychotic or neurotic." There are steady changes of equilibrium, of alliance, of defense. Neither is any of these schematic relations total. As noted, never is the superego completely abolished; we are rather speaking about "more or less."

What are now the concrete and specific implications of this general statement?

The superego has six major functions: (1) the ego ideal—i.e., an ideal image and code of ideal actions, (2) self-criticism and self-punishment, (3) self-approval, self-care, self-protection, (4) stabilization of mood and affects, (5) self-observation, and (6) the protection of outer reality's boundaries.[15]

If it is true that the major defensive efforts are directed against the superego, we would expect not only the instability and even apparent disappearance of many of these functions, but a return of them in warped, twisted, distorted, regressive form—the famous *"return of the repressed or denied."*

The Return of the Denied Ego Ideal

I believe this can be found foremost in that narcissism that was vested in the ego ideal and now returns as the narcissistic gratification reclaimed in the drug-induced intoxication. Specifically it can be stated: "I am as good, as grand, as full, rich and strong—as my wishes bid me to feel because I am protected. My inner judge has been silenced. I am close to an ideal state because I am one with the protector and thus have eliminated the voice of my conscience and of every limit-setting authority."

Self-Punishment

The second part of this "return of the denied superego" lies therein that criticism, retaliation, and punishment are being invited by provocative action, externally, and usually accepted and submitted to. The "protector" thus changes back into "the monkey on my back"—into the confining, enslaving, imprisoning master. The superego, denied, reasserts its claims—smotheringly, paralyzingly—and often fatally.

The "Loving and Beloved Superego"

It is often forgotten that the superego is not solely the ideal-setting, self-observing, and self-condemning part of one's inner life, but very centrally the approving and protecting inner agency.[16] This implies that the defense against the superego as protector, soother, and care giver has immediately the consequence that there is a constant sense of unprotectedness and hurt. This leads to the frantic search for outer "protectors and forgivers," protectors most specifically that would undo the narcissistic injury, the chronic shame, and forgive the guilt.

Several leading explorers of this area have recently stressed the deficit in the self-caring function in these patients.[17, 18] We may now assume that what is referred to in this is just this protective, assuring, approving side of the superego that falls victim to the general regression and splintering of this structure caused by the major defensive effort directed against it.[19]

Discontinuities of Ego-States

It can also now be assumed that it is denial of the superego-induced affects that is ultimately accountable for the strange flip-flop phenomena, the peculiar switches from one extreme to the other, the utter emotional unreliability. The superego is known to act as the mood and affect stabilizer.[20] If it is temporarily and recurrently made "inoperative," life in all, and behavior and attitudes in particular, take on that especially disrupted, chaotic quality noticed before.

Self-Observation

Of particular importance is the return of repressed *self-observation* in form of the vast prevalence of shame over guilt. Here I can give only a few excerpts from a much larger work.[15]

Over the years I have been surprised to see how important various shame affects are in much of pathology, particularly again in compulsive drug use. It is even more the hidden, denied, unconscious shame than the conscious one that lures behind much of symptomatology as an important factor.

Since shame is a form of contempt against oneself, it is understandable that an attitude of contempt against others is frequently a form of reversal: "Instead of my despising myself, I direct withering ridicule or cold scorn against others." Contempt, arrogance, and haughtiness are most typically understood as masks of hidden shame.

What is the feeling of shame? It is seeing oneself exposed in any form of weakness and failure to the looks of someone else or to the "inner eye" of one's conscience, exposed and looked at with cold disregard, with contempt. It is followed by a wish to wipe out the stain, either by a furious counterattack, or by hiding oneself, really or symbolically, by wanting to disappear or by freezing up, "turning into stone." It is less known that shame is also the fear to look. One wishes not to know and covers one's eyes.

Chronic severe depersonalization is another mask of shame: "I observe myself and I am not myself any more—not this disgusting, weak being." The correlation of continuous estrangement with shame is so regular that I suggest that chronic severe states of depersonalization reflect underlying unconscious shame exactly as chronic depression expresses unconscious guilt.

Spite, paranoid fears, compulsive forms of wanting to be mysterious and to mystify others, grandiose ambitions, hiding of all feelings behind a rigid, frozen mask of being unmoved and cold—all may be characteristic ways of dealing with hidden shame, and all are ubiquitous in these patients, as aspects of the return of the repressed.

Limitations

It has been repeatedly mentioned that the addict specifically fights against limits and limitations. It appears now that an important symbol for the superego is precisely such limit, such enclosure and confining structure: the *claustrum*. As I said at the beginning, we find in surprisingly many compulsive drug users a more or less severe *claustrophobia*, although one has to hasten to add that this symptom alone is of course not specific for these patients. It is also significant that this claustrophobia usually is displaced further to metaphorical enclosures. Many feel stifled, smothered, uncomfortably hemmed in by human warmth, by physical or emotional closeness (including intensive psychotherapy), and either have to beat a frightened or angry retreat or have to "burst out" as soon as somebody gets too close; any gesture of such closeness is experienced as a suddenly concrete threat of being engulfed and swallowed up by the other. They, moreover, have to escape any commitment (e.g., marriage), show not enough perseverance in tasks, and are perpetually peregrinating (compulsive travellers).

The oral meaning of such a claustrum is easily recognizable, but it is equally easily overlooked what cardinal importance the equation of such a "devouring claustrum" with the superego and all its representations and representatives really has. It appears that this equation forms part of a *central fantasy* of great specificity.

With this equation, "claustrum = superego = devouring (i.e., also: = orally experienced mother and her interior)," we have not yet reached all that is now opening up to our understanding: ". . . any state of anxiety is physiologically accompanied by feelings of being closed in; and thus reversely, an external closeness (or the idea of it) facilitates the mobilization of the entire anxiety syndrome." [21] Since every intense affect (excitement, rage, etc.), when repressed, appears as anxiety in consciousness, it also becomes equated with an undifferentiated global tension over which all control has been lost and which has left the person helpless and overwhelmed, a tension reawakening an original truly and severely traumatic state, hence the feeling of enclosure and the imperative of breaking out.

Thus we are forced to assume that "the idea of a claustrum or of a claustrophobia" may be "behind all other phobias—and even behind all other symptomatic neuroses," as Leo Rangell suggested.[22] Even the word "anxiety" itself expresses a physical construction and confinement: "angustiae" being a narrow, boxed-in place.

On all levels this anxiety is accompanied by a series of usually aggressive actions which would liberate the self from these various concentric bounds. Yet this liberation and bursting-out itself raises many new specters: condemnation in the form of guilt and shame, aloneness because of the separation from the enclosing, protective, shielding claustrum, and so forth.[6]

Relief from such anxiety can only come from protection, yet this protection would be sought primarily again in external structures, in outside controls and limitations in the hope that somebody else would take over, constrain him, and thus shield him against this dark overwhelming part within him. The tragic paradox, of course, is that all such protection against this devastating anxiety is bound to become once more just a new claustrum and, therefore, a renewed source of terror.

The system of phobic fears is now opposed by the *antiphobic protective system* described before. What is now this magical "protector" who is just as compulsively sought, as the phobic object is avoided? It is more and more likely that the phobic and the antiphobic objects are very closely related to each other. If the phobic equation is *"over-stimulation and helpless exposure = anxiety = claustrum = superego = all limitations,"* the protective system must resemble this archaic "syllogism."

The drug now is part and parcel of such a protection system; it is *equally compulsively sought, as a phobic object may be compulsively avoided.* It is the photographic negative of a phobia.

But I reiterate: Each of these features of the "return of the repressed or denied superego" is, in and by itself, not very specific. Only their conglomeration and their combination with the strictly parallel defenses directed against outer reality, insofar as it reflects these six superego aspects, is of that highest specificity we have been looking for.

How the genesis of these more or less specific psychodynamics can be understood is a topic for another time.[23] Suffice it to say that except for cases where an organic factor is decisive (above all, "minimal brain damage") the psychopathology described corresponds to a fairly specific family constellation, marked by a pentad of characteristics: (1) severe traumatization in the form of child abuse, other violence, or incest; (2) radical inconsistency and absence of hierarchical structure; (3) secretiveness, mendacity, and other forms of deception; (4) intrusiveness; and (5) parental substance abuse. Not all five are usually present, but several of them typically are.

REFERENCES

1. HOLTON, G. 1973. Thematic Origins of Scientific Thought. Kepler to Einstein. Harvard Univ. Press, Cambridge, Mass.
2. KRIS, E. 1938. *In* 1975. Selected Papers. L. M. Newman, Ed. pp. 348, 349. Yale Univ. Press, New Haven, CT.
3. WURMSER, L. 1978. The Hidden Dimension. Psychodynamics in Compulsive Drug Use. Jason Aronson. New York.
4. KRYSTAL, H. 1974. The genetic development of affects and affect regression. Ann. Psychoanal. **2:** 98–126.
5. WURMSER, L. 1974. Psychoanalytic considerations of the etiology of compulsive drug use. J. Am. Psychoanal. Assoc. **22:** 820–843.
6. WURMSER, L. 1979. Phobic core in the addictions and the paranoid process. Internat. J. Psychoanal. Psychother. **8:** 311–336.
7. KOHUT, H. 1971. The Analysis of the Self. International Universities Press, New York.
8. TRUNNELL, E. E. & W. E. HOLT. 1974. The concept of denial or disavowal. J. Am. Psychoanal. Assoc. **22:** 769–784.
9. FREUD, S. 1940. An Outline of Psycho-Analysis. Standard Edition, Vol. 23: 139–207. Hogarth Press. London.

10. FREUD, A. 1965. Normality and Pathology in Childhood: Assessments of Development. Works of A. Freud. Vol. 6: 223. International Universities Press. New York.
11. FREUD, S. 1924. Neurosis and Psychosis. Standard Edition. Vol. 19: 149–156. Hogarth Press, London.
12. WAELDER, R. 1951. The structure of paranoid ideas. In 1976. Psychoanalysis. Observation, Theory, Application. pp. 207–228. International Universities Press. New York.
13. RANGELL, L. 1974. A psychoanalytic perspective leading currently to the syndrome of the compromise of integrity. Internat. J. Psycho-Analysis 55: 3–12.
14. RANGELL, L. 1976. Lessons from Watergate: A derivative for psycho-analysis. Psychoanal. Q. 45: 37–61.
15. WURMSER, L. 1981. The Mask of Shame. Johns Hopkins Univ. Press. Baltimore, MD.
16. SCHAFER, R. 1960. The loving and beloved superego in Freud's structural theory. Psychoanal. Study of the Child 15: 163–188.
17. KHANTZIAN, E. 1977. The Ego, the Self, and Opiate Addiction. Theoretical and Treatment Considerations. NIDA Research Monograph 12: 101–117. Govt. Printing Office, Washington, D.C.
18. KRYSTAL, H. 1977. Self- and Object-Representation in Alcoholism and Other Drug-Dependence. NIDA Research Monogaph 12: 88–100. Govt. Pinting Office, Washington, D.C.
19. WAELDER, R. 1930. The principle of multiple function. In 1976. Psychoanalysis: Observation, Theory, Application. pp. 68–83. International Universities Press. New York.
20. JACOBSON, E. 1971. Depression. pp. 77, 78. International Universities Press. New York.
21. FENICHEL, O. 1944. Remarks on the Common Phobias. In 1954. Collected Papers. Vol. 2: 283. W. W. Norton. New York.
22. RANGELL, L. 1979. Personal communication.
23. WURMSER, L. 1979. The sharing of defenses—The addict and his family. Internat. Psycho-Analytic Assoc. Meeting, New York, 1979.

METHADONE AND OPIATE DRUGS: PSYCHOTROPIC EFFECT AND SELF-MEDICATION

Gerald J. McKenna

Department of Psychiatry
Veterans Administration Medical Center, Brentwood
Los Angeles, California 90073

Department of Psychiatry
University of California, Los Angeles School of Medicine
Los Angeles, California 90024

The concept of drug use as self-medication has been extant for many years but has received considerably more attention in the last decade. This, of course, coincides with the influx of large numbers of mental health professionals into the drug dependence field and renewed efforts to explain the phenomena of drug use and to better understand the complex nature of drug dependence. Attempts have been made to provide a unifying theory of drug dependence, and individual investigators have approached the problem from one or another theoretical viewpoint, each providing a partial explanation for drug dependence.

Wikler in his 1953 paper, "Psychiatric Aspects of Drug Addiction," [1] discussed a multi-etiological basis of "drug addiction" and three formulations of the psychiatric aspects of drug addiction. He notes several different groups using narcotic drugs for differing reasons: "neurotic individuals" seeking relief from anxiety; "psychopaths" seeking a state of elation; "normal individuals" seeking relief from physical pain; and "psychotic individuals" seeking relief from depressive feelings. Since this paper is particularly concerned with this latter group, who seem to use narcotic drugs (in this case, methadone) in the self-treatment of various psychotic symptoms, it will be useful to review some of the relevant literature prior to and subsequent to our initial observations in 1973. Many of the earlier clinical observations on the antipsychotic actions of morphine and methadone have later been more firmly founded in pharmacologic theory with the discovery and investigation of the actions of endorphins. This will be briefly discussed later in this paper and is being more thoroughly discussed in other presentations at this conference.

In a 1971 paper, "The Psychotic Heroin Addict," [2] Wellisch *et al.* cite Nyswander's writing [3] that opiates had been used in Europe to treat manic depressive psychosis and melancholia prior to the introduction of neuroleptic drugs. Others have provided anecdotal reports [3] of similarly using morphine to attempt symptomatic control of severe psychotic symptoms in an age when the psychopharmacologic armamentarium of psychiatry contained only a few drugs, including opiates, barbiturates, and other sedatives such as chloral hydrate. These drugs were used to initially calm very disturbed patients but were not used in an ongoing manner to control psychotic symptoms.

Wellisch *et al.*[2] report that in treating over 1500 patients in their drug detoxification section: "among these patients have been numerous individuals who were using heroin for its tranquilizing and 'antipsychotic' properties." They cite Chein's finding [5] of 22 out of 52 addicts studied were psychotic or borderline psychotic. They also report on several patients who effectively used heroin as

44

0077–8923/82/0398–0044 $1.75/0 © 1982, NYAS

self-medication for psychotic symptoms. They describe a pattern "of many cases in which overtly psychotic individuals remained ambulatory and functional on self-maintained dosages of heroin, only to have their psychoses become overt during or shortly after withdrawal." At the end of their paper they state, "it is our clinical opinion that methadone posseses little, if any, antipsychotic effect, unlike morphine or heroin." It has been our observation, as will be discussed later, that methadone does possess powerful antipsychotic effects.

Other authors in the early '70s described the action of methadone and other narcotics on certain affective states. Both Wurmser [6] and Khantzian [7] reported the calming effects that methadone appeared to exert on rage and aggression in patients on methadone maintenance.

In 1978 Verebey et al.[8] reviewed the work on the existence and possible functioning of endorphins in the brain. Linking these with the pharmacologic properties of opioid drugs, they suggested possible uses of these drugs in treating mental illness. They suggest using methadone as the primary pharmacologic agent in treating selected schizophrenics and others with a psychotic disorder who cannot be treated with the usual neuroleptics because of severe side effects or certain medical conditions. We will return to this important paper and concept later in the discussion since it does appear to have clinical relevance despite some obvious drawbacks.

Also in 1978, Berken et al.[9] describe a woman who had been unresponsive to a variety of treatments, including ECT, neuroleptics, antidepressants, minor tranquilizers, and psychotherapy. When all treatment attempts seemed to have failed she was induced onto methadone maintenance. This treatment better controlled her "rage" than other treatments. They also note the calming effects of methadone on other patients "with a history of rage, current aggressive rage, or repressed rage who joined the program. . . ."

There are a number of other articles in the literature describing various psychopathological disorders in patients on methadone maintenance.[10–20] These articles illustrate the complexities of patients on methadone maintenance and the various mental disorders that either precede or accompany drug dependence in these individuals.

CASE EXAMPLES

In three separate methadone maintenance programs we have observed patients who had first used opioid drugs, primarily heroin, to self-treat pre-psychotic and psychotic symptoms. When they were later on methadone maintenance, this drug served a similar purpose. Several case examples are presented here from a 1973 study conducted at the Boston City Hospital Drug Treatment Program. They will illustrate both the Mental Disorders and the Personality Disorders that often are present simultaneously in such patients.

Method. The three patients were followed clinically for 2½ to 5 years in the Drug Treatment Program and inpatient psychiatric unit of Boston City Hospital. Their charts were extensively reviewed, the staff having contact with them over the years were interviewed, and the patients themselves were extensively interviewed by this author. Concurrence of diagnostic impressions was obtained by independent reviews and interviews by at least two other psychiatrists using the DSM-II diagnostic criteria in use then. We shall later retrospectively review these patients using DSM-III criteria.

Case 1

Al was a 30-year-old divorced man born of Eastern European parentage in a Boston industrial suburb. His father was a heavy drinker and often unpredictable in his behavior toward his wife and the patient. Al recalls frequent fights between his parents and remembers being terrified of his father's outbursts of temper. He felt intimidated by his father and avoided him whenever possible. His first few years of school appeared satisfactory and he formed friendships without difficulty. As he progressed in grade school, though, he experienced a significant change in his peer relationships. He felt scapegoated and ineffective in dealing with the "class leaders." He became increasingly defensive yet continued trying to please his adversaries and maintain a relationship with them. When he transferred to high school, he associated with children of ethnically different backgrounds, which met with parental disapproval. He again found himself feeling inferior and involved in relationships similar to those he had experienced in grammar school. Shortly thereafter he began associating exclusively with black students.

In retrospect he feels that he was indentifying with those looked down upon by peers of his own ethnic background. Temporarily he felt better about himself, began dating black girls, but was finally jilted by one black girlfriend with a subsequent plunge in his self-esteem. Having failed at all his attempts to form meaningful relationships within any group, he now became fascinated with the idea of becoming a "dope fiend." He read extensively about drug addiction, told peers he was addicted and even marked his arms with pinpricks to validate his charade.

He first used heroin in 1955 after joining the Air Force; he experienced a euphoria he had not previously known, felt good about himself for the first time in his memory and thereafter sought narcotics on weekend passes. During the next ten years he became progressively more involved with narcotics (mainly paregoric and dilaudid), had frequent arrests and hospitalizations, but continued drug-seeking behavior when not in confinement. He experienced periods of euphoria alternating with depression when not using narcotics, but had no definite psychotic episodes. He began methadone maintenance in 1968 and in July 1970 made his first attempt at detoxification. It was noted during the hospitalization that he experienced mood swings varying from elation, with flight of ideas, to profound depression. He completed detoxification and was discharged in September 1970. He began using heroin almost immediately and subsequently reentered the methadone maintenance program. From 1970 until 1972 he remained on methadone maintenance and seemed stable during that time.

In February 1972 he was hospitalized for detoxification from 150 mg of methadone. He was detoxified over the next three weeks. When his methadone dose had been decreased to 30 mg, he noted the onset of feelings of elation. These progressed through stages of increased energy, loquaciousness, flight of ideas, and finally the paranoid delusion that he was a prophet sent to save the world, and he felt endowed with extraordinary powers. His psychosis exacerbated following total withdrawal from methadone and he was transferred to the general psychiatry unit and started on thorazine, which was increased to 1600 mg per day. He remained on this dose for 1½ months and his hypomania decreased somewhat. His flight of ideas and delusions of grandeur continued, although abated. It was decided that his past history and present symptomatology represented a manic-depressive psychosis and he began treatment with lithium carbonate. Lithium successfully interrupted his hypomania but he felt increasingly depressed, spontaneously stopped taking lithium after two months and entered a deep depression. Al describes this period as the worst in his life. He suffered assaults of suicidal ideas and felt that some uncontrollable force inside of him was driving him to suicide. There were times when he felt a similar urge to homicide. Panicked by his depression and preoccupation with death he sought relief by taking street thorazine, heroin, and large amounts of alcohol. For a period of two months he was lost to follow-up but returned to the unit in July and was reinduced to 110 mg methadone maintenance and 150 mg amitryptyline daily with a gradual decrease in depressive symptoms and subsequently discontinued the amitryptyline but remained on methadone.

In late 1972 Al was slowly detoxified from methadone at his request and begun on lithium carbonate 1800 mg per day. He did well for the next 8 months and was able to remain free of other drug use. He later left the region with the plan to continue on lithium.

Case 2

John is a 33-year-old divorced white male born in a working class town near Boston. He had a mild physical deformity at birth which limited his later ability to compete with his peers in athletics or other strenuous exercise. His father, a physical fitness and athletic buff, rejected John because of his lack of physical ability. John recalls a "miserable" early life, felt he was the weakest in any group, and was scapegoated in early childhood and during his school years. He was given nicknames such as "dumbo" and "buck teeth," and chronically felt humiliated in peer interactions.

His parents divorced when John was five years old; he lived with his mother after that and has had little contact with his father since. He describes his mother as "naive," having old world ideas, and restricting his physical activities. Neither parent had a drug or alcohol problem.

John did well scholastically in grammar school but was always unpopular. He avoided close relationships and says, "If I got close to someone, I'd end up getting stabbed in the back."

By the eighth grade he "changed tactics" and turned to crime. He says, "I felt I couldn't get anywhere with my classmates so I took to breaking and entering; I was getting recognition for getting into trouble."

In high school he was absent from classes most of the time, was arrested in 1954 and sent to a juvenile reformatory. Following his release one year later he entered a local trade school and did well scholastically. Nevertheless he remembers feeling chronically anxious and agitated and says, "I just couldn't sit still." These feelings progressed, reaching a peak in late high school. He began drinking heavily and using marijuana but felt these drugs did nothing for him. In 1958 he first tried morphine and stated later that "it calmed me down, everything looked beautiful, and I had a new energy." He relates that the morphine changed his relationship with people, allowing him to be now talkative, and able to share his feelings.

From 1958 to 1964 he continued a life of searching for opiates. When he was not using the drugs he had a recurrence of previous feelings of anxiety and depression. He began using street methadone in 1964, felt more controlled with this drug than with other opiates, and stopped using morphine and heroin. He was married in 1964, but divorced in 1966. The relationship was functioning as long as he continued methadone, but when he began self-detoxifying, the relationship began to distintegrate. He attempted self-treatment with barbiturates, tranquilizers, and amphetamines, but could not control his feelings of depression. When his wife left him, John returned to using street methadone, supplementing his dose with valium. His depression cleared, but as he raised his daily dose of methadone beyond 150 mg per day he experienced feelings of uncontrollable anger and paranoia. He sought psychiatric treatment, was detoxified rapidly on a psychiatric ward, experienced an initial withdrawal reaction, and then entered a progressive depression. Three weeks after detoxification he attempted suicide by hanging himself from a rafter in his room.

For the next five years John was in the methadone maintenance program with three inpatient hospitalizations for detoxification at his request. He was never able to become methadone-free without experiencing symptoms of anxiety and severe depression. He was finally placed on a combination of methadone and amitryptline, and valium, which appeared to stabilize him fairly well.

It should be pointed out that at various times it was suggested to John that he be treated with tranquilizers and antidepressants alone, but he refused. He felt that he has tried various combinations of tranquilizers on his own but feels the need to continue using opiates, and whenever he is not in a formal drug treatment program he returns to opiate use with the attendant problems of procuring drugs on the street.

Case 3

Simon was born in Boston in 1946. His parents divorced when he was an infant and he spent the first two years of his life in an orphanage.

He was placed in his grandparents' home at age two, and had a distant relationship with them. He recalls being embarassed by his grandmother in front of his friends because he was enuretic. His grandparents kept his mother's identity secret; though she lived nearby and frequently visited, Simon was told that she was his older sister.

He did well in grammar school, appeared to socialize normally until the fourth grade when the family moved to avoid contact between Simon and his mother. He began a difficult period of adjustment at school, had frequent fights and missed his mother, the person with whom he had the closest relationship. When he was in the sixth grade, his mother found out his whereabouts and there ensued a struggle for the next several years between the mother and grandparents over custody of the child. He discovered his mother's identity at age 13 and went to live with her. His mother and stepfather drank heavily; following a fight between Simon and his stepfather, he was forced to return to his grandparents. For the next year he was constantly in trouble, engaging in car theft, breaking and entering, and drinking heavily. He was sent on court order to live on a farm in Maine and remained there for two years, described as the best in his life. He returned to live with his grandparents for some unclear reason, but was unhappy and soon returned to criminal activity. He attended three different high schools while back in Boston, was expelled from each, and labeled as a troublemaker.

At age 15 he was introduced to drugs by an addict he met while in a juvenile detention center. Upon his release from the center he obtained diluadid from a physician and intraveneously used an opiate for the first time. He says, "I really liked the way it made me feel, there wasn't a problem in the world; it supplemented all the love I had missed."

He continued to use, supporting his habit by breaking and enterings, robbing drug stores, stealing prescriptions, writing bad checks, and using stolen credit cards. From 1960 to 1968 his life was dominated by drug seeking, frequent arrests and jail sentences, a disastrous stint in the Marine Corps, and an equally disastrous marriage to avoid a jail sentence. In 1968 he began methadone maintenance in Boston and was injecting up to 300 mg of take-home and street methadone tablets each day.

In 1970 he was first admitted to the general psychiatry service for detoxification. He remained on the ward for five months and describes the experience as "the worst detoxification ever." He was detoxified over a six-week period and shortly thereafter underwent a psychotic decompensation. He experienced auditory hallucinations and paranoid delusions. He was treated with stelazine, artane, and psychotherapy, with symptomatic improvement. He was discharged on stelazine but was lost to follow-up. According to Simon he stopped the phenothiazines after six weeks. His psychosis returned and he began using methadone. In 1971 he again began methadone maintenance treatment. In the succeeding two years Simon made one more attempt at detoxification and again developed symptoms of a paranoid psychosis which lasted for seven months. He was then reinduced onto 60 mg per day of methadone with subsequent clearing of his psychotic symptoms.

These three patients each meet the DSM-III diagnostic criteria for an Axis I diagnosis of Substance Use Disorder, Opioid Dependence, and the latter two cases meet the criteria for the Axis II diagnosis of Antisocial Personality. The first case meets some of the criteria for Antisocial Personality and could be given the Axis II designation Antisocial Traits. In addition and central to our theme, case 1 meets the criteria for Bipolar Disorder, Mixed; case 2, the criteria for Major Depression, Recurrent; and case 3, the criteria for Schizophrenic Disodrer, Paranoid Type.

Reviewing these histories reveals some interesting phenomena. Each patient actively searched for a drug that would relieve dysphoric symptoms and found that opioid drugs accomplished this better than other classes of drugs. Interestingly, none of these patients spoke of using drugs in order to achieve a euphoric state. Their use of opiates was intended to help them lead quasi-normal lives. In each case, methadone had a definite psychotropic effect. The methadone was more effective in relieving the symptoms of Bipolar Disorder and Schizophrenic Disorder than in relieving the symptoms of the Major Depression. This is consistent with the reports of the high incidence of depression among patients on methadone alone.[10, 11] In fact, the second case presented had more relief of depressive symptoms than would be expected but eventually necessitated tricyclic treatment along with methadone.

In the Cambridge Hospital Drug Treatment Program we conducted retrospective and concurrent chart reviews for patients on the program beginning July 1971 and ending September 1974. Patients with histories and/or diagnoses of a psychotic disorder were reviewed in detail. Staff familiar with the patients were interviewed and, when possible, patients were interviewed. With the exception of one month, there was always at least one patient with a psychotic diagnosis in the methadone maintenance program, and at most times approximately 10% of the patients had a history of non-drug-related psychosis. The two most common diagnoses were Schizophrenic Disorder and Borderline Personality Disorder with psychotic decompensation.

We are currently reviewing patients on methadone maintenance in the Drug Treatment Program of the Veterans Administration Medical Center Brentwood. Preliminary findings again point to a small but consistent percentage of patients with histories of psychotic disorders. Though we do not yet know, we anticipate finding that some of these used opiates as self-medication for their psychotic disorders.

DISCUSSION

Clinical evidence has been presented supporting the concept that opioid drugs are used by some individuals to self-treat dysphoric psychological symptoms. Evidence shows that methadone appears to reduce symptoms usually associated with psychotic disorders. A 1980 report by Judd et al. dismisses this notion. They report on six patients, five of whom were not receiving neuroleptics, who were administered 10 mg intramuscular methadone or placebo. Described results include negative schizophrenic symptomatology, such as emotional withdrawal, motor retardation, and blunted affect. They conclude that "methadone HCL does not exert a specific antipsychotic effect in schizophrenic patients but instead accentuates emotional withdrawal and decreases motor activity. These results may well be due to the single-dose design, which does not replicate the homeostatic effect of longer term methadone or neuroleptic treatment.

While the early observations on the psychotropic effects of methadone and other opioid drugs were clinical, there appears to be mounting theoretical evidence to give further credence to the clinical observations and clinical theory. Most of the theoretical advances have occurred because of the intensive work that has been done since the discovery of the endorphins. The existence of these endogenous opioid peptides has opened the horizons of new research in the biochemical basis of schizophrenic disorders and should ultimately impact significantly on our understanding of the mechanisms involved in opioid drug dependence.

In 1977 and 1978 Gold et al.[22, 23] reported on the dopamine-blocking action of methadone as evidenced by the increase in serum prolactin following administration of methadone. They point out that neuroleptic agents such as haloperidol inhibit the enzyme dopamine-stimulated adenylate cyclase. Methadone and other opioid drugs apparently do the same. They postulate that for this reason "opiate agonists may be antipsychotic in man." Kleber and Gold in 1978 documented well the various uses of psychotropic drugs in the treatment of narcotics addicts on methadone maintenance. They administered lithium carbonate to a group of patients on methadone maintenance with a history of recurrent depression but no history of manic or hypomanic episodes. They allowed the patients to decrease their methadone dose while on the lithium trial and found that the methadone dose decreased significantly ($p < 0.01$) during the trial. They provide support for the hypothesis that methadone is antipsychotic and antimanic and suggest an endorphin hypothesis for the mechanism of action of lithium. They also document the use of neuroleptics in schizophrenic patients maintained on methadone as a result of their opiate dependence. They state, "With the recent developments in opiate receptor and peptide identification reexamined clinical data suggest that opiate receptor activity and opiates may be psychotomimetic and antipsychotic respectively." The antipsychotic properties of methadone are hypothesized on the basis of opiate agonist receptor activity, i.e., interference with the postsynaptic action of dopamine, the mechanisms espoused for the antipsychotic actions of traditional neuroleptic drugs.

In 1978 Verebey et al. suggested the therapeutic uses of opioid drugs in the treatment of certain mental disorders. They advocated the use of methadone particularly in the treatment of selected schizophrenic patients, while cognizant of the disparate results of various researchers in determining the role of the endorphins in the etiology of schizophrenia, a controversy that still exists. They suggested candidates for treatment with methadone, including patients with schizophrenic disorders who have been unresponsive to treatment with traditional neuroleptics, those with especially aggressive behavior unresponsive to neuroleptics, and those with early tardive dyskinesia who cannot discontinue neuroleptic treatment without serious psychotic deterioration. We echo those recommendations today and support their trial recommendations. The most serious argument against such use relates to the political polarization surrounding methadone and the introduction of an addicting drug in the treatment of nonaddicted schizophrenic patients.

In addressing both the arguments for and against using methadone or L-acetylmethadol in the treatment of certain "treatment resistant" patients with schizophrenic or bipolar disorders, there are a number of considerations. First, there are a number of patients at every center who do not respond to any dose of neuroleptic drug. These patients daily continue to suffer from the symptoms of the disorder, without apparent hope of relief. Treatment with opioid agonists might result in symptomatic relief and the possibility of a more normal existence. They would become dependent on the opioid drug, but that might well be preferable to experiencing unabated psychotic symptoms with their attendant dysfunction. There again, the personality traits so often associated with drug-dependent individuals may not develop since the associated behaviors have no need to exist. The experience with large numbers of opiate-dependent servicemen returning from Viet Nam has certainly destroyed the myth that opioid dependence is necessarily connected with further opioid dependence or related behavioral characteristics.

The argument that opioid drugs have antipsychotic properties but do not produce the disabling complications of tardive dyskinesia has been questioned. In a 1980 article by Wasserman and Yahr,[25] choreic movements in a patient on methadone maintenance were reported. They logically conclude that if methadone blocks the postsynaptic dopamine receptor in a manner similar to the neuroleptics, there may develop supersensitivity of the striatal dopamine receptor resulting in the subsequent development of choreic and, presumably, other pseudo-parkinson symptoms in patients on methadone maintenance. This possibility must be carefully examined. The authors correctly point out that it took many years of continuous use of neuroleptics before the serious complication of tardive dyskinesia was discovered and that the same phenomenon may be true of methadone treatment. This prospect should not, however, preclude the use of opioid drugs on a trial basis for the treatment of neuroleptic-resistant patients with schizophrenic disorders. It may also be feasible and desirable to use opioid drugs in the treatment of certain depressive disorders, as described by Kleber,[24] or in the treatment of certain patients with Bipolar Disorder who have developed nephropathy or other serious complications of lithium carbonate treatment.

Last, there are the political considerations. Methadone maintenance treatment has been controversial since its inception. Without reviewing this long-standing controversy, which involves valid clinical, historical, and political arguments, let us say that times do change and perhaps the concept is more acceptable today than heretofore.

CONCLUSION

Evidence has been presented to support the hypothesis that some opiate-dependent individuals use opioid drugs to self-treat prepsychotic and psychotic symptoms. These symptoms were later alleviated by methadone maintenance treatment. This has been observed in three methadone maintenance programs with which we have been involved and has been reported anecdotally by many other professionals involved in methadone maintenance programs. The theoretical basis of these clinical observations has been discussed. The conclusion that methadone does act as a psychotropic drug is presented and recommendations that methadone or longer acting opiate agonists be used on a trial basis in the treatment of certain patients with psychotic disorders is made.

REFERENCES

1. WIKLER, A. & R. W. RASOR. 1953. Psychiatric aspects of drug addiction. Am. J. Med. **14:** 566–570.
2. WELLISCH, M. A., G. R. GAY, D. R. WESSON & D. E. SMITH. 1971. The psychotic heroin addict. J. Psychedelic Drugs **4**(1): 46–49.
3. NYSWANDER, M. 1956. The Drug Addict as a Patient. p. 58. Grune & Stratton. New York.
4. STRAKER, M. 1981. Personal communication.
5. CHEIN, I., D. L. GERARD, R. S. LEE & E. ROSENFELD. 1964. The Road to H. p. 311. Basic Books. New York.
6. WURMSER, L. 1972. Methadone and the craving for narcotics: Observations of patients on methadone maintenance in psychotherapy. *In* Proc. 4th National Methadone Conf. **4:** 525–528.
7. KHANTZIAN, E. J. 1972. A preliminary dynamic formulation of the psychopharmacologic action of methadone. *In* Proc. 4th National Methadone Conf. **4:** 371–374.
8. VEREBEY, K., J. VOLANKA & D. CLOUET. 1978. Endorphins in psychiatry, an overview & hypothesis. Arch. Gen. Psychol. **35:** 877–888.
9. BERKEN, G. H., M. M. STONE & S. K. STONE. 1978. Methadone in schizophrenic rage: A case study. Am. J. Psychiatry **135**(2): 248–249.
10. WEISSMAN, M. M., F. SLOBETZ, B. PRUSOFF, M. MEZRITZ & P. HOWARD. 1976. Clinical depression among narcotics addicts maintained on methadone in the community. Am. J. Psychiatry **133:** 1434–1438.
11. WOODY, G. E., C. P. O'BRIEN & K. RICKELS. 1975. Depression and anxiety in heroin addicts: A placebo-controlled study of doxepin in combination with methadone. Am. J. Psychiatry **132:** 447–450.

12. McKenna, G. J. 1979. Fitting different treatment modes to patterns of drug use. *In* Working With The Impulsive Person. H. Wishnie & J. Nevis-Olesen, Eds. pp. 113–123. Plenum Press. New York.
13. McKenna, G. J. & E. J. Khantzian. 1980. Ego functions and psychopathology in narcotics and polydrug users. Int. J. Addictions 15(2): 259–268.
14. Weissman, M. M., M. Pottenger, H. Kleber, H. L. Ruben, D. Williams & W. D. Thompson. 1977. Symptom patterns in primary & secondary depression. A comparison of primary depressives with depressed opiate addicts, alcoholics, and schizophrenics. Arch. Gen. Psychiatry 34(7): 854–862.
15. Spensley, J. 1976. Doxepin: A useful adjunct in the treatment of heroin addicts in a methadane program. Int. J. Addictions 11(1): 191–197.
16. Salzman, B., M. Kurian, A. Demirjian, E. Morant, S. Dowell, I. Miller & W. Roya. 1973. The paranoid schizophrenic in a methadone maintenance program. 5th National Conf. on Methadone Treatment, New York, Proc. 2: 1304–7.
17. Fisch, A., V. D. Patch, A. Greenfield, A. E. Raynes, G. McKenna & M. Levine. 1973. Depression and self-concept as variables in the differential response to methadone maintenance combined with therapy. 5th National Conf. on Methadone Treatment, New York, Proc. 1: 440–6.
18. Fisch, A., V. D. Patch, A. Greenfield, A. E. Raynes, G. McKenna & M. Levine. 1973. Internal indicators for the management and prognosis of patients in a methadone maintenance program (Internal States Self-Report Scale). 5th National Conf. on Methadone Treatment, New York, Proc. 1: 433–9.
19. McKenna, G. J. 1979. Psychopathology in drug dependent individuals: A clinical review. J. Drug Issues 9(2): 197–205.
20. Treece, C. & B. Nicholson. 1980. DSM-III personality type and dose levels in methadone maintenance patients. J. Nervous Mental Dis. 168(10): 621–628.
21. Judd, L. L., D. S. Jarowsky, D. S. Segal, D. C. Parker & L. Y. Huey. 1981. Behavioral effects of methadone in schizophrenic patients. Am. J. Psychiatry 138(2): 243–245.
22. Gold, M. S., R. K. Donabedian, M. Dillard, F. W. Slobetz, C. E. Riordan & H. D. Kleber. 1977. Antipsychotic effect of opiate agonists. Lancet (2): 398–399.
23. Gold, M. S., D. E. Redmond, R. K. Donabedian, F. K. Goodwin & I. Extein. 1978. Increase in serum prolactin by exogenous and endogenous opiates: Evidence for antidopamine and antipsychotic effects. Am. J. Psychiatry 135(11): 1415–1416.
24. Kleber, H. D. & M. S. Gold. 1978. Use of psychotropic drugs in treatment of methadone maintained narcotic addicts. *In* Recent Developments In Chemotherapy of Narcotic Addiction. Ann. N.Y. Acad. Sci. 311: 81–98.
25. Wasserman, S. & M. D. Yahr. 1980. Choreic movements induced by the use of methadone. Arch. Neurol. 37: 727–728.

Discussion of the Paper

E. J. Khantzian (*Harvard Medical School, Cambridge, MA*): Dr. McKenna, thank you for a very useful and convincing discussion on the antipsychotic action of opiates. I think you have developed some very convincing and provocative thoughts about how these drugs might seriously be considered useful in treating very disturbed individuals.

Perhaps I might just briefly comment on our early psychoanalytic formulation of psychoses, particularly schizophrenia. It used to be emphasized that there was an introversion of the libido, that is, a pulling away of our libido or our love investment in the external world and investing it on the self. This accounted for the peculiarities and particularly withdrawn ways of psychotic individuals. Modern theory, putting it more in structural terms, would emphasize that one of the major malignant influences is the disorganizing influence of rage on the ego that accounts for the disorganization and fragmentation that one observes with very disturbed people and then, secondarily, patients elaborate their own symptoms as a defense to hold themselves together.

I am also reminded of Sheard's work in Connecticut when he worked with felons and administered Lithium to them to study its effects on aggressive behavior and compared such individuals receiving lithium with control groups. He was able to rather convincingly demonstrate a diminution in aggressive behavior as documented by the number of tickets the inmates would get if they manifested any kind of aggression and at the same time he was able to demonstrate an increase in depression in this population of people.

Again, I suspect that the antipsychotic action of these drugs might really reside in their antiaggression action. Also, one of the things we stress with manic patients more than we used to is not only their engaging and charming qualities but also their very aggressive qualities. Certainly, we see it with schizophrenic patients.

G. J. McKenna: I think that may be true. But, returning to Dr. Jaffe's comment from this morning, we are looking at a drug that may not have just one specific action, but may act across a wide spectrum, one of which may target specific anti psychotic actions because of the endorphin system or its interaction with the endorphin system.

A. Corbascio (Oakland, CA): A comment that I would like to make is related to a letter that I received from a patient who committed suicide in a mental institution in California. He wrote among other things, that a drug user is a psychotic patient who is trying empirically to adjust his mental chemistry by trial and error. This search is obstructed by the pharmacological ignorance of the doctors and by the overwhelming prejudice of society.

J. H. Jaffe (University of Connecticut School of Medicine, Farmington): You seem to recommend the use of opiate drugs for certain psychiatric disorders, the converse of what we had with the phenathiazines. With the phenathiazines we found a class of drugs that had specific therapeutic actions, and only later did we discover some very serious side effects and disadvantages such as tardive dyskinesias.

With the opioids, we already known and have known for years about the very serious side effects of the category of drugs. Even if one takes away the illicit aspects, it is not convenient to be obliged to take a drug indefinitely even if the drug were totally free of other side effects; but the fact is, they are not.

Even if there are therapeutic benefits when the opioids are first given, we do not know to what degree tolerance develops to these therapeutic effects. Before we suggest with enthusiasm that the opioids should be used for psychiatric disorders, we ought to be certain that we do not see rapid tolerance to the postulated therapeutic actions. So far, nobody has documented except with anecdotal evidence that there are even brief therapeutic effects. We have little evidence for persistent therapeutic effects, and I think the question of tolerance is one that has to be answered before we talk seriously about opiates as therapeutic agents.

McKenna: Well, again in some of the patients that we followed at both Boston City and Cambridge Hospitals, we, in fact, felt that the therapeutic effects lasted over a period of years. At least the patients were not exhibiting or experiencing psychotic symptoms during the time they were on methadone. At that time we were trying to encourage them to seek treatment in the mental hygiene clinics, but they refused. They preferred an identity as an addict to one as a schizophrenic. I do agree with you that careful clinical studies need to be carried out before opiates are encouraged in the treatment of psychotic patients. I think we can begin with patients who have not previously been addicted, but who are terribly dysphoric because of their psychoses and for whom continued treatment with traditional antipsychotic agents is contraindicated.

Khantzian: Leon, I wondered if you might comment on how you might explain the action of the opiate effects on super ego problems and how such drugs might preclude or mitigate the development of psychoses?

L. Wurmser (*University of Maryland, Baltimore*): The only really important issue is the centrality of very deep intense anxiety. The rage that you describe would not in all likelihood be so disintegrating were it not for the terror of it. I did not talk about the traumatization, but, what adds a kind of foil to my presentation is the child abuse that so many, although not all, drug addicts have suffered. Again, the ultimate thing is the severe panic that they are involved in.

The super ego problems which I moved into the center as the kind of last common pathway in our culture for a compulsive drug user, again, point back to anxiety in our culture, namely, about being disapproved of within ourselves and outside of ourselves. In psychosis it is characteristic for anxiety to assume a mattively disintegrating quality, anxiety that is indeed strongly related to aggression. So I think that is the common feature; I would presume that if we really looked at what the chemical effects are in response to, all the linkages that we described this morning, it may have to do with these very primitive archaic anxiety states.

INTRODUCTORY REMARKS

Robert B. Millman

Departments of Public Health and Psychiatry
Cornell University Medical College
New York, New York 10021

The impetus for my interest in this area derives from two sources. The first is anecdotal in nature. During the mid- to late 1960s, the incidence of acute psychotic reactions, or "bad trips" secondary to the use of psychedelic drugs was quite high. These drugs, particularly LSD, but also including mescaline and marijuana, were often used by naive and unprepared people in unfamiliar or otherwise inappropriate settings. Clinically, the psychotic reaction was no different from so-called functional psychotic states of an acute nature, though generally of shorter duration.

These states were generally treated with reassurance and minor or major tranquilizers by professionals as well as nonprofessionals, with reasonably good results. On the Lower East Side of New York, when these drugs were not available to nonprofessionals, opioids were used, particularly heroin. It was common knowledge that when someone was having an extremely violent psychotic episode, if they were held down and forced to insufflate a small and unknown amount of heroin, the episode would be terminated more rapidly than by any other pharmacologic means. Administration of heroin was considered the most effective way to terminate an acute psychotic episode. I must say with some chagrin, that I discussed this treatment with several psychopharmacologists but they advised that opioids had not been proven useful in psychiatric illness and I did not pursue it further.

The other line of evidence derives from various workers' experience with methadone patients. Some patients who were withdrawn from methadone developed psychotic symptoms. In other cases, when methadone doses were lowered, psychotic symptoms would develop; when the higher dose was reinstated, the symptomatology would defervesce. There is much evidence that a variety of patients self-medicate themselves for varied symptomatology, including apparent functional psychosis, with opioids. Patients clearly describe psychotic symptoms as well as symptoms related to intense anxiety that were controlled by heroin use. Many of them claimed that from their first exposure to heroin, they felt as if a missing part of themselves had been replaced and that they had been waiting for the drugs all their lives.

These observations are not new, of course: there is a rich history of the use of opioids in mental illness going back to Homer. Opioids have been used successfully for psychotic illness, mania and depression, anxiety and almost every other constellation of psychiatric symptomatology. Why these agents fell out of favor and why they are now so interesting to basic scientists and clinicians alike, is worth brief consideration. Perhaps the perils and pain of opiate addiction and the subsequent governmental regulation of these controlled substances did much to stifle research in these areas. In recent years, physicians have even been loathe to prescribe opiates in appropriate dosages for pain. They have been afraid that patients would become addicts or that their prescribing practices would be questioned by governmental authorities. I see some of the patients with intractable pain at the New York Hospital; one of my main functions is to convince the attending physicians to use opiates or to increase the dosage, and that these severely ill people will not become street addicts.

I suspect that the renewed interest in this area is also a function of the exciting discoveries relating to opioid receptors and neurotransmitters and the appreciation of the limits of the presently used antipsychotic agents.

One of the tasks confronting us is to systematize the wealth of clinical observations in this area. This panel and the one that follows will consider the question of which patients or illnesses might be treated effectively with these agents and whether they are superior to conventional therapeutic modes. Perhaps in examining the differential response of patients to opioids, light will be shed on some of the mechanisms underlying emotion, cognition, and psychopathology, as well as the addictive processes.

OPIATES AND SEVERELY DISTURBED PATIENTS

Bernard Salzman

Deparment of Psychiatry
New York University Medical Center
New York, New York 10016

The variations noted in the symptomatology of morphine cases are due to idiosyncracies of the individual and of the surroundings, training, occupation and purposes in life.

In one with a previously defective brain the action of morphine will often conceal the defects or intensify them. [Crothers.[1]]

Although published in 1902, these passages reflect a continuing debate over the relative roles of agent (opiate) and host (individual psychopathology and environment) in the etiology of opiate abuse. Recently restating this, Meissner [2] points out, "the presence of addiction does not necessitate correlative psychological impediments or vulnerabilities as causal determinants. . . . Furthermore, it is not yet known in what manner personality variables may be altered or modified by the pharmacological effects of the drug."

Historically the seemingly inexorable clinical course and centrality of opiate use and behavior generated a number of theories concerning the relationship between drugs and psychosis. Crothers defined morphinism as a form of psychosis,[1] while a later author theorized that the psychosis pre-existed and caused the addiction.[3] Legeive posited a psychosis as part of the abstinence syndrome.[4] In his discussion of the etiology of drug addiction,[5] Glover described the psychopathology of addiction as a "transition state," between neurosis and psychosis. Although pre-supposing a distinct form of antecedent psychopathology in addiction, he correctly delineated the severe character pathology in many opiate abusers.

We are therefore faced with the confounding problem, of an agent (opiates), which alters the manifestation of the psychopathology of the host, and this psychopathology alters the action, use, and effect of the agent. Furthermore, the adaptive lifestyle and chronicity accompanying the use of opiates creates in this population the illusion of homogeneity in a psychopathologically heterogeneous population.

As a group, opiate abusers resemble a comparable psychiatric population, with a skewing toward increased psychopathology.[6] Within this population are the severely disturbed and underdiagnosed functional psychosis and borderline patients. The incidence of the severe psychopathology has been altered by the particular population observed and the setting of the observation.[7–9] Furthermore, the rapid increase in the incidence of heroin addiction following World War II and particularly since 1970 has created a larger, more heterogeneous population under observation.

In order to circumvent these compounding variables, I have adopted a model suggested by Griffith Edwards,[10] who attempted to separate those behavioral factors due to pharmacological effects of the drug and concomitant behavior (pathogenic), from the influence of individual psychopathology and environment (pathoplastic). It is the resultant of these sets of factors, together

0077–8923/82/0398–0058 $1.75/0 © 1982, NYAS

with the particular drug used and the chronicity of its use that accounts for the plasticity of the behavior of drug users.

The psychotic and borderline patient will be observed in three settings; an in-patient psychiatric service; a private consultation, and a methadone maintenance program. The level of observations will be descriptive and phenomonological, dealing predominately with the pathoplastic aspect of patients' behavior.

INPATIENT SERVICE

The inpatient service studied is in a large, municipal hospital (Bellevue). Patients are distributed to the various wards, on a rotating basis, making the population typical of all the other inpatient services. As a result of decreased psychiatric beds, criteria for admission are more stringent, limited to those who are actively psychotic or dangerous to self or others. The particular service is limited to males. With regard to opiate abuse, the patients are admitted under two relevant conditions: firstly, those who have met the psychiatric criteria, who have abused or are addicted to heroin, but who are not a member of a formal treatment program; and secondly, those patients referred from a maintenance program, who have met the psychiatric criteria for admission.

Patients in the heroin-abusing group, like their drug-free counterparts, are admitted actively psychotic. Frequently, they present with auditory and visual hallucinations, disorganized, and frightened. Some of the patients have had psychiatric intervention in early childhood, prior to onset of dysocial behavior or drug taking. Although their drug history is often similar to their nonschizophrenic counterparts, there is a subpopulation with late onset heroin abuse, in which heroin use begins frequently after the age of 20, with or without an antecedent drug history. The patients' abuse, addiction, and abstinence periods parallel the presence or absence of psychotic symptoms. In a similar uncharacteristic manner, their drug history includes multiple self-initiated detoxifications and long periods of abstinence. Not infrequently a psychotic heroin abuser, although not actively addicted at the time, will request methadone instead of a neuroleptic drug.

Case 1

Benjamin, a 38-year-old Black male, presented himself with a history of auditory "voices all around my body," and visual hallucinations, "a woman turned into a fire hydrant." The symptoms began three months ago, and were partially attenuated by alcohol.

The patient first began using heroin 15 years ago. During the period of heroin use, he was married and spent three years in the military service. Auditory hallucinations first began about ten years ago, four days after the patient "licked a heroin habit." He was admitted to the hospital and was treated successfully with Thorazine.

In the intervening years he claims to have been symptom-free, but changed jobs frequently and wandered, "trying to develop my lifestyle." The patient was discharged on Thorazine and referred to a mental health facility.

Patients admitted on methadone maintenance, enter with similar symptoms, but related to secondary drug abuse, usually of the CNS depressant family. On close observation the sequence of events begins with paranoid anxiety and hallucinations, precipitated by separation or estrangement from a symbiotic partner. A secondary drug is utilized for symptom relief, ineffectively, and leads to further ego disorganization and psychosis.

Case 2

Juan, a 46-year-old hispanic male, was admitted from a methadone maintenance program because he heard voices commanding him to "kill people" and "set fires." He complained of seeing "animal-like shapes" on the walls at night. Juan had been in psychiatric hospitals since childhood. He began using heroin about 27 years ago, converting to methadone eight years ago when his "habit" became too expensive. During the years of heroin use he claims to have been free of hallucinations or other symptoms. Over a number of years he voluntarily reduced his dose to 10 mg at which first he "did not feel good" and began to abuse secondary substances, such as LSD and cocaine. A year ago, he was admitted under similar circumstances at a methadone dosage of 5 mg. The patient complained that increasing his dose to 20 mg made him too tired, and preferred to be managed on Mellaril 50 mg twice a day. Following discharge he returned to his methadone maintenance, where he remains in good standing.

The clinical course of the two sets of patients are different. The heroin abuse group, although appearing less sensitive to neuroleptics, have a clinical course similar to their nonabusing counterparts. The methadone maintenance patients recover quickly, with a course similar to that of a "toxic psychosis." This latter group quickly assumes a "pseudo-psychopathic" appearance, although retaining elements of a thought disorder.[11] The shorter, clinical course of this group, together with response to relatively low doses of neuroleptics suggests circumstantial evidence of the antipsychotic actions of opiates.

The clinical course of the drug abuser with borderline personality reflects the impulsivity, drastic mood swings, and irritability characteristic of this diagnosis.[12] These patients are admitted for massive overdoses or serious and dramatic suicide attempts. The drug use histories are marked by "storms" of drug use, that is, large amounts of drugs singularly or in bizarre combinations over a short period of time. These patients appear to have an almost infinite drug tolerance, constantly astounding emergency room personnel by their recovery. Invariably these storms are precipitated by real or threatened estrangement from parent or partner. In a more subtle manner, their own adaptive success threatens separation and leads to a paroxysm of drug use.

Unlike schizophrenics, they often function at high levels inter-ictally, only to sabotage themselves with the use of drugs. Their drug patterns are therefore intermittent and disproportionately large, with frequent periods of quiescence. The inpatient course of the borderline is marked by rapid recovery and vehement "claustrophobic" demand for discharge, in order to re-engage the object of their acted-out rage. Within a few months they return, unchastened, and lacking insight, for the next act in their almost certainly fatal drama.

Case 3

Kevin is a 25-year-old white male transferred from the medical hospital following a massive overdose. The patient was "on a run of heroin and amphetamine" and, upon stopping, felt very depressed. Although he denied a clear precipitant, he decided to take his own life. In a period of a few hours he took: ten Valium (10 mg), five Quaaludes and 2.5 cc of parenteral Valium.

When the patient was 11 years old his brother died of a heroin overdose, which was followed a month later by his father's suicide. He has abused multiple drugs and alcohol, intermittently since the age of 14, with multiple overdoses. He perceives this use of drugs as a form of self-punishment, an attempt to expatiate the death of his father. Currently he is involved in a symbiotic relationship with an older homosexual, and claims, somewhat grandiosely, he is a road manager of a "rock group." Three weeks after this admission, during a period of relative drug abstinence, he was readmitted, because of feelings of despair and suicide. The patient unilaterally terminated follow-up therapy after three weeks.

Private practice represents a second point of observation for the population of disturbed opiate abusers. Patients are invariably brought or forced into therapy by parents or spouse, a resource often not available to either inpatient or methadone maintenance addicts. Although their level of functioning is generally higher, they demonstrate comparable levels of psychopathology and in fact, if seen in terms of social class expectation, greater degrees of deviation.[13]

Drugs users with functional psychoses, make up only a small percentage of patients seen in private practice. They often lack the resources and organization to attend private treatment. Abused drugs in general play an uncovering or precipitant role with regard to psychiatric symptoms. This is classically seen with marijuana, hallucinogens, and central nervous system depressants. Opiate abuse or re-use is generally a sign of an early ongoing psychotic process, in an attempt at direct symptom relief. Although patients are generally vague in their description of opiate effect, it is thought by them to alleviate anxiety or its derivative hallucinations and delusions. At the time of interview, it is the renewed drug use and not the psychological symptoms that becomes the focus of the patient's attention. Frequently schizophrenic patients disorganize during a period of estrangement from a symbiotic partner, or during a transitional stage within a formal addiction program. The most common example of the latter being during the detoxification stage of methadone maintenance, particularly if that stage is precipitous.[14] A second example could be during the shift from the rehabilitation to the re-entry phase within a therapeutic community.[15] In a stable symbiotic relationship with person or program, these patients are frequently asymptomatic, while others are capable of functioning, while actively abusing heroin.

Formal treatment with these patients is often difficult. Replacement of opiates with conventional neuroleptics is perceived by them as inadequate and unacceptable. Frequently these patients return to a formal addiction program to re-establish an acceptable symbiotic relationshp, shifting away from the mental health system.

It would be a gross understatement to describe the borderline psychotic drug user as the most difficult, volatile, and dangerous patient in private practice. Within my personal experience, one patient died of heroin overdose, another shot himself in the head, and three others have survived near fatal overdoses. Invariably brought to therapy by parents, occasionally on the brink of jail sentences, the borderline is a reluctant patient. Their history of drug abuse is long and sporadic. It is marked, as mentioned, by use of unusually large amounts of opiates, as if they were insatiable. Their drug-taking takes place in the setting of an estranged, albeit, intact family. Their fathers, characteristically, are extremely successful, aloof, and unobtainable. Their mothers are emotionally unstable, labile, and inconsistent. It is with the emotionally unstable mother that they secretly identify. The drug storms frequently occur uncannily on the eve of the parents' departure for vacation, and, at times, continue for months following their return. The drug use ritually plays out rage and the wish for re-engagement with the departing parent. Drug bouts are terminated by periods of guilt and expatiation. The latter periods are marked by self-inforced detoxification and periods of relative abstinence. Between episodes, these patients often function initially at a high level, although their interpersonal life varies from abstinence to symbiotic attachment. Their relationship with therapy parallels their drug use patterns, frequently terminating during periods of abstinence, to return with drug re-use, usually on an emergency basis. The patients frequently eschew conventional neuroleptics and antidepressants, although they have been effective in low dose regimes. In those who remain in a therapeutic relationship, change does occur after four or five years, with maturation and luck.

The third point of observation is a methadone maintenance program. The programs are highly structured, rigidly regulated, and ambulatory. Strong emphasis is placed on the "police function" of the clinic, tending to create a high degree of conformity. The staff remains, by and large, stable with well-circumscribed areas of function. The counselors' task includes both police functions and practical counseling. By and large, they are paraprofessionals, with no or little psychological training. They see behavior with little understanding of either antecedents or causology. The programs are characterized by overall stability, predictability with minimal expectations. The use patterns of methadone reflect similar characteristics of dose stability and predictability of effect.

Within this setting, patients with functional psychosis often go undetected, their more blatant psychotic aspects attenuated by the drug effect and the stability of clinic environment. Disordered thinking and logic in the service of "manipulation" are seen as an expected part of addict behavior and ignored. Overt symptoms of hallucinations, hostility, and paranoia overwhelm the under-prepared counselors, and lead to immediate intervention. As mentioned previously, the psychotic breakthrough usually occurs following the sequence of symptoms, secondary drug abuse, and disorganization. Recovery following short-term hospitalization is rapid, with the patient rapidly returning to the clinic. Having returned and been labeled "severely disturbed," their status within the clinic changes. With the professional assistance, they become special patients, their behavior re-interpreted, and in many cases their survival in the program secured. Only a small number of patients will accept long-term concomitant neuroleptics, but they can function marginally within the clinic setting. By and large, schizophrenic patients, if not screened out initially, survive longer in methadone maintenance programs than those patients with more behaviorally oriented character disorders. Of the patients in our original methadone program for disturbed addicts, 18% have died.[16] The majority of the remaining are currently on another methadone program, but some have gone through periods of complete abstinence. Over time, the stable environment of the clinic, its psychological nonintrusiveness, and the antipsychotic effect of the methadone create an idealized setting for these patients.

The patients with a borderline personality have a totally different prognosis within a methadone program. The rigid structure and restrictive rules of the program become like the internalized objects of their psyche, an object of all-out war. The affective storms, with or without secondary drug abuse, leads to increased police interaction with the clinic, leading to rapid and premature discharge from the program. The borderline patient frequently interacts with angry and paranoid interchanges, particularly toward the nurses and administration. Their course is also marked by paroxysms of secondary drug abuse and overdoses, not infrequently fatal. The use of the methadone is less clear with this group of patients. The affective attacks and use of secondary drugs appear less affected by a stable methadone dose. The movement of these patients in and out of methadone programs seems not to affect their psychopathology or their drug use patterns.

The natural drug history of the severely disturbed opiate abuser reflects a unique mixture of pathogenic and pathoplastic effects. Of the many possible effects of opiates, there appears to be one mode of action that approximates the effects of neuroleptics. Both acute and chronic administration of opiates appears to attenuate psychotic anxiety in the schizophrenic addict. This affect appears itself attenuated, however, in chronic administration, such as methadone maintenance, with recurrent evidence of symptom breakthrough. This suggests some form of biological tolerance; however, it may be that, in a manner similar to those patients on chronic neuroleptic maintenance, the patients' chaotic life circumstances overrides the pharmacologic benefits of the drug. Atypical opiate use patterns best reflect the intermittent nature of the nuclear illness, where the opiate serves a most immediate need for symptom relief.

The use patterns in borderline patients are less clear. During periods of "affective storms," their opiate needs appear insatiable, and only partially relieved by the drug. This ability to exquisitely control drug use, interepisodically, is both atypical and reflects the dominance of pathoplastic factors. It also suggests a set of biological processes different than the way in which schizophrenics are affected, and it invites further investigation.

Finally, it should be mentioned that other, nonspecific factors may lead to the attenuation of psychotic symptoms in this population. Specifically, a stable environment, such as symbiotic relationship or a multi-dimensional drug rehabilitation program, diminishes symptom manifestations. More importantly, chronicity, in many schizophrenic patients, changes symptoms from their florid to deficit forms.

REFERENCES

1. CROTHERS, T. D. 1902. Morphinism and Narcomania from Other Drugs. W. B. Saunders Company. Philadelphia, PA.
2. MEISSNER, W. W. 1980. Addiction and paranoid process: Psychoanalytic perspectives. Int. J. Psychoanal. Psychother. 8: 273–310.
3. WILLIAMS, E. H. 1922. Opiate Addiction. p. 11. Macmillan. New York.
4. LEGEIVE, B. 1924. Delirium beim Morphinismus. Z. Gesamte Neurol. Psychiatr. 89: 558.
5. GLOVER, E. 1956. On the etiology of drug addiction. In On the Early Development of the Mind. International Universities Press. New York.
6. DeLEON, G. 1974. Phoenix House: Psychopathological signs among male and female drug-free residents. Addict. Dis. 1: 135.
7. GERARD, D. L. & C. KORNETSKY. 1955. Adolescent opiate addiction: A study of control and addict. Psychiatr. Q. 29: 457.
8. PFEFFER, A. Z. & D. C. RUBLE. 1948. Chronic psychoses and addiction to morphine. Arch. Neurol. Psychiatr. 56: 665.
9. HEKIMIAN, L. J. & S. GERSHON. 1968. Characteristics of drug abusers admitted to a psychiatric hospital. J. Am. Med. Assoc. 205: 125.
10. EDWARDS, G. 1974. Drugs, drug dependence and the concept of plasticity. Q. J. Studies Alcohol 35: 176–195.
11. GELLER, M. 1980. Sociopathic adaptation in psychiatric patients. Hosp. Community Psychiatry 31(2): 108–112.

12. GROVES, J. E. 1981. Borderline personality disorder. N. Engl. J. Med. **305**(5): 259–262.
13. KAUFMAN, E. 1978. The relationship of social class and ethnicity to drug abuse. *In* A Multicultural View of Drug Abuse. D. Smith *et al.*, Eds.: 158–163. G. K. Hall/Schankman, Cambridge, Mass.
14. PFEFFER, A. Z. 1947. Psychosis during withdrawal of morphine. Arch. Neurol. Psychiatry **58:** 221–226.
15. ROHRS, C. 1981. (Psychiatric Consultant, Project Return.) Personal communication.
16. SALZMAN, B. & W. FROSCH. 1972. Methadone maintenance for the psychiatrically disturbed. *In* Proc. 4th Nat. Conf. on Methadone Maintenance. pp. 117–119. National Association for the Prevention of Addiction to Narcotics. New York.

TREATMENT OF MIXED ABUSERS IN METHADONE MAINTENANCE: ROLE OF PSYCHIATRIC FACTORS *

A. Thomas McLellan, George E. Woody,
Bradley D. Evans, and Charles P. O'Brien

Department of Psychiatry
Philadelphia Veterans Administration Medical Center
and University of Pennsylvania
Philadelphia, Pennsylvania 19104

INTRODUCTION

The majority of published work on the etiology and treatment of drug dependence has focused upon the opiate addict. However, the population of "mixed substance abusers" now comprises between 5 and 25 percent of drug abuse patients,[1, 2] and little more than anecdotal observations are available regarding their treatment. By "mixed abuse" we mean the regular (at least three times weekly), concurrent or consecutive use of drugs from more than one class of chemicals: opiates (heroin, hydromorphone, methadone), stimulants (amphetamine, cocaine, methylphenidate), depressants (barbiturates, alcohol, benzodiazepines), or hallucinogens (LSD, PCP, cannabis).

The question of how to treat patients with mixed abuse is important on both practical and theoretical grounds. At present two conceptually different approaches are available. The drug-free therapeutic community (TC) attempts to promote detoxification and abstinence in a structured, peer-oriented community setting, using group "encounter" therapy.[3] Methadone maintenance (MM) attempts to stabilize opiate use through substitution of the synthetic opiate methadone and to gradually withdraw the opiate (often over a period of years), simultaneously developing family, job, and social supports in that context.[4]

From a practical perspective the treatment of mixed abusers in either of these modalities has been problematic. They have the poorest post-treatment oucomes and the worst record of behavior problems during therapeutic community treatments, often disrupting treatment activities and dropping out prematurely.[5, 6] Treatment within a methadone maintenance modality is often inappropriate or illegal since many mixed abusers have not had sufficient opiate abuse to meet FDA admission requirements. Thus, the practical treatment options available for the mixed abusers are often limited.

From a theoretical perspective, there is reason to believe that methadone maintenance, for those mixed abusers who qualify, would be more effective than drug-free treatment. For example, there is evidence that mixed abusers present with a greater range and severity of psychiatric problems than opiate addicts.[5, 7, 8] Independent work at this clinic and others suggests that the psychiatric status of drug abuse patients at admission is the most significant factor in predicting post-treatment outcome.[9] In this regard, emerging evidence from

* This work was supported by Health Service Research & Development Projects 284 and 525 from the Veterans Administration.

65

0077–8923/82/0398–0065 $1.75/0 © 1982, NYAS

clinical and laboratory studies with the endorphins indicates that both endogenous and exogenous opiates (including methadone) may have antidepressant, antianxiety, and antipsychotic effects.[10-13] Thus, methadone maintenance may be a more effective treatment than drug-free therapy for this population of patients.

With this in mind, we undertook the present study to compare the relative effectiveness of methadone maintenance and drug-free therapy in the treatment of mixed drug abusers. We have selected opiate–stimulant abusers, opiate–depressant abusers, and an opiate-only group, under the hypothesis that methadone maintenance will be differentially effective with these mixed abusers.

METHOD

Subjects. Subjects were selected *retrospectively* from a larger pool of 282 male veterans who had been treated for drug dependence at the Philadelphia or Coatesville VA Medical Centers during 1978. All of these subjects had received a comprehensive evaluation at admission to treatment and at six-month follow-up as part of a larger study.[14] Each of the patients had received a minimum of 15 inpatient days or 15 outpatient visits in either the drug-free, therapeutic community (TC) or methadone maintenance (MM) rehabilitation programs.

Treatment Programs. The drug abuse treatment network of the Veterans Administration in the Philadelphia area consists of two inpatient drug abuse programs (one conventional TC, one combined alcohol and drug abuse TC) at the Coatesville VA Medical Center, and one outpatient methadone maintenance clinic at the Philadelphia VA Medical Center. This treatment network has enjoyed cooperative referral arrangements since 1970. Once admitted to either hospital, patients are assigned to rehabilitation treatment based upon their personal requests, the clinical judgment of the treatment team, or administrative considerations such as bed census and patient-visit criteria.

(*a*) *The Therapeutic Community Program.* The TC program is an intensive, 60-day, 30-bed program involving both personal and social treatment. Individual and group (encounter) therapies in addition to the social structure of a self-governing community are the primary therapeutic tools. Family therapy as well as educational and vocational counseling are also offered. The program is directed by a social worker and includes a staff of two psychologists, two social workers, two nurses, and four rehabilitation technicians. Limited use of psychotropic medications is permitted when indicated by the attending physician.

(*b*) *The Methadone Maintenance Program.* The MM program is a research and treatment program which offers methadone plus individual counseling and vocational guidance to an active census of 275 patients. The use of adjunctive psychotropic medications is also permitted within this program and is supplemented by regular sessions of individual counseling by the rehabilitation technicians. The staff consists of three psychiatrists, one psychologist, two social workers, two nurses, and eight rehabilitation technicians.

PROCEDURE

Subject Selection and Matching

Since we wanted to compare treatment outcomes in subjects who *could* have been assigned to either the TC or MM programs we selected only those subjects who met or surpassed the minimum FDA requirements for methadone treatment. These included a minimum of three years of physical dependence on opiates, and two or more prior unsuccessful detoxifications. One hundred and seventeen subjects were selected retrospectively in this manner, thus all subjects were legally eligible for either TC or MM treatment.

These subjects were further divided into three drug-use classes based upon the nature of their non-opiate drug use. Opiate–stimulant (OS) subjects reported three or more years of regular stimulant (amphetamine, methylphenidate, cocaine) use but less than two years of regular depressant use. *Note:* The operational definition of "regular use" used in the present study is a frequency of three or more occasions per week. Opiate–depressant (OD) subjects reported three or more years of regular depressant (barbiturates, benzodiazepines, sedative-hypnotics) use but less than two years regular stimulant use. Opiate-only (OO) subjects reported less than two years of regular use of either stimulants or depressants. Alcohol and marijuana use were recorded but were not used in the grouping criteria. Initial analyses of these drug use patterns indicated a tendency ($p < 0.12$) toward greater alcohol use by the OD and OO groups, and greater marijuana use ($p < 0.15$) by the OS group. No differences in frequency of use were statistically significant.

Once these three drug-use classes were differentiated, subjects within each group were divided and matched into those who had been treated in the TC and those who had been treated in MM. Subjects were matched on the basis of age, race, years of drug use, number of prior treatments, and psychiatric severity. Psychiatric severity was judged using the Addiction Severity Index psychiatric scale [15] (see *Data Collection*). Psychiatric severity was used as a matching criterion since prior work has shown it to be the best general index of overall status at treatment admission and a good predictor of treatment response.[9] In the course of this matching procedure 13 subjects were eliminated leaving 104 subjects: 15 pairs of OS subjects, 15 pairs of OD subjects, and 22 pairs of OO subjects.

Data Collection

All data collected during the study were obtained using the Addiction Severity Index (ASI) [15] at admission to treatment and again at follow-up, six months later. The ASI is a structured, 30–40 minute, clinical research interview designed to assess problem severity in six areas commonly affected by addiction. It is important to note that problem severity in each area is assessed independently and six areas are included: medical, legal, substance abuse, employment, family, and psychiatric problems. In each of the areas, objective questions are asked measuring the number, extent, and duration of problem symptoms in the patient's lifetime and in the past 30 days. The patient also supplies a subjective report of the recent (past 30 days) severity and importance of the problem area. The interviewer assimilates the two types of information to produce a rating (0–9) reflecting the extent to which treatment is needed by the patient in each area. These 10-point ratings have been shown to provide reliable and valid general estimates of problem severity for both alcoholics and drug addicts,[15] and the individual items offer a comprehensive basis for clinical and experimental assessment.

All ASI follow-up interviews were done six months following treatment admission by an independent research technician, either in person or over the phone. No information from secondary sources was used and all data were closely monitored to preserve confidentiality. The validity of the follow-up data was maintained through built-in consistency checks within the ASI and through spot checks on subsamples of the population assessing the ASI data against urinalysis, pharmacy, and criminal justice system records.

Outcome Criteria

It was important for the aims of this study to have general measures of treatment outcome, since single item measures can be inherently unreliable.[16] We therefore constructed criterion composites or factors from sets of single items within each of the ASI problem areas. Several items from each problem area were intercorrelated to exclude those that were unrelated, and the remaining items were standardized and tested for conjoint reliability using Cronbach's formula.[17] A set of 4 to 6 objective items from each ASI problem area was selected using this procedure, and each set showed a standardized reliability coefficient of 0.73 or higher. Seven composites or factors (medical problems, employment, drug use, alcohol use, legal status, family problems, and psychiatric function) were constructed in this manner and scores on each were calculated for all patients at admission and follow-up. This method has been employed effectively by Luborsky and Mintz in their studies of outcome from psychotherapy.[18, 19]

RESULTS

Admission Comparisons

TABLE 1 presents a comparison of the demographic characteristics and general status of the six groups at the time of treatment admission. Comparisons are presented for each of the areas covered by the ASI showing the global severity rating (0, no problem; 9, maximum severity) as well as several representative items in each area. As can be seen, within each drug-use class the TC and MM groups are very well matched. No pair of groups differed on more than three items ($p < 0.05$ by t-test) with the obvious exceptions of the drug use variables, which were not compared. Further, there were no consistent trends between any of the TC-MM pairs with regard to overall severity at the time of admission.

Comparisons among the three drug-use classes (collapsing across treatment groups) revealed a significantly ($p < 0.05$) higher proportion of Black subjects in the OO group than in the other two categories. This is consistent with the clinical impression shared by most workers, that Black drug abusers are less prone to regular, mixed drug abuse than their white counterparts. Analyses of the remaining demographic items showed no significant ($p < 0.10$) differences among the three drug-use classes. However, analyses of the rankings of patient status measures at the time of treatment admission revealed a general trend toward better overall status in the opiate-only class ($x^2 = 20.6$, df $= 4$, $p < 0.01$). Chi-square or one-way ANOVA analyses were then performed on 25 of the admission ASI variables and 17 were found to differ significantly at $p < 0.05$ or less. Ten of these comparisons indicated that the opiate-only class had a

TABLE 1

BACKGROUND CHARACTERISTICS OF THE DRUG-FREE THERAPEUTIC COMMUNITY (TC) AND METHADONE MAINTENANCE (MM) GROUPS

Variable	Opiate–Stimulant Abusers		Opiate–Depressant Abusers		Opiate-Only Abusers	
	TC	MM	TC	MM	TC	MM
N	16	16	18	18	22	22
Age	32	30	31	30	33	33
Race (% Black)	32	28	50	52	59	64
Yrs education	11	12	12	12	12	12
Previous treatments	5	5	6	5	4	4
Medical severity †	2.8	2.6	3.2	3.0	1.9	1.8
Previous Hosp.	2	3	4	3	3	2
% w/Chronic prob.	33	40	34	29	40	23 *
Employment severity †	5.6	5.9	6.1	5.5	4.6	4.5
% w/Skill or trade	80	67 *	40	63 *	68	58
% Worked past 3 yrs	65	68	42	48	55	48
Substance abuse severity †	6.3	6.8	7.0	6.4	6.0	5.6
Yrs alcohol abuse	1.5	1.8	5.0	3.4	2.6	2.2
Yrs opiate use	9	11	8	6	12	10
Yrs stimulant use	7	8	1	1	1	1
Yrs depressant use	2	1	9	7	1	0
Legal severity †	4.0	4.2	5.0	4.2	4.0	4.4
Arrests	6	5	9	4	6	4
Months incarcerated	27	29	20	14 *	24	24
Family†social severity	5.3	4.9	4.4	3.7	3.7	3.6
% Divorced/separated	27	20	31	33	23	27
% Never married	40	33	27	27	36	18 *
% Living alone	33	27	18	22	18	18
Psych. severity	4.5	4.4	5.1	4.7	3.3	2.3
% Prev. hosp.	33	40	29	23	18	11
% Sign. depressed	43	38	73	66	51	44
% Suicide attempts	7	18 *	27	21	9	5
% Hallucinated	36	22 *	21	7 *	0	8
Maudsley neuroticism	32	34	30	27	18	20
Shipley C.Q.	88	85	76	79	88	91
Beck Depression Inventory	11	13	21	19	17	15

† ASI Severity Scores: 0, no problem; 9, maximum severity.
* Significant difference between TC and MM groups, $p < 0.05$ by paired t-test.

significantly better status than the other groups. Further, the OO class was not significantly worse than the other classes on any variable. The results were particularly clear in the psychiatric status variables where the OO class showed significantly better admission status ($p < 0.05$) than the other groups on 4 of the 8 measures. No consistent differences in overall status were observed between the OS and the OD patients.

OUTCOME COMPARISONS BETWEEN TREATMENT PROGRAMS

Comparisons of admission to follow-up improvement, as well as adjusted comparisons of six-month outcomes were calculated for the two treatment programs and these results are presented for each of the drug-use classes individually.

Opiate–Stimulant Subjects

Admission and follow-up results are presented for all OS subjects, divided into the two treatment programs, in TABLE 2. Considerable disparity is seen in the performance of patients in the two treatment programs. As seen, the methadone maintenance subjects showed more improvement in more criterion areas and at generally higher levels of significance than the matched patients

TABLE 2

OPIATE–STIMULANT SUBJECTS

Criteria †	Therapeutic Community N = 16		Methadone Maintenance N = 16		ANCOVA Analysis of 6-Month Scores ‡
	At Admission	At 6 Months	At Admission	At 6 Months	
Medical factor	11.2	12.9	9.0	9.7	
Days Med. Prob.	9	10	7	7	
Employment factor	20.4	8.7 **	31.3	6.1 **	*
Days Worked	3	9	2	12 **	
Money Earned	54	277 *	68	371 **	*
Welfare Support	62	38	71	47 *	
Alcohol use factor	15.4	16.1	20.5	10.6 *	**
Days Intoxicated	4	5	7	2 *	
Money Spent on Alcohol	7	6	8	3 *	
Drug use factor	109.1	61.0 *	197.4	38.2 **	**
Days Opiate Use	11	5 *	15	3 **	
Days Depr. Use	2	1	3	2	
Days Stim. Use	10	2 **	8	2 *	
Money Spent on Drugs	148	72 *	230	70 **	*
Legal status factor	66.2	21.0 *	86.3	16.4 **	*
Days Comm. Crime	6	4	15	6 *	
Illegal Income	160	58 *	130	14 *	*
Family rel. factor	13.0	10.6	15.9	11.9	
Days Fam. Prob.	10	9	12	8	
Psychological factor	15.4	14.3	17.0	12.7 *	*
Days Psych. Prob.	12	10	14	7 *	*

* $p < 0.05$; ** $p < 0.01$.
† All data reflect the 30-day periods prior to admission and follow-up (6 month).
‡ Admission score was the covariate in each analysis.

from the therapeutic community program. MM patients from this drug-use class showed significant improvements in all criterion areas except medical status and family relations. While the TC patients showed clear gains in employment and some improvement in drug use, they showed only minor improvement in legal status and no significant change in medical status, alcohol use, family relations, or psychological function.

Analyses of covariance (ANCOVA) on the six-month outcome status variables for the two programs showed results which were similar to the improvement data and these are presented in the last column of TABLE 2. In each of these analyses, the admission criterion score was used as the only covariate since the subjects were matched on virtually all other relevant variables. The follow-up outcome measures showed *better adjustment in the MM subjects* on all but three of the 21 comparisons, and these differences were significant ($p < 0.05$ or less) on ten of those comparisons. Thus, these treatment results indicate greater and more pervasive improvements, as well as generally better six-month outcomes in the OS subjects who were treated in methadone maintenance, than in matched OS subjects treated in the therapeutic community.

Opiate–Depressant Subjects

TABLE 3 presents admission and follow-up data for the OD subjects treated in each of the two rehabilitation programs. Again, there was an overall difference in the performance of the two treatment programs but *opposite* to that seen in the OS class. The TABLE 3 analyses of admission to follow-up improvement indicate that 11 variables showed significant improvement in the TC subjects as compared with seven significant changes in the MM subjects. Neither group showed evidence of significant improvement in medical condition or family relations, and only minor improvements were shown by the TC subjects in alcohol use. TC subjects showed somewhat less improvement than the MM subjects in drug use, somewhat more improvement in employment and legal status and clearly greater improvement in psychiatric function.

The between-programs analyses of covariance on the six-month outcome data substantiated the results of the within-program analyses. As can be seen in the last column of TABLE 3, the follow-up status of the TC patients was better than that shown by the MM patients on all but three of the 21 measures; significantly so ($p < 0.05$ or less) on ten variables. These results indicate *generally greater improvement and better six-month outcomes among OD subjects treated in the Therapeutic Community* than matched OD patients treated in methadone maintenance.

Opiate-Only Subjects

The within- and between-program comparisons for the OO subjects are presented in TABLE 4. In the case of these subjects, no clear differences in levels of improvement or in six-month follow-up status are evident between the two treatment programs. Within-program comparisons indicate 11 variables that showed significant ($p < 0.05$ or less) improvement for the TC subjects and 13 significantly improved criteria for the MM subjects. The MM subjects showed somewhat more improvement than the TC subjects in the area of medical status

TABLE 3

OPIATE–DEPRESSANT SUBJECTS

Criteria †	Therapeutic Community N = 18		Methadone Maintenance N = 8		ANCOVA Analysis of 6-Month Scores ‡
	At Admission	At 6 Months	At Admission	At 6 Months	
Medical factor	15.1	10.3	10.2	7.1	
Days Med. Prob.	12	8	7	5	
Employment factor	29.2	4.0 *	21.5	10.6 *	*
Days Worked	2	10 *	6	8	*
Money Earned	65	285 *	117	211 *	
Welfare Support	59	48	68	106	*
Alcohol use factor	25.0	15.9	16.7	9.9	
Days Intoxicated	6	2	4	2	
Money Spent on Alcohol	24	9 *	13	10	
Drug use factor	114.5	35.3 **	140.1	80.1 **	*
Days Opiate Use	14	8	17	6 **	*
Days Depr. Use	17	8 **	13	10	
Days Stim. Use	3	1	3	1	
Money Spent on Drugs	70	24	131	54 **	
Legal status factor	76.4	8.2 **	91.8	32.8 **	**
Days Comm. Crime	8	1 *	14	7 *	*
Illegal Income	188	10 *	169	81	*
Family rel. factor	9.8	6.8	12.7	10.9	
Days Fam. Prob.	7	5	9	8	
Psychological factor	18.9	9.3 **	19.4	16.2	**
Days Psych. Prob.	20	6 **	9	8	*

* $p < 0.05$; ** $p < 0.01$.
† All data reflect the 30-day periods prior to admission and follow-up (6 month).
‡ Admission score was the covariate in each analysis.

while the TC subjects showed greater improvement in employment and family relations. The remaining areas showed approximately equal levels of improvement between the two programs. These OO subjects showed the greatest improvements in the areas of drug use, employment, and legal status and this is consistent with previous reports from this clinic regarding the major results of drug abuse treatment.[20]

Between-program analyses of the follow-up data also showed few significant outcome differences between the two rehabilitation programs. The adjusted outcome status of the MM patients was better on 12 of the 21 comparison variables but the difference was significant on only the drug-use variable. Correspondingly, the TC subjects showed better outcome status on 9 of the 21 comparisons, significantly so in two cases. These results do not suggest any general trend toward better outcomes for either treatment program although the *subjects from this drug-use class, regardless of treatment program, showed generally better six-month outcomes than the OS or OD subjects.* This impression was confirmed by analyses of covariance between drug-use classes (collapsed across treatment program), using the admission criterion score as the covariate in each analysis. Results of these analyses indicated nine variables on which the OO subjects showed significantly ($p < 0.05$ or less) better status than the other subjects, ten variables on which there was no significant difference ($p > 0.10$) and only one variable (illegal income) where the OO subjects had significantly poorer outcome ($p < 0.05$) than the other subjects. Thus, opiate-only subjects showed generally better outcomes than other drug-use subjects but approximately equal levels of improvement and similar six-month adjustments when treated in either the therapeutic community or the methadone maintenance programs.

DISCUSSION

Mixed abuse of drugs from pharmacologically different classes continues to present therapeutic and management problems for treatment personnel within the substance abuse field. The widely documented evidence of greater psycho-

TABLE 4

OPIATE-ONLY SUBJECTS

Criteria †	Therapeutic Community		Methadone Maintenance		ANCOVA Analysis of 6-Month Scores ‡
	At Admission	At 6 Months	At Admission	At 6 Months	
Medical factor	5.6	6.2	7.7	5.8	
Days Med. Prob.	4	4	6	3 *	
Employment factor	27.0	4.0 **	32.0	8.6 **	
Days Worked	4	11 *	6	10	
Money Earned	135	316 *	156	213	
Welfare Support	34	25	96	77	*
Alcohol use factor	17.3	6.5 *	20.3	8.3 *	
Days Intoxicated	4	1	5	1 *	
Money Spent on Alcohol	10	2 *	19	2 *	
Drug use factor	164.7	49.9 **	210.7	41.6 **	*
Days Opiate Use	18	3 **	22	3 **	
Days Depr. Use	4	2	5	2	
Days Stim. Use	4	3	4	2	
Money Spent on Drugs	205	32 **	251	40 **	
Legal status factor	94.6	18.0 **	88.7	20.1 **	
Days Comm. Crime	15	4 *	12	3 *	
Illegal Income	249	80 *	270	105 *	
Family rel. factor	7.0	5.6	12.7	14.0	*
Days Fam. Prob.	7	4 *	9	10	
Psychological factor	6.5	6.4	7.0	4.1 *	
Days Psych. Prob.	3	4	7	5	

* $p < 0.05$; ** $p < 0.01$.
† All data reflect the 30-day periods prior to admission and follow-up (6-month).
‡ Admission score was the covariate in each analysis.

pathology among mixed abusers [5, 7, 8] and the growing evidence for psychotropic action of the opiates [10-13] suggested the possibility that methadone maintenance (MM) might be more effective than drug-free therapeutic community (TC) treatment for those mixed abusers who would qualify. In an attempt to examine this issue we compared MM and TC treatment in groups of mixed opiate–stimulant (OS) and opiate–depressant (OD) abusers and in a comparison group of opiate-only (OO) subjects. All subjects were male veterans who had been treated for drug abuse in the Philadelphia area as part of a larger treatment evaluation study.[14] Only patients who met the minimum FDA requirements for MM treatment were included in the study, thus *each subject could have been treated in either modality*. Subjects from each of the drug-use classes were divided into those who had been treated in MM or TC and then matched on the basis of age, race, years of drug use, number of prior treatments, and a global measure of psychiatric severity. This resulted in 16 matched pairs of OS subjects, 18 matched pairs of OD subjects, and 22 pairs of OO subjects who were evaluated on 21 variables from seven criterion areas at admission and again at six-month follow-up.

The overall results indicated that the two mixed abuse classes, regardless of treatment program, showed significantly greater incidence of psychopathology and generally worse status on most areas than the opiate-only class at the time of treatment admission and again at follow-up. This finding is consistent with the reported literature on mixed abusers and our own clinical experience, indicating generally poorer function in most areas and less potential for post-treatment adjustment than the traditional opiate addict. It should be recognized that a major covariate within this study was the greater proportion of Black subjects in the OO class. Our experience, and that of other workers, suggest that as a group, the greater proportion of Black drug abuse patients are opiate-only users and at the same time are more psychologically intact than their white counterparts. It is quite possible that there are some causal connections in these relationships, but without definite proof, it is sufficient to note that these factors are covaried and that some of the generally poorer status seen in the mixed abusers may be a partial function of the racial composition as well as the drug preference.

Comparisons of treatment efficacy within the drug-use classes yielded remarkable differences. For example, OS patients who were treated in MM showed much greater improvement and clearly better outcomes than the matched OS patients who received treatment in the TC modality. Conversely, OD patients who received TC treatment showed greater improvement and better outcomes than matched OD patients treated in MM. Finally, consistent with our prior data,[9] there were no general differences in rates of improvement or in post-treatment outcomes for opiate-only patients treated in either MM or TC.

Prior to discussion and interpretation of these findings, it is important to clarify the limitations of the study. Perhaps the major qualification to the results is the lack of our experimental design. The present data were collected retrospectively as part of a larger treatment evaluation study and the patients were not randomly assigned to the two treatment programs. This raises the possibility that the treatment groups were not equal on important variables prior to treatment. We attempted to address this retrospectively in two ways. First, we took care to match the patients on those variables which have historically been important in determining treatment outcome. The TABLE 1 data indicate that with few exceptions the matched groups were equal in terms of demographic, background, and current status factors. Secondly, we utilized analyses of covariance to statistically equate the treatment groups on each of the comparisons. While this alone is not a sufficient substitute for a randomized design, the procedure does permit a conservative analysis of outcome between groups.[6] Taken together, the matching and the analysis of covariance procedures compensate substantially for the lack of an experimental design and permit cautious interpretation of the findings, although experimental replication is indicated.

The lack of random assignment to treatments also raises the possibility that one of the treatment groups received more favored, better prognosis patients. We do not feel this is likely in the present study for two reasons. First, despite the fact that the groups were not assigned randomly, they were assigned in the same way and in approximately the same proportion to each of the treatment programs. All patients were assigned to treatment on the basis of their personal choice, the clinical judgment of the admission staff, administrative considerations, and simple choice. This reduces the possibility of differential assignment strategies. Secondly, if differential assignment was in effect, it does not, by itself, explain the differential performance of the three drug patterns in the two programs. The fact that neither program was generally more effective *across* all drug-pattern groups suggests that neither program received generally favored patients.

A final qualification to the present study is the follow-up procedure. For reasons of time and expense in our ongoing project, we adopted a procedure in which patients were contacted six months after admission to treatment. For this reason, the time between treatment discharge and follow-up was not equal for all patients. We have examined the relationships between time out of treatment and outcome status on all criterion measures, and no significant ($p < 0.10$) correlations were shown for any of the groups. Similar follow-up procedures have been used in previous studies [6, 21, 22] and we are satisfied that the procedure employed did not significantly or differentially distort the results.

Given the present results and the design limitations, we would like to interpret the data in a manner that is consistent with certain known facts and with the clinical pictures presented by these patients.

The Opiate–Stimulant Group

We are not surprised by the results of the treatment comparison in the OS group. We have studied this population of stimulant abusers extensively, and, coupled with the reports of others, we conclude that the psychopathological symptoms of hypersensitivity, dependence, paranoia, mania, and schizophrenia are characteristic of these patients, often long after successful detoxification.[23, 24] It is not yet clear whether the stimulants actually cause or simply reveal these symptoms, or whether the duration and intensity of stimulant use is related to the duration of the psychopathology. Nevertheless, these OS patients often experience a range and intensity of these symptoms as they enter the TC for rehabilitation. Since the philosophy of the TC program inhibits the use of psychotropic medication, these patients can be uncomfortable from the outset. In addition, the pressures of the new interpersonal living arrangements, the patient government, and especially the encounter therapy of the group sessions may prove too much for many of these patients, leading to increased anxiety or early termination and an unfavorable treatment response.

The relatively better performance of the OS group in the MM program may be a function of several factors. First, the therapy provided by the counselors was individual and supportive, thus potentially less threatening and more engaging to this group of patients than group encounter. Secondly, the daily methadone maintenance regimen provided a regular schedule, thereby stabilizing their lives to some extent. Further, the philosophy of the program was such that regular psychotropic medicines were provided when necessary. The daily methadone schedule provided a vehicle for their prescription (taken with or mixed in the methadone), thereby insuring compliance. Finally, there is clinical and some experimental evidence for the direct antianxiety, antipsychotic actions of methadone.[12, 13] Several stimulant abusing patients have presented with psychotic symptoms that they (and often their families) claim are abated during methadone stabilization. While the strength and range of methadone's neuroleptic action remains to be determined, it is well tolerated without the extrapyramidal side effects of traditional neuroleptics.

The Opiate–Depressant Group

The differential performance shown by the OD subjects in the two treatment programs was directly opposite to the results seen in the OS subjects. However, the results of several studies with this population suggest that they often present a different clinical picture than their OS counterparts. Our experience with depressant or sedative abusers indicates that they often exhibit clear evidence of depressive spectrum disease, even following detoxification.[23] Again, it is not possible to determine at this time whether the psychiatric symptoms are the impetus for depressant abuse or its result. Given this clinical picture, we might have expected the methadone maintenance regimen to show better results, under the assumption of a regulatory and antidepressant effect of the methadone. However, it has also been our experience that patients who abuse depressants and sedative hypnotics (including the benzodiazepines) have serious problems with depression even when on methadone. In these patients, the depressant effect of the sedatives can predominate over the reported antidepressant effects of methadone, or there may be a methadone-sedative interaction that accentuates depression. We speculate that under these conditions, it may be especially difficult to stabilize these patients, thus reducing the likelihood of improvement.

The inpatient and drug-free status of the TC may be particularly important for these patients. For example, our earlier work has indicated the significant tendency toward suicidal ideation and suicidal attempts among the depressant users.[23] While this may be a joint function of greater depression and the subsequent danger of accidental overdose, we suggest that an inpatient setting may be a more conservative and therapeutic modality in which to treat these patients. Secondly, we have evidence suggestive of cognitive impairment in the depressant-abusing population,[8] which may require a sustained period of stable drug-free treatment in order to recover normal function and restore judgment. Again, we must emphasize that these suggestions are *post hoc* speculations, but we feel they are consistent with the data, with our clinical experience and with relevant experimental work in the field.

The Opiate-Only Group

The clinical picture presented by the majority of our OO subjects is generally much different than that seen in either of the mixed abuse classes. The majority of our OO patients have a stable pattern of drug use, clear problems of unemployment and crime, but few psychiatric symptoms other than mild-moderate depression and sociopathy.[23] As reported in previous studies,[9, 20] we have seen marked treatment effects in these patients in both the TC and MM programs. We consider these patients to have the best general prognosis since they have often developed skills that can be applied to employment and they have few psychiatric symptoms which would interfere with interpersonal relations. Thus, we were not surprised to see equal amounts of improvement in these two groups.

The Role of Psychiatric Factors in Rehabilitation

We have speculated regarding the reasons for the differential results seen in the MM and TC programs with the OS and OD groups, and we have concentrated upon psychiatric factors to account for the results. It may be argued that differences between the two programs in other factors such as job referral or the quality of special training of the treatment staffs may be equally important. We think that the psychiatric factors are the most important aspects in determining the appropriate match of patients and treatments and in predicting the post-treatment outcomes.[9] In the present study, as in previous work reported from this group, the groups that showed the greatest overall benefit from treatment were those (MM in the OS patients, TC in the OD patients) that showed significant improvement in psychiatric status. Clearly, a wide range of factors in each treatment had an impact on the patients who entered, but, especially for these mixed abuse patients in whom drug use and psychological symptomatology are particularly intertwined, we feel that psychiatric factors are most important. It remains for further, more refined studies to investigate the specific aspects within each treatment modality and within each drug-use class that interact to produce the favorable and unfavorable treatment responses shown in the present study.

ACKNOWLEDGMENT

The cooperation and support of Dr. Keith A. Druley and his staff at the Substance Abuse Treatment Unit of the Coatesville VA Medical Center are gratefully acknowledged.

REFERENCES

1. NIDA Statistical Series. 1981. Q. Rep. **2**(8, May).
2. Veterans Administration Annual Report. 1979. [1980]. U.S. Government Printing Office, Washington, D.C.
3. DeLeon, G. & M. S. Rosenthal. 1979. Therapeutic communities. *In* Handbook on Drug Abuse. R. L. DuPont, A. Goldstein & J. O'Donnell, Eds. pp. 39–47, NIDA, Washington, D.C.

4. LOWINSEN, J. & R. MILLMAN. 1979. Clinical aspects of methadone maintenance treatment. Ref. 3, p. 49–56.
5. MCLELLAN, A. T., J. MACGAHAN & K. A. DRULEY. 1978. Changes in drug abuse clients—1972–1978: Implications for revised treatments, Am. J. Drug Alcohol Abuse 6(2): 151–162.
6. SIMPSON, D. D., L. J. SAVAGE, M. R. LLOYD & S. B. SELLS. 1979. Evaluation of drug abuse treatments based on the first year after DARP, Services Research Monograph Series, DHEW Pub. No. ADM-78-701, NIDA, Washington, D.C.
7. ZUCKERMAN, M., S. SOLA, J. MASTERSON, et al. 1975. MMPI patterns in drug abusers before and after treatment in therapeutic communities. J. Consult. Clin. Psychol. 43: 286–296.
8. GRANT, I. & L. JUDD. 1976. Neuropsychological and EEG disturbances in poly-drug users. Am. J. Psychiatry 133: 1039.
9. MCLELLAN, A. T., C. P. O'BRIEN, L. LUBORSKY & G. E. WOODY. 1981. Certain kinds of substance abuse patients do better in certain kinds of treatments. Problems of Drug Dependence 1980, NIDA Research Monograph 34. U.S. Government Printing Office, Washington, D.C.
10. COMFORT, A. 1977. Morphine as an antipsychotic. Lancet (2).
11. GOLD, M., R. K. DONABEDIAN, M. DILLARD, et al. 1977. Antipsychotic effects of opiate agonists. Lancet (2).
12. SALZMAN, B. 1982. Opiates and Severely Disturbed Patients. Ann. N.Y. Acad. Sci. 398. This volume.
13. BERKEN, G. 1982. Methadone: An effective agent in managing intractable pain as a symptom of psychotic anger. Ann. N.Y. Acad. Sci. 398. This volume.
14. MCLELLAN, A. T., C. P. O'BRIEN, R. KRON, et al. 1980. Matching substance abuse patients to appropriate treatments: A conceptual and methodological approach. Drug Alcohol Depend. 5:189–195.
15. MCLELLAN, A. T., L. LUBORSKY, G. E. WOODY & C. P. O'BRIEN. 1980. An improved evaluation instrument for substance abuse patients: The Addiction Severity Index. J. Nerv. Ment. Dis. 168(1): 26–33.
16. NUNNALLY, J. 1967. Psychometric Theory. McGraw-Hill. New York.
17. CRONBACH, L. J. & L. FURBY. 1980. How should we measure "change"—or should we? Psychol. Bull. 74.
18. LUBORSKY, L. 1980. Predicting the outcomes of psychotherapy—Findings of the Penn Psychotherapy Project. Arch. Gen. Psychiatry 37: 471–481.
19. MINTZ, J. & L. LUBORSKY. 1979. Measuring the outcomes of psychotherapy: Findings of the Penn Psychotherapy Project. J. Consult. Clin. Psychol. 47:
20. MCLELLAN, A. T., L. LUBORSKY, G. E. WOODY, et al. 1982. Is substance abuse treatment effective? Four different perspectives. J. Am. Med. Assoc.
21. BALE, R., W. VAN STONE, J. KULDAU, et al. 1980. Therapeutic communities vs. methadone maintenance. Arch. Gen. Psychiatry 37.
22. BAKER, S. L., T. LOREI, H. MCKNIGHT & J. DUVALL. 1977. The Veterans Administration comparison study: Alcoholism and drug abuse—Combined and conventional treatment settings. Alcoholism: Clinical and Experimental Research, 1.
23. MCLELLAN, A. T., G. E. WOODY & C. P. O'BRIEN. 1979. Development of psychiatric illness in drug abusers. N. Engl. J. Med. 301: 1310–1314.
24. ELLINWOOD, E. H. 1967. Amphetamine psychosis I: Description of the individuals and process. J. Nerv. Ment. Dis. 144: 273–283.

THE POPPY: THERAPEUTIC POTENTIAL
IN CASES OF DEMENTIA WITH DEPRESSION

D. Wilfred Abse, William J. Rheuban,
and Salman Akhtar

Saint Albans Hospital
Radford, Virginia 24143

Department of Psychiatry
University of Virginia School of Medicine
Charlottesville, Virginia 22901

Through advances in medicine, the human life span has lengthened with a consequent increase in the population of geriatric patients with dementia and depression. The choice of psychotropic medication for these patients poses special problems owing to their increased susceptibility to adverse drug reactions.[1-3] The side effects of major tranquilizers, e.g. extra-pyramidal restlessness, parkinsonism, and hypotensive episodes, may complicate the clinical picture of an elderly, agitated patient. However, the main clinical problem with these drugs is that there is often *mental hebetude* even though target symptoms have abated. The patients appear overdrugged, and relatives often refer to them as "zombies," and are discomforted in their presence. Many of these patients display rapid clinical improvement following discontinuation of maintenance doses of psychotropic drugs,[4] calling in question the advisability of long-term medication for psycho-geriatric patients.

As for tricyclic medication for the depressed aged patient, there is a lowered threshold for toxic confusion, glaucoma, urinary retention, cardiovascular embarrassment, and parkinsonism.[5] This may at time seriously limit their use in the elderly.

OPIATES AND THE GERIATRIC PATIENT WITH DEMENTIA AND DEPRESSION

Few reports exist on the use of opiates in the treatment of the depressed and confused elderly patient. In their 1960 study,[6] Abse and Dahlstrom found that depressed and agitated geriatric patients receiving deodorized tincture of opium showed cheerful mood, increased mental competence, and interest in people and surroundings. During the past 27 years, the senior author has treated many cases of senile dementia with suitably adjusted dosage of opium-related compounds. The results have often been superior to those obtained previously in the same patients with other medications, including phenothiazines and tricyclic antidepressants. Not only the target symptoms (depression, confusion, paranoid ideation, etc.) abated, but a cheerful and cooperative mood appeared, rendering the patient amenable to rehabilitative measures.

The following two cases illustrate the value of opiates in the clinical management of the depressed and confused elderly patient.

Case 1. An 87-year-old wealthy man suffered from agitation, confusion, and disturbed sleep. At night he repeatedly got up to check the doors of his large

79

0077–8923/82/0398–0079 $1.75/0 © 1982, NYAS

house, which he thought was about to be robbed by burglars. During the day, he was depressed with fluctuating confusion and agitation. The senior author, who had been consulted by the family physician, confirmed a diagnosis of cardiovascular degeneration, including cerebral arteriosclerosis, and was of the opinion that the patient might live for another six months. His medicines included a small regular dose of digitalis, and he had been on sedatives and tranquilizers. These, however, had all been ineffective or else had rendered the patient stuporous. An opiate (liquor morphine bimecatis) when given in this case succeeded in establishing a mildly euphoric condition. The previously difficult-to-manage patient became responsive to his caretakers and his interest in life around him revived, including interest in his business affairs. He slept well and, as it happened, lived comfortably for another two years.

Case 2. An 86-year-old widow was hospitalized in an agitated, depressed, and confused state. Living alone for five years following the death of her husband, she had become anxious and depressed, to the point of needing medical attention for some time prior to admission. One of her sons had taken her into his home for the past three months and, although a little improvement at first took place, her symptoms again worsened. She suffered marked insomnia, anorexia, weight loss, and agitation. A variety of psychotropic medications, including major tranquilizers and antidepressants, in adequate doses were ineffective in relieving her symptomatology.

On admission, the patient was cooperative but agitated and depressed, with marked orofacial dyskinesia, which the patient attributed to ill-fitting dentures. She was oriented, but her recent memory was severely impaired. She did report at times becoming rather confused. She often repeated during the initial interview that she would prefer to be dead rather than incapacitated as she was. Physical examination revealed grade II arteriosclerotic fundi changes and slight pitting edema over both legs.

A number of tests, SMA-6, CBC, VDRL, urinalysis, T3, T4, B12, folate levels, 24-hour urine for heavy metals, chest and skull X-rays, and EEG, were unremarkable. A CAT scan revealed evidence of cerebro-atrophy. An EKG revealed prolonged QT intervals and ST and T wave changes with poor R wave progression. A cardiology consult for abnormal EKG recommended digitalization, which was accomplished on 0.125 units q.o.d. This did not produce improvement in her psychological symptoms. The patient was then placed on doxepin HCl 25 mg t.i.d., later increased to 50 mg t.i.d. She showed only minimal response. After two weeks of treatment, however, this medication had to be stopped since she developed marked orthostatic hypotension. She was then placed on deodorated tincture of opium. On this medication, she improved gradually, requiring, on discharge, 20 drops orally b.i.d. and 35 drops orally q.h.s. The patient was then transferred to a minimal care nursing facility. Though not able to take full care of herself, she was more responsive, cheerful, and sleeping regularly. She is doing so well at the time of this writing (two months after transfer) that she is planning to return to her son's household.

COMMENT

Several considerations are apt to restrain medicinal use of opiates. The possibility of serious side effects, e.g., respiratory depression, and the potential for addiction are two most important deterrents to their use. Jaffe [7] many years ago opined that the fear of addiction is out of proportion to the actual frequency of its occurrence. In the cases of opium-treated dementias with which we are concerned, this fear seems especially misplaced. In our experience, while the chronic brain syndrome patient does once again become symptomatic if taken off the opiates, he does *not* require increasing doses of it over time. In this regard, the operant conditioning experiment of Nichols [8] is of special interest. He demonstrated that rats who administer morphine to themselves become addicted whereas rats who receive the drug passively do not. He also found that older rats develop less "opiate-directed behavior" than young rats do; this implies an inverse relationship between opiate addiction and age.

The favorable response of the depressed and demented geriatric patients to opiates needs replication in controlled, double-blind trials. Such confirmation may imply that certain chronic brain syndromes result from the deficiency of the recently discovered endogenous morphine-like substances [9, 10] and that opium serves as a supplemental source for such patients. Karl Verebey *et al.*[11] in a 1978 review of recent knowledge of endogenous opioid peptides, proposed that the level of functional endorphins is related to psychological events, with a normal level needed for psychological homeostasis. It seems likely that in some patients suffering organic dementia with depression that part of the pathogenesis lies in a disturbance of this homeostasis, since some of them respond favorably, even dramatically, to the administration of the deodorated tincture of opium. On the other hand, some patients with similar symptoms accompanying organic dementia do not respond.

Some of these nonresponders to deodorated tincture of opium alone, do respond favorably to a combination of tricyclic medication and deodorated tincture of opium, and I have found it possible to reduce the dosage of tricyclic medication considerably and to administer, with this reduced dose of a tricyclic, 10–15 drops of deodorated tincture of opium, t.i.d., with a subsequent favorable response, that is, diminution of confusion, agitation, depression, and paranoid ideation. Of course, it is known that the hypothalamic and limbic dysfunctions occurring in depression involve the monoamines and that tricyclic antidepressants block neuronal re-uptake of them.[12] I have found that some senile dementia patients with depressive symptomatology do better with tricyclic medication by day and deodorated tincture of opium at night.

REFERENCES

1. JONES, T. H. 1962. Chlordiazepoxide (Librium) and the geriatric patient. J. Am. Geriatr. Soc. **10:** 259–263.
2. WEBB, W. L., JR. 1971. The use of psychopharmacological drugs in the aged. Geriatrics **26:** 94–103.
3. COLE, J. O. 1976. Phenothiazines. *In* Drug Treatment of Mental Patients. L. L. Simpson, Ed. Raven Press. New York.
4. RASKIND, M. & R. EISDORFER. 1976. Psychopharmacology of the Aged. *In* Drug Treatment of Mental Patients. L. L. Simpson, Ed. Raven Press. New York.
5. PRANGE, A. J. 1975. Antidepressants. *In* American Handbook of Psychiatry. 2nd edit. Vol. 5. D. X. Freedman & J. E. Dyrud, Eds. Basic Books. New York.
6. ABSE, D. W. & W. G. DAHLSTROM. 1960. The value of chemotherapy in senile mental disturbances. J. Am. Med. Assoc. **174:** 20036–42.

7. JAFFE, J. H. 1968. Opiate dependence and the use of narcotics for the relief of pain. Modern Treatment 5: 1121–35.
8. NICHOLS, J. R. 1965. How opiates change behavior. Sci. Am. 212: 80–88.
9. HUGHES, J. 1975. Isolation of an endogenous compound from the brain with pharmacological properties similar to morphine. Brain Res. 88(2): 295–308.
10. KOSTERLITZ, H. W. & J. HUGHES. 1975. Some thoughts on the significance of enkephalin, the endogenous ligand. Life Sci. 17(1): 91–6.
11. VEREBEY, K., J. VOLAVKA & D. CLOUET. 1978. Endorphins in psychiatry. Arch. Gen. Psychiatry 35: 877–88.
12. GLASS, R. M. & D. X. FREEDMAN. 1981. Psychiatry. J. Am. Med. Assoc. 245(21): 2218–20.

METHADONE: AN EFFECTIVE AGENT IN MANAGING INTRACTABLE PAIN AS A SYMPTOM OF PSYCHOTIC ANGER

Gilbert H. Berken,* Melvin M. Stone,
and Shirley K. Stone

*Hollywood Memorial Hospital
Hollywood, Florida 33021*

I would like to begin this talk by giving a brief account of the experiences that led us to consider methadone as a psychoactive medication.

During an 11-year period of treating opiate addicts, the Hollywood Memorial Hospital clinical staff noted that a relatively small number of their patients, which varied between 10% and 15%, demonstrated a specific behavioral profile.

As a group, the patients with this profile represented the most difficult management problems. They demonstrated numerous suicide attempts, self-mutilation, accident involvements, impulsive overt rage reactions, and often attacks upon others, including homicidal acts. Threats of violence and verbal intimidation were common. They reported chaotic fantasies generally associated with violence toward a family member or friend. Minimal stress caused severe mood swings and unpredictable behavior. Self-hatred and depression were almost always found within this group.

These patients were enrolled in a methadone maintenance program, and as stabilization on methadone progressed, certain behavioral changes were documented. The requirements for psychotropic medication were decreased whether originally prescribed by a physician or self-prescribed by the patient. The patient's recognition of the onset of overt rage was a major change. The range of mood swings decreased and gradually the frequency of mutilation decreased. The homicidal and suicidal behaviors diminished or appeared extinguished.

In any given patient in this group, tapering of his or her methadone dose, early in the treatment, would result in a return to the behavioral profile noted on his or her admission to the program. As we continued to document how this group responded, it became apparent over time that the methadone functioned as a psychoactive agent that helped to "normalize" the behavior of these patients.

These observations agreed with Dr. Khantzian who proposed that methadone is "also effective because it has a stabilizing, anti-aggression action in the central nervous system" in 1972 at The Fourth National Conference on Methadone.[1] The ability of narcotic agents to function as anti-aggressive agents was also noted among several psychiatric patients.

This led to the collaboration of the authors in reviewing the potential of methadone to function as a psychoactive agent in patients where conventional management proved ineffective. It was mutually determined that the clinicians' observations were compatible, and agreement was reached on the methodology of treatment.

* Address for correspondence: 158 North Federal Highway, Dania, Florida 33004.

0077–8923/82/0398–0083 $1.75/0 © 1982, NYAS

In an earlier case study, Ms. A, a 19-year-old woman, had been severely mutilating herself and had made several significant attempts at suicide.[2] Methadone was used successfully as the principal agent to control her psychotic rage.

Based upon the successful use of methadone as a therapeutic agent to control schizophrenic rage, a second patient with an equally frustrating course using conventional psychotropic medications was placed on methadone as a primary treating agent for intractable migraine pain of 11 years duration. In December 1978, the following case was discussed with the medical director of an area methadone clinic. It was agreed that, based upon current federal guidelines, methadone could be used for the treatment of intractable migraine, and the treating psychiatrist could provide methadone by prescription with regular reports made to the methadone clinic.

CASE STUDY

Ms. B, a 50-year-old Caucasian female hospital patient, was referred by her internist and has been under the care of the treating psychiatrist since December 1972. The reason for referral was, "persistent cephalgia of unknown etiology. The patient also has a tendency towards seizures and has to be carefully monitored."

The patient was found to have a severe depression with evident suicidal ideation. She experienced a series of convulsions secondary to an underlying seizure disorder and possible drug withdrawal. The patient's sleep EEG on this admission demonstrated a convulsive tendency; however, a repeat sleep EEG produced a normal pattern. The clinical impression was that the persistent cephalgia of two years duration was a depressive equivalent. The patient's discharge medication included a major tranquilizer, a tricyclic antidepressant, anticonvulsants, and analgesics. In early 1973 following a second hospitalization, lithium carbonate was added to control significant mood swings.

In July 1975, the patient was readmitted to the hospital where an EEG demonstrated an abnormal study, "indicating a focal condition in the left temporal region with irritative features." The patient was severely depressed. She complained that she could not function at home and blamed this upon the severity of her headaches. An EMI scan and brain scan were interpreted as normal. The patient experienced long period of dysfunction when faced with stress within her life.

The patient was hospitalized again in the latter part of 1976. A diagnosis of migraine headaches was made. A significant problem was the patient's tendency to abuse medication. She had become confused and bewildered, and burned her face while trying to light a cigarette on the electric element on her stove. The patient's husband agreed to monitor her medication and dispense it to her on a regular schedule.

In mid-1977, the patient was hospitalized again following the laceration of her right wrist with tendon and nerve injury. Her suicidal preoccupation had become more violent and her covert anger frequently became expressed during episodic abuse of alcohol. Her internist also noted that the patient had "a great deal of subdued anger and rage kept in check."

It had become apparent through the course of therapy that the patient's primary symptomatology was that of a schizophrenic condition and that her rage and hostility were expressed primarily in the disabling migraine headaches. She experienced progressive deterioration over five years, during which time suicidal preoccupation and attempts had become a regular part of her existence.

Correspondence with the Bureau of Drugs Division of Methadone Monitoring of the United States Food and Drug Administration determined that, "if it is necessary in the physician's medical judgement, a patient may be narcotized to prevent the recurrence of a chronic and severely painful condition." In December 1978, the patient was evaluated in the hospital by the medical director of the methadone program. It was believed that Ms. B's condition warranted the administration of methadone on an outpatient basis.

The patient was started on 10 mg methadone twice a day. This was increased in two weeks to a schedule of 20 mg twice daily, which has become her maintenance dose. The patient stated that she experienced a significant headache-free period. When she did experience a migraine headache, it would usually abate in three or four days and could be controlled by the use of Empirin with codeine.

The patient's husband continued to monitor and dispense her medication and stated emphatically the methadone was a significant benefit to his wife. He noted that she was more alert and less overtly depressed, and she was undertaking her household responsibilities in a more effective manner than she had for several years.

Ms. B has been taking methadone for approximately three years with a marked improvement in her general level of function and with no suicidal attempts or preoccupation. She seems satisfied that she has headache-free periods, that her migraine episodes are less severe, and that suicide as an available alternative has not been necessary.

With this patient, the need for conventional psychotropics was not supplanted by the introduction of methadone. A major tranquilizer and tricyclic antidepressant have been continued in her management. Without these medications, the patient progressively becomes more paranoid, preoccupied with resentments concerning her husband and family, and her manifest anger becomes more apparent. The methadone contributed to a reduction of perceived pain and led to improved function and greater stability.

DISCUSSION

The experience with Ms. A and Ms. B correlated well with the observations made of the 10% to 15% subgroup within the methadone program. Equally, the return of their anger and self-hatred with reduction in dosage suggests that the level of methadone should be carefully monitored. Frequently doses as high as 175 mg per day may be required to adequately control these patients.

Detoxifying these patients is generally unwise and quickly results in a return to their morbid, rageful personalities.

Of interest, though, is that Ms. A was successfully detoxified from methadone in 1976; and her behavior since suggests that she had become a more mature woman who displayed greater self-control. It is the shared opinion of the three clinicians who worked with Ms. A that without the interim benefit of methadone she would have successfully terminated her life by suicide.

CONCLUSION

Our experience with these two patients suggests that methadone can be an effective "normalizing" psychoactive agent where overt psychotic rage or intractable pain is present as a constant symptom of rage.

This provides the clinician with an additional tool when attempting to manage severely dysfunctional patients who do not respond favorably to more conventional treatment methods. It is our hope that the beneficial effects of methadone on behavior will result in additional research that could further explain what has been observed clinically.

REFERENCES

1. KHANTZIAN, EDWARD J. 1972. A Preliminary Dynamic Formulation of the Psychopharmacologic Action of Methadone. Proceedings of the 4th National Conference on Methadone, San Francisco, January, 1972. p. 373. The National Association for the Prevention of Addiction to Narcotics. New York.
2. BERKEN, G., M. STONE & S. STONE. 1978. Methadone in Schizophrenic Rage: A Case Study. Am. J. Psychiatry 135(2): 248.

METHADONE TREATMENT OF PENTAZOCINE ABUSE

Jerrold S. Maxmen *

Department of Psychiatry
College of Physicians & Surgeons
Columbia University
New York, New York 10032

Pentazocine (Talwin), the N-allyl derivative of the narcotic analgesic phena-zocine, is a moderately strong analgesic and a weak narcotic antagonist. The standard 30 mg intramuscular (i.m.) dose provides slightly more relief from moderate to severe pain than does the standard 50 mg oral dose. On a mg-per-mg basis, its potency parenterally is one-third of morphine's, and orally is about equal to codeine's. In terms of analgesic potency, a 30 mg i.m. dose of pentazo-cine is equivalent to a 10 mg dose of morphine and a 75 mg dose of meperidine.[1]

The side effects of pentazocine are similar to morphine-like analgesics. Psychotomimetic reactions—most commonly hallucinations (usually visual), mood alteration, disorientation, and depersonalization—occur in 1.4% of parenteral recipients and in 1% of oral recipients.[2] Unlike other narcotics, pentazocine can induce initial insomnia.[3]

PENTAZOCINE ABUSE

Although the true incidence of pentazocine misuse remains unknown, it appears to have a definite, albeit low, potential for abuse and dependence. Jasinsky has concluded that it has less abuse potential than nalorphine or cyclazocine.[4] Rarely is pentazocine the first drug of abuse; most patients have previously or are concurrently abusing either hypnosedatives, alcohol, or heroin.[2] Chambers found that 5.4% of 1,494 narcotic-dependent subjects abused penta-zocine, and 11 of these 80 patients (13.75%) were "addicted" to it. Thus, 0.7% of the 1,494 were "addicted" to pentazocine.[5] Nearly all cases of pentazocine dependence result from parenteral administrations, typically between 300 and 960 mg i.m. daily. There are scattered reports, however, of its oral misuse.[2,6]

A not unusual finding is that medical personnel are especially susceptible to pentazocine abuse, frequently being unaware of or minimizing its potential for dependency.[6,7] Another particularly addiction-prone group are middle-class housewives, many of whom have been placed on pentazocine by misguided physicians seeking to relieve menstrual cramps, migraine headaches, and so on. (Even when pentazocine is given appropriately for the treatment of chronic pain, the physician must warn the patient against using the drug in *anticipation* of pain rather than in the *relief* of pain.) Street addicts are a third high-risk group, and also the fastest growing one; from 1973–75 to 1978, there was a sevenfold increase in its illegal use in Chicago.[8] Other data suggest that about three to six million doses annually are being diverted on the streets.[9] Most often, street addicts mix 50 mg crushed tablets of both pentazocine and tripelennamine to produce a euphoria similar to that of a heroin–cocaine mixture.[8,10]

* Address for correspondence: 30 Fifth Avenue #6E, New York, N.Y. 10011.

0077–8923/82/0398–0087 $1.75/0 © 1982, NYAS

The development of euphoria or tolerance or mild withdrawal symptoms are the three major "causes" for pentazocine-dependency. A study of 30 of these patients at the Mayo Clinic revealed that the duration of abuse ranged from one month to three years.[6] Moreover, since the drug rarely produces significant toxicity, even at four times the recommended maximum daily therapeutic dose (viz., 600 mg orally and 360 mg parenterally), patients are likely to increase their dose without medical approval.

Abrupt withdrawal of pentazocine-addicted patients is relatively mild, usually consisting of "drug-seeking" behaviors, restlessness, diarrhea, nausea, cramps, rhinorrhea, and insomnia.[4, 6, 11]

THE ROLE OF METHADONE

Being a mild narcotic antagonist, pentazocine precipitates withdrawal symptoms when given to those on methadone maintenance. On the other hand, methadone has been used frequently with relative safety to alleviate abstinence symptoms in pentazocine-dependent patients. But, since withdrawal from pentazocine is generally mild, is the administration of methadone for these patients effective, necessary, or advisable? And if so, under what circumstances?

These questions are difficult to answer because there are no studies—not to mention well-designed ones—in this area, even though the drug (i.e., pentazocine) has been marketed in the United States since 1967. Nonetheless, some *tentative* guidelines, based on the literature and on clinical experience, can be drawn. To do so, one can look at three different, albeit related, clinical circumstances: uncomplicated withdrawal—acute phase; uncomplicated withdrawal—chronic phase; complicated withdrawal.

Uncomplicated Withdrawal—Acute Phase

When methadone is employed under these conditions, initially 5 mg every 6 hours is given, and then gradually tapered off within 5 to 20 days. Although the substitution of a stronger narcotic (i.e., methadone) for a weaker one (i.e., pentazocine) potentially replaces one addiction for another,[11] this fear seems unwarranted because methadone administration in these circumstances is relatively brief. Yet from a strictly physiologic standpoint, methadone is unnecessary for acute uncomplicated withdrawal, since major abstinence symptoms without methadone are mild and usually disappear within one to seven days of pentazocine being stopped. Furthermore, methadone is not innocuous; it too has side effects as well as addiction potential. Indeed, without resorting to methadone at all, small doses of antianxiety agents (e.g., diazepam) have been used successfully to quell anxiety and restlessness, which are at times the most stressful symptoms of pentazocine-withdrawal.[11] But even though, for the most part, the use of methadone for acute uncomplicated withdrawal seems inadvisable, there may be three exceptions, or at least caveats, to this guideline.

First, because these patients are often polydrug abusers, and frequently lie about or underestimate their drug-taking, the clinician should be alert to abstinence symptoms from other drugs, most often hypnosedatives, alcohol, or narcotics. Second, those addicted to relatively large amounts of pentazocine will have more severe abstinence symptoms, and therefore, methadone-aided withdrawal may alleviate such discomfort.

Third, and perhaps most important, the use of methadone for acute uncomplicated withdrawal may be advisable for psychological reasons. Pentazocine-dependent patients are notoriously uncooperative. In a study of 30 hospitalized pentazocine-abusers, only 30% were deemed "cooperative;" 67% invoked denial, 27% were felt to be manipulative and demanding or secretly used drugs while in the hospital, and 27% signed out early. In this study, those with the most severe withdrawal symptoms were most likely to leave the hospital prematurely.[6] Consequently, although there is no solid evidence proving that methadone-aided pentazocine-withdrawal enhances cooperation, clinical experience suggests that with potentially "difficult" patients, the use of methadone may increase compliance. Parenthetically, if the family will directly tell the patient, and mean it, that they will not allow him home until hospital treatment is completed, the odds for success are greatly improved.

Uncomplicated Withdrawal—Chronic Phase

Even after acute withdrawal is finished, drug-seeking behavior is commonly employed, and often secretly at that. Many of these patients have major, and more frequently, minor affective disorders, which go undiagnosed either due to physician neglect or because the patient does not stay around long enough for proper assessment in a *drug-free* state (which is another reason to avoid methadone during uncomplicated—acute withdrawal). Consequently, to alleviate their dysphoria, patients readily seek out a pentazocine-induced euphoria soon after discharge. So whenever possible, a careful search for an underlying mood disorder in a drug-free state should be conducted to see if antidepressants would be helpful. If it appears that they are not indicated, the advisability of substituting methadone for the usual three to six months following withdrawal is contingent on at least some of the following considerations:

First, if the patient has abused pentazocine *parenterally*, and if relapse appears probable—a conclusion based more on the patient's past history than on his current statements—orally administered methadone will be medically safer. Inflammation, sclerosis, fibrosis, and ulceration often occur at the sites of pentazocine-injections [12] (FIGURE 1). In addition, all the usual risks of the illicit use of needles are reduced with oral methadone substitution. Second, persistent craving for pentazocine, even after active withdrawal, is an ever-present danger, especially in apparently "responsible" patients. For example, Raskin reports that a 28-year-old physician, after abusing pentazocine intravenously (i.v.) for a year, continued to crave it seven days following an unsettling drug-free withdrawal period. Yet one hour after the employment of 10 mg of methadone, his drug-craving ceased abruptly. During the subsequent six months his methadone (initially 10 mg twice daily) was gradually tapered and then discontinued with no evidence of further drug abuse (of any kind).[13] On the other hand, after an extensive search of the world's literature, Wendel reported two out of three cases in which methadone substitution was ineffective. Given the unreliability of pentazocine-dependent patients and the absence of controlled studies, he cautions against replacing a stronger narcotic with a weaker one [7]; so does the American Medical Association's Department of Drugs.[11] This concern, although merited, may derive more from broad philo-

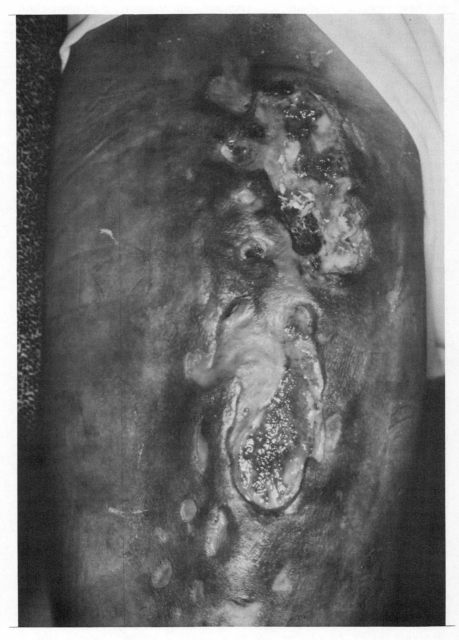

FIGURE 1. Massive fibrosis, sclerosis, and ulceration at pentazocine injection sites on the anterior right thigh.

sophical and theoretical objections than from strictly medical and humanistic considerations.

The third, and perhaps once again the most important, factor rests with a psychiatric assessment of the patient accompanied by active social interventions. Potential suppliers of pentazocine—be they the patient's physician(s) or pharmacist(s)—should be alerted. Careful monitering by the patient's family and physician, along with regular screening of urines, are highly advantageous. If drug-seeking behavior seems apparent or even likely, especially with a history of parenteral abuse, then oral methadone for a three to six month period seems worth trying. For even in Wendel's report cited above, it is not clear if the failure of methadone-substitution meant that the patients became addicted to methadone or relapsed onto pentazocine.[7]

Complicated Withdrawal

Although an admittedly arbitrary distinction, in this context "complicated withdrawal" refers to problems besides drug-craving that persist after the acute abstinence phase, or to the emergence of atypical symptoms during acute withdrawal, as vividly illustrated in the following case: (Although this patient has been reported previously,[14] this presentation introduces new material regarding her neurological and sleep problems.)

A 47-year-old working mother of two was initially admitted to the dermatology service for the debridement and grafting of massive skin ulcerations (FIGURE 1) caused by four years of i.m. self-injected pentazocine averaging 600 mg a day divided between 15 to 20 doses. When the dermatologists abruptly terminated her pentazocine, she abruptly left the hospital. Threatening to commit her to a state hospital, the patient's family "forced" her into the nearest community mental health center, where her drug was gradually discontinued over five days with moderate ease. This occurred despite the patient's agitation, irritation, demands for more pentazocine, and complaints of arm and leg pains, the latter symptoms being what launched her 16-year history of codeine, meperidine, and then pentazocine abuse. With emotional support from the staff, her uncooperativeness and complaints of pain abated. Nevertheless, repeated myoclonic jerks and moderate pain constantly awoke her, mainly from stage 2 sleep. Concurring with the nurses' reports, the patient slept fitfully for a mere two hours a night.

In order to arrest her insomnia, on different occasions she was orally given (a) perphenazine 8 mg with benzotropine 1 mg, (b) chlorpromazine 100 mg with benzotropine, (c) flurazepam 30 mg, (d) flurazepam 60 mg, and (e) paraldehyde 8 cc. Although she had taken all of these medications previously except paraldehyde without difficulty, now, 30 to 60 minutes after ingesting each of them, for the first time in her life she became markedly confused and disoriented. What's more, she developed athetoidlike movements in her distal arms and legs lasting 20 seconds, stopping for 10 seconds, starting again, and alternating like this until they, and the delirium, ceased after 90 to 120 minutes.

There was no electroencephalographic nor clinical evidence of a seizure. Even though convulsions have been described in patients given large i.v. doses of pentazocine,[15] there are no reports of seizures erupting during abstinence. Because her athetoidlike movements occurred not only too early, but also with hypnosedatives and antiparkinsonian drugs, it is unlikely that they were an extrapyramidal dyskinesia. Nevertheless, the possibility of pre-existing minor neurological impairment could not be ruled out. As an infant, she allegedly stopped breathing for several minutes and turned "blue" after a quarter stuck in her throat and had to be removed by a doctor. Although her mother had a "spinal, degenerative disease"—probably amyotrophic lateral sclerosis—the patient had no previous signs of this illness.

Whatever the pathogenesis of her bizarre symptoms—whether or not they were related to long-term pentazocine abuse—she was finally given 15 mg of methadone at bedtime (h.s.) and slept for 12 hours without aches, athetoidlike movements, or delirium. Although her myoclonic jerks persisted and her sleep recordings on methadone revealed excessively long (30%) and intense REM periods occurring almost immediately after dropping off, she reported having "the best sleep in weeks." This apparent disinhibition of the REM system may be unrelated to methadone. Although the effects of methadone and chronic pentazocine abuse on sleep's infrastructure are unknown, heroin and morphine markedly *decrease* REM and *delay* its onset.[3]

Over the next 22 months, her methadone was reduced to 7.5 mg at h.s., she abstained from the use of any other drugs, she slept well, and for the first time in 16 years, she was free of aching extremities.[14] It could be that she was susceptible to a complicated withdrawal due to some covert, pre-existing neurological difficulty. This case suggests, however, that methadone may alleviate some complicated pentazocine-withdrawal states where other less addictive medications (e.g., diazepam) prove ineffective. In these circumstances, the (continued) use of methadone should be based solely on pragmatic considerations.

CONCLUSION

As reports of increasing pentazocine abuse escalate,[8] the necessity of knowing precise guidelines for methadone substitution with pentazocine-dependent persons is growing. Meanwhile, the indications for methadone should be based on the patient's idiosyncratic and overall behavioral and psychiatric status.

Based on the above case history and on the one of Raskin's [13] mentioned above, it may well be that if methadone vitiates drug-craving and complicated withdrawal states at all, its effectiveness becomes apparent after a *single* dose. So when double-blind, controlled studies are being performed, researchers might wish to see if the immediate response to methadone is a good predictor of long-term outcome.

But for now, given our ignorance of this subject, pragmatic and clinical, not philosophical or theoretical, reasons should guide the treating physician.

REFERENCES

1. SADOVE, M. S. 1971. A look at narcotic and nonnarcotic analgesics. Postgrad. Med. **49:** 102–105.
2. BROGDEN, R. N., T. M. SPEIGHT & G. S. AVERY. 1973. Pentazocine: A review of its pharmacological properties, therapeutic efficacy and dependence liability. Drugs **5:** 6–91.
3. MAXMEN, J. S. 1981. A Good Night's Sleep: A Step-By-Step Program for Overcoming Insomnia and Other Sleep Problems. W. W. Norton. New York.

4. JASINSKY, D. R., W. R. MARTIN & R. D. HOELDTKE.   1970.   Effects of short- and
long-term administration of pentazocine in man. Clin. Pharmacol. Ther. **11:**
385–402.
5. CHAMBERS, C. D., J. A. INCIARDI & R. C. STEPHENS. 1971. A critical review of
pentazocine abuse. Health Services and Mental Health Administration Reports
86: 627–653.
6. SWANSON, D. W., R. L. WEDDIGE & R. M. MORSE. 1973. Hospitalized pentazocine abusers. Mayo Clinic Proc. **48:** 85–93.
7. WENDEL, H. A. 1971. Management of pentazocine dependency. N. Engl. J.
Med. **284:** 504.
8. LAHMEYER, H. W. & R. G. STEINGOLD. 1980. Medical and psychiatric complications of pentazocine and tripelennamine abuse. J. Clin. Psychiatry **41:** 275–278.
9. ANNEXTON, M. 1978. Pentazocine reclassified in Illinois. J. Am. Med. Assoc.
240: 2234, 2240.
10. SHOWALTER, C. V. & L. MOORE. 1978. Abuse of pentazocine and tripelennamine.
J. Am. Med. Assoc. **239:** 1610–1612.
11. AMERICAN MEDICAL ASSOCIATION'S DEPARTMENT OF DRUGS. 1973. Use and
misuse of pentazocine: A follow-up. J. Am. Med. Assoc. **225:** 1530–1531.
12. PARKS, D. L., H. O. PERRY & S. A. MULLER. 1971. Cutaneous complications of
pentazocine injections. Arch. Dermatol. **104:** 231–235.
13. RASKIN, N. N. 1970. Methadone for the pentazocine-dependent patient. N. Engl.
J. Med. **283:** 1349.
14. MAXMEN, J. S., P. M. SILBERFARB & E. PLAKUN. 1975. Pentazocine abuse and
problems of withdrawal. Br. J. Psychiatry **126:** 370–371.
15. ALARCON, R. D., S. D. GELFOND & G. S. ALARCON. 1971. Parenteral and oral
pentazocine abuse. Hopkins Med. J. **129:** 311–318.

DISCUSSION OF THE PAPER

H. D. KLEBER (*Yale Medical School, New Haven, CT*): I do not know whether we have anyone here from the FDA, but I gather that what we have been hearing in regard to using tincture of opium to treat senile dementia is illegal. As far as I understand, you cannot use maintenance narcotics other than methadone for treating nonpain conditions. This was not pain. Therefore, as I understand FDA rules, it would not be legal and yet, I am sure it is practiced by many physicians. Likewise in theory you are supposed to withdraw pentazocine and Darvon and any other narcotic drug also with methadone by FDA rules even though it may fly in the face of good medical practice. Are any representatives here or anyone else who has other thoughts about the legal status?

R. B. MILLMAN (*Cornell University Medical College, New York*): Let's discuss the issue of legality or illegality and let's consider the use of tincture of opium, for example, in senile dementia.

J. H. JAFFE (*University of Connecticut School of Medicine, Farmington*): When the only regulations that existed concerning methadone were those of the FDA, it would have been "not indicated" and the risk would have been largely a medicolegal one. This would have been a rather minimal risk because these are older drugs for which there is no package insert. Therefore, it would have been a very gray area.

However, in 1974 legislation was introduced and passed in Congress giving the DEA purview over maintenance issues concurrent with that of FDA. In this legislation they attempted to define with great detail the kinds of opiates that could be used for maintenance treatment and I believe, therefore, there are Federal laws specifying how one could, in what situations one could maintain people on opiates, which opiates can be used, and which opiates are illegitimate for maintenance. It is not clear whether these laws could prevent long-term opioid use in those not initially opioid dependent, since after a few months all patients would be dependent.

I think that Dr. Kleber has raised an interesting issue. I think that the era of the 1950s under Mr. Anslinger are past. Presently Federal regulators seem somewhat less zealous in seeking to prosecute doctors who are practicing legitimately.

I am not sure that the risk of prosecution is a significant issue at the present time, but, it could get to be one. Clarification, at some point, would be helpful.

J. S. MAXMEN *(Columbia University, College of Physicians and Surgeons, New York):* The situation occurred when we were using methadone for the treatment of the pentazocine-abusing patient. There was no legal indication for what we were doing. What happened was, that we wrote to the FDA and said, "We don't know what else to do at this point; we would like to try methadone because there have been some case reports in the literature that indicate beneficial effects."

We then received a letter from the FDA saying that "You can go ahead and use methadone for this one person only."

JAFFE: As I helped to write that little piece in the package insert about methadone about 13 years ago, I know something about the origin of that caution and about pentazocine.

The issue was not legality. The issue was not even pharmacology so much as a medicolegal consideration at the time. In 1968, pentazocine was largely uncontrolled and people did get dependent on pentazocine. The risk there was not that methadone would not work in suppressing withdrawal. There is no reason why it should not. Methadone seems to suppress both withdrawal from both mu and kappa receptors.

The real question was what would be the medicolegal position of a physician taking somebody who was on pentazocine, a drug that was not controlled at the time, and putting the person into a methadone maintenance program with no evidence that they had been dependent on a schedule II narcotic? Could the physician not find himself in considerable difficulty if he had a litigious patient who would say, "I was really only using this drug (pentazocine) with no problem. I could get it and it was not illegal and now you have put me on a drug that requires a methadone maintenance clinic and now I am addicted." If then when the patient tries to get off the methadone, they use heroin, the patient might try to attribute all subsequent difficulties to the physician who first used the methadone. Further, as you correctly put it, the syndrome is mild enough that the use of methadone is often not required.

So the advice was given that it is probably more appropriate to simply reduce the pentazocine than to switch on to the methadone. It had very little to do with the pharmacology. Methadone would be perfectly adequate and would work, but it is still uncertain as to what might happen to somebody who had never really been dependent on an opiate that requires methadone, if, having come to you for treatment, he/she leaves with that requirement.

MAXMEN: Then there are really two questions. The first is whether or not this litigious patient will end up suing you for putting him/her on a strong opiate. And second the question that Dr. Kleber raised is whether or not you are in violation of some Federal law and the government would sue. I think they are two separate questions.

JAFFE: They are. I am simply talking about 1968 when that warning was put into the package insert for pentazocine. At that time there was no Federal law of this kind.

So even if you were to take away the problem whether it was illegal, you might still have the problem as long as you have two different opiates and radically different schedules of control as to whether or not you might have a problem with a patient who says: "You overtreated me. You put me on methadone and that made me dependent on a narcotic."

MILLMAN: I always wondered who wrote those package inserts, and I also wanted to know whether you got paid for it.

JAFFE: I got a modest fee.

E. J. KHANTZIAN (*Harvard Medical School, Cambridge, MA*): I at first was inclined to not comment because I was wondering what these legalistic concerns had to do with the subject of this conference, but I think it begins to get to the heart of the matter.

In Massachusetts it is even a little more ridiculous in that there is a law on the books that says that if you are going to maintain an addict on a controlled substance, you must report it to the Department of Mental Health, and the Commissioner of Mental Health, and you will then not be in violation of state statutes.

Now this statute was around in the books in the early 1970s so people would not be on more than one methadone maintenance program at a time, although the law did not specifically mention it.

It has put a lot of doctors in a sense of false security because they think by reporting it to the Commissioner they are not in violation of any laws when in fact they are in violation of Federal statutes.

I think this kind of ambiguity and inconsistency reflects a mental blindness—almost an illness—that we have in our culture about opiates. I think you know Musto's book is about that—we created this illness about the whole subject matter. In fact, the subject matter of this conference is the very important fundamental discoveries about the endogenous and exogenous opiates that regulate behavioral CNS functions. I also suspect we should address these legalistic issues, because there is not yet a climate where we can think and talk about using opiates in a rational way.

PART IV. THE USE OF EXOGENOUS OPIATES AND OPIATE ANTAGONISTS
IN THE TREATMENT OF MENTAL DISEASES

INTRODUCTORY REMARKS

Joel Solomon

Department of Psychiatry
State University of New York, Downstate Medical Center
Brooklyn, New York 11217

We know that psychiatric disorders represent a heterogeneous group of conditions. One way that heterogeneity is expressed is through its diagnostic classification. Another way that it is expressed is through treatment responses; some of the things that we heard today and are going to hear this afternoon and throughout the conference have to do with treatment responses to specific medications: the opiates and opiate antagonists.

From another perspective we know that drug-dependent people are also a very heterogeneous group. In some of these people the psychiatric pathology is quite predominant, often precipitating and certainly contributing to the drug-seeking behavior and ultimate drug dependence. These people also are often successfully treating their psychiatric disorder. The difficulty, of course, is the institution within which the psychiatric disorder is being treated, the street institution as opposed to the formal psychiatric establishment that also treats psychiatric disorders.

The papers presented in this section examine the interface between the use of specific exogenous opiates and opiate antagonists in the treatment of various mental disorders.

NALOXONE AND NALTREXONE IN MENTAL ILLNESS AND TARDIVE DYSKINESIA *

Jan Volavka, Brian Anderson, and Gabriel Koz

New York University at Manhattan Psychiatric Center
Ward's Island
New York, New York 10035

INTRODUCTION

Since the discovery of endorphins, a number of hypotheses relating these substances to mental illness have been formulated; these hypotheses are discussed in other papers in this volume. The administration of opioid antagonists has been used as a tool to test some of these hypotheses. This strategy is based on the displacement of endorphins from the receptors; the functions that are affected by endorphins are thus altered. Unfortunately, opioid antagonists have many other effects besides the displacement of endorphins. These confounding effects will be discussed later.

NALOXONE AND NALTREXONE IN SCHIZOPHRENIA

Swedish investigators have observed increased endorphin cerebrospinal (CSF) levels in chronic psychotic patients; they reported that these high levels decreased after successful treatment with conventional antipsychotic drugs.[1] These findings led to the hypothesis that increased endorphin levels may be involved in the pathophysiology of psychoses. It seemed logical to test this hypothesis by the administration of an opioid antagonist. The same Swedish group has therefore conducted the first therapeutic trial of an opioid antagonist in schizophrenia.[2] They administered 0.4 mg of naloxone to chronic schizophrenic patients in a single-blind study. Few of these patients have reported a reduction of hallucinations. Several experiments using mostly low doses of naloxone (0.4–1.8 mg) gave negative results,[3-5] although Davis et al.[6] reported a decrease of unusual thought content after naloxone. The Swedish investigators were unable to replicate their own findings when they used a double-blind design and a higher dose (0.8 mg) of naloxone.[7] Emrich et al.[8] reported that 4 mg of naloxone had some antipsychotic activity, but a replication study by the same authors using a higher dose of naloxone (24.8 mg) yielded equivocal results.[9] However, several investigators using a dose of 10 mg naloxone i.v. report consistently positive results.[10-12] The study of Berger et al.[11] used 14 subjects; 8 of these 14 patients were reported earlier.[10] Lehmann et al.[12] used 6 subjects. These studies [10-12] suggest that there is a subpopulation of schizophrenics that responds to naloxone by a reduction of hallucinations and perhaps by other symptom reduction.

If such a subpopulation of naloxone responders exists, we expect that its members would respond consistently. Thus, once a patient responds to naloxone, he will respond to repeated injections of naloxone, but not to placebo. This

* This work was supported in part by Grant MH34558 from the U.S. Public Health Service to J.V.

0077–8923/82/0398–0097 $1.75/0 © 1982, NYAS

procedure was employed with negative results in a potential responder in an early study,[5] and its use was formally proposed later.[13, 14] More recently, a group of Russian investigators used this technique with apparent success.[15] Using repeated injections of naloxone (0.3 mg/kg s.c.) and placebo, they uncovered 3 consistent naloxone responders among 7 patients resistant to neuroleptics.

It has been suggested that the stiffness elicited in the rat by the intracerebral administration of β-endorphin may be similar to schizophrenic catatonia.[16] This daring analogy led some investigators to expect an amelioration of catatonic schizophrenia after naloxone. The studies of naloxone in catatonia yielded mixed results. One catatonic patient failed to respond to 1.4 mg of naloxone,[17] a study of three catatonics was equivocal,[8] and another investigator reported an improvement in 8 of 9 patients with catatonic stupor in an open pilot study.[18] These results await replication.

In summary, it is possible that a subpopulation of schizophrenic patients responds to naloxone by clinical improvement. The effective therapeutic dose of naloxone seems to be 10–20 mg. Two-phase experiments consisting of screening for naloxone response and then repeated placebo–naloxone crossovers should be used to identify the consistent responder. Another approach consists in the use of biological screening tests for endorphin hyperactivity as proposed by Davis et al.[13] Measures of pain sensitivity, respiratory rate, pupillary diameter, somatosensory evoked potentials, and plasma and CSF endorphin levels might be the variables measured in such screening tests. ACTH plasma levels were also proposed as predictors of clinical response to naloxone.[12]

The main disadvantages of naloxone are the short duration of action and the lack of an oral form. Naltrexone is an orally effective opioid antagonist. Its duration of action is up to 72 hours after a single oral dose of 120–200 mg.[19, 20] Two uncontrolled trials showed no beneficial effects of naltrexone administered to schizophrenics for 2–8 weeks at the daily doses of 50–800 mg.[21–23] A trial using a double-blind crossover design showed no advantage of 100 mg naltrexone for 2 weeks over placebo in 10 schizophrenics.[7] An open study [24] using 5 schizophrenics as subjects showed equivocal results with naltrexone.

Naltrexone trials in mental disease did not yield promising results. Naltrexone has more agonist activity than naloxone, it has more side effects, and its future in mental health research is uncertain.

NALOXONE IN TARDIVE DYSKINESIA

Tardive dyskinesia is a syndrome marked by involuntary movements of facial, lingual, mandibular, and other muscles. Its pathophysiology is not clearly understood. Most of the prevailing theories implicate aberrations of the dopaminergic nigro-striatal system. Over the past 5 years, it has become increasingly obvious that the endorphin systems interact with the dopaminergic ones.[25] Naloxone was shown to interact with the dopaminergic system in animals. It enhanced the rate-reducing effect of chlorpromazine on schedule-controlled behavior in pigeons,[26] and it blocked the stereotypy induced by apomorphine in the rat.[27, 28] These observations tend to predict that a single dose of naloxone might decrease tardive dyskinesia.

To explore the possibility that endorphins play a role in the pathophysiology of tardive dyskinesia, Bjorndal et al.[29] treated eight tardive dyskinetic patients with single doses of a synthetic Met-enkephalin analogue of morphine and of 0.8 mg of naloxone. The Met-enkephalin analogue reduced tardive dyskinesia in patients who were treated concurrently with high doses of neuroleptics. Morphine had a similar, although weaker effect. The authors state conservatively that naloxone had no effect. However, their data (Figure 1) suggest a slight decrease of tardive dyskinesia after naloxone.

We are currently studying the effects of a single dose of naloxone (10 mg i.v.) on tardive dyskinesia in a double-blind, placebo-controlled crossover experiment. Two raters administer a standardized rating scale for the assessment of involuntary movements (AIMS) before the injection, and at 20, 40, 60, 120, and 360 minutes after the injection of naloxone and placebo (each subject has two experimental sessions). Patients with moderate or severe tardive dyskinesia are the subjects. At the time of this writing, sessions were completed in 10 subjects. Naloxone elicited a nonsignificant *increase* of tardive dyskinetic movements. In 5 of these subjects, samples for β-endorphin and ACTH were drawn before and at 30 and 60 minutes after the injection. The radioimmunoassays for β-endorphin in these 5 subjects indicate a significant increase of β-endorphin at 30 minutes after the injection. The pre-naloxone and post-naloxone averages were 6.2 and 8.9 picomoles/liter, respectively; $t = 3.58$, $p < 0.05$ (t-test for matched pairs). The analogous averages for pre-placebo and 30-minute post-placebo tests are 7.4 and 6.4 picomoles/liter ($t = 1.50$, not significant). This experiment is in progress; additional data are being acquired.

NALOXONE IN AFFECTIVE DISORDERS

Endorphin excess may underlie euphoria and mania.[30, 31] Judd *et al.*[32] demonstrated an antimanic effect in 12 manic patients who received naloxone (20 mg) and placebo i.v. Naloxone elicited a feeling of lethargy which peaked within 15 minutes after the end of the infusion; the return to baseline occurred within two hours. This time course is shorter than that reported for the improvement of schizophrenic symptoms.[10, 12] This difference suggests a different mechanism of action of naloxone in schizophrenia and mania.

In addition to the schizophrenic patients reviewed earlier, the group of Russian investigators [15] also studied one manic patient using the two-phase crossover design described above and a dose of 0.3 mg/kg of naloxone. This patient was found to respond consistently to naloxone. Other investigators employed naloxone doses of 6 mg or less in several manic and hypomanic patients without success.[9, 33] A recent study employing 20 mg of naloxone s.c. has failed to demonstrate any antimanic effect in 10 patients.[34]

In summary, a single dose of naloxone (20 mg or more) may have antimanic effects. Most of the data on naloxone effect in mania come from a group of investigators at the University of California at San Diego. Their innovative and carefully executed studies await replication.

The effects of naloxone in depression have not been thoroughly studied. Low doses of naloxone (up to 6 mg) were tried in small patient samples, and no consistent antidepressant effects were noted.[9, 33, 35] We should point out that low doses of naloxone were also found ineffective in schizophrenia, whereas doses of 10–20 mg yielded some promising results. High doses of naloxone have apparently not been tried in depression.

The Mechanism of Naloxone Action in Mental Illness

Naloxone was originally assumed to have no other activity than the antagonism of opioids. This assumption is incorrect at the doses employed in the promising psychopharmacological studies (i.e., 10–30 mg). High doses of naloxone were repeatedly shown to have *agonist* effects *in vivo* and *in vitro*.[36] Those observations bring up the possibility that some of the psychoactive effects of high naloxone doses may be due to the agonist (i.e., morphine-like) rather than antagonist effects of this drug.

Furthermore, the assumption that naloxone acts selectively on opiate receptors may not be valid. The existence of a nonopiate naloxone receptor has been suggested. Two naloxone binding sites were demonstrated in the brain: type I with high affinity for naloxone (a site available to dihydromorphine) and type II with low affinity for naloxone (not available to dihydromorphine).[37, 38] It is possible that high doses of naloxone activiate the nonopiate, low-affinity receptor. The functions of this receptor are unclear; it is unlikely that it is a part of any endorphin system.

Another way in which the naloxone effects in psychoses might have bypassed any opiate receptors is by interacting with antipsychotic medication. In several positive studies using high doses of naloxone,[10, 15, 32] some patients were maintained on antipsychotic drugs. As mentioned above, naloxone potentiates certain effects of chlorpromazine in pigeons;[26] and numerous other studies demonstrating interactions between naloxone and the drugs that affect the dopaminergic system were summarized elsewhere.[36] It is conceivable that some antipsychotic effects of naloxone in patients were due to potentiation of their concurrent antipsychotic treatment. It is interesting that only one out of 10 patients in the negative study reviewed above[34] was receiving a neuroleptic drug concurrently with naloxone.

In summary, the naloxone effect alone cannot automatically be accepted as a proof of endorphin involvement. Naloxone has psychological,[32, 39] neurophysiological,[40] and endocrinological[41] effects in normal man. We should expand our knowledge of naloxone effects in normal subjects if we want to understand its action in mental illness.

Acknowledgment

Mr. Tom Cooper of the Rockland Research Institute performed the radioimmunoassays for β-endorphin.

References

1. Terenius, L., A. Wahlström, L. Lindström & E. Widerlöv. 1976. Neurosci. Lett. **3:** 151–162.
2. Gunne, L.-M., L. Lindström & L. Terenius. 1977. J. Neural. Transm. **40:** 13–19.
3. Janowsky, D. S., D. Segal, F. Bloom, A. Abrams & R. Guillemin. 1977. Am. J. Psychiatr. **134:** 926–927.
4. Kurland, A. A., O. L. McCabe, T. E. Hanlon & D. Sullivan. 1972. Am. J. Psychiatr. **134:** 1408–1410.

5. VOLAVKA, J., A. MALLYA, S. BAIG, J. PEREZ-CRUET. 1977. Science (N.Y.) **196:** 1227–1228.
6. DAVIS, G. C., W. E. BUNNEY, E. G. DE FRAITES, J. E. KLEINMAN, D. P. VAN KAMMEN, R. M. POST & R. J. WYATT. 1977. Science (N.Y.) **197:** 74–77.
7. GUNNE, L.-M., L. LNIDSTRÖM & E. WIDERLÖV. 1979. *In* Endorphins in Mental Health Research. G. Usdin, W. E. Bunney & N. Kline, Eds.: 393–406. Macmillan. London.
8. EMRICH, H. M., C. CORDING, S. PIRÉE, A. KÖLLING, D. V. ZERSSEN & A. HERZ. 1977. Pharmakopsychiatr. Neuropsychopharmakol. **10:** 265–270.
9. EMRICH, H. M., C. CORDING, S. PIRÉE, A. KÖLLING, H. J. MÖLLER, D. V. ZERSSEN & A. HERZ. 1979. *In* Endorphins in Mental Health Research. G. Usdin, W. E. Burney & N. Kline, Eds.: 452–460. Macmillan. London.
10. WATSON, S. J., P. A. BERGER, H. AKIL, M. J. MILIS & J. D. BARCHAS. 1978. Science (N.Y.) **201:** 73–76.
11. BERGER, P. A., S. J. WATSON, H. AKIL & J. D. BARCHAS. 1981. Am. J. Psychiatr. **138:** 913–918.
12. LEHMANN, H., N. P. V. NAIR & N. S. KLINE. 1979. Am. J. Psychiatr. **136:** 762–766.
13. DAVIS, G. C., M. S. BUCHSBAUM & W. E. BUNNEY. 1979. Schizophrenia Bull. **5:** 244–250.
14. VEREBEY, K., J. VOLAVKA & D. CLOUET. 1978. Arch. Gen. Psychiatr. **35:** 877–888.
15. LIDEMAN, R. R., G. P. PANTELEEVA, M. Y. CUCULKOVSKAYA, F. E. VARTANIAN & B. S. BELYAEV. 1980. Zh. Nevropat. Psikhiat. **80:** 231–237. (In Russian.)
16. BLOOM, F., D. SEGAL, N. LING & R. GUILLEMIN. 1976. Science (N.Y.) **194:** 630–632.
17. ABRAMS, A., D. BRAFF, D. JANOWSKY, S. HALL & D. SEGAL. 1978. Pharmakopsychiatr. Neuropsychopharmakol. **11:** 177–179.
18. SCHENK, G. K., P. ENDERS, M. P. ENGELMEIER, T. EWERT, S. HERDEMERTEN, K. H. KÖHLER, E. LODEMANN, D. MATZ & J. PACH. 1978. Arzneimittel-Forsch. **28:** 1274–1277.
19. RESNICK R. B., J. VOLAVKA, A. M. FREEDMAN & M. THOMAS. 1974. Am. J. Psychiatr. **131:** 546–650.
20. VOLAVKA, J., R. B. RESNICK, R. S. KESTENBAUM & A. M. FREEDMAN. 1976. Biol. Psychiatr. **11:** 679–685.
21. MIELKE, D. H. & D. GALLANT. 1977. Am. J. Psychiatr. **134:** 1430–1431.
22. SIMPSON, G. M., M. H. BRANCHEY & J. LEE. 1977. Curr. Ther. Res. **22:** 909–913.
23. GITLIN, M. & M. ROSENBLATT. 1978. Am. J. Psychiatr. **135:** 377–378.
24. RAGHEB, M., S. BERNEY & T. BAN. 1980. Int. Pharmacopsychiatr. **15:** 1–5.
25. VOLAVKA, J., L. C. DAVIS & Y. H. EHRLICH. 1979. Schizophrenia Bull. **5:** 227–239.
26. MCMILLAN, D. E. 1971. Psychopharmacologia **19:** 128–135.
27. COX, B., M. ARY & J. LOMAX. 1976. Pharmacol. Exp. Ther. **196:** 637–641.
28. HENDERSON, G. L. & R. WESTKAEMPER. 1975. Proc. Wash. Pharmacol. Soc. **18:** 204–207.
29. BJORNDAL, N., D. E. CASEY & J. GERLACH. 1980. Psychopharmacology **69:** 133–136.
30. BELLUZI, J. D. & L. STEIN. 1977. Nature (Lond.) **266:** 556–558.
31. BYCK, R. 1976. Lancet **1:** 72–73.
32. JUDD, L. L., D. S. JANOWSKY, D. S. SEGAL & L. Y. HUEY. 1980. Arch. Gen. Psychiatr. **3:** 583–586.
33. DAVIS, G. C., W. E. BUNNEY, M. S. BUCHSBAUM, G. DE FRAITES, W. DUNCAN, J. C. GILLIN, D. P. VAN KAMMEN, J. KLEINMAN, D. L. MURPHY, R. M. POST, V. REUS & R. J. WYATT. 1979. *In* Endorphins in Mental Health Research. G. Usdin, W. E. Bunney & N. Kline, Eds.: 393–406. Macmillan. London.

34. DAVIS, G. C., I. EXTEIN, V. I. REUS, W. HAMILTON, R. M. POST, F. K. GOODWIN & W. E. BUNNEY, JR. 1980. Am. J. Psychiatr. 137: 1583–1585.
35. TERENIUS, L., A. WAHLSTRÖM & H. AGREN. 1977. Psychopharmacology 54: 31–33.
36. SAWYNOK, J., C. PINSKY & F. S. LaBELLA. 1979. Life Sci. 25: 1621–1632.
37. LEE, C. Y., T. AKERA, S. STOLMAN & T. M. BRODY. 1975. J. Pharmacol. Exp. Ther. 194: 583–592.
38. SQUIRES, R. F. & C. BRAESTRUP. 1978. J. Neurochem. 30: 231–236.
39. JONES, R. T. & R. I. HERNING. 1979. In Endorphins in Mental Health Research. G. Usdin, W. E. Bunney & N. Kline, Eds.: 484–491. Macmillan. London.
40. VOLAVKA, J., B. JAMES, D. REKER, V. POLLOCK & D. CHO. 1979. Life Sci. 25: 1267–1272.
41. VOLAVKA, J., J. BAUMAN, J. PEVNICK, D. REKER, B. JAMES & D. CHO. 1980. Psychoneuroendocrinology 5: 225–234.

[NOTE: This paper will be discussed with the next one, which is by Ervin Varga *et al.*]

THE EFFECT OF CODEINE ON INVOLUTIONAL AND SENILE DEPRESSION

Ervin Varga,* A. Arthur Sugerman, and Jeffrey Apter

Carrier Foundation
Belle Mead, New Jersey 08502

INTRODUCTION

Before the introduction of electroconvulsive therapy for the treatment of depression, opium extracts were widely used for this purpose. The so-called "laudanum cure" was a course of treatment that was started with 16 mg of tincture of opiate and was increased over 22 days by 3 mg per day. On that ceiling, the dose plateaued for a couple of days and then gradually decreased by 2 mg per day. This treatment was especially recommended for agitated depression. The laudanum cure was used even in the 1950s before antidepressant drugs were introduced for those patients for whom electroconvulsive therapy was contraindicated or where no consent was available. The textbook descriptions [1, 2] and anecdotal reports describe the laudanum cure as an effective treatment not only because it suppressed the agony of the agitated depression, but also because after two months of treatment, the depressive symptoms disappear.

During the years of my psychiatric residency training in Europe, I myself witnessed such cures. I remember one case clearly, in which a severely agitated and depressed man in his 60s responded to this treatment after a couple of weeks and was doing fine when discharged on no medication.

More recently, Abse and Dahlstrom [3] tried to use opiates in senile mental disturbances, and found no specific effect.

Lehmann *et al.*[4] in an open study administered Demerol hydrochloride (Winthrop) together with Dexedrine Sulfate (Smith Kline & French) and found evidence of some improvement; however, it was not clear as to from what.

A more recent study of methadone and morphine in depression by Extein [5] found no good evidence of antidepressant efficacy when single i.v. doses of morphine and methadone were used; but Extein recommended further investigation of possible antidepressant affects of opioids, endorphins, and analogs in depression and in other psychiatric disorders.

The present study aimed to investigate the usefulness of codeine, a well-known and commonly used opiate, in the treatment of depression—depression that has not responded to standard methods of drug therapy.

We started to select patients who were aged 30 and above. Although addiction has apparently never occurred in patients who were treated for depression or schizophrenia with opioids, we found it preferable to avoid any involvement of young patients who had any addictive problem.

* Address for correspondence: Carrier Foundation, P.O. Box 147, Belle Mead, NJ 08502.

0077–8923/82/0398–0103 $1.75/0 © 1982, NYAS

PATIENTS AND METHODS

We selected those patients who failed to respond to antidepressant, tricyclic and/or monoamine oxidase inhibitors, and psychotherapy, and who were also unsuitable for or unwilling to have electroconvulsive therapy. Both male and female patients were selected, and they met the research diagnostic criteria for major depressive disorder. Therefore, patients with a history of drug addiction or alcoholism were excluded. All the patients signed a consent form before beginning the treatment. They were warned of the possible side effect: constipation, which they had anyhow due to agitated depression, and which they would have on tricyclic antidepressants also.

The initial dose of codeine sulfate was 30 mg, 3 times a day, which was increased gradually to 45 mg, 3 times a day in the second week, and if necessary, 60 mg 3 times a day in the third week, at the discretion of the treating psychiatrist, the investigator.

The patients completing three or more weeks were included in the final analysis.

DISCUSSION

In the first group, we had eight patients. All of them were above 70 years of age; six were female and two were male. All of them suffered from prolonged depression lasting longer than the minimum of six months. All of them received various tricyclic antidepressants, and no improvement was documented. We added codeine to the last-used tricyclic antidepressant. Only one patient showed improvement on the combination—the other seven did not. Finally, five accepted electroconvulsive treatments. Two of the patients improved on monoamine oxidase inhibitors. All of them had more severe constipation once codeine was added. None of them experienced even temporary euphoria, but all of them got some relief from the temporary sedative effect of the codeine. The only patient who did show improvement was eventually discharged on codeine and nortriptyline and was doing fine after the discontinuation of both, six weeks after her discharge.

The second group of patients received only codeine. Here we used the open study design described earlier, with blind evaluations and rating scales (Hamilton and Zung).

We could collect only four patients—all of them failed to respond to codeine. One of them developed a severe allergic reaction to codeine on the second day; the other three suffered from marked constipation and somnolence, but no euphoria. They all remained depressed, and three of them eventually accepted and improved on electroconvulsive treatment after codeine was discontinued.

None of our patients developed dependence on codeine. Our study found no antidepressant effect of codeine in severe intractable depression; however, on electroconvulsive treatment and monoamine oxidase inhibitors, most patients eventually got better.

SUMMARY

The authors studied the effect of codeine on 12 severely depressed patients who failed to respond to tricyclic antidepressants. They all were in involution. Eight patients received codeine in combination with other tricyclic antidepressants and only one of them showed improvement. Four depressed patients received codeine alone and none of them improved. The patients were kept on codeine up to three weeks. The dose was gradually increased from 90 mg/day to 180 mg/day. All patients suffered from severe constipation—more than what they had on tricyclic antidepressant medication. All of the patients experienced a sedative effect. None of them had euphoria and none of them developed dependence. After the failure of codeine, the patients finally accepted electroconvulsive therapy or monoamine oxidase inhibitors, and with one exception, all improved.

REFERENCES

1. KRAEPELIN, E. 1905. Die psychiatrische Klinik. p. 11. Barth, Leipzig.
2. WEYGANDT, W. 1935. Lehrbuch der Nerven—und Geistes—Krankheiten. p. 507. Verlagsbuchhandlung, Halle, Marhold.
3. ABSE, D. W. & W. G. DAHLSTROM. 1960. The value of chemotherapy in senile mental disturbances. Controlled comparison of chlorpromazine, reserpine-pipradol and opium. J. Am. Med. Assoc. **174:** 2036–2042.
4. LEHMANN, H. E., J. V. ANANTH, K. C. GEAGEA & T. A. BAN. 1971. Treatment of depression with dexedrine and demerol. Curr. Ther. Res. **13:** 42–49.
5. EXTEIN, I., D. PICKAR, M. S. GOLD, *et al.* 1981. Methadone and morphine in depression. Psychopharmacol. Bull. **17:** 29–33.

NALOXONE AND NALTREXONE IN MENTAL ILLNESS

by Jan V. Volavka

CODEINE IN THE TREATMENT OF INVOLUTIONAL AND SENILE DEPRESSION

by Ervin Varga

———◆———

DISCUSSION OF THE PAPERS

K. VEREBEY (*State University of New York, Downstate Medical Center, Brooklyn*): I would like to make a comment about the pharmacological considerations of codeine versus other opiate agonists such as methadone.

Codeine, just like morphine, is poorly and erratically absorbed by various individuals. It is very difficult to tell how much of this drug is absorbed by each patient. In future experiments blood level measurements must be incorporated into the protocol to insure adequate bioavailability of codeine. Another problem with codeine is that it is a weak opiate agonist. I feel that by accepting these negative results we do not do justice to the possible effectiveness of codeine or other opiate agonists when we do not even know the bioavailability.

J. SOLOMON (*State University of New York, Downstate Medical Center, Brooklyn*): That is a point well taken.

J. J. KAUFMAN (*Johns Hopkins, Baltimore, MD*): A number of mental diseases are well characterized by their neurochemical aberrations. Over the past 10 years careful analysis of blood and urine samples allowed quantitation of the neurotransmitters and their metabolites. Thus it was possible to determine if there were deficiencies or excesses.

The way one uses drugs to try to treat patients with such mental disorders is to try to titrate their body chemistry to get it back to normal. When one is using opiates or opiate antagonists it would enhance the value of the studies considerably if the clinical patients could be tested more thoroughly, because it is very difficult to get consent in many places. It would be helpful to do a careful profile of the neurotransmitters and their metabolites before, during, and after treatment. This profile should include not only the regular neurotransmitter but also the normal neuro-endocrine peptides. This way with one's very valuable patients a spectrum could be generated that might help unravel what is happening. Currently the physician is dosing, dosing, and dosing and simultaneously looking at a number of psychological parameters that are sometimes harder to characterize well than are the objective neurochemical parameters.

I would like to throw this open because it has been an interest of ours for many years. We started with the late Dan Effron when he was at the National Institute of Mental Health trying to figure out what was happening to the neurochemistry of patients and how the drugs affected the patterns. We then became involved with the opiates trying to look similarly for neurochemical effects. Now is the time for physicians having clinical populations to mesh together the subjective, behavioral, and objective neurochemical effects of opiates.

106

H. M. EMRICH *(Max Planck Institute for Psychiatry, Munich, FRG)*: I would like to comment to Dr. Volavka's paper. It is interesting that in the studies using high dosage of naloxone there is an antipsychotic effect in three studies, whereas with naltrexone such an effect is not observed. This could be due to the fact that the very short half-life of naloxone induces, as you showed, an increase of endorphins. As a result of a very short blockade of opiate receptors the endorphins would reach their receptors. This would fit the concept that practically all drugs and procedures that have antipsychotic efficacies, for example, neuroleptics, electroconvulsion, and stress, (e.g. cold water stress, rotational stress) induce an increase and not decrease of endorphin activity in the brain.

J. V. VOLAVKA *(New York University School of Medicine, New York)*: I agree.

POSSIBLE ANTIDEPRESSIVE EFFECTS OF OPIOIDS: ACTION OF BUPRENORPHINE

H. M. Emrich, P. Vogt, and A. Herz

Max-Planck Institute for Psychiatry
D-8000 Munich 40, Federal Republic of Germany

INTRODUCTION

The euphorogenic and anxiolytic properties of opiates [1] and of endorphins [2] prompt questions as to the possibility that a defectively operating endorphinergic system may represent a causative factor in the pathogenesis of endogenous depression. Though from biochemical and pharmacological data the evidence in support of this hypothesis is weak (cf. ref. 3) it, nevertheless, requires additional evaluation. However, irrespective of the presence of a hypothetical constitutional deficit of endogenous morphinomimetic substances compensated for by an exogenous supply in the therapy of depressed patients, the question arises if, independently from such a possible type of metabolic dysfunction in depression, there may exist direct pharmacodynamic therapeutic effects of opioids in depressive syndromes. Since anxiety and sleep disturbances, in addition to melancholia, make up an integral part of the psychopathology of depression, from their profile of action, it may be anticipated that opioids could be highly effective, therapeutically, in depressive illness.

Indeed, since the time of Emil Kraepelin [4] the "opium cure" has been recommended for the treatment of depressed patients, employing slowly increasing and later decreasing dosages of tinctura opii [5] and of other opiates.[6] Interestingly, according to reports of that time, although a standardized evaluation of the therapeutic efficacy was, and is, lacking, this treatment was effective and did not result in opiate addiction, possibly, since the doses applied were comparatively low. Later, Fink et al.[7] applied the mixed agonist/antagonist cyclazocine (1.0–3.0 mg) in 10 severely depressed patients and observed a strong antidepressive effect, in particular concerning the items "depressed mood" and "apathy." A further clinical evaluation of possible beneficial effects of opiates has been deferred, possibly owing to the psychotomimetic effects of cyclazocine and, furthermore, in view of the fact that the discovery of tricyclic antidepressants and of MAO-inhibitors opened a new era in the pharmacotherapy of depressive syndromes. Interestingly, immediately after the discovery of the endorphins, which shed new light onto the possible psychotropic effects of an activation of opiate receptors, new attempts were initiated in the evaluation of the possible antidepressive effects of opioids. Kline et al.[2] were the first to perform clinical trials in different types of psychiatric disorders (schizophrenia, depression, neuroses) by use of β-endorphin infusions (1.5–6.0 mg) and observed in two depressed patients, in an open design, positive effects of this treatment. Angst et al.,[8] also in an open trial, investigated the possible antidepressive action of infusions of 10 mg of β-endorphin and detected a switch to hypomania/mania in three of six depressed patients. Subsequently, double-blind trials as to the possible antidepressant efficacy of β-endorphin have been

108

0077–8923/82/0398–0108 $1.75/0 © 1982, NYAS

performed by two groups.[9, 10] Gerner *et al.*[9] reported a significant improvement 2 to 4 hours after β-endorphin infusions, as compared to placebo treatment in 10 depressed patients, whereas Pickar *et al.*[10] found no significant change in 4 depressed patients after β-endorphin therapy. The application of the synthetic enkephalin analogue FK 33-824 in 10 depressed patients produced a sizable improvement in 3 of the patients and a tranquilizing effect in 4 of them.[11]

Interestingly, the investigation as to the possible value of opioids in antidepressive therapy were not confined to endogenous morphinomimetic substances or their derivatives but were—in line with the attempts performed prior to the studies of Fink *et al.*[7]—also undertaken with opiates, such as morphine and other opium alkaloids in clinical therapeutic trials. Gold *et al.*,[12] for example, presented data suggestive of a potential antidepressant and anxiolytic/antipanic effects of opiates. On the other hand, Extein *et al.*[13] reported only a slight antidepressive effect of 5.0 mg morphine in 10 patients with major depressive disorders (open study), whereas in a double-blind investigation in 6 depressed in-patients, 5.0 mg methadone proved not different in effect from placebo.

Another basis from which to speculate as to possible antidepressive properties of opioids lies in the fact that electroconvulsion, which is certainly one of the most efficacious and rapidly acting somatic treatments in depression, possesses endorphin-activating properties. As shown by Belenky and Holaday [14] in animal experiments, electroconvulsion induces a spectrum of vegetative, naloxone-reversible changes, which apparently reflect an EC-effected activation of particular endorphinergic systems. Similar conclusions may be derived from the estimation of plasma β-endorphin immunoreactivity in depressed patients before and after electroconvulsion, which exhibits a highly significant increase after this procedure.[15] Interestingly, these endorphin-mobilizing properties are not confined to electroconvulsion but also are exhibited by other physical methods used in the past in the treatment of psychotic disorders (e.g. cold-water stress,[16] insulin coma,[17] rotational stress [cf. ref. 18]). Additionally, the stressful procedure of hemodialysis, which in some cases apparently exerts antidepressant effects,[19] unequivocally induces an elevation of plasma β-endorphin immunoreactivity,[20] an effect which is possibly also exhibited by sham-dialysis. Therefore, some of the controversial results concerning the action of hemodialysis in different types of psychoses may be explained in terms of an nonspecific stress effect of this procedure.

Investigations as to a possible antidepressant effect of the opiate mixed agonist/antagonist buprenorphine [21] are suggested not only by the total body of evidence concerning the possible antidepressive effect of opioids, reviewed above, but also by the observations that it, as shown by Mello and Mendelson,[22] has highly positive subjective effects in opiate addicts. Furthermore, the finding that buprenorphine has mood-improving effects in postoperative patients [23] and the very important fact that this strong analgesic substance is devoid of psychoto-mimetic effects and has a very low abuse potential [24, 25] suggests the performance of clinical trials with the aim of developing a new opioid substance with a strong antidepressant potency and a high degree of drug safety.

METHODS

The study was performed by use of a double-blind $A_1/B/A_2$-design ($A_{1/2}$ = placebo; B = buprenorphine). Ten patients who met the research diagnostic criteria [26] for major depressive disorder gave their informed consent to participate in the study. The duration of the three therapeutic phases varied between: A_1: 1–7 days, B: 5–8 days; A_2: 0–4 days. The patients were free of conventional thymoleptic drugs. Before the beginning of the trial, a wash-out period of 4 days was performed. During the buprenorphine treatment phase, two sublingual tablets (0.2 mg per day) were given at 8:30 and 16:30 h. Psychopathological evaluation was performed by a trained psychiatrist every two days in the afternoon by use of the IMPS [27] and the Hamilton scale for depression.[28] Additionally, the global impression of depression and, as a screening of side effects, the symptoms "nausea," "vomiting," "dizziness," and "euphoria" were evaluated by use of the VBS (Verlaufs-Beurteilungs-Skala).[29]

RESULTS

The mean results of the Hamilton-scores before (A_1), during (B_1; B_2; B_3) and after (A_2) buprenorphine treatment are depicted in FIGURE 1. The data

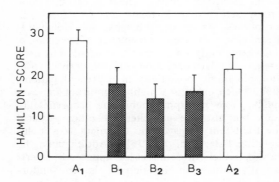

FIGURE 1. Averaged Hamilton-scores of 10 depressed patients before (A_1), during (B_1-B_3), and after (A_2) buprenorphine treatment. Bars: SEM; for details see text.

B_1–B_3 represent the average values of the Hamilton-score at the beginning of the blind buprenorphine treatment (B_1), in the middle of buprenorphine treatment phase (B_2), and at the end of buprenorphine treatment (B_3). A_2 represents the average data of the Hamilton-scores at the end of the second placebo treatment period. As can be seen in FIGURE 1, there is a strong reduction in the Hamilton-scores during the phases B_1–B_3 in comparison with the placebo phases A_1, and, to a lesser degree, also in comparison with the second placebo phase A_2. These differences are highly significant ($p \leq 0.02$, Wilcoxon-test).

An evaluation of the single data of individual patients (data not shown) reveals that about 50% of the patients responded very strongly to buprenorphine, whereas the other 50% were, apparently, nonresponders. Since practically all of the patients included in the study were nonresponders to conventional thymoleptic therapy, this is a significant result. Most of the patients experienced some degree of slight nausea, dizziness and sedation (vomiting in one case) in the course of the study, but these side effects, with the exception of the one case of vomiting, never became a problem during therapy.

DISCUSSION

As shown in the present investigation, the mixed opiate agonist/antagonist buprenorphine exhibits antidepressant properties in cases not responding to conventional thymoleptic therapy. This is a remarkable finding, since for this type of patient, an inevitable consequence would be the application of electro-convulsion, a somatic type of therapy which, in view of some of its side effects [30] and therapeutic risks [31] is not a desirable choice in the treatment of psychiatric patients. Therefore, the intriguing possibility has to be considered that the type of therapy indicated here may represent a way of mimicking by chemical means the neurobiologically therapeutic effects of electroconvulsion; one can thus speculate that other physical and/or chemical means of inducing endorphin activation (e.g. inhibition of enkephalinases) may, also, in the future, play a therapeutic role in the treatment of endogenous depression.

REFERENCES

1. MARTIN, W. R., Ed. 1977. Drug Addiction. I. Morphine, Sedative-Hypnotic and Alcohol Dependence. Handbuch der Experimentellen Pharmakologie, Vol. 45. Springer. Berlin-Heidelberg-New York.
2. KLINE, N. S., C. H. LI, H. E. LEHMANN, A. LAJTHA, E. LASKI & T. COOPER. 1977. β-Endorphin-induced changes in schizophrenic and depressed patients. Arch. Gen. Psychiatry **34:** 1111–1113.
3. EMRICH, H. M. 1981. A possible role of opioid substances in depression. *In* Typical and Atypical Antidepressants, Vol. 1: Clinical Practice. E. Costa & G. Racagni, Eds.: 77–84. Raven Press. New York.
4. KRAEPELIN, E. 1901. Einführung in die Psychiatrische Klinik. Joh. Ambrosius Barth-Verlag. Leipzig.
5. KRAEPELIN, E. 1927. Psychiatrie I. Joh. Ambrosius Barth-Verlag. Leipzig.
6. WEYGANDT, W. 1935. Lehrbuch der Nerven- und Geisteskrankheiten. Marhold-Verlagsbuchhandlung. Halle.
7. FINK, M., J. SIMEON, T. M. ITIL & A. H. FREEDMAN. 1970. Clinical anti-depressant activity of cyclazocine—a narcotic antagonist. Clin. Pharmacol. Ther. **11:** 41–48.
8. ANGST, J., V. AUTENRIETH, F. BREM, M. KOUKKOU, H. MEYER, H. H. STASSEN & U. STORCK. 1979. Preliminary results of treatment with β-endorphin in depression. *In* Endorphins in Mental Health Research. E. Usdin, W. E. Bunney, Jr. & N. S. Kline, Eds.: 518–528. Macmillan. London.
9. GERNER, R. H., D. H. CATLIN, D. A. GORELICK, K. K. HUI & C. H. LI. 1980. β-Endorphin. Intravenous infusion causes behavioral change in psychiatric inpatients. Arch. Gen. Psychiatry **37:** 642–647.
10. PICKAR, D., G. C. DAVIS, S. C. SCHULZ, I. EXTEIN, R. WAGNER, D. NABER, P. W. GOLD, D. P. VAN KAMMEN, F. K. GOODWIN, R. J. WYATT, C. H. LI & W. E. BUNNEY, JR. 1981. Behavioral and biological effects of acute β-endorphin injection in schizophrenic and depressed patients. Am. J. Psychiatry **138:** 160–166.
11. RÜTHER, E., G. JUNGKUNZ & N. NEDOPIL. 1981. Clinical effects of the synthetic analogue of methionine enkephalin FK 33–824. IIIrd World Congress of Biological Psychiatry, Stockholm. (Abstract)
12. GOLD, M. S., A. L. C. POTTASH, D. R. SWEENEY, H. D. KLEBER & D. E. RED-MOND. 1979. Rapid opiate detoxification: Clinical evidence of antidepressant and antipanic effects of opiates. Am. J. Psychiatry **136:** 982–983.
13. EXTEIN, I., D. PICKAR, M. S. GOLD, P. W. GOLD, A. L. C. POTTASH, D. R. SWEENEY, R. J. ROSS, R. REBARD, D. MARTIN & F. K. GOODWIN. 1981. Methadone and morphine in depression. Pharmacol. Bull. **17:** 29–33.

14. BELENKY, G. L. & J. W. HOLADAY. 1979. The opiate antagonist naloxone modifies the effects of electroconvulsive shock (ECS) on respiration, blood pressure and heart rate. Brain Res. **177:** 414–417.
15. EMRICH, H. M., V. HÖLLT, W. KISSLING, M. FISCHLER, H. LASPE, H. HEINEMANN, D. V. ZERSSEN & A. HERZ. 1979. β-Endorphin-like immunoreactivity in cerebrospinal fluid and plasma of patients with schizophrenia and other neuropsychiatric disorders. Pharmakopsychiatr/Neuro-Psychopharmakol. **12:** 269–276.
16. BODNAR, R. J., D. K. KELLY, M. BRUTUS & M. GLUSMAN. 1980. Stress-induced analgesia: Neural and hormonal determinants. Neurosci. Biobehav. Rev. **4:** 87–100.
17. HÖLLT, V., R. PRZEWLOCKI & A. HERZ. 1978. Radioimmunoassay of β-endorphin. Basal and stimulated levels in extracted rat plasma. Arch. Pharmacol. **303:** 171–174.
18. MILLAN, M. J. 1981. Stress and endogenous opioid peptides: A review. *In* The Role of Endorphins in Neuropsychiatry. H. M. Emrich, Ed. Modern Problems in Pharmacopsychiatry. **17:** 49–67. Karger. Basel.
19. SCHEIBER, S. C., I. COHEN, H. YAMAMURA, R. NOVAL & L. BEUTLER. 1981. Dialysis for schizophrenia: An uncontrolled study of 11 patients. Am. J. Psychiatry **138:** 662–665.
20. HÖLLT, V., G. HILLEBRAND, B. SCHMIDT & H. J. GURLAND. 1979. Endorphins in schizophrenia: Hemodialysis/hemoperfusion are ineffective in clearing β-leu⁵-endorphin and β-endorphin from human plasma. Pharmakopsychiatr/Neuro-Psychopharmakol. **12:** 399–406.
21. LEWIS, J. W. 1980. Buprenorphine—a new strong analgesic. *In* Problems in Pain. C. Peck & M. Wallace, Eds.: 87–89. Pergamon Press. Oxford.
22. MELLO, N. K. & J. H. MENDELSON. 1980. Buprenorphine suppresses heroin use by heroin addicts. Science **207:** 657–659.
23. HARCUS, A. H., A. E. WARD & D. W. SMITH. 1980. Buprenorphine in postoperative pain: Results in 7500 patients. Anaesthesia **35:** 382–386.
24. JASINSKI, D. R., J. S. PEVNICK & J. D. GRIFFITH. 1978. Human pharmacology and abuse potential of the analgesic buprenorphine. Arch. Gen. Psychiatry **35:** 501–516.
25. MELLO, N. K., M. P. BREE & J. H. MENDELSON. 1981. Buprenorphine self-administration by rhesus monkey. Pharmacol. Biochem. Behav. **15:** 215–225.
26. SPITZER, R. L., J. ENDICOTT & E. ROBINS. 1978. Research Diagnostic Criteria (RDC) for a Selected Group of Functional Disorders. 3rd edit. New York Biometrics Research, New York State Psychiatric Institute. New York.
27. LORR, M., C. J. KLETT, D. M. MCNAIR & J. J. LASKY. 1962. Inpatient Multidimensional Psychiatric Scale. Consulting Psychologists Press. Palo Alto, CA.
28. HAMILTON, M. 1960. A rating scale for depression. J. Neurol. Neurosurg. Psychiat. **23:** 56–62.
29. EMRICH, H. M., C. CORDING, S. PIRÉE, A. KÖLLING, D. V. ZERSSEN & A. HERZ. 1977. Indication of an antipsychotic action of the opiate antagonist naloxone. Pharmakopsychiatr/Neuro-Psychopharmakol. **10:** 265–270.
30. BRENGELMANN, J. C. 1959. The Effect of Repeated Electroshock on Learning in Depressives. Springer, Berlin-Göttingen-Heidelberg.
31. WEINER, R. D. 1979. The psychiatric use of electrically induced seizures. Am. J. Psychiatry **136:** 1507–1517.

A POSSIBLE OPIOID RECEPTOR DYSFUNCTION
IN SOME DEPRESSIVE DISORDERS

Irl Extein
Fair Oaks Hospital
Summit, New Jersey 07901

Clinical Psychobiology Branch
National Institute of Mental Health
Bethesda, Maryland 20014

A. L. C. Pottash and Mark S. Gold
Regent Hospital
New York, New York 10021

Psychiatric Diagnostic Laboratories of America
Summit, New Jersey 07901

Opioid receptors were discovered and characterized in the mammalian brain in the past decade, leading to the identification of endogenous opioid peptides (endorphins) in the brain.[1] The discovery of endorphins, which are thought to function as neuromodulators in the human brain, sparked interest in the possible role of endorphins in depressive illness.[2] The high concentration of opioid receptors and endorphins in limbic and hypothalamic regions, and their interaction with noradrenergic and dopaminergic systems, suggest involvement of endorphin systems in depression, as also suggested by certain clinical observations. These include anecdotal reports from the prepsychotropic era of the efficacy of opiates in depression, reports of the appearance—in some detoxified opiate addicts—of depression responsive to opiates and antidepressants,[3] and reports of improvement in some depressed patients following β-endorphin.[4] These observations, as well as the euphoric, analgesic, and calming effect of opiates, suggest that decreased functional activity in endorphin systems may be involved in the pathophysiology of depression. Because of technical difficulties in measuring endorphins, as well as the obvious difficulties in directly measuring opioid receptors in human brain, the possibility of alterations in endorphin systems in depressed patients has been difficult to investigate directly.

We have utilized two neuroendocrine challenge paradigms to investigate indirectly hypothesized decreased brain endorphin activities and/or decreased opioid receptor sensitivities in depressed patients. In the first study, we administered the opioid agonist morphine to depressed patients and controls and measured the prolactin response. Because the increased prolactin secretion in response to morphine is mediated through opiate receptor stimulation,[5, 6] it may indirectly reflect changes in opioid receptors in depression. In the second study, we administered the opioid antagonist naloxone to depressed patients and controls and measured the cortisol response. Adrenocorticotropic hormone (ACTH) and β-endorphin both derive from the same peptide precursor, pro-opiocortin.[1] Cortisol is secreted in response to ACTH. Thus, cortisol secretion following naloxone[7] probably parallels endorphin secretion in response to a blockade of endorphin receptors, and may indirectly reflect changes in endorphin systems in depression.

113

0077-8923/82/0398-0113 $1.75/0 © 1982, NYAS

METHODS

Study 1

This study was an open investigation in 10 inpatients with major depressive disorder as classified by the Research Diagnostic Criteria (RDC) [8] (9 unipolar, 1 bipolar; 5 male, 5 female; mean age $= 44 \pm 5$). The control group was comprised of two normal volunteers and four inpatients with personality disorders (2 male, 4 female; mean age $= 33 \pm 8$). All subjects gave written informed consent to participate. Patients with recent neuroleptic use were excluded, and patients received no medication except flurazepam for at least 1 week prior to the study. After an overnight fast, subjects were at bedrest for placement of an indwelling venous catheter through which 5 mg of morphine were infused at 9:00 a.m. Samples of blood were obtained via the catheter before, and 30, 60, 90, 120, and 180 min after, morphine infusion for assay of serum prolactin (PRL) in duplicate by radioimmunoassay. We calculated the maximum prolactin response (Δ prolactin) for each patient by subtracting the baseline prolactin level from the maximum prolactin level after morphine infusion.

Each subject filled out an adjective checklist self-rating scale before the infusion and at the time of each blood drawing. Drug abusers were excluded.

Study 2

Subjects in this study consisted of 9 normal volunteer controls (9 male, 0 female; mean age $= 27 \pm 2$) and 19 depressed inpatients (10 male, 9 female, mean age 32 ± 4). Of the depressed patients, 14 met RDC for major depression (13 unipolar, 1 bipolar). Three had minor depression by RDC, and 2 schizo-affective disorder, depressed type by RDC. All subjects gave written informed consent to participate in this study. Patients with endocrine disease or substance abuse were excluded. All were free of all medications except flurazepam and acetaminophen for at least one week prior to testing. Subjects were at bedrest after an overnight fast for placement of an indwelling venous catheter through which 20 mg of naloxone (Endo Labs) was infused. Blood samples were taken -15, 0, 15, 30, 45, 60, 75, and 105 minutes after naloxone infusion for assay of cortisol in duplicate by radioimmunoassay. The maximum cortisol response (Δ cortisol) for each patient was calculated by subtracting the baseline cortisol level from the maximum cortisol level after naloxone infusion. Statistical comparisons in both studies 1 and 2 was performed by the 2-tailed t-test, and data is presented as mean $\pm$ standard error (SE).

RESULTS

Study 1

Morphine infusion produced only small, nonsignificant antidepressant and antianxiety effects in both the depressed and control groups, but produced marked, significant increases ($p < 0.05$) in serum prolactin levels 30, 60, 90, 120, and 180 minutes after infusion in the control subjects. There was no

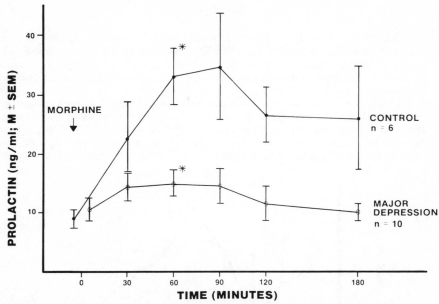

FIGURE 1. Serum prolactin levels following infusion of 5 mg of morphine in patients with major depression and controls. * Prolactin levels in depressed patients significantly less than in controls ($p < 0.01$ by t-test).

significant difference in the increase in prolactin levels in the patients with personality disorders compared with the normal volunteers. In the patients with major depressive disorder, morphine infusion produced only small, nonsignificant increases in serum prolactin (FIGURE 1). Mean baseline prolactin level of 9.0 ± 1.4 ng/ml in the control group did not differ from that of 10.5 ± 1.9 ng/ml in the depressed group. Mean prolactin levels in the depressed group were significantly lower than those in the control group at 60 ($p < 0.01$), 90 ($p < 0.02$), 120 ($p < 0.02$), and 180 ($p < 0.05$) minutes (FIGURE 1). The mean maximal prolactin response of 7.2 ± 2.7 ng/ml in the depressed group was significantly lower than that of 31.9 ± 9.5 ng/ml in the control group ($p < 0.01$). There was no significant correlation between maximal prolactin responses and baseline prolactin levels. The control subjects and the depressed patients did not differ significantly in age or sex distribution.

Study 2

Cortisol concentrates in serum following naloxone infusion are presented in FIGURE 2. Mean baseline cortisol levels of 15.8 ± 1.7 μg% in controls and 12.6 ± 1.1 in depressed patients did not differ significantly. Mean Δ cortisol of 5.0 ± 1.5 μg% in the controls did not differ significantly from that of 6.7 ± 1.6 in the depressed patients. The mean Δ cortisol in the unipolar patients also did not differ from that of controls.

DISCUSSION

The results of Study 1 show a blunted prolactin response to morphine in major depression, suggestive of alterations in endorphin systems or opioid receptors in this disorder. The results of Study 2 show no changes in cortisol response to naloxone in depression, and provide no evidence for possible changes in endorphin systems in depression.

With regard to the blunted prolactin response to morphine, both exogenous opioids and endogenous opioid peptides are potent stimulators of secretion of the pituitary hormone prolactin in animals [9-11] and man.[4-6, 12, 13] Morphine in the dosage range we used has been reported to produce large and reliable increases in serum prolactin in normal subjects.[5] Prolactin secretion is controlled

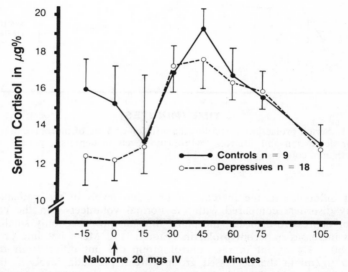

FIGURE 2. Cortisol response to naloxone in depression. Serum cortisol levels following infusion of 20 mg of naloxone in depressed patients and controls.

in part by the dopaminergic tuberoinfundibular tract, which exerts an inhibitory effect over the secretion of prolactin.[6] Serotonergic neurons have a stimulatory effect on prolactin secretion, and other neurotransmitters and neuromodulators, including norepinephrine and epinephrine, have been reported to modulate prolactin secretion as well.[6] Researchers have located opioid receptors on dopaminergic neurons.[1] When these opioid receptors are activated, they inhibit the dopaminergic tonic inhibition of prolactin secretion. Such opioid receptor activation would therefore allow increased secretion of prolactin after administration of opioids [11] (FIGURE 3).

Thus the absent or blunted increase in serum prolactin occurring after morphine infusion in our patients with major depressive disorder may reflect abnormalities in central endorphin, dopamine, serotonin, or other neuroregulatory systems. Possible abnormalities in endorphin systems that could account for a blunted prolactin response to morphine in major depression include an opioid receptor deficit, an excess of endogenous opioid antagonist, or elevated endorphin levels with compensatory down-regulation of opioid receptors. Although there was no significant difference in baseline prolactin levels between the control subjects and the patients with major depressive disorder, subtle changes in baseline prolactin secretion or diurnality might partially explain the blunted prolactin response to morphine exhibited by the patients with major depressive disorder. Halbreich and associates reported increased secretion of prolactin in depressed patients during the afternoon and evening.[11] An increased prolactin secretion at some time of the day in the patients with major depressive disorder could conceivably have decreased the sensitivity of the prolactin system to stimulation. Possibly the use of psychotropic medication by some of the depressed patients in the 6 weeks before the study may have influenced their prolactin response to morphine. If this were the case, however, one would probably expect a significant difference between mean baseline prolactin levels of patients with major depressive disorder and those of control subjects, or correlation between maximal prolactin responses and baseline prolactin levels. We observed neither of these. Researchers should explore other factors that might influence prolactin response to morphine in depression, such as corticosteroid or thyroid axis abnormalities or pharmacokinetic changes.

While we observed significant miosis, we noted only a small, nonsignificant subjective antidepressant effect in the depressed patients. This lack of antidepressant response to morphine parallels the lack of neuroendocrine response in depressed patients. Perhaps higher doses of morphine or other opioids are needed to stimulate prolactin secretion in depressed patients than in control subjects. Preliminary work shows elevation of serum prolactin in depressed patients after infusion of 5 mg of methadone, which is about twice as potent as morphine.[15]

Despite the lack of change in cortisol response to naloxone (FIGURE 4) in depression in Study 2, further exploration of the involvement of endorphins in depression, and in changes in the hypothalamic-pituitary-adrenal (HPA) axis in depression, seems of interest. The decrease in plasma cortisol following opiates and methadone,[15] as well as the increase in cortisol following naloxone,[7] are interesting in view of the known hypersecretion of cortisol and the failure of suppression of cortisol on the dexamethasone suppression test in patients with

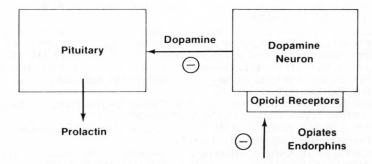

FIGURE 3. Opioids increase serum prolactin. Possible mechanism of increased prolactin secretion following the administration of opioids.

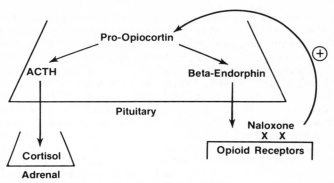

FIGURE 4. The opioid antagonist naloxone increases serum cortisol. Possible mechanism of increased cortisol secretion following the administration of naloxone.

major depression.[16] Since ACTH and β-endorphin have a common precursor,[1] the relationship between these two in depression needs to be explored. The strategy used here in Study 2 measured brain endorphin systems function indirectly. This strategy has been demonstrated to be sensitive to the presumed endorphin deficit in detoxified methadone addicts.[17] However, other, more direct measures may be sensitive to endorphin dysfunction in depression and the involvement of endorphins in HPA dysfunction in depression.

In conclusion, the neuroendocrine strategies reported here provide some indirect support for opioid receptor dysfunction in major depression.[1–4, 18, 19] Other neuroendocrine strategies, as well as more direct methods for evaluating endorphin systems in depressed patients need to be pursued.

REFERENCES

1. SNYDER, S. H. 1978. The opiate receptor and morphine-like peptides in the brain. Am. J. Psychiatry 135: 645–652.
2. PICKAR, D., I. EXTEIN, P. W. GOLD, R. SUMMERS, D. NABER & F. K. GOODWIN. (In press.) Endorphins and Affective Illness. In Endorphins and Opiate Agonists in Psychiatric Research: Clinical Implications. N. S. Shah & A. G. Donald, Ed. Plenum Press. New York.
3. GOLD, M. S., A. L. C. POTTASH, D. R. SWEENEY, H. D. KLEBER & D. E. REDMOND. 1979. Rapid opiate detoxification: Clinical evidence of antidepressant and antipanic effects of opiates. Am. J. Psychiatry 136: 982–983.
4. KLINE, N. S., C. H. LI, H. E. LEHMANN, A. LAJTHA, E. LASKI & T. COOPER. 1977. Beta-endorphin induced changes in schizophrenic and depressed patients. Arch. Gen. Psychiatry 43: 1111–1113.
5. TOLIS, G., R. DENT & H. GUYDA. 1978. Opiates, prolactin, and the dopamine receptor. J. Clin. Endocrinol. Metab. 47: 200–203.
6. BOYD, A. E. & S. REICHLIN. 1978. Neural control of prolactin secretion in man. Psychoneuroendocrinology 3: 113–130.
7. VOLAVKA, J., D. CHO., A. MALLYA & J. BAUMAN. 1979. Naloxone increases ACTH and cortisol levels in man. N. Engl. J. Med. 300: 1056–1057.
8. SPITZER, R. L., J. ENDICOTT & E. ROBINS. 1978. Research diagnostic criteria rationale and reliability. Arch. Gen. Psychiatry 35: 773–782.

9. FERLAND, L., K. FUXE, P. ENEROTH, J. A. GUSTAFSSON & P. SKETT. 1977. Effects of methionine enkephalin on prolactin release and catecholamine levels and turnover in the median eminence. Eur. J. Pharmacol. **43:** 89–90.
10. GOLD, M. S., E. E. REDMOND, JR., R. K. DONABEDIAN, F. K. GOODWIN & I. EXTEIN. 1978. Increase in serum prolactin by exogenous and endogenous opiates: Evidence for antidopamine and antipsychotic effects. Am. J. Psychiatry **135:** 1415–1416.
11. EXTEIN, I., F. K. GOODWIN, A. J. LEWY, R. I. SCHOENFELD, L. R. FAKHURI, M. S. GOLD & D. E. REDMOND. 1979. Behavioral and biochemical effects of FK33–824, a parenterally and orally active enkephalin analogue. *In* Endorphins in Mental Health Research. E. Usdin, W. E. Bunney, Jr. & N. S. Kline, Eds. : 279–292. Macmillan Press. London.
12. GOLD, M. S., R. K. DONABEDIAN, M. DILLARD, F. W. SLOBETZ, C. E. RIORDAN & H. D. KLEBER. 1977. Antipsychotic effect of opiate agonists. Lancet (2): 398–399.
13. GRAFFENRIED, B. V., E. D. POZO, J. RAUBICEK, E. KREBS, W. POLDINGER, P. BURMEISTER & L. KERP. 1978. Effects of the synthetic enkephalin analogue FK33–824 in man. Nature **272:** 729–730.
14. HALBREICH, U., L. GRUNHAUS & M. BEN-DAVID. 1979. Twenty-four-hour rhythm of prolactin in depressive patients. Am. J. Psychiatry **36:** 1183–1186.
15. EXTEIN, I., D. PICKAR, M. S. GOLD, P. W. GOLD, A. L. C. POTTASH, D. R. SWEENEY, R. J. ROSS, R. REBARD, D. M. MARTIN & F. K. GOODWIN. 1981. Methadone and morphine in depression. Psychopharmacol. Bull. **17:** 29–33.
16. CARROLL, B. J., M. FEINBERG, J. F. GREDEN, J. TARIKA, A. A. ALBALA, R. F. HASKETT, N. M. JAMES, Z. KRONFOL, M. STEINER, J. B. DE VIGNE & E. YOUNG. 1981. A specific laboratory test for the diagnosis of melancholia. Arch. Gen. Psychiatry **83:** 15–22.
17. GOLD, M. S., A. L. C. POTTASH, I. EXTEIN & H. D. KLEBER. 1980. Anti-endorphin effects of methadone. Lancet (2): 972–973.
18. GOLD, M. S. & R. BYCK. 1978. Endorphins, lithium, and naloxone: Their relationship to pathological and drug-induced manic-euphoric states. *In* The International Challenge of Drug Abuse. R. D. Peterson, Ed. NIDA Research Monograph 19. pp. 192–209. U.S. Govt. Printing Office, Washington, D.C.
19. VEREBEY, K., J. VOLAVKA & D. CLOUET. 1978. Endorphins in psychiatry. Arch. Gen. Psychiatry **35:** 877–888.

THE USE OF ANTIDEPRESSANTS WITH METHADONE IN DEPRESSED MAINTENANCE PATIENTS *

George E. Woody, Charles P. O'Brien, A. Thomas McLellan,
Martin Marcovici, and Bradley D. Evans

*Drug Dependence Treatment Unit
Philadelphia Veterans Administration Medical Center
and Department of Psychiatry
University of Pennsylvania
Philadelphia, Pennsylvania 19104*

BACKGROUND

The motivation for much of the work on the use of tricyclic antidepressants with methadone for the treatment of depressed opiate addicts originates from the self-medication theory. This theory postulates that some proportion of drug-seeking behavior in addicted people originates from a desire to relieve psychological distress via the direct pharmacological action of the abused drug. This theory is best expressed by Wurmser [1] and by Khantzian [2] who provide it with a psychodynamic framework, and who also supply case reports to illustrate how addicted individuals will respond to psychological stress with drug-seeking behavior.

Recent work investigating the psychiatric aspects of opiate addiction has demonstrated that high levels of psychopathology are present in addicts. Rounsaville *et al.* recently completed a large study in which approximately 750 opiate addicts were evaluated psychiatrically using the Schizophrenia and Affective Disorders—Lifetime interview (SADS-L), with both the Diagnostic and Statistical Manual III (DSM-III) and Research Diagnostic Criteria (RDC) diagnoses being made. Of their sample, 85% had experienced a diagnosable psychiatric illness by DSM-III criteria in addition to opiate addiction at some time in their lives. Interestingly, depressive illnesses, and not sociopathy, were the most common psychiatric disorders found. Approximately 30% of those interviewed had a current depressive illness, and approximately 50% had experienced a depressive episode at some time in their lives.[3] Almost identical findings were obtained in studies done using the SADS-L in comparable population samples in Philadelphia [4] and Boston.[5] Next to depression, sociopathy was the most common problem, occurring in approximately 45% of those interviewed when diagnosed using DSM-III criteria, and in 20%–25% when diagnosed using the more stringent RDC criteria. Alcoholism and anxiety disorders were found in 10%–15% of the samples and a large number of less common problems, including schizophrenia, were found in smaller proportions of those interviewed.

These psychiatric illnesses, and especially depression, are problems that would appear to lend themselves to relief via illicit opiate use. Opiates have powerful anxiety-reducing and mood-elevating effects, and thus the high levels

* This work was supported in part by the National Institute of Drug Abuse (Grant 1 RO1 DA01983).

0077–8923/82/0398–0120 $1.75/0 © 1982, NYAS

of depression in this population would appear to make the patients especially vulnerable for acting out urges to obtain the immediate relief that would result from self-medicating by intravenous opiate use.

THE PREVALENCE AND COURSE OF DEPRESSION

We have had a special interest in studying depression, particularly in reference to the role it may play in encouraging self-medication and in contributing to the various disabilities seen in opiate addicts. Several years ago we compared the prevalence of depression found in methadone-maintained addicts with that found in a general population in an attempt to get a clear idea of the prevalence of depression in addicts as compared to the population at large. Although we had no comparison group with similar demographic characteristics, a community survey of depressive illnesses in New Haven, CT done by Weissman and Myers provided a reference point.[6,7] The population they studied represented a cross-section of the community population and included all ethnic, racial, and socioeconomic groups. A systematic sample of 1,095 households was selected in 1967 and one adult (over 18 years old) was interviewed at random in each household in 1969 and again in 1975. Of those interviewed, 31% were in social classes I and II, 10% were non-white, 43% were males, and the average age was approximately 48. Depressive illness was studied using the SADS-L and RDC in 1975: 16% of the 400 males studied by Weissman and Myers in 1967 and 12% of males studied in 1969 reported depressive symptoms on a self-report scale that measures depressive symptoms,[8] and which is similar to the Beck Depression Inventory (BDI). When evaluated by using the SADS-L in 1975, 6.8% of their sample had a current depressive illness and 26.6% either had a current illness or had experienced a past depressive episode. The comparison between depressive illnesses in the community sample and in our addict sample is shown in TABLE 1, which summarizes and highlights the much greater prevalence of depressive illnesses in the addict sample.

TABLE 1

SUMMARY OF PERCENT DEPRESSIVE ILLNESS IN COMMUNITY AND METHADONE SAMPLES
(Current and Past)

	Community Sample (percent) (n = 400)	Addicts on Methadone (percent) (n = 400)
Current		
Major	4.3	17.5
Minor	2.5	17.5
Major & minor	6.8	30.0
Lifetime		
Major	19.9	45.0
Minor	9.2	25.0
Major & minor	26.6	50.0

Rounsaville *et al.* recently focused on the course of depressive illness in methadone-maintained patients and found that most depressions improved within one year. This study showed that the proportion of patients who were depressed at any one time remained fairly constant; however, different individuals were suffering depressive symptoms at different times. In this study, as in those cited above, higher levels of drug use were found in the more symptomatic depressed patients than in those without depression.[9] One possible interpretation of these results is that the depressed patients are self-medicating and using more drugs in an attempt to relieve their symptoms.

Clinical observations indicate that the type of depression seen in addicts is usually of mild to moderate intensity and not the delusional and markedly slowed-down type that is seen commonly on psychiatric inpatient units. It is often precipitated by situational factors, especially loss, and usually responds to interpersonal interactions. It usually has an anxiety component and is more prevalent at intake to a methadone program than it is one or more months after treatment has begun. In one recent study, BDI scores were elevated in about 60% of addicts who applied for methadone treatment, but when those remaining in treatment were examined one month later, only 30% continued to have elevated scores.[10] Part of this improvement probably reflects the suppression of opiate withdrawal symptoms seen at intake by methadone maintenance, as some symptoms of depression and opiate withdrawal are similar. Relief of the acute distress which motivated patients to seek treatment by the counseling and other program services probably accounts for another proportion of this improvement.

TRICYCLIC TREATMENT RESULTS

Several issues related to depressive illness and its relation to drug abuse have interested us, and the one of special interest for this presentation is: Can these depressions be treated successfully with tricyclic antidepressants? To the extent that patients use opiates, stimulants, or other abuseable drugs in response to depressive or other psychological symptoms, it seems reasonable to implement a treatment that would reduce the frequency and intensity of these symptoms and, with it, one additional motive for illicit drug use. With this in mind, we started working with doxepin in an attempt to find a nonabuseable antidepressant that could be an effective antidepressant with this patient group. Doxepin hydrochloride was chosen because it comes in a liquid form and it can be mixed with methadone, thus insuring compliance. Also, it has sedative as well as antidepressant effects, which we felt were important in view of the common occurrence of anxiety in these depressions.

We first studied the efficacy of doxepin in depressed patients who were applying for methadone treatment. After giving informed consent, patients were evaluated using a variety of measures, and then randomly assigned to receive either doxepin or placebo. The process was completed within the first week of methadone treatment. An attempt was made to treat only those patients with depressive symptoms that had been persistent and that appeared to be distinct from withdrawal-induced depressive symptoms. The drop-out rate from this study was high with only 24 of 35 patients who started completing one month of therapy. End point analyses were done on the 24 patients who completed one or more months of treatment and the results are seen in TABLE 2.

TABLE 2

	Pretreatment Mean (N = 35)	Adjusted Mean		F Ratio	Level of Significance
		Doxepin Group (N = 13)	Placebo Group (N = 11)		
Hamilton Depression Rating Scale (Range: 0–62)*					
Sleep disturbance	1.45	0.49	1.04	2.51	n.s.
Somatization	0.95	0.48	0.70	0.97	n.s.
Anxiety/depression	1.00	0.39	0.89	7.67	.025
Retardation/apathy	0.79	0.38	0.44	0.12	n.s.
Anxiety cluster	1.48	0.72	1.09	1.70	n.s.
Total score (Index)	0.87(18.3)	0.34(7.1)	0.72(15.1)	4.25	.06
Beck Depression Inventory (Range: 0–39)*					
Total score	9.10	3.64	10.27	14.41	.005
Zung Depression Scale (Range: 1–4)*					
Retarded depression	2.57	2.34	2.53	0.47	n.s.
Anxious depression	2.01	1.52	2.06	14.84	.005
Total score (Index)	2.28(58)	1.99(50)	2.32(58)	3.52	.10
Patients monthly report					
Craving for heroin (N = 17) (Range: 1–5)*	2.24	0.29	1.30	5.89	.05
Nervousness (N = 10) (Range: 1–5)*	3.00	2.32	3.69	6.54	.025

* Higher scores indicate more pathology.

As seen, the results favor the doxepin over the placebo group. Both groups improved but the doxepin-treated patients did significantly better than those who received placebo, especially on the measures of anxious depressive symptoms. The average dosage used was 100 mg/day. All medication was given at one time along with the daily methadone. Patients were started on 25 or 50 mg of doxepin or its placebo equivalent and were gradually increased to their maintenance dose. No significant sedation or other adverse affects were seen. Patients receiving doxepin reported less use of amphetamines than the placebo group, but these results were not confirmed by urine test reports. There were no differences in methadone dose between the groups.[11]

At about the same time, Kleber *et al.* did a similar study in which they used imipramine hydrochloride, a nonsedating tricyclic. Only patients who had been stabilized on methadone and who were moderately or severely depressed were selected for their study in an attempt to make sure that the diagnosis of depression was not confounded with signs of opiate withdrawal. Before and after treatment measures showed that all patients improved, and that there were no significant differences between the treated and control groups. In each group 22 patients continued for one or more months and the doses used were 150–200 mg/day, given in a single dose with the daily methadone. Thus they found no evidence that imipramine was a useful treatment for the depression seen in addicts. As in our study, the drop-out rate was high, with only about half of those who started completing the 4 month study period.[12]

Currently we are in the process of doing a second study in which we are comparing doxepin, desipramine hydrochloride, and placebo in depressed patients who are stabilized on methadone. A preliminary analysis of pretreatment and one month data on that sample of our subjects who were the most depressed is shown in TABLE 3. The major treatment effect seen in this analysis is that all patients are getting better. There is a suggestion that the doxepin patients are showing more improvement than those receiving either desipramine or placebo, but the difference is not large. There is no suggestion that the desipramine patients are doing better than the placebo group.

Goldstein, McBride, and Westy at the University of Miami have also been doing a similar project in which depressed methadone-maintained addicts are randomly assigned to receive either doxepin or placebo. I spoke to Mr. McBride prior to this meeting and received his permission to mention their results, and they are as follows: They have done preliminary analyses on 44 patients, 22 in each group. Patients were evaluated using the following criteria: Beck, Hamilton Depression, Raskin Covi, POMS, and the SCL-90. Some of these measures were repeated weekly over a period of 12 months. Their preliminary analyses indicate that there is more improvement in those patients receiving doxepin than in the placebo group. The difference in improvement between the groups is not large on any single measure, but it is consistent across all measures and throughout the period of observation. As in the other studies, both the placebo and the drug group improved, but the placebo group took 12–16 weeks to get to the same point that the doxepin group reached within 4 weeks. The variability of measures was less with the doxepin than with the placebo group, also suggesting a medication affect. There were no differences in retention, urine test results, or in methadone dose between the groups. The doses used were approximately 100 mg per day, similar to the other doxepin studies.[13]

TABLE 3

N	Sinequan Intake	Sinequan 4 Weeks 10	Norpramine Intake	Norpramine 4 Weeks 10	Placebo Intake	Placebo 4 Weeks 10	Ancova 4 Weeks
BECK	18	* 12	15	* 8	19	* 13	$p < .06$ Nor.
Hamilton depression	26	** 13	22	* 10	24	** 11	
Hamilton anxiety	21	* 12	19	* 10	21	** 8	$p < .06$ Plac.
Raskin	11	7	10	6	10	6	
COV1	8	6	9	6	8	5	
SCL–90	144	* 130	135	* 110	147	136	$p < .03$ Nor.
Physical symptoms	12	** 1	9	4	10	* 3	$p < .06$ Sin.
Methadone dose	48	* 44	36	38	46	46	
Proportion dirty urines	.96	* .40	.54	.55	.40	.50	$p < .03$ Sin.

* = $p < .05$; ** = $p < .01$.

Conclusions and Discussion

Our conclusions from these data are as follows. There seems to be reasonably good evidence that doxepin is a useful adjunct for the treatment of depressed methadone-maintained addicts. The doxepin appears to work at lower doses than are typically used for the treatment of depression in nonaddicts, suggesting that there may be a potentiation of its antidepressant effect by methadone, or that its antidepressant effect is influenced by its antianxiety effects, and thus the antidepressant effects could be secondary to a reduction in anxiety. The main effect appears to be on reducing the psychiatric symptoms and not on reducing the drug abuse. There is no evidence that the nonsedating antidepressants are useful in this population, as both Kleber's results with imipramine, and our preliminary results with desipramine, do not show any differences favoring drug over placebo.

Programs vary in their philosophy regarding ancillary medicines and their willingness to use them. Some programs have blanket restrictions against the use of any ancillary medicines and others will try a variety of ancillary medicines, provided they do not appear to have a significant abuse potential. If one chooses to use doxepin, it has the singular advantage of being prepared in a liquid form, and thus it can be mixed with the methadone in a single daily dose. It is probably best to start at a very low dose such as 25 or 50 mg and slowly increase to the 75 or 125 mg range over a period of 1–3 weeks depending on clinical response. When dosages are increased slowly in this way, the chances of causing over-sedation or other adverse affects are minimized.

We have used doxepin for 8 years and feel that it has a low abuse potential even in this population. Of course, any drug that is prescribed to drug addicts is subject to abuse, at least in the sense that the patients will test it to see if they can get high. However, the absence of a visible market for doxepin after a long period of time would tend to argue against any significant abuse potential for this drug. This absence of significant abuse is very evident when we compare the situation with doxepin to that seen with diazepam. We have observed marked differences in the level of drug-seeking behavior that patients will exert to get prescriptions for these two substances, with diazepam being the object of considerable drug-seeking behavior and having a street value.[14] Amitriptyline hydrochloride is another sedative tricyclic which also may be helpful in treating the depression seen in addicts. However, there is clear evidence that amitriptyline can be abused and thus, it should probably be avoided with this population.[15]

In summary, the evidence available at this time indicates that doxepin is probably a useful adjunct for treating the depressive illnesses that are seen in addicts. There is no information regarding what type of depression responds best; i.e., major depressive disorder, intermittent depressive disorder, or minor depressive disorder, as the studies done to date have used only the more global measures of symptom severity, rather than the RDC subtypes. These more finely grained treatment studies could be the subject of future work.

Acknowledgments

We are indebted to Beverly Pomerantz and Alicia Bragg for their excellent technical assistance.

REFERENCES

1. WURMSER, L. 1972. Drug abuse: Nemesis of psychiatry. Am. Scholar (Summer): 393–407.
2. KHANTZIAN, E. J., J. E. MACH & A. F. SCHATZBERT. 1974. Heroin use as an attempt to cope: Clinical observations. Am. J. Psychiatry **131:** 160–164.
3. ROUNSAVILLE, B. J., M. M. WEISSMAN, H. D. KLEBER & C. H. WILBER. 1982. The heterogeneity of psychiatric diagnosis in treated opiate addicts. Arch. Gen. Psychiatry. **39**(2): 161–166.
4. WOODY, G. E., C. P. O'BRIEN, A. T. MCLELLAN, L. LUBORSKY & A. T. BECK. 1981. Psychotherapy for opiate addiction, does it add anything to drug counseling? (Presented to NIDA.)
5. TREECE, C. & E. KHANTZIAN. 1981. Psychiatric diagnosis of opiate dependent patients. (Presented to NIDA.)
6. WEISSMAN, M. W. & J. H. MYERS. 1978. Affective disorders in a U.S. urban community. Arch. Gen. Psychiatry **35:** 1304–1311.
7. WEISSMAN, M. W. & J. H. MYERS. 1978. Rates and risks of depressive symptoms in a United States urban community. Acta Psychiatr. Scand. **57:** 219–231.
8. GURIN, G., J. VEROFF & S. FELD. 1960. Americans View Their Mental Health: A Nationwide Interview Study. New York, Basic Books, Inc., New York, N.Y.
9. ROUNSAVILLE, B. J., M. M. WEISSMAN, K. CRITS-CHRISTOPH, C. H. WILBER & H. D. KLEBER. 1982. Diagnosis and symptoms of depression in opiate addicts: Course and relationship to treatment outcome. Arch. Gen. Psychiatry. In press.
10. MINTZ, J., A. T. BECK, G. E. WOODY & C. P. O'BRIEN. 1980. Depression in treated narcotic addicts. Ex-addicts, non-addicts and suicide attempters. Am. J. Drug Alcohol Abuse 7(1).
11. WOODY, G. E., C. P. O'BRIEN & K. RICKELS. 1975. Depression and anxiety in heroin addicts: A placebo-controlled study of doxepin in combination with methadone. Am. J. Psychiatry **132:** 4, 447–450.
12. KLEBER, H., M. WEISSMAN & B. ROUNSAVILLE. 1981. Verbal communication.
13. MCBRIDE, D. 1981. Personal communication.
14. WOODY, G. E., C. P. O'BRIEN & R. GREENSTEIN. 1975. Misuse and abuse of diazepam: An increasingly common medical problem. Int. J. Addictions 10(5): 843–848.
15. STIMMEL, B. 1978. Ann. N.Y. Acad. Sci. **311:** 99–109.

PART IV. THE USE OF EXOGENOUS OPIATES AND OPIATE ANTAGONISTS IN THE TREATMENT OF MENTAL DISEASES: GENERAL DISCUSSION

J. SOLOMON (*State University of New York, Downstate Medical Center, Brooklyn*): I wonder whether Dr. Volavka has any idea about variables that might predict which patients will respond to methadone or other opiates? I mean clinical variables: symptoms, duration of symptoms, family history or course of the illness, for example.

J. V. VOLAVKA (*New York University School of Medicine, New York*): I do not really have any predictive variables. I think that from what we know so far, patients who have episodes of explosive rage would be those who might be the best candidates for methadone treatment.

I was very interested to see Dr. Extein's slide showing the increase in cortisol after naloxone administration. We published similar data in 1979. It is possible that endorphins exert a tonic inhibitory effect on the release of ACTH, probably through the hypothalamus. We published that model in 1980. I think that that model is somewhat similar to the one that he is proposing. I am no longer so sure that this model is true because I have since read many papers describing other effects of naloxone that are not mediated through the opiate receptor at all. So, I am not exactly retracting the model, but I am not enthusiastic about explaining this strictly on the opiate receptor level. As far as the effect on prolactin goes, I would be very much inclined to say that this may be a direct effect on the dopamine receptor. It may be that we do not have to bother with the opiate receptor for an explanation.

QUESTION: Could I just follow that up? I would like to ask Dr. Volavka about dosage effects. The receptor work *in vitro* showed that after very low doses of naloxone it specifically displaced stereospecific isomers of morphine, but, when whole body experiments were done doses of naloxone as large as 20 mg were administered intravenously. What concentrations might occur at the receptors? And won't they start affecting other systems?

VOLAVKA: Well, obviously, I do not know. Avram Goldstein is saying that 10 milligrams is more than sufficient to saturate all the opiate receptors in man. Maybe Dr. Way, or someone else more qualified than I, could comment on this. I certainly think that at the dose level of 20 milligrams it is increasingly difficult to ascribe the whole spectrum of effects of naloxone to action on opiate receptors alone.

E. L. WAY (*University of California School of Medicine, San Francisco*): I would like to comment on Dr. Volavka's views about the negative effects of naloxone. In general I agree, but I would not necessarily give up yet on saying that most of the changes that were examined are not related to the endorphin system. Of course, with any drug, if you give enough, it is going to produce a lot of nonspecific effects; but even 10 milligrams of naloxone may not be enough to saturate all the opiate receptors. We are finding more and more about subtypes of opiate receptors and they have varying degrees of affinity for naloxone.

The other thing that we know is that a common effect of morphine is inhibition of neurotransmitter release. Opioids decrease the release of acetylcholine, of norepinephrine, of dopamine, of serotonin and of substance

P, apparently by a calcium-dependent process. So, presumably, all these systems can be affected very selectively by the endorphin systems and naloxone could still affect the responses of these varied neurotransmitters via the endorphin system.

E. FEIGELSON (*State University of New York, Downstate Medical Center, Brooklyn*): The prolactin effect on major depression is interesting from a number of standpoints, particularly as a possible biological marker in major depression. I wonder if anyone here knows whether it normalized when the depression got better?

D. R. SWEENEY (*Fair Oaks Hospital, Summit, NJ*): I really cannot answer that question specifically, but my best expectation would be that it would. In terms of the other neuroendocrine measurements that we do in depressive disorders, the thyrotoprin-releasing hormone test as well as the dexamethasone suppression test, when a patient recovers, these abnormalities normalize and, in fact, there is some literature to indicate that a failure to normalize is predictive of relapse or of a quicker relapse than occurs in patients who normalize.

I think that all of the neuroendocrine responses that we measure in affective disorder are essentially state variables that will normalize if the patient recovers from the depressive illness.

W. ABSE (*University of Virginia, Charlottesville*): I wanted to make a comment about the patients with organic brain disease, the elderly patients who receive DTO, deodorized tincture of opium. It is very important to watch out for constipation, which can be severe. That is truthfully the greatest problem in the treatment, so I am glad of the chance to mention this since it has not been mentioned before. It can be a very considerable complication. There is one other point that I would like to comment on. Some 20 years ago at the University of North Carolina where I was working, people were interested in some of the opiate effects on elderly people at the psychiatric unit for whom the drug was euphoric. Also, these researchers investigated cheerful, young adults who were being given various drugs and opiates to see their reactions. Healthy, cheerful students who received opiates became depressed after they had had a dose, which was the opposite of what was happening with the older people with impaired nervous systems.

A BIOCHEMICAL AND NEUROPHYSIOLOGICAL COMPARISON OF OPIOIDS AND ANTIPSYCHOTICS

Doris H. Clouet

New York State Division of Substance Abuse Services
Department of Psychiatry
SUNY Downstate Medical Center
Brooklyn, New York 11217

The hypothesis that endogenous opioids play a role in the normal and pathological functioning of the nervous system is supported both by clinical evidence of the efficacy of opioid agonists or antagonists in treating mental illness (described in other papers in this Conference), and by studies indicating a possible relationship between opioid levels in cerebrospinal fluid and psychiatric diagnoses.[1, 2]

Such data are suggestive, but lack critical information concerning the physiological bases for linking endogenous opioids (EO) and behavior. An alternative procedure is inferential; i.e., if certain criteria are met, the inference is strong that there is a relationship between EOs and mental functioning. In this procedure, the neurochemical and neurophysiological effects produced by opioid administration are compared to those produced by drugs known to be effective in treating psychosis, the antipsychotic neuroleptic drugs. If common neurochemical pathways are altered in the same brain neuronal systems in the same direction by both opioids and neuroleptics, then the inference is that similar behavioral responses should be produced.

ENDOGENOUS AND EXOGENOUS OPIOIDS

The discovery of EOs in brain and other nervous tissue was preceded by the discovery of opiate receptors in the central and peripheral nervous systems.[3-5] The localization of opiate receptors in brain areas known to be involved in responses to the administration of narcotic drugs [medulla (respiration), limbic system (mood, stress responses), pain pathways (analgesia), gastrointestinal tract (constipation), and the hypothalamic-hypophyseal system (pituitary trophic hormone effects)] suggested that these tissues were exposed to natural opioids. Hughes and his collaborators identified in the brain two related penta-peptides, methionine- and leucine-enkephalin.[6] A number of endocrinologists were able to show that β-lipotropin, already recognized as a pituitary hormone, contained the Met-enkephalin sequence of five amino acids, and that β-LPH was hydrolyzed to an active opioid, β-endorphin.[7-9]

It soon became apparent that there were at least two chemical families of EOs of different origin and with different functions, although all peptides contained the sequence Try-Gly-Gly-Phe-X at their N-terminals. The endorphin family includes the large precursor, pro-opiocortin,[10] β-LPH, and β-endorphin. The second chemical family of EOs is the enkephalin family. Both Met-

0077-8923/82/0398-0130 $1.75/0 © 1982, NYAS

enkephalin and Leu-enkephalin are derived from a large peptide precursor containing both sequences,[11] with the generation of intermediates by processing.[12] Hexa- and hepta-peptides with one or two basic amino acids attached to the carboxyl end of enkephalin, and a heptapeptide: Met-enkephalin·Arg·Phe, seem to be naturally occurring intermediates.[13]

Peptides from each family seem to act both as neurotransmitters and as neurohormones. The pentapeptide enkephalins are localized in nerve terminals and are released from neurons upon stimulation. They have a short half-life, and thus act as neurotransmitters. Leu- and Met-enkephalins and related small peptides are released from the adrenal medulla into blood, thus acting in this situation as neurohormones.[14] Beta-endorphin is released from the pituitary gland into blood,[15] thus acting hormonally. Beta-endorphin may also act as a neurotransmitter in a discrete pathway in brain.[16] Both endorphins and enkephalins produce biochemical and pharmacological responses, including tolerance, dependence, and abstinence, similar to those produced by narcotic analgesic drugs when the EOs are administered to man or animals.[17, 18] The pharmacology of narcotic analgesic drugs such as morphine, methadone, heroin, and etorphine have been described many times.[19, 20] The EOs plus the narcotic drugs are members of the class "opioids."

There are multiple types of opioid binding sites defined by the relative affinities for various opioid ligands. Both the μ site which binds benzomorphan drugs preferentially and the δ site have specific ligands that have little affinity for any other site: d-Ala[2], mePhe[4], Gly-OH[5] enkephalin and d-Ala[2], d-Leu[5] enkephalin, respectively.[21] The κ binding site does not have a specific ligand, but can be measured by ethylketazocine binding in the presence of μ and δ ligands.[21] The σ binding site binds N-allylnorcyclazocine specifically in the presence of cyclazocine, and can be displaced by phencyclidine.[22] Enkephalins have the greatest affinity for the δ receptor, while β-endorphin binds to μ and δ sites. Brain areas and peripheral nervous tissue have distinct distribution patterns of various binding sites,[23] although interconversion of μ and δ sites has been reported.[24]

Neuroleptic Drugs

There are many chemical families of neuroleptic drugs, among them: phenothiazines (chlorpromazine), butyrophenones (haloperidol), and benzamides (sulpiride). These drugs have structural features in common with dopamine (DA) and have the property of blocking DA receptors.[25] These drugs also have effects on other neurotransmittory systems, either by a direct action (receptor binding) or by indirect mechanisms. In addition to DA receptor binding, antipsychotic drugs also bind to α_2-noradrenergic receptors and to muscarinic receptors (TABLE 1). The extrapyramidal effects of neuroleptics have been related to low affinity for the muscarinic receptor.[27]

The multiplicity of DA receptors in the central nervous system has been defined by the relative affinities of DA, its agonists, and antagonists.[28] Only one DA receptor is coupled to adenylate cyclase (the D_1 receptor) and is localized on membranes of neurons postsynaptic to DA neurons. The D_2 receptor is more sensitive to neuroleptics than to DA. The behavioral effects of DA antagonists correlate with their affinities to the D_2 site. Some of the D_3 sites are presynaptic, and are probably autoreceptors.[24] The D_2 receptors are

TABLE 1

RECEPTOR BINDING AFFINITIES AND BEHAVIORAL EFFECTS OF SOME NEUROLEPTICS *

Drug	Dopaminergic		α_2 Noradrenergic		ACh-Muscarinic	
	K_1	Anti-psychotic	K_1	Seda-tive	K_1	Extra-pyramidal
Clozepine	120	+	17	+	0.3	+
Thoridazine	15	+ +	5.4	+ + +	1.5	+ +
Chlorpromazine	10	+ + + +	5.2	+ + +	10	+ + +
Haloperidol	1.4	+ + + +	12	+	500	+ + + + +
Fluphenazine	0.9	+ + + + +	10	+	125	+ + + +

* The affinity constants (K_1) are nM. The behavioral effects are rated + to + + + + + for increasing responses.

related to schizophrenia both by neuroleptic binding affinities and by the elevation of D_2 densities in the brains of schizophrenics.[28]

ELECTROPHYSIOLOGICAL COMPARISON

The most common response of neurons to the application of opioids topically or systemically is a naloxone-sensitive inhibition of neuronal activity.[28] This inhibition has been found in cortex, hypothalamus, caudate nucleus and other limbic areas, sympathetic ganglia, and spinal cord.[28] However, iontophoresis of opioids onto some neurons produces a naloxone-sensitive excitation. Pyramidal cells in the hippocampus exhibit this response.[29] The excitation seems to be produced by the inhibition of inhibitory synaptic potentials produced by interneurons, i.e., by disinhibition.[29] The DA neurons in the zona compacta of the substantia nigra that have axons extending to terminals in the striatum also respond to opioids by a naloxone-sensitive excitation.[30] This inhibition is also due to disinhibition, produced in this case by inhibition of γ-aminobutyric acid (GABA) inhibitory neurons that impinge on the DA cell bodies in the substantia nigra.[30] The mechanism by which opioids depress impulse transport is by increasing the duration of the after-hyperpolarization of the presynaptic cell increasing the period in which calcium enters the cell, thus preventing the neuron from reducing its free intracellular calcium concentration.[31] This effect is not limited to DA neurons. Cholinergic,[32] glutaminergic,[29] and noadrenergic[33] neurons are also depressed by opioids. Tolerance develops in most of these effects on chronic opioid use.

Neuroleptic drugs impair DA neurotransmission by blocking postsynaptic D_2 receptors,[34] and, at much higher concentrations, by acting at presynaptic DA autoreceptors to stimulate DA release.[35] DA produces a prolonged inhibitory postsynaptic potential that is blocked by neuroleptics.[34] Chronic treatment with neuroleptics produces a DA supersensitivity that includes supersensitive responses of caudate neurons to iontophoretically applied DA.[36] This supersensitivity is accompanied by an increase in the number of D_2 receptors.[37]

Thus, there is electrophysiological evidence that neuroleptics and opioids act on the nigrostriatal DA system to block impulse transmission (FIGURE 1).

Opioid effects are inhibited by narcotic antagonists and neuroleptic effects are reversed by DA agonists such as apomorphine.[3] The mechanisms of inhibition and the sites of action at the synapse, however, are different.

A Neurochemical Comparison

The administration of morphine and other opioids to laboratory animals increases the rate of DA biosynthesis in the striatum.[39, 40] DA stimulation of adenylate cyclase in ruptured synaptosomes from rat striatum is not inhibited by the addition of morphine or levorphanol.[41] In the same preparation, haloperidol produces an inhibition of DA-stimulated adenylate cyclase activity.[41] The administration of β-endorphin [42] or enkephalin [43] has the same effect on the rate of DA biosynthesis in the striatum. The administration of neuroleptics also stimulates DA metabolism in the nigrostriatal pathway.[44] Upon chronic administration of either class of drug, tolerance develops both to the increased rate of DA turnover and to the inhibition of transmission.[41, 44] The postsynaptic DA receptor becomes supersensitive in tolerant animals.[41, 45]

In the limbic DA system, opioids and neuroleptics also enhance the turnover of DA.[46] In both the nigrostriatal pathway and in the nucleus accumbens septi, the stimulation of DA neurons is due to a regulatory feedback activity. GABA neurons that control a slow rate of spontaneous firing of DA neurons in the substantia nigra are affected by muscarinic neurons in the striatum. Neuroleptics, opiates, and endorphins increase the turnover of acetylcholine in the striatum and also in limbic areas [47, 48] by blocking the postsynaptic DA receptor. Since acetylcholine is inhibitory to GABA neurons, the excitation of muscarinic receptors decreases GABA release on DA cell bodies in the substantia nigra, thus diminishing the inhibition of DA firing. A similar feedback loop seems to operate in the nucleus accumbens septi.

In another DA pathway, the pathway in which the hypothalamic A-12 neurons impinge on releasing-factor neurons, both neuroleptics [49] and opioids [50]

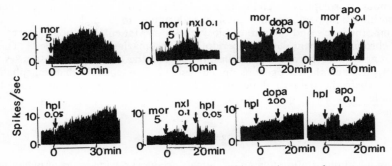

FIGURE 1. The effect of morphine and haloperidol on the rate of spontaneous firing of nigrostriatal dopamine neurons. The integrated record of firing rate expressed as spikes/sec is shown on the ordinates. Morphine at a dose of 5 mg/kg or haloperidol at a dose of 0.05 mg/kg were injected subcutaneously. The effects of the opioid antagonist, naloxone at a dose of 0.1 mg/kg is shown. The effect of dopamine agonists, therefore haloperidol antagonists, dopa and apomorphine is shown for doses of 200 mg/kg and 0.1 mg/kg, respectively.

antagonize the inhibition produced by DA. Since there is no feedback loop in this system, DA neurons are inhibited. Both classes of drugs, therefore, enhance the release of pituitary trophic hormones that are under DA inhibitory control: prolactin and growth hormone and, possibly, ACTH. Thus, prolactin release from the anterior pituitary is increased by the administration of neuroleptics, opiates,[51] β-endorphin, and Met-enkephalin.[52]

In the locus coeruleus, noradrenergic agonists including norepinephrine and clonidine act to decrease neuronal firing.[53] Some neuroleptics are α_2 receptor antagonists (TABLE 1) and increase the firing rate of these neurons, while opiates and β-endorphin act to decrease the firing rate in the same cells.[54] Aside from the minor activity of some neuroleptics at muscarinic and α_2-adrenergic sites, the action of antipsychotic drugs is exclusively on DA neurotransmission. As mentioned earlier, opioids act on DA, NE, serotonergic, muscarinic, and glutaminergic neurons.

From the biochemical data we conclude that neuroleptics produce very similar effects on DA systems (nigral, limbic, and hypothalamic neurons). They also act similarly in associated systems. These similarities persist during chronic drug use, when tolerance develops. Any behavioral response mediated by DA neuronal pathways may be produced by either class of drugs.

Since exogenously applied opioids are presumed to act on receptors for endogenous opioids, do endogenous opioids produce the same biochemical effects as exogenous opioids? Most evidence suggest the answer to this question is: "Yes, to a degree." Endogenous opioids are present in nervous tissue in picogram amounts. Presumably these levels are controlled by mechanisms acting on the rates of biosynthesis and catabolism. The active enkephalins have a very short halflife, so that both peptide availability and the short duration of action limit its activity. Beta-endorphin has a longer halflife in circulating blood, but its level is well below that required for activity when applied exogenously. One might predict that the responses to exogenous and endogenous opioids is qualitatively similar, but quantitatively very different.

The fact that there are endogenous opioids, and that there are no endogenous neuroleptics, makes another biochemical relationship possible: the effect of exogenous neuroleptics on endogenous opioids. In both man and animals, daily haloperidol treatment elevates plasma endorphins to a high level.[55] In rat striatum, the levels and the rate of biosynthesis of Met-enkephalin are increased after chronic treatment with haloperidol, chlorpromazine, or pimozide.[56] These data suggest that there is a relationship between the biochemical responses to neuroleptics and the endogenous opioid system. It is possible that enkephalins act to repair the damage done at the DA synapse by postsynaptic receptor blockade.

BEHAVIORAL COMPARISON

Opioid administration to man or animals produces a wide range of behavioral and autonomic responses including: changes in pain perception, motor behavior, and mood, and reinforcement of opioid-seeking behavior, as well as those due to pituitary hormones and autonomic changes in respiration, temperature control, and rate of blood flow.[57] Subjective effects in man include: a feeling of well being, euphoria, relaxation, mental clouding, and, on intravenous injection, a "rush." [58] Tolerance to some of these effects occurs on chronic opiate use. The suggestion has been made that opiate addicts use opiates as a form of self-medication for mental disorders,[59] seeking effects such as tranquillization, reduction of rage and aggression, reduction of paranoia and feelings of inadequacy, and a reduction of aggression and anxiety.[58] Most brain areas have been involved in these effects. The brain "reward" system has been considered a pleasure pathway, and has been localized in man and animals by localizing the pathways for self-electrostimulation.[64] By lesioning brain centers and measuring the effect on rates of self-stimulation, the reward pathway has been traced from the frontal cortex, through the caudate nucleus and the medial forebrain bundle to the ventral midbrain (hypothalamus and thalamus), the ventral tegmentum, and the substantia nigra.[65] These are all DA pathways. In addition, another reward pathway starts at the enterorhinal cortex and passes through the hippocampus-thalamus to the locus coeruleus.[64] This is an NE pathway that is primarily involved in memory but is also related to self-stimulation.[64] Hypothalamic self-stimulation is suppressed by morphine and chlorpromazine at doses at which alertness and motor coordination are retained.[65] These data can be interpreted in two ways: either the drugs produce enough euphoria that hypothalamic self-stimulation is no longer rewarding, or, the drugs reduce pleasure-seeking behavior at doses that do not decrease their physical appearance. Another form of pleasure-seeking, opiate self-administration, seems to involve the same DA pathways, since lesions in the cortical-caudate-nigra pathway and in the cortical-hippocampus pathway decreases morphine reinforcing activity.[66]

Neuroleptic administration to man produces antipsychotic effects ranging from reduction of agitation, ideas of persecution, irritability, indifference to environment, and so on.[60] Since the antipsychotic effects are due to antagonism at DA receptors, the sites of action in brain of these drugs is limited to DA pathways, which are, however, the major components of the reward pathway.[60] The antipsychotic effects of neuroleptics in man are not apparent after the first dose, and increase with the duration of treatment. The effects seem to be related to the supersensitivity of DA receptors previously described. Since the mesolimbic and mesocortical DA systems do not develop tolerance to the same degree as the nigrostriatal DA pathway, some of the effects that do not diminish with continuing treatment may be ascribed to these areas.[60]

Both neuroleptics and opioids act on the hypothalamic–hypophyseal system to enhance or decrease the release of pituitary hormones under DA regulation. Many peptide hormones from the hypothalamus or pituitary exert a direct effect on the central nervous system in addition to their neuroendocrine effects. For example: ACTH and its 4–10 segment act on midbrain limbic structures to improve mental performance by increasing the attention span.[63] Thyrotropin-releasing-hormone potentiates DOPA-induced hyperactivity and antagonizes the sedative effects of depressants, thus behaving like an antidepressant drug.[62]

There is a temporal disassociation between the therapeutic effects of neuroleptics and their effect on prolactin release or other biochemical responses.[63] It is possible that neuroendocrine defects play inherent or secondary roles in mental illnesses, and that these defects are ameliorated by chronic neuroleptic treatment. It is well known that a subpopulation of depressed patients have a hypersecretion of cortisol from the adrenal gland, a phenomenon not due to stress or therapeutics.[67] A pituitary-adrenal disinhibition has been suggested to be an intrinsic part of the depressed state. This disinhibition is detected by a dexamethasone suppression test in which the subpopulation escapes suppression in less than 24 hours.[68] Although the involvement of hypothalamic or hypophyseal endorphins in this condition has not been investigated as yet, such an involvement would not be surprising.

Another relationship between opioids and neuroleptics is introduced by the finding that a derivatve of γ-endorphin with the N-terminal tyrosine missing [(des Tyr) γ-endorphin (DTγE)] has neuroleptic-like activity.[69] In both open and double-blind trials, the daily intramuscular injection of DTγE improved psychotic symptoms in a few days. Since all opioid activity disappears when the N-terminal Tyr is removed, this activity of DTγE cannot be considered opiate-like. The phenomenon may be an example of a hypothetical sequence of events that has been suggested both for pro-opiocortin and for a "large" enkephalin precursor: that successive processing of the big peptide by proteolytic action produces peptides of intermediate lengths with varying pharmacological activities that regulate or modify a sequence of biological events.

Another group of behaviors associated with endorphins is the appetitive behaviors. In genetically obese mice or rats, eating misbehavior is abolished by small doses of naloxone.[71] The levels of β-endorphin are elevated over normal in both species in the pituitary but not in the hypothalamus.[71] However, the high levels of endorphin in the pituitaries of obese mice emerge at 4–6 months of age, while obesity develops at 3 months, suggesting that the high levels of endorphins are a consequence of the obesity.[72] Another behavior, associated with copulation, is decreased by the intraventricular injection of β-endorphin.[73]

An often neglected facet of opioid action, their effects on autonomic functions, may also contribute to antipsychotic activity. In acute schizophrenia, patients exhibit abnormal functioning of the autonomic nervous system: higher basic heart rate, low responsivity to stimuli, low arousal response to stress, and slow habituation.[69] Chronic unmedicated schizophrenics also show these abnormalities. Opioid antagonists would seem to offer the best chance of returning these systems to normal.

The results of behavioral studies suggest that some human behavior can be associated with DA pathways that, in animals, are usually associated with motor activity or analgesia. Pleasure pathways demonstrated by self-administration of opioids in animals have been shown to occur via the same DA areas (nucleus accumbens septi, substantia nigra, etc.) involved in analgesia and locomotion.[74] Thus, the animal equivalent of euphoria may be ascribed to these DA neuronal pathways. Since both opioids and neuroleptics alter DA neurotransmission to some extent, if a condition is ameliorated by neuroleptics, it should respond to at least one class of opioids. A caveat must be added: that opioids produce other effects not associated with DA neurotransmission that may not be beneficial to the mental condition.

Conclusions

The preponderance of evidence from electrophysiological, neurochemical, and behavioral studies supports the hypothesis, or at least, is not incompatible with the hypothesis, that opioids and neuroleptics are both useful in treating psychoses, since both classes of drugs produce similar responses in the various DA neuronal pathways in the central nervous system. Because these pathways comprise the major part of the pleasure, or reward, pathway system, both classes of drugs should produce behavioral effects. However, since opioids have additional actions in other neuronal pathways in the central and peripheral nervous systems, it is possible that an adverse or antitherapeutic response to opioids could limit the usefulness of opioids in treating mental illness.

The hypothesis that endogenous opioids are involved in mental illness gains a degree of support from evidence that exogenous opioids can improve psychotic symptoms. It also gains support from the biological evidence that neuroleptics and exogenous opioids act as the same neuronal site, the DA synapse, to suppress neurotransmission through the synapse, albeit through different mechanisms. The present data are not strong enough to force the conclusion that endogenous opioids act either as causal factors or as ameliorating factors in schizophrenia or other mental illnesses.

REFERENCES

1. RIMON, R., L. TERENIUS & R. KAMPMAN. 1980. Arch. Psychiatr. Scand. **61:** 395.
2. TERENIUS, L., A. WAHLSTRÖM & H. ÅGREN. 1977. Psychopharmacology **54:** 31–33.
3. TERENIUS, L. 1973. Acta Pharmacol. Toxicol. **32:** 317–320.
4. PERT, C. B. & S. H. SNYDER. 1973. Science **179:** 1011–1014.
5. SIMON, E. J., J. M. HILLER & I. EDELMAN. 1973. Proc. Natl. Acad. Sci. USA **70:** 1947–1949.
6. HUGHES, J., T. W. SMITH, H. W. KOSTERLITZ, L. B. FOTHERGILL, B. A. MORGAN & H. R. MORRIS. 1975. Nature **258:** 577–580.
7. LI, C. H. & D. CHUNG. 1976. Proc. Natl. Acad. Sci. USA **73:** 1145–1148.
8. LING, N., R. BURGUS & R. GUILLEMIN. 1976. Proc. Natl. Acad. Sci. USA **73:** 3942–3946.
9. BRADBURY, A. F., W. F. FELDBERG, D. G. SMYTH & C. R. SNELL. 1976. *In* Opiates and Endogenous Opioid Peptides. H. W. Kosterlitz, Ed.: 9–18. North-Holland. Amsterdam.
10. EIPPER, B. A., R. E. MAINS & D. GUENZI. 1976. J. Biol. Chem. **251:** 4121–4126.
11. STERN, A. S., R. V. LEWIS, S. KIMURA, J. ROSSIER, L. D. GERBERT, L. BRINK, S. STEIN & S. UDENFRIEND. 1979. Proc. Natl. Acad. Sci. USA **76:** 6680–6683.
12. STERN, A. J., B. N. JONES, J. E. SHIVELY, S. STEIN & S. UDENFRIEND. 1981. Proc. Natl. Acad. Sci. USA **78:** 1962–1966.
13. HEXUM, T. D., H.-Y. T. YANG & E. COSTA. 1980. Life Sci. **27:** 1211–1216.
14. LIVETT, B. G., D. M. DEAN, L. E. WHELAN, S. UDENFRIEND & J. ROSSIER. 1981. Nature **289:** 317–319.
15. TESCHEMACHER, H., T. BREIDENBACH, A. KONIG, M. LUCKHARDT & S. DAVIES-OSTERKAMP. 1979. *In* Exogenous and Endogenous Opioid Agonists and Antagonists. E. L. Way, Ed.: 307–308. Pergamon Press. New York.
16. BLOOM, F. E., E. BATTENBERG, J. ROSSIER, N. LING & R. GUILLEMIN. 1978. Proc. Natl. Acad. Sci. USA **75:** 1591–1595.
17. LOH, H. H., L. F. TSENG, E. WEI & C. H. LI. 1976. Proc. Natl. Acad. Sci. USA **73:** 2895–2898.
18. CATLIN, D. H., K. K. HUI, H. H. LOH & C. H. LI. 1978. Adv. Biochem. Psychopharmacol. **18:** 341–350.
19. JAFFE, J. & W. R. MARTIN. 1975. *In* Pharmacological Basis of Therapeutics. L. S. Goodman & A. Gilman, Ed. : 273–275. Macmillan Press. New York.
20. CLOUET, D. H., ED. 1971. Narcotic Drugs: Biochemical Pharmacology. Plenum Press. New York.
21. PATERSON, S. J., J. MAGNAN, A. TAVANI & H. W. KOSTERLITZ. 1981. *In* Advances in Exogenous and Endogenous Opioids. H. Takagi, Ed.: 13. Kodansha Ltd. Tokyo.
22. ZUKIN, S. R., A. MARGOLIS & R. S. ZUKIN. 1981. *In* Advances in Exogenous and Endogenous Opioids. T. Takagi, Ed. Kodansha Ltd. Tokyo.

23. QUIRION, R., R. P. HAMMER, M. HERKENHAM & C. B. PERT. 1981. Proc. Natl. Acad. Sci. USA **78:** 5881–5885.
24. BOWEN, W. D., S. GENTLEMAN, M. HERKENHAM & C. B. PERT. 1981. Proc. Natl. Acad. Sci. USA **78:** 4818–4822.
25. BARTHOLINI, G. 1981. *In* Handbook of Biological Psychiatry, Part IV. H. M. van Praag, Ed.: 767–804. Marcel Dekker, Inc. New York.
26. SNYDER, S. H., D. GREENBERG & H. YAMAMURA. 1974. Arch. Gen. Psychiatry **31:** 58–61.
27. BARTHOLINI, G., H. STADLER & K. G. LLOYD. 1975. *In* Cholinergic Mechanisms. P. Waser, Ed.: 411–418. Raven Press. New York.
28. SEEMAN, P. 1981. Pharmacol. Rev. **32:** 229–313.
28a. BRADLEY, P. B., R. J. GAYTON & L. A. LAMBERT. 1978. *In* Centrally Acting Peptides. J. Hughes, Ed.: 215–229. Macmillan Press. London.
29. SIGGINS, G. R. & W. ZEIGLGANSBERGER. 1981. Proc. Natl. Acad. Sci. USA **78:** 5235–5239.
30. IWATSUBO, K. & D. H. CLOUET. 1977. J. Pharmacol. Exp. Ther. **202:** 429–436.
31. MORITA, K. & R. A. NORTH. 1981. *In* Advances in Endogenous and Exogenous Opioids. H. Takagi, Ed.: 43. Kodansha Ltd. Tokyo.
32. KONISHI, S. 1979. Nature **282:** 515–517.
33. KORF, J., B. S. BUNNEY & G. K. AGHAJANIAN. 1974. Europ. J. Pharmacol. **25:** 165–169.
43. SEEMAN, P. 1977. Biochem. Pharmacol. **26:** 1741–1748.
35. MILLER, J. C. & A. J. FRIEDHOFF. 1979. Biochem. Pharmacol. **28:** 688–690.
36. SKIRBOLL, L. R. & B. S. BUNNEY. 1979. Life Sci. **25:** 1419–1434.
37. MULLER, P. & P. SEEMAN. 1977. Life Sci. **20:** 1951–1958.
38. CLOUET, D. H., G. J. GOLD & K. IWATSUBO. 1975. Br. J. Pharmacol. **54:** 541–548.
39. CLOUET, D. H. & M. RATNER. 1970. Science **168:** 854–855.
40. SESAME, H. A., J. PEREZ-CRUET, G. DICHIARA, A. TAGLIAMONTE, P. TAGLIAMONTE & G. L. GESSA. 1972. J. Neurochem. **19:** 1953–1957.
41. IWATSUBO, K. & D. H. CLOUET. 1975. Biochem. Pharmacol. **24:** 1499–1503.
42. VAN LOON, G. R. & C. KIM. 1978. Life Sci. **23:** 961–966.
43. FERLAND, L., K. FUXE, P. ENEROTH, J. A. GUSTAFSSON & P. SKETT. 1977. Europ. J. Pharmacol. **46:** 89–90.
44. ANDEN, N. E. 1972. J. Pharm. Pharmacol. **24:** 905–911.
45. SCHWARTZ, J. C., J. COSTENTIN & M. P. MARTRES. 1978. Neuropharmacol. **17:** 665–668.
46. WESTERLINK, B. H. C. & J. KORF. 1975. Eur. J. Pharmacol. **33:** 31–37.
47. RACAGNI, G., D. L. CHENEY, G. ZSILA & E. COSTA. 1975. Neuropharmacology **15:** 723–731.
48. MORONI, P., D. L. CHENEY & E. COSTA. 1975. Neuropharmacology **17:** 191–198.
49. RUBIN, R. T. & S. E. HAYS. 1979. *In* Catecholamines-Basic and Clinical Frontiers. E. Usdin, Ed.: 1890–1892. Pergamon Press. Oxford, England.
50. DEYO, S. N., R. M. SWIFT, R. J. MILLER & V. S. FANG. 1980. Endocrinology **106:** 1469–1474.
51. MEITES, J., J. F. BRUNI, D. A. VAN VUGT & A. F. SMITH. 1979. Life Sci. **24:** 1325–1329.
52. DUPONT, A., L. CUSAN, M. GARON, F. LABRIE & C. H. LI. 1977. Proc. Natl. Acad. Sci. USA **74:** 358–361.
53. CEDARBAUM, J. M. & G. K. AGHAJANIAN. 1978. Life Sci. **23:** 383–387.
54. AGHAJANIAN, G. K. 1978. Nature **276:** 5684–5691.
55. HOLLT. Personal communication.
56. HONG, J. S., H-Y. T. YANG, J. C. GILLIN, A. M. DIGIULIO, W. FRATTA & E. COSTA. 1979. Brain Res. **160:** 192–195.
57. JAFFE, J. H. & D. H. CLOUET. 1981. *In* Handbook and Biological Psychiatry. Part IV. H. M. van Praag, Ed.: 278–308. Marcel Dekker, Inc. New York.

58. VEREBEY, K., J. VOLAVKA & D. H. CLOUET. 1978. Arch. Gen. Psychiatry **35:** 877–888.
59. KHANTZIAN, E. J., J. E. MACK & A. F. SCHATZBERG. 1974. Am. J. Psychiatry **131:** 160–164.
60. CROW, T. J. 1981. *In* Handbook of Biological Psychiatry. Part IV. H. M. van Praag, Ed.: 3–80. Marcel Dekker, Inc., New York.
61. RIGTER, H. & H. VANRIEZEN. 1981. *In* Handbook of Biological Psychiatry. Part IV.: 469–510. Marcel Dekker, Inc., New York.
62. PLOTNIKOFF, N. P., A. J. PRANGE, G. R. BREESE, M. S. ANDERSON & I. C. WILSON. 1972. Science **178:** 417–418.
63. MELTZER, H. Y. & V. S. FANG. 1976. Arch. Gen. Psychiatry **33:** 279–286.
64. ROUTTENBERG, A. 1979. Fed. Proc. **83:** 2446–2453.
65. OLDS, M. E. 1976. Neuropharmacol. **15:** 117–131.
66. GLICK, S. D. & R. D. COX. 1978. Psychopharmacology **57:** 283–288.
67. BROWN, W. A. & C. B. QUALLS. 1981. Psychiatr. Res. **4:** 115–128.
68. CARROLL, B. J. 1972. *In* Depressive Illness: Some Research Studies. B. Davis, B. J. Carroll & R. W. Mowbray, Ed.: 87–104. C. C Thomas. Springfield, IL.
69. VERHOEVEN, W. M. A., H. M. VAN PRAAG, J. M. VANREE & D. DEWIED. 1979. Arch. Gen. Psychiatry **36:** 294–298.
70. ZAHN, T. P., W. T. CARPENTER & T. H. MCGLASHAN. 1981. Arch. Gen. Psychiatry **38:** 251–258.
71. MARGULES, D. L., B. MOISSET, M. J. LEWIS, H. SHIBUYA & C. B. PERT. 1978. Science **202:** 988–991.
72. ROSSIER, J., J. ROGERS, T. SHIBASAKI, R. GUILLEMIN & F. E. BLOOM. 1979. Proc. Natl. Acad. Sci. USA **76:** 2077–2080.
73. MEYERSON, B. J. & L. TERENIUS. 1977. Eur. J. Pharmacol. **42:** 191–192.
74. BELLUZZI, J. D. & L. STEIN. 1977. Nature **266:** 556–558.

ANTIMANIC, ANTIDEPRESSANT, AND ANTIPANIC EFFECTS OF OPIATES: CLINICAL, NEUROANATOMICAL, AND BIOCHEMICAL EVIDENCE

Mark S. Gold,*† A. Carter Pottash,*†
Donald Sweeney,* David Martin,† and Irl Extein *

*Fair Oaks Hospital
Summit, New Jersey 07901
† Psychiatric Diagnostic Laboratories of America
Summit, New Jersey 07901

Preclinical biochemical and behavioral studies [1, 2] have suggested the endogenous opioid peptides, endorphins, and exogenous agonists may have antipsychotic, antimanic, antipanic, and antidepressant effects.[3-5] At least four strategies have been used in studying the possible role of endorphins in humans. First is the use of narcotic antagonists (e.g., naloxone) that displace morphine and endogenous opioid-like compounds from opiate receptors. Narcotic antagonists have been used in efforts to treat psychiatric illnesses such as schizophrenia and mania. Second, studies have been conducted and are underway to administer β-endorphin to humans and then to study the behavioral and biochemical changes that are produced. Third, assays have been developed for β-endorphin in urine, plasma, and cerebrospinal fluid to study basal levels in psychiatric patients and the effects of pain, stress, diurnal variation, and activity on β-endorphin activity. Finally, investigators have stimulated the release of β-endorphin by pain, stress, and electrodes implanted in those areas of the brain rich in opiate receptors.

A great deal of effort in the past 5 years relates to the synthesis, degradation, and mapping of opiate receptors, and the relationship of endorphins to other neurotransmitter systems. However, while endorphins have anatomical distribution suggesting possible involvement in psychiatric illnesses, they have not been systematically studied or administered to patients in a double-blind placebo-controlled design to test the hypothesis that opiate agonists have antipsychotic and antidepressant effects. Therefore the physiologic roles of the various endorphins as neurotransmitters have yet to be clearly defined. While we have much to learn about endorphins in psychiatry, the possible implications for clinical medicine seem great because of the extensive effects of narcotic analgesics on behavior and physiology. Could changes in endorphins be associated with psychiatric illnesses? Could specific alterations in endorphin function produce any of the symptoms of psychiatric illness? Could opiate addicts have preexisting opioid system deficits or deficiencies secondary to opiate abuse? Is methadone or other exogenous opiates sufficiently endorphinomimetic to be used in clinical research trials in psychiatry?

In the past, morphine was extensively used in treating manic and other psychoses.[3] Comfort [7] has stated that morphine "can claim to be regarded as the first specific antipsychotic to be subjected to experimentation." Although others

140

0077–8923/82/0398–0140 $1.75/0 © 1982, NYAS

have suggested antipsychotic effects of opiate analgesics,[4] there have been no clinical trials of opiates in the era of modern pharmacology. This is due to the fear of addiction and presence of effective nonaddicting antipsychotics and lithium. Opiates have anxiolytic effects which relate to abuse by musicians and performers. We have presented phenomenological and behavioral data which has demonstrated marked similarities between human opiate withdrawal and naturally occurring panic states.[9–11] We have suggested that this may reflect a common central noradrenergic (NE) hyperactivity.[12, 13] This locus coeruleus (LC) hyperactivity hypothesis is also supported by our primate studies which demonstrated striking behavioral similarities between opiate withdrawal, electrical stimulation of the LC, pharmacological activation of the central noradrenergic system by piperoxane or yohimbine, and reversal of these anxiety-panic states with clonidine, morphine, or endorphins.[14–17] These data suggested that naturally occurring panic states might result from a functional deficit in endorphin-mediated inhibition of ascending NE activity.[18–21] Opiates (e.g., heroin and methadone) would be expected to provide a self-regulated treatment for this state, which would only manifest itself upon discontinuation of chronic opiate administration.[5] This would be a possible fifth strategy for investigating endorphin function in man. Finally, addicts might have a pre-existing or drug-induced endorphin abnormality whereas panic-anxiety patients might have a naturally occurring endorphin-LC dysfunction, which could be identified by diagnostic studies of methadone programs and post-detoxification follow-up studies.[5, 9, 22–25]

If endorphins have antidepressant effects then it might be expected that methadone programs would have an over representation of patients with major depression [5, 9] and methadone detoxification might be associated with the re-emergence of major depressive syndromes.[9] We have also studied the hypothesis that endorphin abnormalities might be present in mania and depression using neuroendocrine challenge paradigms. This hypothesis has been evaluated by a number of research groups.[26–29]

We have additional clinical evidence for the antipsychotic, antidepressant, and antipanic effects of opiate agonists as a result of our experience with the previously described procedure for rapid opiate detoxification with clonidine.[30] We have treated 200 individuals addicted to methadone, heroin, or synthetic opiates by discontinuing opiates and administering clonidine to suppress the signs and symptoms of opiate withdrawal.[30, 31] Clonidine markedly reduces opiate withdrawal symptoms and enables addicts who have been maintained for years on 100 mg/day of methadone or less to discontinue use of opiates and clonidine in fewer than 14 days without significant withdrawal symptoms.[32–35] We have followed these patients for at least 4 weeks, in some cases for 24 months. Within 120 days of abrupt methadone discontinuation, 8 of these opiate addicts had significant depressive episodes, 5 had episodes of panic-anxiety, and 3 had acute mania that required treatment. We will describe 3 of these patients, one who developed a significant depressive episode, another who developed a panic-anxiety disorder, and another who developed an acute mania, to illustrate the natural history of the phenomenon and the similarities of these episodes to naturally occurring major depressive and panic-anxiety episodes as defined by the Research Diagnostic Criteria.[36]

CASE REPORTS

Case 1

Mr. A, a 25-year-old married man, had a 2-year history of unsuccessful attempts to detoxify from methadone and a 9-year history of episodic opiate use. He was admitted to the clonidine study and detoxified from 50 mg/day of methadone. Mr. A was able to return to work within a week of his hospital discharge, but approximately 2 weeks later he complained of difficulty falling asleep, a 2.7-kg weight loss, decreased libido, energy, concentration, no appetite, and a depressed mood. He failed to keep a scheduled appointment for follow-up and evaluation of these complaints. Five weeks after Mr. A's discharge from the hospital, his wife found him with a large kitchen knife, tearful, and expressing the desire to die. When he was admitted to a psychiatric hospital, he stated that he was unable to work for the previous week and that he was "hearing voices in my head saying I'm no good and should die." He had a quinine-positive urine and said he had transient symptom relief after heroin use. Mr. A's family gave a history of two previous depressive episodes, one of which resulted in psychiatric hospitalization (diagnosis of psychotic depression) and treatment with ECT. He was not addicted to opiates at this time. He expressed the desire to return to the methadone program. Methadone was administered and he was discharged from the hospital after 30 days. Mr. A returned to work on a maintenance dose of 25 mg/day of methadone.

Case 2

Mr. B, a 25-year-old married professional man, was successfully detoxified with clonidine from addiction to hydromorphone after an intermediate stabilization of 35 mg/day of methadone. He said he had used cocaine and amphetamine in the past, but they made him "too nervous to function." He had had no previous psychiatric hospitalizations or treatment but gave a history of episodic nervousness and feelings of impending doom when he was not taking opiates. Mr. B did well after hospital discharge, he returned to work immediately, and his urine specimens were negative for opiates. He had no complaints of any physical or psychic discomfort for weeks, but he then noted the abrupt onset of one to three "attacks" of nervousness, sweating, irritability, and fear: he said he sometimes felt like he should "run away somewhere, or hide, or do something, but I didn't know really what to do." These symptoms were not clearly relatable to environmental events or changes. He began to "lose confidence in myself" but continued working. There were no neurovegetative signs of symptoms of depression, although he said he was depressed. Medical consultation and evaluation failed to find evidence of a medical syndrome that would explain his symptoms. He was given low doses of imipramine (25 mg p.o. t.i.d.) and reported that his attacks disappeared within weeks. He also said he had obtained a prescription for clonidine and was taking 0.2 mg of clonidine with his imipramine.

Case 3

Mr. C was a 32-year-old physician who had a 14-month history of morphine abuse and addiction. He had a history of marijuana and methaqualone

(Quaalude) abuse. He had no previous psychiatric treatment but gave a history of a short-lived depression during his freshman year of college. This depression was described as being "paralytic," but after "sleeping for 5 days" the episode remitted. The patient also gave a history consistent with 2 days of grandiosity and complete insomnia after taking amphetamines during his first year of medical school. Recently the patient was successfully detoxified as an inpatient after a comprehensive evaluation. He refused naltrexone but joined an A.A. program and left the hospital. Approximately three weeks after discharge the patient's wife called to say her husband had begun to act in an "atypical" manner. He became unable to sleep, hypersexual, and lost his appetite. He stayed at his office working on a manuscript "exposing" his colleagues. He refused to be interrupted in his work by patient appointments or his nurses and office staff. He told his wife he was uncomfortable with his house and bought a new house. He was hospitalized and treated with lithium carbonate.

DISCUSSION

The association between opiate addiction and psychopathology has a long history, which is now partially supported by empirical data. For example, opiate addicts have been shown to have high rates of depression,[37–43] antisocial personality characteristics,[44] schizophrenia or schizotypical features,[45–47] manic symptomatology,[8, 44, 48] and alcoholism.[49] The major problem to date, in the studies of psychopathology in opiate addicts, is that the assessment of psychopathology has usually been with symptom or personality scales. Diagnostic techniques, particularly the more recently improved measures and neurobiological testing,[50–53] have rarely been applied to the opiate addict. The result is that there has been a gap between general psychiatric practice and the treatment of opiate abusers. This gap is reflected in the fact that opiate addicts like other drug abusers are usually treated in separate unidimensional specialty clinics, like patients with tuberculosis had been treated in the past. The isolation of the addict in separate "programs" and from doctors and hospitals transmits a profound message to these people and isolates them from recent developments in psychiatric diagnostic practice, which leads to misdiagnosis and mistreatment.[54] For example, the opiate addict who has agorophobia might benefit from monoamine oxidase (MAO) inhibitors, as a bipolar patient might benefit from lithium; or the addict who has a major depression by ratings and biological testing would benefit from treatment with a tricyclic antidepressants. We can only conclude after frequently observing the post-detoxification emergence of major psychopathology that many opiate addicts have been self-medicating and could be treated with alternative treatments.

As part of this study, we have also seen the patients described above and 7 other patients who had signs and symptoms of primary major depressive disorder (one with psychotic features), 2 with acute mania, and another 4 who had complaints consistent with the diagnosis of panic state. These patients had symptoms and courses similar to those of the patients described above. Six depressed patients were successfully treated with tricyclics and the other 2 were readmitted to the methadone program. Three panic patients were successfully treated with TCAs, one with an MAO inhibitor, and one was readmitted to the methadone program. The 2 manic patients were treated acutely with haloperidol and ultimately maintained on lithium alone. One of these manic patients was also readmitted to a methadone program. The clinical observations presented here support the notion that for some patients methadone maintenance does not merely help control opiate abuse, but also serves as a psychotropic maintenance program [5] for depressive, manic, psychotic, and panic states.[9]

PANIC AND ANXIETY

The pattern of signs and symptoms exhibited by patients withdrawing from opiates and by patients experiencing spontaneous attacks of panic-anxiety is similar, and this pattern is also observed in humans after the administration of drugs such as piperoxane or yohimbine, which markedly activate the noradrenergic nucleus locus coeruleus, and after abrupt discontinuation of chronic clonidine administration. These similarities suggest a possible common endorphin–noradrenergic mechanism mediating the syndromes of opiate withdrawal and panic anxiety. This had suggested to us that clonidine could be used in methadone withdrawal, and methadone in clonidine withdrawal. However, there are no reports of direct and quantitative comparison of these two syndromes.

Ten opiate addicts (8 males, 2 females) and 10 patients with histories of frequent attacks of panic anxiety (4 males, 6 females) were studied. The test battery included vital signs, the Addiction Research Center Inventory for Weak Opiate Withdrawal, the Speilberger State Anxiety Inventory, and analog self-rating scales for anxiety, fear, irritability, unpleasantness, anger, and euphoria. This battery was administered to opiate addicts twice daily during a baseline period of methadone maintenance, then every 6 hours for 36 hours after the abrupt discontinuation of methadone. For the panic-anxiety patients, the battery was administered twice daily for 7 medication-free days and immediately upon the onset of a panic attack. All patients had at least 2 spontaneous panic attacks during the study period.

The 2 groups did not differ during the baseline period. During withdrawal or panic, both groups showed significant increases in heart rate, blood pressure, temperature, tremulousness, anorexia, insomnia, restlessness, and gastrointestinal discomfort ($p < 0.01$). The opiate withdrawal patients demonstrated a significantly greater elevation of anger and irritability than did the panic-anxiety patients, who in turn, demonstrated a significantly greater elevation of fear ratings ($p < 0.01$). All opiate withdrawal patients responded to treatment with clonidine with a rapid decrease in symptoms. Three of the panic anxiety patients with previous unsuccessful responses to imipramine were given clonidine during a panic-anxiety attack. Two of these three patients showed nearly complete alleviation of panic symptoms, while the third patient showed a significant, but partial, response to clonidine.

These findings again suggest a common neurobiological mediation of opiate withdrawal and panic anxiety. Theoretical implications of these results have been discussed,[10] but include the use of opiates by physicians to treat intractable panic and anxiety states.

Clonidine is an efficacious nonopiate treatment for opiate withdrawal; however, it does not prevent readdiction or modify the numerous factors that are related to opiate use and addiction.[30, 31] One of these factors may be an underlying psychopathology or a vulnerability to major psychoses or panic-anxiety states in patients maintained on opiates. If opiate agonists are effective or somewhat effective in the treatment or self-medication of major psychoses or panic states, then discontinuation of maintenance treatment might be expected to result in an exacerbation of the previously controlled syndrome. This may explain the clinical data reported here on the post-detoxification emergence of panic states, major depression mania, and psychosis. Although psychological and social factors or drug-induced changes might be invoked to explain the emergence of severe psychiatric symptomatology after clonidine detoxification, neurobiologic explanations invoking a pre-existing illness may be more parsimonious.

DEPRESSION

The discovery of opioid receptors and endogenous opioid peptides (endorphins) in the brain has kindled interest in the possible role of endorphin systems in psychiatric disorders.[34, 55, 56] The analgesic, anxiolytic, euphoric, and calming effects of exogenous opiates suggest that decreased functional activity in endogenous opioid peptide systems could be linked to the pathophysiology of depression. Opiate receptors and endorphins are widely distributed in limbic and hypothalamic areas thought to be involved in depression. Endogenous opioid peptides may modulate noradrenergic and dopaminergic neuronal systems that are implicated in the etiology and pharmacotherapy of depression.

There are anecdotal reports from the prepsychotropic era of the efficacy of opiates in treating depression. We have observed and reported here significant depression in opiate addicts after detoxification. Some of these patients have been successfully treated with opiates and tricyclic antidepressants, suggesting that opiate discontinuation resembles the discontinuation of effective psychopharmacologic maintenance treatment. Administration of β-endorphins has ameliorated depressive symptoms in some patients.[56] These data support the hypothesis that endogenous opioids influence the maintenance of pathological mood states.

We used a neuroendocrine challenge paradigm to study *in vivo* endogenous opioid systems in depressed patients. The normally pronounced increase in serum prolactin produced by morphine [57] was markedly blunted in patients with major depressive disorder.

Both exogenous opioids and endogenous opioid peptides are potent stimulators of secretion of the pituitary hormone prolactin in animals [58] and man.[3, 27, 59] Morphine in the dosage range we used has been reported to produce large and reliable increases in serum prolactin in normal subjects.[57] Prolactin secretion is controlled in part by the dopaminergic tuberoinfundibular tract, which exerts an inhibitory effect over the secretion of prolactin.[60] Serotonergic neurons have a stimulatory effect on prolactin secretion; and other neurotransmitters and neuromodulators, including norepinephrine and epinephrine, have been reported to modulate prolactin secretion as well.[58-60] When opioid receptors located on dopaminergic neurons [55] are activated, they inhibit the dopaminergic tonic inhibition of prolactin secretion. Such opioid receptor activation would therefore allow increased secretion of prolactin after administration of opioids.[58] The mean maximal prolactin response of 7.2 ± 2.7 ng/ml in the depressed group was significantly lower than that of 31.9 ± 9.5 ng/ml in the control group ($p < 0.01$).

Thus the absent or blunted increase in serum prolactin occurring after morphine infusion in our patients with major depressive disorder may reflect abnormalities in central endorphin, dopamine, serotonin, or other neuroregulatory systems. Possible abnormalities in endorphin systems that could account for a blunted prolactin response to morphine in major depression include an opioid receptor deficit, an excess of endogenous opioid antagonist, or elevated endorphin levels with compensatory down regulation of opioid receptors. This might suggest a role for endorphin testing in depression and a possible use of endorphins in the treatment of intractable depression.

The mood effects produced by the acute and chronic use of narcotic analgesics offer some support for these neuroendocrine data and suggest that endorphins may play a role in affective disorders. In one outpatient study, cyclazocine, a mixed agonist–antagonist, was found to be an antidepressant.[61] When patients who are depressed were given acute infusions of naloxone, no effect was seen on depressed mood.[62] These clinical data reported here are also in agreement with our previously described hypothesis for bipolar affective illness.[8]

We have previously described the self-medication of schizophrenic patients with opiates in a methadone maintenance program[5] and the theoretic and clinical data suggesting the antipsychotic efficacy of opiate antagonists.[3, 5] These schizophrenic patients were well known to us and were not detoxified from methadone maintenance. We did not observe the emergence of a schizophrenic of schizophrenic-like psychosis after rapid detoxification in the sample of patients reported here. What we did observe was the appearance of significant depression and mania, with and without psychotic features, and panic episodes that were virtually identical to naturally occurring depressive and panic episodes.[36] In addition, these patients were successfully treated with opiates, tricyclic antidepressants, or a combination of tricyclic antidepressants and clonidine, which suggests that opiate discontinuation in these patients was similar to the discontinuation of an effective psychopharmacologic maintenance treatment.

SUMMARY

These clinical data may offer some support for the hypothesis that opiates have antidepressant, antimanic, and antipanic effects. This hypothesis should be studied directly by double-blind studies of the effects of exogenous and synthetic endogenous opioid peptides in patients with major depressive illness, panic and anxiety states, schizophrenia, and schizo-affective illness. These clinical data support our studies in nonhuman primates and man which suggest a common LC or NE hyperactivity may underly both drug withdrawal and spontaneous panic states.[63, 64] Whether endorphin deficiency or derangements account for the postulated NE hyperactivity needs additional study and we will discuss our preliminary work later. Failure of endorphins to terminate bursts in LC firing rate and NE release may be responsible for both of these types of panic states.[6, 65–67] In addicts, this mechanism could exist prior to opiate use, or abuse of potent exogenous endorphinomentic compound may cause an endorphin-abnormality.[68] Both of these possibilities would be compensated by continuous opiate maintenance.

Methadone maintenance is a complicated psychiatric, psychological, and social phenomenon. Further studies are necessary to evaluate the role of opiate maintenance in treating or suppressing the emergence of underlying psychopathology. Previous psychiatric hospitalization or treatment for a schizophrenic or affective illness may contraindicate absolutely the use of clonidine or other rapid detoxification methods. These data suggest the possibility of substituting a nonaddicting psychotropic medication for opiates in some patients who are self-medicators. The clinical data support other data suggesting the potential antipsychotic, antidepressant, and antianxiety/antipanic effects of the endogenous opioids, endorphins, and exogenous opioids, endorphins, and exogenous opiates.[56, 69-74] These and other data suggest potential utility for opioid agonists and endorphin testing in psychiatric treatment and diagnosis.

REFERENCES

1. GESSA, G. L. & A. TAGLIAMONTE. 1975. Effect of methadone and dextromoramide on dopamine metabolism. Neuropharmacology **14:** 913–920.
2. GOLD, M. S., D. E. REDMOND, JR., R. K. DONABEDIAN, *et al.* 1978. Increase in serum prolactin by exogenous and endogenous opiates: Evidence for antidopamine and antipsychotic effects. Am. J. Psychiatry **135:** 1415–1416.
3. GOLD, M. S., R. K. DONABEDIAN, M. DIELARD, *et al.* 1977. Antipsychotic effect of opiate agonists. Lancet 2: 398–399.
4. VEREBEY, K., J. VOLAKA & J. CLOUET. 1978. Endorphins in psychiatry. Arch. Gen. Psychiatry **35:** 877–888.
5. KLEBER, H. D. & M. S. GOLD. 1978. Use of psychoropic drugs in treatment of methadone-maintained narcotic addicts. Ann. N.Y. Acad. Sci. **311:** 81–98.
6. GOLD, M. S., A. L. C., POTTASH & I. EXTEIN. 1980. Antiendorphin effect of methadone. Lancet 2: 973.
7. COMFORT, A. 1977. Morphine as an antipsychotic relevance of a 19th century therapeutic fashion. Lancet 2: 448–449.
8. GOLD, M. S. & R. BYCK. 1978. Endorphins, lithium and naloxone: Their relationship to pathological and drug-induced manic-euphoric states. NIDA Monogr. **19:** 192–209.
9. GOLD, M. S., A. L. C. POTTASH, D. R. SWEENEY, *et al.* 1979. Rapid opiate detoxification: Clinical evidence of antidepressant and antipanic effects of opiates. Am. J. Psychiatry **136:** 982–983.
10. SWEENEY, D. R., M. S. GOLD, N. RYAN, *et al.* 1980. Opiate withdrawal and panic anxiety. APA Abstract :123.
11. GOLD, M. S., A. L. C. POTTASH, D. R. SWEENEY, *et al.* 1980. Clonidine decreases opiate withdrawal related anxiety: Possible opiate noradrenergic interaction in anxiety and panic. Substance and Alcohol Actions Misuse **1:** 239–246.
12. GOLD, M. S., R. BYCK, D. R. SWEENEY, *et al.* 1979. Endorphin-locus coeruleus connection mediates opiate action and withdrawal. Biomedicine :1–4.
13. GOLD, M. S. & H. D. KLEBER. 1979. A rationale for opiate withdrawal symptomology. Drug and Alcohol Dependence 4: 419–424.
14. REDMOND, D. E., Y. H. HWANG, J. BAULU & M. S. GOLD. 1979. Evidence for the involvement of a brain norepinephrine system in anxiety. *In* Catecholamines: Basic and Clinical Frontiers. E. Usdin, I. Kopin & J. Barchas, Eds. Vol. **2:** 1693–1695. Pergamon Press. New York.
15. GOLD, M. S., D. E. REDMOND, *et al.* 1977. Pharmacological activation and inhibition of noradrenergic activity alter specific behaviors in non human primates III. Neurosci. Abstracts **783:** 250.
16. REDMOND, D. E., JR., M. S. GOLD & Y. H. YWANG. 1978. Enkephalin acts to inhibit locus coeruleus mediated behaviors. Soc. Neurosci. Abst. **4:** 413.
17. GOLD, M. S. & A. L. C. POTTASH. 1981. Clonidine and lofexidine: Evidence for an endorphin-norepinephrine connection mediating opiate withdrawal. *In* Advance and Substance Abuse Behavioral and Biological Research. Vol. 3.

18. GOLD, M. S., D. E. REDMOND, H. D. KLEBER, *et al.* 1979. NE hyperactivity in opiate withdrawal supported by clonidine reversal of opiate withdrawal. Am. J. Psychiatry **136:** 100–102.
19. GOLD, M. S., A. L. C. POTTASH & D. R. SWEENEY. 1980. Opiate withdrawal using clonidine. J. Am. Med. Assoc. **243:** 343–346.
20. GOLD, M. S., A. L. C. POTTASH, I. EXTEIN, *et al.* 1980. Clonidine in acute opiate withdrawal. N. Engl. J. Med. **302:** 1421–1422.
21. SWEENEY, D. R., M. S. GOLD, A. L. C. POTTASH, *et al.* 1980. Neuro-Biological Theories. *In* The Handbook of Stress and Anxiety: Current Knowledge, Theory and Treatment. I. L. Kutash & L. B. Schlesinger, Eds. Jossey Bass. San Francisco, CA.
22. GOLD, M. S., R. K. DONABEDIAN, D. E. REDMOND, JR., *et al.* 1978. Antipsychotic effect of opiate agonists? New Research Program **23:** 3. American Psychiatric Association, Washington, D.C.
23. ROUNSAVILLE, B. J., M. M. WEISSMAN, P. H. ROSENBERGER, *et al.* 1979. Detecting depressive disorders in drug abusers: A comparison of screening instruments. J. Affect. Dis. **1:** 255–267.
24. WEISSMAN, M. M., F. SLOBETZ & B. PRUSOFF. 1976. Clinical depression among narcotic addicts maintained on methadone in the community. Am. J. Psychiatry **133:** 1434–1438.
25. ROUNSAVILLE, B. J., P. ROSENBERGER, C. H. WILBER, *et al.* 1980. A Comparison of the SADS/RDC and the DSM III: Diagnosing drug abusers. J. Nerv. Ment. Dis. **168:** 90–97.
26. EXTEIN, I., A. L. C. POTTASH, M. S. GOLD, D. R. SWEENEY, *et al.* 1980. Opiate receptor deficit in major depressive disorder? Am. J. Psychiatry **137:** 375–376.
27. GOLD, M. S., A. L. C. POTTASH, D. A. MARTIN, *et al.* 1980. Opiate-endorphin test dysfunction in major depression. Soc. Neurosci. Abst. **255:** 759.
28. EXTEIN, I., A. L. C. POTTASH, M. S. GOLD, *et al.* 1980. Blunted prolactin response to morphine in major depressive disorder. Int. Soc. Psychoneuroendocrinol. Abstr. :76. Florence, Italy.
29. GOLD, M. S., A. L. C. POTTASH, I. EXTEIN, *et al.* 1981. Endorphin dysfunction in panic anxiety and primary affective illness. *In* Endorphins and Opiate Antagonists in Psychiatric Research: Clinical Implications. N. S. Shah & A. G. Donald, Eds. Plenum Pub. Corp. New York. In press.
30. GOLD, M. S., D. E. REDMOND & H. D. KLEBER. 1978. Clonidine blocks acute opiate withdrawal symptoms. Lancet 2: 599–602.
31. GOLD, M. S., D. E. REDMOND & H. D. KLEBER. 1978. Noradrenergic hyperactivity in opiate withdrawal supported by clonidine reversal of opiate withdrawal. Am. J. Psychiatry **136:** 100–102.
32. GOLD, M. S., A. L. C. POTTASH, D. R. SWEENEY, *et al.* 1980. The effect of methadone dosage no clonidine detoxification efficacy. Am. J. Psychiatry **137:** 375–376.
33. GOLD, M. S. & A. L. C. POTTASH. 1981. The neurobiological implications of clonidine HCl. Ann. N.Y. Acad. Sci. **362:** 191–202.
34. GOLD, M. S. & H. D. KLEBER. 1981. Clinical utility of clonidine in opiate withdrawal: A study of 100 patients. Psychopharmacology of Clonidine. H. Lal & S. Fielding, Eds.: 299–306. Alan R. Liss, Inc. New York.
35. KLEBER, H. D., M. S. GOLD & C. E. RIORDAN. 1980. The use of clonidine in detoxification from opiates. Bull. Narcotics **32:** 1–10.
36. SPITZER, R. & E. ROBINS. 1978. Research diagnostic criteria rationale and ability. Arch. Gen. Psychiatry **35:** 773–782.
37. DORUS, W. & E. C. SENAY. 1980. Depression, demographic dimensions, and drug abuse. Am. J. Psychiatry **137:** 699–704.
38. LEHMAN, E. X. & G. G. DEANGELIS. 1972. Adolescents, methadone and psychotherapeutic agents. *In* Narcotics. Proc. 4th Natl. Conf. Methadone

Treatment. : 55–58. National Association for the Prevention of Addiction to Narcotics. New York.

39. ROBINS, P. R. 1974. Depression and drug addiction. Psychoanal. Q. **48:** 375–386.

40. ROUNSAVILLE, B. J., M. M. WEISSMAN, P. H. ROSENBERGER, *et al.* 1979. Detecting depressive disorders in drug abusers: A comparison of screening instruments. J. Affect. Dis. **1:** 255–267.

41. STEER, R. A. & E. KOTZKER. 1980. Affective changes in male and female methadone patients. Drug Alcohol Depend. **5:** 116–122.

42. WIELAND, W. F. & S. SOLA. 1970. Depression in opiate addicts measured by objective tests. *In* Proc. 3rd Natl. Conf. Methadone Treatment. National Association for the Prevention of Addiction to Narcotics. New York.

43. WEISSMAN, M. M., F. SLOBETZ, B. PRUSOFF, *et al.* 1976. Clinical depression among narcotic addicts maintained on methadone in the community. Am. J. Psychiatry **133:** 1434–1438.

44. CRAIG, R. J. 1979. Personality characteristics of heroin addicts: A review of the empirical literature with critique—Part II. Int. J. Addict. **14:** 607–626.

45. SHEPPARD, C., D. FIORENTINO, L. COLLINS, *et al.* 1969. Comparison of emotion profiles as defined by two additional MMPI profile types in male narcotic addicts. J. Clin. Psychol. **25:** 186–188.

46. HEKIMIAN, L. J. & S. GERSHON. 1968. Characteristics of drug abusers admitted to a psychiatric hospital. J. Am. Med. Assoc. **205:** 75–80.

47. ZIMMERING, P., J. TOOLAN, R. SAFRIN, *et al.* 1952. Drug addiction in relation to problems of adolescence. 108th Ann. Meet. American Psychiatric Association. Atlantic City, NJ.

48. FLEMMENBAUM, A. 1974. Affective disorders and chemical dependence: Lithium for alcohol and drug addiction. Dis. Nerv. Syst. **35:** 281–286.

49. BELENKO, S. 1979. Alcohol abuse by heroin addicts: A review of research findings and issues. Int. J. Addict. **14:** 965–975.

50. EXTEIN, I., A. L. C. POTTASH & M. S. GOLD. 1980. The TRH test in depression. N. Engl. J. Med. **302:** 923–924.

51. GOLD, M. S., A. L. C. POTTASH, I. EXTEIN & D. R. SWEENEY. 1981. Diagnosis of Depression in the 1980's. Bench and Bedside Series. J. Am. Med. Assoc. **254:** 1562–1564.

52. POTTASH, A. L. C., M. S. GOLD & I. EXTEIN. 1981. The use of the clinical laboratory in inpatient psychiatry. Inpatient Psychiatry: Diagnosis and Treatment. (In press.)

53. EXTEIN, I., A. L. C. POTTASH, M. S. GOLD & F. K. GOODWIN. 1981. Relationship of TRH test and dexamethasone suppression test abnormalities in unipolar depression. Psychiatry Res. **4:** 49–53.

54. LING, W., E. D. HOLMES, G. R. POST, *et al.* 1973. A systematic psychiatric study of the heroin addicts. *In* Proc. 5th Natl. Conf. Methadone Treatment. pp. 429–432. National Association for the Prevention of Addiction to Narcotics. New York.

55. SNYDER, S. H. 1978. The opiate receptor and morphine-like peptides in the brain. Am. J. Psychiatry **135:** 645–652.

56. KLINE, N. W., C. H. LI, H. E. LEHMANN, *et al.* 1977. β-Endorphin induced changes in schizophrenic and depressed patients. Arch. Gen. Psychiatry **34:** 1111–1113.

57. TOBIS, G., R. DENT & H. GUYDA. 1978. Opiates, prolactin, and the dopamine receptor. J. Clin. Endocrinol. Metab. **47:** 200–203.

58. GOLD, M. S., D. E. REDMOND, JR. & R. K. DONABEDIAN. 1978. Increase in serum prolactin by exogenous and endogenous opiates: evidence for anti-dopamine and antipsychotic effects. Am. J. Psychiatry **135:** 1415–1416.

59. GRAFFENRIED, B. V., E. D. POZO, J. ROUBICEK, *et al.* 1978. Effects of the synthetic enkephalin analogue FK33–824 in man. Nature **272:** 729–730.

60. GOLD, M. S., D. E. REDMOND, JR. & R. K. DONABEDIAN. 1979. The effects of opiate agonist and opiate and opiate antagonists on serum prolactin in primates: Possible role for endorphins in prolactin regulation. Endocrinology 105(1).

61. FINK, M., J. SIMEON, T. M. ITIL, et al. 1970. Clinical antidepressant activity of cyclozacine: a narcotic antagonist. Clin. Pharmacol. Ther. 11: 41–48.

62. DAVIS, G. C., W. E. BUNNEY, JR., E. G. DE FRAITES, et al. 1977. Intravenous naloxone administration in schizophrenia and affective illness. Science 197: 74–77.

63. GOLD, M. S., A. L. C. POTTASH, I. EXTEIN, et al. 1981. Neuroanatomical sites of action of clonidine in drug withdrawal syndromes. In Psychopharmacology of Clonidine. H. Lal & S. Fielding, Eds.: 285–298. Alan R. Liss, Inc. New York.

64. GOLD, M. S. & A. L. C. POTTASH. 1980. Clonidine: Complete acute and chronic antiopiate withdrawal effects. In Advances in Substance Abuse: Behavioral and Biological Research. N. K. Mello, Ed. JAI Press, Inc., Greenwich, CT. In press.

65. GOLD, M. S., A. L. C. POTTASH, I. EXTEIN, et al. 1981. Lack of ACTH response to Naloxone in methadone addicts: Evidence for endorphins dysfunction. Drug Alcohol Depend. : 257–262.

66. GOLD, M. S. & A. L. C. POTTASH. 1981. Endorphins, locus coeruleus, clonidine and lofexidine: A mechanism for opiate withdrawal and new nonopiate treatments. In Advances in Alcohol and Substance Abuse. Vol. 1 (1): 33–52.

67. GOLD, M. S., A. L. C. POTTASH, I. EXTEIN, et al. 1982. Methadone induced endorphin dysfunction in addicts. : 476–482. NIDA Monogr. Committee on Problem Drug Dependence.

68. GOLD, M. S., A. L. C. POTTASH & I. EXTEIN. 1981. ACTH response to naloxone in Methadone addicts. Int. Soc. Psychoneuroendocrinol. Abstracts.

69. EXTEIN, I., A. L. C. POTTASH & M. S. GOLD. 1982. Cortisol response to naloxone in depressed patients and controls. Int. Soc. Psychoneuroendocrinol. Abstracts.

70. EXTEIN, I., D. PICKAR, M. S. GOLD, et al. 1981. Methadone and morphine in depression. Psychopharmacol. Bull. 17: 29–33.

71. MIRRIN, S. M., R. E. MEYER & B. McNAMEE. 1976. Psychopathology and mood during heroin abuse: Acute vs. chronic. Arch. Gen. Psychiatry 33: 1503–1508.

72. EXTEIN, I., F. K. GOODWIN & A. J. LEWY. 1979. Behavioral and biochemical effects of FK 33–824; A parenterally and orally active enkephalin analogue. In Endorphins in Mental Health Research. E. Usdin, W. Bunney, Jr. & N. Kline., Eds.: 279–292. The Macmillan Press Ltd. London.

73. COHEN, M. R. & D. PICKAR. 1981. Pharmacological challenges to the endogenous opioid system in affective illness. J. Clin. Psychopharmacol. 1: 223–231.

74. PICKAR, D., I. EXTEIN, P. GOLD, et al. 1982. Endorphins and affective illness. In Endorphins and Opiate Antagonists in Psychiatric Research: Clinical Implications. N. S. Smith & A. G. Donald, Eds. Plenum Press. New York.

CHRONIC USE OF
OPIOIDS AND ANTIPSYCHOTIC DRUGS:
SIDE EFFECTS, EFFECTS ON ENDOGENOUS
OPIOIDS, AND TOXICITY *

Mary Jeanne Kreek and Neil Hartman

The Rockefeller University
New York, New York 10021

There is increasing enthusiasm, supported both by anecdotal clinical observations and various pieces of scientific information, to consider the use of natural opiates or opioids, including narcotic drugs, endogenous opioid peptides, and their synthetic congeners, in the management of specific types of psychiatric disorders. It is essential to identify the potential risks of such treatment, and to compare these risks with those encountered during chronic treatment with clinically accepted agents. Potential "risks" of a therapeutic agent such as opioids include undesirable side effects, alterations of normal physiological function, including alterations in hormonal levels, adverse reactions, and also direct drug toxicity. The side effects, the interactions with endogenous opioids, and the toxicity of opioids, antipsychotic agents, and antidepressant drugs will be the topic of this discussion.

However, another area of potential risk, not to be discussed in detail, but clearly relevant to chronic opioid use, is the predictable development of tolerance to physical dependence on the drug, which may be related to the subsequent development of addiction. There is also the potential risk that any perturbation in normal physiology that might occur during chronic treatment with an opioid might return to normal very slowly or even be irreversible following cessation of treatment, and that these alterations might, in fact, be related to the processes of tolerance, dependence, and addiction. Tolerance, physical dependence, and addiction do not develop during chronic treatment with most of the antipsychotic or antidepressant drugs currently used for the management of the specific psychiatric disorders that might alternatively (or more successfully) be managed by chronic opioid treatment. If an opioid were found to be very effective in the management of any specific disorder, and if chronic treatment were indicated, the development of tolerance and physical dependence might *not* be considered to be major risks. "Addiction" would not be recognized unless treatment were discontinued. However, potential problems related to the development of tolerance, dependence, and addiction must be carefully considered prior to instituting short- or long-term treatment with opioids.

Information concerning the side effects, adverse reactions, and toxicity of any drug is often fragmentary. Many side effects of chronic usage of a drug do not appear until after years of treatment, and a large number of patients under treatment is required to detect side effects of low or moderate frequency in their occurrence. Some so-called "side effects" of drugs are really well-known

* This work was supported by grants from the National Institute on Drug Abuse (DA–01138) and New York State Division of Substance Abuse Services (C–148039 and C–148087). Dr. Kreek is a recipient of a Research Scientist Award (DA–00049) from the Health and Human Services—American Drug Abuse and Mental Health Association—National Institute on Drug Abuse.

0077–8923/82/0398–0151 $1.75/0 © 1982, NYAS

specific effects other than the desired effect. This is certainly true of many of the opioid "side effects." Some side effects are predictable and dose related, others unpredictable but still dose related, and still other side effects are idiosyncratic responses. Another problem encountered in detecting and then estimating the prevalence of side effects and adverse reactions to a drug is that most drugs are given to patients with diseases. Whether these diseases are organic or functional, their presence makes the differentiation of drug-related effects difficult.

In addition to illicit use (usually of the short-acting narcotic, heroin) by narcotic addicts, opiates are administered on a chronic basis primarily for the relief of pain, or for the maintenance treatment of addiction. Side effects of opioids are difficult to assess in both heroin addicts and patients receiving narcotics on a chronic basis for pain relief because of the difficulties in performing studies in such patients. Also, since many of the so-called "side effects" of opiates are simply well-known narcotic effects, the effects of short-acting narcotics such as heroin, morphine, or meperidine are, in part, quite different from those of long-acting narcotics such as methadone.

It is possible to conduct prospective and retrospective studies to determine the side effects, alterations in normal physiology (including interactions between exogenous and endogenous opioids), and toxic effects of opioids in former narcotic addicts in chronic methadone treatment. Many of the observations made from such studies have provided important clues as to the possible roles of endogenous opioids in normal physiology. After oral administration of methadone, there are minimal peak effects coincident with peak plasma levels of methadone, and stable effects with sustained levels of drug through the remainder of the 24-hour dosing interval.[1-4] This relatively steady state of perfusion with increased levels of opioid cannot be achieved by intermittent administration of short-acting narcotics.

Prospective, retrospective, and special studies have been carried out in methadone-maintained patients. After 6-months of chronic methadone treatment, tolerance has developed to many, but not all, of the acute and subacute narcotic effects initially experienced by patients (TABLE 1).[5] Stabilization is

TABLE 1

CLINICAL SIDE EFFECTS OBSERVED DURING CHRONIC METHADONE TREATMENT

	Duration in Treatment	
	> 6 months *	> 3 years †
1. Increased sweating	47%	48%
2. Constipation	57%	17%
3. Libido abnormalities	26%	22%
4. Abnormalities in sexual performance	?	14%
5. Sleep abnormalities (insomnia)	23%	16%
6. Appetite abnormalities	19%	4%
7. Nervousness, tenseness	21%	—
8. Headaches	12%	—
9. Body aches and pains	11%	—
10. Chills	10%	—
11. Weight gain	?	?

* Yaffee et al.[5]
† Kreek.[1]

not yet fully achieved, however, so that some symptoms more commonly associated with narcotic abstinence such as nervousness, headaches, body aches, and chills are still observed. After 3 years or more of chronic high-dose methadone treatment, full stabilization has been achieved.[6–10] Tolerance has developed to most of the acute and subacute narcotic affects, but tolerance does not develop to the ability of methadone to prevent the signs and symptoms of narcotic withdrawal or the symptoms of drug hunger. Increased sweating is observed in around 50% of all such patients while constipation, persistent abnormalities in libido and sexual performance, and insomnia are each experienced by around 20% of patients. None of these side effects have been documented to result from significant injury to any organ system.

Around 50%–60% of all heroin addicts and patients entering methadone treatment have biochemical evidence of chronic liver disease; over 50% of patients in chronic methadone treatment have persistent liver function test abnormalities (TABLE 2).[6, 7, 9] Nevertheless, in prospective and retrospective

TABLE 2

ABNORMAL LIVER FUNCTION TEST VALUES IN
METHADONE MAINTENANCE PATIENTS *

	Study Group	Abnormal Tests		Duration of Treatment (months)	Reference
		On Admission	During Treatment		
1.	Adults ($N = 53$) (prospective study)	57%	51%	36–66	6
2.	Adults ($N = 1357$) (retrospective study)	63%	52%	3–72	1

* Abnormal liver function was defined as a plasma SGOT level greater than 30 units. No evidence of hepatotoxicity of methadone was found.

studies there has been no evidence of hepatotoxicity due to methadone. Patients with normal liver function at time of admission to methadone treatment do not develop abnormalities of liver function except in the setting of acute viral hepatitis or chronic alcohol abuse. Neither liver function tests nor clinical status were shown to deteriorate during methadone treatment in patients with liver function abnormalities at time of admission to treatment, except in patients known to be alcohol abusers.

The etiology of chronic hepatic dysfunction observed in methadone-maintained patients is of two types: sequelae of earlier acute infection with hepatitis B virus or non-A non-B virus, and various types of alcohol-induced liver disease (TABLE 3).[6, 7, 9, 11, 12] It has been shown that 10%–12% of adult and adolescent methadone-maintained patients are chronic carriers of hepatitis B antigen, and that approximately 50% of all patients have hepatitis B core antibody.[6, 9] In a study of maintained patients, all with chronic liver disease, over 96% had some marker of prior hepatitis B infection.[12] The percentage of patients with chronic sequelae due to hepatitis non-A non-B virus is unknown.

It has been shown that, contrary to earlier belief, substantial numbers (about 20%) of street heroin addicts are also chronic abusers of alcohol.[6, 7, 9, 11] In

TABLE 3

HEPATITIS B ANTIGENEMIA AND ANTIBODIES IN
METHADONE-MAINTAINED PATIENTS*

Study Groups	% of Patients in Study Groups			Duration in Treatment	Reference
	Hepatitis B Antigen	Core Anti-body	Surface Anti-body		
1. Adults ($N = 50$) (prospective study; MMT)	12%	46%	ND	36–66 months	12
2. Adolescents ($N = 51$) (prospective study; MMT)	10%	ND	ND	3–36 months	†
3. Adults ($N = 46$) (consecutive cases with chronic liver disease undergoing biopsy; heroin users and MMT)	11%	96%	78%	—	12

* MMT, methadone maintenance treatment; ND, not done.
† Kreek *et al.* (in progress).

clinical studies from this laboratory, we found that 25–35% of adult and adolescent methadone-maintained patients are chronic abusers of alcohol, and that in this group of patients, progressive liver disease may occur.

A variety of biochemical and physiological alterations have been observed. Two types of abnormalities commonly observed are alterations in serum protein levels and immunological indices (TABLE 4).[6, 7, 9, 15–17] Some of these alterations, such as elevations in levels of serum albumin may be a direct effect of opioid treatment.[16] Others, such as elevated levels of globulins, are more likely due to chronic liver disease or a long history of injection of diverse foreign materials. Thyroid binding globulin levels are also elevated, leading to apparent elevations in T_4 levels. Elevated IgG and IgM levels are observed in patients for years after cessation of parenteral drug abuse. Biological false positive test results for syphilis reflecting abnormal IgM levels are also observed. Lymphocytosis occurs in approximately 20% of patients in methadone treatment for three years or more; abnormal percentages of B cells and abnormal T cell rosette formation have been reported. It has been suggested that some of these alterations in immune function may be due to direct or indirect opioid effects.

In our prospective studies of the physiological effects of chronic methadone treatment, we have observed normal to elevated, rather than depressed, levels of serum albumin in patients at time of admission to methadone treatment, with greater numbers of patients having elevated levels of serum albumin after three years or more of methadone treatment (TABLE 5).[6–8] These findings of persistent elevations in serum albumin levels are novel and especially unusual in a population with a high prevalence of chronic liver disease and alcohol abuse. Subsequent studies in adults as well as in adolescents have confirmed these earlier findings.[9, 15] In addition, normal to elevated levels of serum albumin

TABLE 4

"SIDE EFFECTS" OF CHRONIC METHADONE USE (?)
BIOCHEMICAL AND PHYSIOLOGICAL ALTERATIONS *
SERUM PROTEIN AND IMMUNOLOGICAL ABNORMALITIES

Alterations Observed	% of Patients Studied
↑ Serum total protein	> 30%
↑ serum albumin	> 20%
↑ serum globulin	> 20%
↑ serum gamma globulin	> 50%
↑ serum α_2-globulin	> 50%
↑ Thyroxine binding globulin	> 50%
↑ serum IgG	30–50%
↑ serum IgM	35–70%
Biological false positive tests for syphilis	> 10%
Lymphocytosis	> 20%
Abnormal % B cells	?
Abnormal T cell rosette formation	?

* Based on studies from our laboratory and other reports in the literature.

have recently been observed in a prospective study of alcoholic methadone-maintained patients. This finding is very provocative since alcohol is known to

TABLE 5

SERUM ALBUMIN LEVELS IN METHADONE MAINTENANCE TREATMENT PATIENTS *

Study Group	Admission to Treatment		During Treatment		Duration of Treatment (months)
	E	D	E	D	
1. Adults (prospective study determined in 47 cases)	17%	4%	32%	2%	36–66
2. Adults (retrospective study determined in 503 cases)	5%	—	21%	—	3–72
3. Adolescents (prospective study determined in 43 cases)	21%	—	21%	—	6–36
4. Adults (28 cases identified as alcohol abusers and followed prospectively for 2 years)	—	—	13%	4%	27–75

* E = Elevated level, greater than 5 g/dl.
  D = Depressed level, less than 3 g/dl.

decrease albumin synthesis. Studies carried out in a rabbit model have shown that chronic administration of methadone results in increased intra- and extra-vascular pools of albumin coupled with accelerated (not depressed) degradation of albumin suggesting sustained increases in albumin synthesis.[16]

In studies performed by other laboratories, it has been shown that several alterations in respiratory physiology occur during early methadone maintenance treatment including decreased sensitivity of the central nervous system receptors to CO_2, alveolar hypoventilation and arterial hypercapnea (TABLE 6).[9, 18-20]

TABLE 6

"SIDE EFFECTS" OF CHRONIC METHADONE USE
BIOCHEMICAL AND PHYSIOLOGICAL ALTERATIONS *
RESPIRATION CONTROL ABNORMALITIES

Prior to development of full tolerance to narcotic effects (2–12 months in treatment)

↓ Sensitivity of CNS chemoreceptors to CO_2
Alveolar hyperventilation
Arterial hypercapnia

Persistent alterations in some patients (early effects that persist more than 12 months in treatment)

↓ Sensitivity of CNS receptors to hypoxia

---

* Based on reports from other laboratories.

Only one alteration in normal respiratory physiology persists during chronic treatment for 12 months or more: a decreased sensitivity of central nervous system receptors to hypoxia.[19] To date, there have been no clinical symptoms reported referable to this alteration. Also it has been shown that the normal hyperventilation of late pregnancy is diminished in methadone-maintained pregnant women.[20] Recently it was suggested that endogenous opioids may play a role in normal pulmonary physiology.

Acute administration of short- or long-acting narcotics or of large amounts of endogenous opioids cause diverse and significant biochemical alterations in normal endocrine and neuroendocrine function. It has been of special interest to determine which of these effects persist during chronic long-term methadone treatment and which effects are no longer seen during chronic treatment because of the development of tolerance.[7-9, 21-37] These findings pertain only to long-acting opioids; there are many endocrine effects to which tolerance does not develop during chronic administration of short-acting narcotics because of their very different pharmacokinetic properties with significant peak levels followed by rapid decline to nadir levels three or four times during each 24-hour period. Many findings concerning the acute or chronic effects of opioids on endocrine function that are made using animal models cannot be extrapolated directly to man because, in animals, the pharmacokinetic properties of most narcotic drugs are significantly different. For instance, methadone, which has been shown to have an apparent terminal half-life in plasma of 24 hours in man when conventional techniques are used (and a much longer half-life of approximately 48 hours when more sensitive stable isotope tracer techniques are used), has a plasma half-life of 90 minutes in the rat.[1, 4, 13, 38-40] Even in apparently carefully executed studies of endocrine function in patients maintained on methadone, it is not always clear whether or not patients with liver disease and/or patients using alcohol or marijuana on a regular basis have been excluded, since these factors can significantly affect endocrine function.[14]

Acute administration of short-acting opiates in animal models causes a reduction in FSH and LH levels, a reduction in glucocorticoid levels, and an increase in prolactin levels. In studies of methadone-maintained patients, several workers have found that plasma levels of FSH and LH may be significantly reduced in some patients during the first year of chronic treatment (TABLE 7).

TABLE 7

"SIDE EFFECTS" OF CHRONIC METHADONE USE
BIOCHEMICAL AND PHYSIOLOGICAL ALTERATIONS*
ENDOCRINE AND NEUROENDOCRINE ALTERATIONS

Prior to development of full tolerance to narcotic effects (2–12 months in treatment)
  ↓ FSH levels
  ↓ LH levels
  Abnormal metyrapone test (hypothalamic reserve)

Persistent alterations in some patients (early effects that persist more than 12 months in treatment)
  ↑ T_4 and T_3 levels secondary to elevated binding protein levels (~50%)
  ↓ Serum testosterone levels (~20–30% of patients)
  ↑ Serum prolactin levels and/or altered diurnal variation in levels (~100% patients)

---

* Based on studies from our laboratory and other reports in the literature.

In both prospective and special studies, it has been shown that levels of these hormones returned to normal after two or more years of chronic methadone treatment. However, we have found that testosterone may remain decreased in around 20–30% of patients after one year of chronic treatment.

It has been well-documented that the acute or subacute administration of narcotics to humans results in a predictable significant reduction in plasma cortisol levels, presumably reflecting a reduction in ACTH levels. It has also been shown that during cycles of subacute or chronic morphine administration in former heroin addicts, both cortisol levels and total urinary excretion of glucocorticoids are reduced. However, our group and others have shown that during chronic long-term methadone administration, plasma cortisol levels are within normal range with a brisk but normal circadian variation.[7, 8, 25, 37] In recent studies to be discussed in more detail, we have also shown that plasma levels of ACTH are normal in patients during chronic long-term methadone maintenance treatment.[37] In early studies reported in 1972 and 1974, we have found that during the first 2 months of chronic methadone treatment, significant alterations of function of the hypothalamic-pituitary adrenal axis *do* exist, as evidenced by abnormal metyrapone test results, indicating reduced hypothalamic-pituitary reserve for release of tropic hormones.[8, 25] We showed that tolerance develops to this effect after three or more months of stabilized methadone treatment.

In 1977 at another New York Academy of Sciences meeting, we reported the very provocative finding of elevated levels of prolactin in significant percentages of methadone-maintained patients, and also, in a highly controlled study of patients maintained on a steady dose of methadone treatment for more than one year, the intriguing finding of altered prolactin release, without or with absolute elevation in prolactin levels.[9] Prolactin levels returned to the normal pattern of diurnal variation following detoxification from methadone. These findings are of considerable interest in attempting to understand both the mechanisms underlying the efficacy of chronic methadone maintenance, and the mechanisms underlying the addictive disease process. Since prolactin is normally under tonic inhibitory control by dopaminergic factors, and possibly by dopamine itself, the finding of persistent responsiveness of prolactin release to peak levels of opioids, even during chronic methadone administration when tolerance has developed to most of the endocrine and neuroendocrine effects of opioids, is very compelling. It suggests that even during long-term treatment, methadone may reduce, antagonize, or block central dopaminergic action. Findings of elevated levels of prolactin in patients maintained on methadone have been made by other groups as well.

We have performed studies to elucidate further the effects of chronic methadone treatment on prolactin release as well as on related peptide and steroid hormones in well-classified subgroups of patients, including otherwise healthy subjects, patients with defined types of chronic liver disease and patients receiving anticonvulsant treatment with phenobarbital and phenytoin, both of which have been shown to lower plasma levels of methadone.[35] One methadone-maintained woman has been followed throughout a normal pregnancy with respect to the effects of methadone on prolactin release. All patients were studied in a metabolic research ward after several days of stabilization during which no other drugs were administered. Normal day–night cycles were established and time of meals and doses of methadone were controlled. Blood specimens were drawn through intravenous catheters before (at 9 am) and at 4 hours (1 pm) and at 10 hours (7 pm) after oral administration of the daily dose of methadone. Plasma levels of methadone were determined by gas-liquid chromatography techniques; peak levels of methadone were observed around four hours after the oral dose. In this group of otherwise healthy maintained patients, plasma levels of FSH and LH were within normal limits and there was a normal diurnal variation in levels. However, peak plasma levels of prolactin occurred in these patients around 4 hours after the oral dose of methadone, the time when peak levels of methadone were also observed. Actual levels of prolactin exceeded the upper limits of normal in some patients only. In all but one patient, the expected diurnal variation of prolactin levels (with highest levels in the morning), was altered with peak levels observed at 1 pm, four hours after the methadone dose. Similar findings were made in patients with chronic liver disease and also in patients receiving anticonvulsant treatment, despite the fact that plasma levels of methadone were much lower in this group.

In the pregnant methadone-maintained patient, plasma levels of methadone were found to become progressively lower during the third trimester of pregnancy.[34] However, peak plasma levels of methadone continued to occur around four hours after oral dosing, and peak plasma levels of prolactin were also observed at that time, even in late pregnancy when prolactin levels were appropriately very high. This responsiveness of prolactin release to peak levels of methadone was thus observed in all subgroups of long-term methadone-maintained patients.

It has been reported that catechol estrogens, along with dopamine, may inhibit prolactin release, whereas estrogenic metabolites of estradiol may facilitate prolactin release. We have carried out studies to determine the effects of chronic methadone treatment on the formation of both catechol estrogens and estrogenic 16-hydroxylated metabolites of estradiol in methadone-maintained patients.[36] Again, in a controlled clinical research setting, sequential studies using radiometric assay techniques were conducted to determine the extent of estradiol metabolism by each pathway.

There were no differences in catechol estrogen formation in otherwise healthy methadone-maintained patients as compared with otherwise healthy unmedicated control subjects. However, catechol estrogen formation was significantly reduced in methadone-maintained patients with chronic liver disease. Further studies are in progress to determine whether catechol estrogen formation is reduced in patients with chronic liver disease who are not receiving methadone.

Significantly increased formation of 16-hydroxylated metabolites of estradiol was found in methadone-maintained patients both without and with chronic liver disease as compared with otherwise healthy control subjects. Since prolactin response to methadone was observed in patients without as well as with chronic liver disease, it is unlikely that reduced peripheral formation of catechol estrogens is a mechanism underlying this phenomenon. However, the findings of increased production of estrogenic metabolites of estradiol in methadone-maintained patients could be of importance.

In reported studies from other laboratories and our own, performed primarily in animals, chronic administration of exogenous opioids or their antagonists have been found either to have no effects or to reduce brain or plasma concentrations of endogenous opioids. In recent studies carried out in the rat, we have shown that chronic administration of methadone (2.5 mg/kg $\times$ 30 days) did not alter levels of β-endorphin in any region of the brain, in the pituitary, or in the plasma.[41] However, chronic administration of the narcotic antagonist, naltrexone (2.0 mg/kg $\times$ 30 days or 4.9 mg/kg $\times$ 36 days), resulted in significantly depressed β-endorphin concentrations in the amygdala, thalamus, and hypothalamus, but not in the pituitary.

It is known that β-endorphin is derived from β-lipotropin and that β-lipotropin and ACTH share a common 31 K precursor. In a variety of studies carried out in animal models and in man, it has been shown that ACTH, β-lipotropin, and β-endorphin are released in parallel with each other both under normal conditions and in stress. Serial metyrapone studies have been performed in patients during and following induction into methadone maintenance treatment. In these early studies, metyrapone was administered in divided doses over a 24-hour period and response was determined by measurement of urinary excretion of 17-hydroxycorticosteroids, which normally rise two- to threefold in response to metyrapone administration because of the blockade of 11-β hydroxylation, which prevents the formation of cortisol by the adrenal cortex. This results in increased release of corticotropin-releasing factor and ACTH, which in turn causes an increase in production by the adrenal of the precursors of cortisol.[8, 25] During the first two months of methadone treatment, at a time when the doses of methadone were being increased, and tolerance was developing to diverse narcotic effects, the response to metyrapone was significantly reduced, indicating suppressed production of corticotropin releasing factor or ACTH in response to chemically induced stress.

However, when the same patients were restudied after three or more months of chronic methadone treatment, the response to metyrapone had become normal, with increased urinary excretion of 17-hydroxycorticosteroids indicating the normal release of increased amounts of corticotropin releasing factor and ACTH in response to stress.

We have recently completed an initial study to determine the effects of long-term administration of methadone on plasma levels of β-endorphin and simultaneously on levels of ACTH and cortisol in man.[37] Eight patients who had received methadone on a daily basis for 2 years or more were studied in a clinical research unit under controlled conditions detailed above. The lower limits of detection of β-endorphin immunoreactivity with the radioimmunoassay used was 7 pg/ml. Plasma levels of β-endorphin were undetectable in one-third of 25 otherwise healthy control subjects, and the mean level of β-endorphin in the remaining control subjects was 12.0 ± 1.9 (SE) pg/ml. Plasma levels of β-endorphin were undetectable in 6 of 8 methadone-maintained patients at time 0, that is, 24 hours after the last dose of methadone, with levels of 19 and 22 pg/ml in the other two patients. At four hours after the methadone dose, around time of peak plasma levels of methadone, plasma levels of β-endorphin were undetectable in 3 of 7 patients with a mean level of 11.3 ± 2.3 (SE) pg/ml in the rest. At eight hours after the methadone dose, plasma levels of β-endorphin were undetectable in 4 of 7 methadone-maintained patients with a mean level of 12.2 ± 1.4 (SE) pg/ml in the others. In this initial study, levels of β-endorphin were not abnormally high in patients maintained on methadone. Although the levels of β-endorphin were undetectable in many patients, similar findings have been made in control subjects in this study as well as in others. Essentially normal levels of β-endorphin were present in those patients with measurable levels of hormones. Methadone, when used on a chronic long-term basis, has no apparent effects on peripheral levels of β-endorphin, according to the results of this initial study.

Plasma levels of ACTH were also determined in these patients using radioimmunoassay techniques. The mean plasma levels of ACTH was 73.1 ± 7.9 (SE) pg/ml at time 0; 88.5 ± 18.1 (SE) pg/ml at four hours; and 84.3 ± 20.7 (SE) pg/ml at eight hours after methadone dose. All of these ACTH levels were within normal limits. Neither ACTH levels nor β-endorphin levels were significantly different at the three time-points studied.

Plasma levels of cortisol were also measured simultaneously in these patients. At time 0, which was at 9 am, the mean plasma cortisol level was 18.3 mg/dl; at four hours the mean level was 6.8; and at eight hours after methadone dose, 7.2 mg/dl. Thus, cortisol levels were within normal limits, and a normal and brisk diurnal variation in these levels was observed.

To summarize what is known about chronic effects of opioids (in particular, methadone), many interesting physiological and biochemical alterations occur, but there are minimal side effects that are clinically detectable in patients during chronic methadone maintenance treatment. Toxicity related to methadone during chronic treatment is extraordinarily rare. To date there has been only one report of a death due to methadone in any methadone-maintained patient. A man who had suffered from severe chronic constipation during methadone maintenance treatment developed complete obstipation, repeatedly refused medical treatment until the day of his death, and died due to complications of complete intestinal obstruction.[42]

Although there have been various reports in animal models of neurotoxicity due to very high doses of methadone, to date there has been only one case reported of a neurological problem specifically linked to chronic methadone treatment.[43] A 25-year-old man who had a seven-year history of heroin addiction and polydrug abuse was admitted to methadone maintenance treatment and within several months began to experience symptoms including light-headedness, dizziness, visual disturbances, speech disturbances, and tremulousness. He was seen by a physician because of these problems, and two months later was seen by other physicians who published this case report. At that time he had chronic movements of the arms, shoulder, and head and his speech was abnormal, with stuttering and difficulties in verbalization. His dose of methadone was slowly reduced and within two months he had reached 0 dose of methadone. No other medications were administered. The choreic movements disappeared and his speech returned to normal. Within six months there was no recurrence of chorea while he remained methadone-free. The findings in this case are similar to those which have been reported following treatment with a variety of anti-psychotic agents. It was suggested by the authors that possibly more cases of this type would be seen. Although this is certainly possible, high dose methadone treatment has been used for over 17 years with approximately 85,000 patients in treatment each year since 1972. Therefore, it is unlikely that neuro-toxicity due to chronic methadone treatment will emerge as a major adverse reaction as it has during chronic use of antipsychotic drugs.

It has been suggested that opioids may be effective in the management of some types of psychiatric disorders. Specifically, it has been suggested that opioids may be used as antipsychotic agents, as antidepressant agents, and also may have a role in the management of panic disorders. The pharmacologic agents usually used to treat these disorders at this time should be considered with respect to their side effects and toxicity. There is no specific information at this time concerning interactions between the various psychotropic drugs and the endogenous opioids.

Antipsychotic neuroleptic drugs such as chlorpromazine and haloperidol are primarily used in the management of thought disorders including a variety of schizophrenic disorders: schizophreniform disorder (if it is not self-limited), brief reactive psychosis (if behavior is dangerous), and also in some cases of atypical psychosis, paranoid disorders, and schizoaffective disorders (TABLE 8). Neuroleptic agents are also indicated for acute management of psychotic de-pressed and manic patients. In the chronic treatment of schizophrenia, some clinicians have recommended the routine concomitant use of anti-Parkinson agents because of the very high prevalence of Parkinson-like syndrome in patients receiving chronic neuroleptic treatment. It has also been suggested that opioids might be effective drugs to use in the management of some of these disorders.

Tricyclic antidepressants such as amitriptyline or imipramine, without or with the addition of neuroleptic agents or other types of psychotropic drugs, are indicated for a variety of affective disorders (TABLE 9). Acute manic episodes may be managed with a neuroleptic followed by chronic treatment with lithium. Major depressive episodes can be managed either with electro convulsant therapy (ECT) or pharmacologically with tricyclic antidepressant without or with acute treatment with neuroleptics. Bipolar disorder is usually managed chronically with lithium although tricyclic antidepressant may be needed in the initial treatment of those patients presenting with depression and neuroleptic agents for agitation. Major depression is usually managed pharmacologically with tricyclic

TABLE 8

THOUGHT DISORDERS AND PHARMACOLOGICAL TREATMENT

Type	Major Features	Treatment
1. Schizophrenic disorders	Delusions; auditory hallucinations; thought disorders; progressive deterioration; duration at least 6 months	a) Neuroleptics (e.g., chlorpromazine, haloperidol, other) b) Often with anti-Parkinson agent c) ECT for resistant cases
2. Schizophreniform disorder	Schizophrenia-like; duration 2 wk–6 mos	Neuroleptics if not self limited
3. Brief reactive psychosis	Psychotic symptoms under stress with no progression	a) Sedative b) Neuroleptics if behavior dangerous
4. Other a) Atypical psychosis	Delusions; progressive dysfunction, e.g. post-partum psychosis	Neuroleptics—some cases
b) Paranoid disorders	Persecutory delusions; no impaired function	Neuroleptics—some cases
c) Schizoaffective disorders	Affective disorder with persistent delusions	Lithium with neuroleptics

antidepressants initially although again, neuroleptic agents may be needed acutely for destructive behavior and lithium therapy has demonstrated efficacy as a prophylactic agent. Cyclothymic disorder may be managed chronically with lithium and finally dysthymic disorder may be treated with psychotherapy alone or in conjunction with tricyclic antidepressants or monoamine oxidase inhibitors. Likewise, both phobic disorders and panic disorder are frequently treated with a combination of imipramine and psychotherapy (TABLE 10).

Side effects, physiological alterations, and toxic reactions due to these various antipsychotic and other psychotropic drugs have been reported extensively but the prevalence of each of these effects is unknown with wide ranges of estimates reported for each effect. These drugs are usually administered on a chronic basis only to patients with significant symptomatology, and often are administered in combination with other drugs, which makes precise delineation of type and prevalence of side effects difficult. However, numerous reports of small and large numbers of patients receiving these drugs have appeared and the clinical side effects as well as toxic reaction observed will be summarized.

The clinical side effects of the tricyclic antidepressant drugs such as imipramine and amitriptyline are usually mild (TABLE 11). They include dry mouth, sweating, dizziness due to hypotension, constipation, disturbed vision, tremor or twitching, hyperactivity, urinary retention, drowsiness, increased sexual desire, palpitations, and blurred vision.[44–52] Of these, the cardiac abnormalities, which have been observed in some patients receiving therapeutic doses, should cause the greatest concern, although apparently the occurrence of these abnormalities becomes significant only when therapeutic doses are exceeded, such as during episodes of drug overdose. Both the phenothiazine neuroleptics and tricyclic antidepressants lower the seizure threshold and must be used with extreme caution in patients with an underlying convulsant disorder. In addition, the anticholinergic effects of neuroleptics and tricyclic antidepressant drugs may increase intraocular pressure and exacerbate glaucoma in some patients.

Clinical side effects or toxic effects of lithium are apparently greater both with respect to prevalence and also potential severity (TABLE 12).[53-70] Thus, close monitoring of doses administered and blood levels of drug achieved are of critical clinical importance. The effects observed include fine or coarse tremor, diarrhea, nausea and vomiting, drowsiness, tinnitus, blurred vision, fatigue, polydypsia and polyuria, vertigo and unsteady gait, and dry mouth. The prevalence of each of these symptoms in different reports varies enormously; however, it seems to be the general concensus that such clinical side effects or toxic effects of lithium are very common during treatment with usual therapeutic doses, and may be expected to occur whenever blood levels of lithium become elevated. In addition there is growing concern about nephrotoxicity and thyrotoxicity in some patients receiving chronic lithium treatment.

Of even greater significance with respect to potential serious morbidity, especially when coupled with the apparent prevalence, are the clinical side effects or toxic effects observed during chronic treatment with antipsychotic, neuroleptic drugs such as chlorpromazine or haloperidol (TABLE 13).[44, 71-82] A variety of movement disorders, some of which resemble Parkinson's syndrome

TABLE 9

AFFECTIVE DISORDERS AND PHARMACOLOGICAL TREATMENT

Type	Major Features	Treatment
1. Manic episode	Mania; with or without dangerous behavior or agitation	Neuroleptic (acutely for agitation or destructive behavior) Lithium (chronic)
2. Major depressive episodes	Depression, with or without self-destructive behavior	a) Tricyclic antidepressant (e.g. amitriptyline or imipramine) b) ECT if severe c) Neuroleptics (acutely for agitation or destructive behavior)
3. Bipolar disorder	Mania; depression	a) Lithium (chronic) b) Tricyclic antidepressant (if in depressed phase) c) Neuroleptic (agitated)
4. Major depression	Chronic episodic depression without mania	a) Tricyclic antidepressant b) Neuroleptic (acutely for destructive behavior)
5. Cyclothymic disorder	Depressive and hypomanic periods with periods of normal mood	a) Tricyclic antidepressant for depression b) Lithium for mania
6. Dysthymic disorder	Depression; anger; with periods of normal mood	a) Psychotherapy alone b) Tricyclic antidepressant c) MAO inhibitors

TABLE 10

PHOBIC DISORDERS, ANXIETY STATES, AND PERSONALITY DISORDERS

Type	Major Features	Pharmacological Treatment
1. Phobic disorders a) Agoraphobia b) Agoraphobia with panic c) Social phobia	Fear of being alone or in public places, with or without panic or fear of specific situation	a) Imipramine b) MAO inhibitors— some cases
2. Panic disorder	Discrete episodes of panic or fear with diverse somatic symptoms	a) Imipramine b) Propranolol if cardio-vascular symptoms predominant
3. Generalized anxiety disorder	Persistent anxiety (more than one month) with autonomic hyperactivity, vigilance, apprehension	Minor tranquilizers
4. Borderline personality disorder	Impulsivity; lack of control of anger; identity problems; affective instability; boredom; physically self-damaging acts; abnormal interpersonal relationships	a) Tricyclic antidepressants b) Neuroleptics (low dose) if "mini psychoses" predominant

may be observed clinically, as well as a variety of other adverse effects. These clinical effects include muscular rigidity and tremor, uncoordinated spasmodic movements, involuntary motor restlessness, abnormal movements of face and mouth, dizziness and weakness, nausea and heartburn, constipation, impaired

TABLE 11

CLINICAL SIDE EFFECTS OF ANTIDEPRESSANT DRUGS
(IMIPRAMINE, AMITRIPTYLINE) *

1. Dry mouth
2. Sweating
3. Dizziness
4. Constipation
5. Disturbed vision
6. Tremor or twitching
7. Hyperactivity
8. Urinary retention
9. Drowsiness
10. Increased sexual desire
11. Palpitations
12. Blurred vision

* Observed during chronic treatment.

TABLE 12

CLINICAL SIDE OR TOXIC EFFECTS OF LITHIUM *

1. Fine or coarse tremor
2. Diarrhea
3. Nausea and vomiting
4. Drowsiness
5. Tinnitus
6. Blurred vision
7. Fatigue
8. Polydypsia and polyuria
9. Vertigo and unsteady gait
10. Dry mouth

* Observed during chronic treatment.

ejaculation, galactorrhea, menstrual abnormalities, drowsiness, impaired vision, and jaundice. These are very serious effects affecting multiple organ systems (TABLE 14).

Central nervous system effects include acute extrapyramidal disorders (such as Parkinson's syndrome), dystonia and akathisia, tardive dyskinesia, and somnolence and sedation. Autonomic nervous system effects include orthostatic hypotension, dryness of mouth and other membranes, nausea and vomiting, urinary retention, and constipation or diarrhea. Skin and eye reactions of a variety of types occur. Hepatic effects include acute drug hepatitis and severe progressive cholestatic hepatitis. Agranulocytosis may occur. Neuroendocrine effects include abnormal menses, elevated prolactin levels, and galactorrhea. It is estimated that some type of serious side effect may occur in up to 90% of patients receiving these drugs.

Tardive dyskinesia is in some respects the most disturbing of these adverse, toxic reactions since it may occur during, but also following, chronic treatment with a neuroleptic agent, and since this syndrome, which is also called the

TABLE 13

CLINICAL SIDE OR TOXIC EFFECTS OF ANTIPSYCHOTIC DRUGS
(NEUROLEPTICS, E.G., CHLORPROMAZINE, HALOPERIDOL) *

1. Muscular rigidity, tremor
2. Uncoordinated spasmodic movements
3. Involuntary motor restlessness
4. Abnormal motor movements of face and mouth
5. Dizziness and weakness
6. Nausea and heartburn
7. Constipation
8. Impaired ejaculation
9. Galactorrhea; menstrual abnormalities
10. Drowsiness
11. Impaired vision
12. Jaundice

* Observed during chronic treatment.

TABLE 14

CLASSIFICATION OF MAJOR SIDE EFFECTS OF ANTIPSYCHOTIC DRUGS

I. Central nervous system effects
   A. Acute extrapyramidal disorders
      1. Parkinson's syndrome
      2. Dystonia
      3. Akathisia
   B. Tardive dyskinesia
   C. Somnolence; sedation
   D. Decrease in seizure threshold
II. Autonomic nervous system effects
   A. Orthostatic hypotension
   B. Dryness of mouth and other mucous membranes
   C. Nausea and vomiting
   D. Urinary retention
   E. Constipation or diarrhea
III. Skin and eye effects (including increased intraocular pressure, retinitis pigmentosa and photosensitivity)
IV. Hepatic effects (including acute hepatitis and progressive cholestatic hepatitis)
V. Agranulocytosis
VI. Neuroendocrine effects (abnormal menses; elevated prolactin levels, galactorrhea)

"buccolingual masticatory syndrome" may be irreversible (TABLE 15). No specific treatment is known, although reinstitution or increase in doses of the neuroleptic agent that was used may be beneficial in some cases. However, since the neuroleptic agent itself is clearly implicated in causing this syndrome, many clinicians would recommend discontinuation of neuroleptic treatment and trial of one of a number of diverse agents which have been used with varying degrees of success. The mechanism underlying this disorder is unclear but it is thought to be related to dopamine receptor hypersensitivity, which may occur during chronic treatment with a neuroleptic agent because of chronic receptor blockade, coupled with over-production of dopamine.

In summary, side effects of the antipsychotic agents are multiple and many of them are severe with respect to their morbidity in a variety of organ systems

TABLE 15

TARDIVE DYSKINESIA
"BUCCOLINGUAL MASTICATORY SYNDROME"

Abnormal movements of face and mouth, involuntary rhythmic movements with smacking, puckering or licking of lips, protrusion of cheek by tongue; also, occasionally rhythmic movement of other parts of body

Occurs following or during chronic treatment

May be irreversible; no specific treatment

Mechanism underlying disorder unclear

? Dopamine receptor hypersensitivity (due to chronic receptor blockade + over production of dopamine)

especially the nervous system. During proper usage, side effects and toxic reactions due to lithium are intermediate in their severity, and the side effects and toxicities of tricyclic antidepressants seem to be relatively mild, as are the effects of chronic opioid treatment. It must be emphasized, however, that tolerance and physical dependence, with potential subsequent addiction, develop to the opioids, but not to these other classes of drugs.

Of great interest with respect to an understanding of the mechanism of action of these various psychotropic drugs, and also possibly of the disorders that have been effectively managed by their chronic administration, is that there is one common "side effect" for all of the antipsychotic drugs, the opiates, and other opioids: elevation in plasma levels of prolactin or prolactin release in response to drug occurs during acute and chronic administration of each of these groups of agents (TABLE 16). Prolactin levels increase and become elevated in response

TABLE 16

COMMON "SIDE EFFECT" OF ANTIPSYCHOTIC DRUGS
OPIATES AND OPIOIDS

Elevation in plasma levels of prolactin:

a) Prolactin levels increase and become elevated in response to acute administration of drug

b) Prolactin levels increase to peak levels in response to peak plasma levels of drug during chronic administration (methadone)

c) Tolerance apparently does not develop to these effects

? Prolactin response (increase in levels) to drug a marker of common effect of antipsychotic drugs, opiates and opioids, i.e., inhibition of central dopamine function

to acute administration of each of these types of drugs; prolactin levels increase to their peak levels in response to the peak plasma levels of drug during long-term chronic administration of one opioid, methadone; and finally tolerance apparently does not develop to these drug effects on prolactin release.

It has been previously suggested by many investigators, in consideration of antipsychotic drug therapy, that elevated prolactin levels may be used to monitor compliance. It has also been suggested that the dopaminergic effect of various antipsychotic drugs may be predicted by prolactin response.[83] However, there is still a controversy as to whether abnormalities in dopaminergic function are the central defects in the various psychiatric disorders such as schizophrenia, in which antipsychotic drugs, with their primary action of inhibition of central dopamine function, are effective. In consideration of the potential role of opioids in the management of these diseases, it is of interest that the one neuroendocrine effect to which tolerance does *not* develop during chronic opioid administration is prolactin responsiveness. Thus, increased levels of prolactin following administration of one of these agents may be a marker of a common effect of antipsychotic drugs, opiates, and opioids, specifically, inhibition of central dopamine function, and such inhibition of central dopamine function may be the major action that makes each of these agents effective in the treatment of the disorders in which they have been proven to be efficacious. Thus, one major, if not sole, abnormality in the various disorders effectively managed by these drugs may be excessive central dopaminergic activity.

ACKNOWLEDGMENTS

The author wishes to thank Dr. Robert A. Schaefer for his many helpful comments and Mr. Jay G. Ruckel and Mrs. Waraporn Wun for assistance in compiling the bibliography and preparing the manuscript.

REFERENCES

1. KREEK, M. J. 1973. Plasma and urine levels of methadone. N.Y. State J. Med. **23:** 2773–2777.
2. KREEK, M. J., M. ORATZ & M. A. ROTHSCHILD. 1978. Hepatic extraction of long- and short-acting narcotics in the isolated perfused rabbit liver. Gastroenterology **75:** 88–94.
3. RUBENSTEIN, R. B., M. J. KREEK, N. MBAWA, R. KORN, C. L. GUTJAHR & W. I. WOLFF. 1978. Human spinal fluid methadone levels. Drug and Alcohol Depend. **3:** 103–106.
4. KREEK, M. J., D. L. HACHEY & P. D. KLEIN. 1979. Stereoselective disposition of methadone in man. Life Sci. **24:** 925–932.
5. YAFFE, G. J., R. W. STRELINGER & S. PARWATIKAR. 1973. Physical symptom complaints of patients on methadone maintenance. Proc. 5th Nat. Conf. Methadone Treatment, Vol. **1:** 507–514.
6. KREEK, M. J., L. DODES, S. KANE, J. KNOBLER & R. MARTIN. 1972. Long-term methadone maintenance therapy: Effects on liver function. Ann. Intern. Med. **77:** 598–602.
7. KREEK, M. J. 1973. Medical safety and side effects of methadone in tolerant individuals. J. Am. Med. Assoc. **223:** 665–668.
8. KREEK, M. J. 1973. Physiologic implications of methadone treatment. Proc. 5th Natl. Conf. Methadone Treatment, NAPAN **2:** 824–838.
9. KREEK, M. J. 1978. Medical complications in methadone patients. Ann. N.Y. Acad. Sci. **311:** 110–134.
10. LONGWELL, B., R. J. KESTLER & T. J. COX. 1979. Side effects in methadone patients: A survey of self-reported complaints. Int. J. Addict. **14**(4): 485–494.
11. BEVERLEY, C. L., M. J. KREEK, A. O. WELLS & J. L. CURTIS. 1980. Effects of alcohol abuse on progression of liver disease in methadone-maintained patients. *In* Proceedings on the 41st Annual Scientific Meeting of the Committee on Problems of Drug Dependence. L. S. Harris, Ed.: 399–401. NIDA Research Monograph series, NIDA, Rockville, MD.
12. NOVICK, D., A. GELB, R. STENGER, S. YANCOVITZ, B. ADELSBERG, F. CHATEAU & M. J. KREEK. 1981. Hepatitis B serologic studies in narcotic users with chronic liver disease. Am. J. Gastroenterol. **75:** 111–115.
13. KREEK, M. J., C. L. GUTJAHR, J. W. GARFIELD, D. V. BOWEN & F. H. FIELD. 1976. Drug interactions with methadone. Ann. N.Y. Acad. Sci. **281:** 350–370.
14. KREEK, M. J. 1978. Effects of drugs and alcohol on opiate disposition and actions. *In* Factors Affecting the Action of Narcotics, M. W. Adler, L. Manara & R. Samanin, Eds.: 717–740. Raven Press. New York.
15. KREEK, M. J. 1981. Metabolic interactions between opiates and alcohol. Ann. N.Y. Acad. Sci. **362:** 36–49.

16. ROTHSCHILD, M. A., M. J. KREEK, M. ORATZ, S. S. SCHREIBER & J. G. MONGELLI. 1976. The stimulation of albumin synthesis by methadone. Gastroenterology **71:** 214–220.

17. MATSUYAMA, S. S., V. C. CHARUVASTRA, J. OUREN, J. SCHWARTZ & L. JARVIK. 1980. Immunoglobulin levels in heroin addicts after treatment with methadone and methadyl acetate. Drug/Alcohol Depend. **6:** 345–348.

18. MARKS, C. & R. GOLDRING. 1973. Chronic hypercapnia during methadone maintenance. Ann. Rev. Respirat. Dis. **108:** 1088–1093.

19. SANTIAGO, R. V., A. C. PULIESE & N. H. EDELMAN. 1977. Control of breathing during methadone addiction. Am. J. Med. **62:** 347–354.

20. METCALFE, J., M. J. DUNHAM, G. D. OLSEN & M. A. KRALL. 1980. Respiratory and hemodynamic effects of methadone in pregnant women. Res. Physiol. **42:** 383–393.

21. BLINICK, G. 1968. Menstrual function and pregnancy in narcotics addicts treated with methadone. Nature **219:** 180.

22. CUSHMAN, P., JR. 1973. Plasma testosterone in narcotic addiction. Ann. J. Med. **55:** 452–458.

23. AZIZI, F., G. V. APOSTOLOS, C. LONGSCOPE, et al. 1973. Decreased serum testosterone concentration in male heroin and methadone addicts. Steroids **22:** 467–472.

24. CUSHMAN, O., JR. & M. J. KREEK. 1974. Methadone-maintained patients: Effects of Methadone on plasma testosterone, FSH, LH and prolactin. N.Y. State J. Med. **74:** 1970–1973.

25. CUSHMAN, P., JR. & M. J. KREEK. 1974. Some endocrinologic observations in narcotic addicts. *In* Narcotics and the Hypothalamus. E. Zimmermann & R. George, Eds.: 161–173. Raven Press. New York.

26. MENDELSON, J. H., J .E. MENDELSON & V. D. PATCH. 1975. Plasma testosterone levels in heroin addiction and during methadone maintenance. J. Pharmacol. Exp. Ther. **192:** 211–217.

27. MENDELSON, J. H., R. E. MEYER, J. ELLINGBOE, et al. 1975. Effects of heroin and methadone on plasma cortisol and testosterone. J. Pharmacol. Exp. Ther. **195:** 296–302.

28. SANTEN, R. J. 1974. How narcotics addiction affects reproductive function in women. Contemp. Obstet. Gynecol. **3:** 93–96.

29. SANTEN, R. J., J. SOFSKY, N. BILIC, et al. 1975. Mechanism of action of narcotics in the production of menstrual dysfunction in women. Fertil. Steril. **26:** 538–548.

30. WEBSTER, J. B., J. J. COUPAL & P. CUSHMAN, JR. 1973. Increased serum thyroxine levels in euthyroid narcotic addicts. J. Clin. Endocrinol. Metab. **37:** 928–934.

31. AZIZI, F., A. G. VAGENAKIS, G. I. PORTNAY, et al. 1974. Thyroxine transport and metabolism in methadone and heroin addicts. Ann. Intern. Med. **80:** 194–199.

32. BASTOMSKY, C. H. & R. R. M. DENT. 1976. Elevated serum concentrations of thyroxine-binding globulin and ceruloplasmin in methadone-maintained patients. Clin. Res. **24:** 655A.

33. RENAULT, P. F., C. R. SCHUSTER, R. L. HEINRICH, et al. 1972. Altered plasma cortisol response in patients on methadone maintenance. Clin. Pharmacol. Ther. **13:** 269–273.

34. CUSHMAN, P. JR. 1972. Growth hormone in narcotic addiction. J. Clin. Endocrinol. Metab. **35:** 352–358.

35. KREEK, M. J. & E. KHURI. 1979. Effects of methadone maintenance on prolactin release. 1979. Abstract of The Endocrine Society Ann. Meet., Anaheim, CA. p. 289.

36. KREEK, M. J., H. L. BRADLOW, R. MILLMAN & E. KHURI. 1981. Effects of chronic narcotic treatment on catechol estrogen formation in man. Endocrinology. In press.

37. KREEK, M. J., S. L. WARDLAW, J. FRIEDMAN, B. SCHNEIDER & A. G. FRANTZ. 1981. Effects of chronic exogenous opioid administration on levels of one endogenous opioid (β-endorphin) in man. *In* Advances in Endogenous and Exogenous Opioids. E. Simon & H. Takagi, Eds.: 354–366. Kodansha Ltd. Publishers. Tokyo.

38. KREEK, M. J. 1979. Methadone disposition during the perinatal period in humans. Pharmacol. Biochem. Behav. **11**(Suppl.): 7–13.

39. ZIRING, B. S., M. J. KREEK & L. T. BROWN. 1981. Methadone disposition following oral versus parenteral dose administration in rats during chronic treatment. Drug Alcohol Depend. **7**: 311–318.

40. NAKAMURA, K., D. L. HACHEY, M. J. KREEK, C. S. IRVING & P. D. KLEIN. 1981. Quantitation of methadone enantiomers in man using stable labeled methadone-$^2H_3$, $^2H_5$, $^2H_8$. J. Pharmacol. Sci. In press.

41. RAGAVAN, V. V., S. L. WARDLAW, M. J. KREEK & A. G. FRANTZ. 1981. Depletion of hypothalamic β-endorphin after chronic naltrexone administration. Clin. Res. **29**: 431A.

42. SPIRA, I. A., R. RUBENSTEIN, D. WOLFF, *et al.* 1975. Fecal impaction following methadone ingestion simulating acute intestinal obstruction. Ann. Surg. **181**: 15–19.

43. WASSERMAN, S. & M. D. YAHR. 1980. Choreic movements induced by the use of methadone. Arch. Neurol. **37**: 727–728.

44. KLEIN, D. F., R. GITTELMAN, F. QUITKIN & A. RIFKIN. 1980. Diagnosis and Drug Treatment of Psychiatric Disorders: Adults and Children. 2nd edit. Williams & Wilkins. Baltimore, MD.

45. GLASSMAN, A. H., E. V. GIARDINA, J. M. PEREL, J. T. BIGGER JR., S. J. KANTOR & M. DAVIES. 1979. Clinical characteristics of imipramine-induced orthostatic hypotension. Lancet **1**: 468–472.

46. LOWRY, M. R. & F. J. DUNNER. 1980. Seizures during tricyclic therapy. Am. J. Psychiatry **137**: 1461–1462.

47. RACY, J. & A. WARD-RACY. 1980. Tinnitus in imipramine therapy. Am. J. Psychiatry **137**(7): 854–855.

48. HORST, D. A., N. D. GRACE & P. M. LaCOMPTE. 1980. Prolonged cholestasis and progressive hepatic fibrosis following imipramine therapy. Gastroenterology **79**: 550–554.

49. YON, J. & S. ANURAS. 1975. Hepatitis caused by amitriptyline therapy. J. Am. Med. Assoc. **232**: 833–834.

50. LANGOU, R. A., C. VAN DYKE, S. R. TAHAN & L. S. COHEN. Cardiovascular manifestations of tricyclic antidepressant overdose. Am. Heart J. **100**(4): 458–464.

51. GAWIN, F. H. & R. A. MARKOFF. 1981. Panic anxiety after abrupt discontinuation of amitriptyline. Am. J. Psychiatry **138**(1): 117–118.

52. TOBIS, J. M. & W. S. ARONOW. 1981. Cardiotoxicity of amitriptyline and doxepin. Clin. Pharmacol. Ther. **29**(3): 359–364.

53. REISBERG, B. & S. GERSHON. 1979. Side effects associated with lithium therapy. Arch. Gen. Psychiatry **36**: 879–887.

54. PRIEN, R. 1980. Update on lithium. Psychopharm. Bull. **16**(4): 13–15.

55. BONE, S., S. P. ROOSE, D. L. DUNNER & R. R. FIEVE. 1980. Incidence of side effects in patients on long-term lithium therapy. Am. J. Psychiatry **137**(1): 103–104.

56. HAGMAN, A., K. ARNMAN & L. RYDEN. 1979. Syncope caused by lithium treatment. Acta Med. Scand. **205**: 467–471.

57. DONALDSON, J. O., M. S. HALE & M. KLAU. 1981. A case of reversible pure-word deafness during lithium toxicity. Am. J. Psychiatry **138**(2): 242–243.

58. POHL, R. B., R. BERCHOU & B. K. GUPTA. 1979. Lithium-induced hypothyroidism and thyroiditis. Biol. Psychiatry **14**(5): 835–837.

59. JEFFERSON, J. W. 1979. Lithium carbonate-induced hypothyroidism. J. Am. Med. Assoc. **242**: 271–272.

60. SCHOENBERG, M., T. O. T. TSO & A. N. MEISEL. 1979. Single case study: Graves's disease manifesting after maintenance lithium. J. Nerv. Ment. Dis. **167**(9): 575–577.

61. PREODOR, D., E. A. WOLPERT, A. GIMBLE & P. C. HOLINGER. 1979. Single case study: Lithium toxicity with hypothyroidism as a possible determinant. J. Nerv. Ment. Dis. **167**(3): 186–188.

62. MIZRAHI, E. M., J. F. HOBBS & D. I. GOLDSMITH. 1979. Brief clinical and laboratory observations: Nephrogenic diabetes insipidus in transplacental lithium intoxication. J. Pediatrics **94**(3): 493–495.

63. FEINBERG, M., M. STEINER & B. J. CARROLL. 1979. Effects of long-term lithium treatment on serum calcium, magnesium, and calcitonin. Psychopharm. Bull. **15**(2). 81–84.

64. DAVIS, B. M., A. PFEFFERBAUM, S. KRUTZIK & K. L. DAVIS. 1981. Lithium's effect on parathyroid hormone. Am. J. Psychiatry **138**(4): 489–492.

65. RICHMAN, A. V., H. L. MASCO, S. I. RIFKIN & M. K. ACHARYA. Minimal-change disease and the nephrotic syndrome associated with lithium therapy. Ann. Intern. Med. **92**: 70–72.

66. WAHLIN, A., W. RAPP & E. H. JONSSON. 1980. Failure of chlorothiazide to improve urinary concentrating capacity in lithium-treated patients. Acta Med. Scand. **207**: 195–196.

67. BUCHT, G., A. WAHLIN, R. WENTZEL & B. WINBLAD. 1980. Renal function and morphology in long-term lithium and combined lithium-neuroleptic treatment. Acta Med. Scand. **208**: 381–385.

68. MOSKOVITZ, R., P. SPRINGER & M. URZUHART. 1981. Lithium-induced nephrotic syndrome. Am. J. Psychiatry **138**(3): 382–383.

69. VESTERGAARD, P. & K. THOMSEN. 1981. Renal side effects of lithium: the importance of the serum lithium level. Psychopharmacology **72**(2): 203–204.

70. COLT, E. W. D., D. KIMBRELL & R. R. FIEVE. 1981. Renal impairment, hypercalcemia, and lithium therapy. Am. J. Psychiatry **138**(1): 106–108.

71. KECHKICH, W. A. 1978. Neuroleptics: Violence as a manifestation of akathisia. J. Am. Med. Assoc. **240**(20): 2185.

72. KLAWANS, H. L., D. K. FALK, P. A. NAUSIEDA & W. J. WEINER. 1978. Gilles de la tourette syndrome after long-term chlorpromazine therapy. Neurology **28**: 1064–1066.

73. ZARRABI, M. H., S. ZUCKER, F. MILLER, R. M. DERMAN, G. S. ROMANO, J. A. HARTNETT & A. O. VARMA. 1979. Immunologic and coagulation disorders in chlorpromazine-treated patients. Ann. Intern. Med. **91**: 194–199.

74. EVANS, D. L., J. F. ROGERS & S. C. PEIPER. 1979. Intestinal dilatation associated with phenothiazine therapy: A case report and literature review. Am. J. Psychiatry **136**(7): 970–972.

75. GOLDMAN, L. S., J. I. HUDSON & W. W. WEDDINGTON. 1980. Lupus-like illness associated with chlorpromazine. Am. J. Psychiatry **137**(12): 1613–1614.

76. MORRIS, H. H., III, W. F. McCORMICK & J. A. REINARZ. 1980. Neuroleptic malignant syndrome. Arch. Neurol. **37**(7): 462–463.

77. GERLACH, J. & H. SIMMELSGAARD. 1978. Tardive dyskinesia during and following treatment with haloperidol, haloperidol + biperiden, thioridazine, and clozapine. Psychopharmacology **59**: 105–112.

78. WEINER, M. F. 1979. Haloperidol, hyperthyroidism and sudden death. Am. J. Psychiatry **136**(5): 717.

79. PECK, V. & L. SHENKMAN. 1979. Haloperidol-induced syndrome of inappropriate secretion of antidiuretic hormone. Clin. Pharm. Ther. **26**(4): 442–444.

80. CUTLER, N. R. & J. F. HEISER. 1979. Leukopenia following treatment with thiothixene and haloperidol. J. Am. Med. Assoc. **242**(26): 2872–2873.
81. MEHTA, D., S. MEHTA, J. PETIT & W. SHRINER. 1979. Cardiac arrhythmia and haloperidol. Am. J. Psychiatry. **136**(11): 1468–1469.
82. MIZRAHI, E. M., D. HOLTZMAN & B. THARP. 1980. Haloperidol-induced tardive dyskinesia in a child with Gilles de la Tourette's disease. Arch. Neurol. **37**(12): 780.
83. DE LA FUENTE, J.-R. & A. H. ROSENBAUM. 1981. Prolactin in psychiatry. Am. J. Psychiatry **138**(9): 1154–1160.

THE INTERACTION OF A TREATMENT PROGRAM USING OPIATES FOR MENTAL ILLNESS AND AN ADDICTION TREATMENT PROGRAM

Herbert D. Kleber

Department of Psychiatry
Yale University School of Medicine
and Substance Abuse Treatment Unit
Connecticut Mental Health Center
New Haven, Connecticut 06508

INTRODUCTION

While there is evidence, historical,[1] clinical,[2] and experimental,[3] suggesting that opiate-type drugs have an ameliorating effect on psychotic symptoms, the case is far from clear for there are contrary findings indicating no such effect.[4,5] Since it has been noted by Voltaire that "a long dispute means both parties are wrong," it may very well be that, whatever effect there is, is not a clear-cut one. A number of variables, including the particular symptomatology of the patient, the duration of his illness, the dose of the drug, and the duration it is given, may all be related to outcome. This paper will not concern itself with the rightness or wrongness of the proposition that opiates do affect schizophrenic or other symptoms. Instead, I will assume that there is some effect and that it is large enough to justify, in some cases at least, the use of opiate-type drugs to treat psychiatric syndromes. In such cases, what would be the best way of administering the drug to achieve optimal results both in terms of the patient and of the larger society? This paper will look at some of the options and the problems associated with each.

The important complications that exist in thinking about the use of these drugs outside of the treatment of narcotic addiction are the current legal status of opiates, and the existence of a large group of individuals who obtain such drugs illicitly. The great monetary value placed on illicit supplies of the drug because of the above factors means that a system that simply makes quantities of the drug available as needed to patients on a take-out or prescriptive basis may create problems elsewhere in society.

THE EXISTING PSYCHIATRIC SYSTEM

With these concerns in mind, let us look first at the existing delivery system for treatment of the psychotic patient. At present a schizophrenic patient who is being maintained on a drug like chlorpromazine is likely to obtain it from a private practitioner or clinic and receive a prescription for at least two to four weeks of the drug, since the chronic psychotic patient is unlikely to be seen on a weekly basis. Where there is concern about compliance with such a regime or other constraining factors, the patient instead may be given a shot of the depot form of a drug like fluphenazine. The patient is expected to return for another shot approximately one month hence.

173

0077–8923/82/0398–0173 $1.75/0 © 1982, NYAS

The prescriptive system works only partially since, as pointed out by Black-well and others,[6,7] the incidence of patients continuing to take the drug after discharge from state hospitals, for example, is no higher than about 50%. However, it is a relatively economic way of dispensing the medication and for a significant number of patients provides them with a drug at relatively low cost and in a manner easily utilized, namely, having the medication at home and only having to come in for refills at prolonged intervals. In thinking about using this system for the giving of opiate drugs to these patients, one should start with the chronic psychotic individual since it is most likely these are the patients who will get such drugs. Because of the danger of addiction or of altering on a lasting basis the endogenous opiate-like neurotransmitters, it is unlikely that opiate drugs would be given to the acute schizophrenic who could be managed readily with the routine neuroleptics, unless the opiates show a remarkably powerful effect. While at some point the dangers of tardive dyskinesia may need to be balanced against the dangers of addiction, more evidence of efficacy for the narcotic would have to be present in order to make the equation come close. Thus it is likely we are dealing with the chronic psychotic patient and perhaps one with tardive dyskinesia. The advantages of using the present system are those that have been enumerated. The system provides a cheap, easily available source of drugs. The patients are not inconvenienced by numerous visits to a clinic and not stigmatized any more than they already are.

The disadvantages are also readily apparent. Since there is no equivalent to the depot phenothiazines for the narcotics, and since even the long-acting form of methadone, LAAM, is not yet readily available, we need to assume a scenario in which the patient has to take one dose of methadone every 24 hours. If one simply gives these patients a prescription to last a week or two, one is left with a situation in which the most vulnerable of patients may be confronted by the most artful of dodgers. The compulsive neediness of the addict in terms of getting his medication at a price he can afford is likely to win out much of the time over the relative fragility of the schizophenic. The problem this creates is not just the one for the larger society of making illicit narcotics more readily available. There is, of course, also the problem of the patients who would be deprived of medication useful to them in the treatment of their illness. Further, since missing doses of the narcotic, once the individual is dependent, would lead to withdrawal, the schizophrenic patients may not only have to do without the drug on days when they get ripped off by addicts or sell their drug for money, but may also have to go through withdrawal on those days. The money aspect cannot be overlooked either since schizophrenics tend to be downwardly mobile socially, and shortage of funds is a perennial problem. The monetary value of the narcotics to them in their lifestyle thus may be significant. While this has some appeal in terms of solving some of the economic problems of schizophrenics, it may encounter public opposition and generate adverse publicity toward such programs.

THE ADDICTION TREATMENT SYSTEM

Let us turn now to the advantages and disadvantages of dispensing the narcotic medication, which presumably would be methadone or LAAM through the addiction treatment system as opposed to the psychiatric treatment system. Even in thinking about this, certain points immediately come to mind. First of all, the philosophic underpinnings between the two systems are very different. Schizophrenic patients are seen as vulnerable, at times fragile, individuals who have difficulty in coping with the stresses of everyday reality and need to receive support and nurturance. The opinion of Szasz to the contrary, they are usually viewed as mentally ill. Narcotic addicts on the other hand, are often viewed as willful deviants, pursuing a hedonistic life style, unwilling to conform their behavior to rules and structure, needing to be confronted about their rule breaking, and more criminal than mentally ill.

The psychiatric treatment system has found that schizophrenic patients are often reluctant to come to treatment, miss appointments, are ambivalent about taking medication, and often drop out only to return when there is a crisis, either of their own volition or by family members' pressure. While similar points could be made for narcotic addicts, it no longer holds when methadone or other narcotics are involved. Once one uses an addicting drug, the nature of the situation changes. Now we have a system where the individual more often than not is dependent upon the treatment program and the treatment program has acquired certain leverage so that it can expel patients, put them on probation, demand certain kinds of conditions of adherence, and so forth. All of these are relatively absent from the normal treatment of the schizophrenic patient. The methadone treatment program, as it is usually carried out, involves patients coming during the first three months on a six or seven day a week basis. Then, as they display clean urines, they are offered some employment or schooling, and attendance at the therapy activities, and get permission to have take-out medication which increases from the weekend bottles to bottles during the week so that at one point the individual may only have to come in twice a week. In a typical treatment program, if the patient is late for the medication without having called to make arrangements, even if staff is still there, the patient will not be medicated. A similar refusal of medication would follow upon the patient refusing to give up a urine specimen when due or appearing intoxicated at the dispensing window. While schizophrenics may be loathe to engage in treatment, one can probably assume that once they have become addicted to a narcotic they will, more likely than not, show up for the medication and not want to be discharged from the program.

Including these patients in a regular methadone maintenance program poses certain questions. Should one impose the same structure on these patients as one does on the addict as far as being late for medication, failure to attend groups, and so on? Should one take urines to see whether they are abusing other drugs? If they are, should they be expelled? There are no easy answers to these questions. Experienced program managers know that a program can be destroyed if perceived by patients as being run in a discriminatory manner. On the other hand, too rigid enforcement might simply drive the psychotic patients away.

Experience with schizophrenic methadone patients has shown that they often have great trouble adjusting to program rules, and paranoid ones in particular can be very disruptive.[8] To avoid this, it may be necessary to have these patients both a part of the program and yet separate. Separate could mean different dispensing hours and different staff, with time being given by the staff from the larger psychiatric system. Since illicit drug use by some methadone program members tends to be associated with higher amounts of such use by other members if the use is tolerated, it is probable that illicit drug use would need to be treated uniformly. To the extent that rules and structure can be a useful part of the treatment of the chronic patient, then utilizing them with the schizophrenic patient would be all to the better; and to the extent that putting them on a narcotic makes it possible, then the patient and the larger society have both benefited. What happens, however, in rural areas where there are no methadone programs or where it is too far to drive? One possibility is to utilize the drug store mechanism suggested several years back for methadone, whereby these patients could go to a pharmacy in their community and get the medication there. Should they have the same take-out privileges as the addict patients? Probably yes because otherwise they are too tightly bound to a program that would not permit them to go away for weekends and in other ways makes it cumbersome to carry out the various facets of daily living. However, if they were in a program that does not permit take-out for the addicts, then they should be treated no differently.

Another potential difficulty has to do with waiting lists. Currently, especially in the Northeast, many methadone programs have waiting lists of up to six months. Financial stringencies and governmental cutbacks do not bode well for the next three to four years at a minimum. What would happen if similar circumstances were to hold when one wanted to treat schizophrenic patients. Would they be given a different priority, would they not have to wait before coming on? If so, does this not perpetuate a blame theory of addiction in which the addict is seen as a willful individual who uses drugs simply to get high, whereas a schizophrenic is seen as an unfortunate victim of either psychological or biochemical problems, not of his own doing?

This brings me to the final point. Perhaps the major disadvantage against having schizophrenics receiving their medication via methadone programs has to do with stigma and possible contagion. Already clinicians who work in consultational-liaison work are well aware that many cancer patients are reluctant to take methadone, and other patients needing to take chronic pain medication are also reluctant to take the drug because it is identified as a drug for addicts, and they do not wish to be so stigmatized. A similar problem would, of course, hold with schizophrenic patients. The problem of contagiousness is also not one that should be lightly dismissed. To the extent that certain features of the addict's lifestyle are transmittable by peer pressure, cultural influence, and other environmental factors, then one would not want to put into that environment individuals who did not have an addiction problem. To sum up, the major drawbacks against medicating schizophrenic patients with methadone through the traditional psychiatric system would be the problem of developing either a dispensing system parallel to that of methadone programs or else increasing the availability of methadone by prescription with the strong possibility of diversion. It has the advantages of not treating schizophrenics in the addict network with possible stigmatizing and contagiousness as well as greater convenience for the schizophrenic patient. Using the existing methadone treatment centers would have the advantage of less cost, fewer possibilities of diversion, and perhaps greater structure in the schizophrenic's life as the same rules are applied to them as to addicts. The disadvantages would be possible stigmatization and contagiousness as well as structural problems. My own opinion is the former difficulties are more problematic than these latter ones. Programs could have separate medication hours, for example, and other innovative approaches to minimize those difficulties.

It is probable that even with some proven usefulness of the narcotics that the number of patients who would be so treated would not be that great. Schizophrenia makes up only about 1% of the country's population, and it is unclear what percentage of that would benefit from narcotic treatment. Therefore, any one center might not have enough to justify a separate system, and there would be marked economies of scale in combining it with the addict treatment program. In such a program, the normal incidence of schizophrenics is less than 2%.[9] There could also be some useful learning on both sides: the addict programs could teach the staff of traditional psychiatric programs about structure in dealing with patients, and conversely the psychiatric program staff could be helpful to the addict programs in improving their skills in diagnosis, psychotherapy, and the use of ancillary psychotropic medication. One can imagine a useful combining of resources with a net result that each system also becomes more knowledgeable and competent in dealing with patients from the other system.

I welcome the possibility that it may be shown that drugs of the opioid class have certain antipsychotic or antimanic effects. New additions to our therapeutic armamentarium are always sought for. I would like to add a note of caution in closing, however, by describing a cartoon I have on my office wall, given me by a patient. It shows a doctor handing some drugs to a patient and saying, "Now this drug will cure your psoriasis, but the side effects may turn you into a frog!"

REFERENCES

1. CARLSON, E. T. & M. M. SIMPSON. 1963. Opium as a tranquilizer. Am. J. Psychiatry **120:** 112–117.
2. BERKEN, G. H., M. M. STONE & S. K. STONE. 1978. Methadone in schizophrenic rage: A case study. Am. J. Psychiatry **135:** 2, 248–249.
3. BERGER, P. A., S. J. WATSON, H. AKIL, et al. 1980. Beta-endorphin and schizophrenia. Arch. Gen. Psychiatr. **37:** 635–640.
4. WIKLER, A. 1952. Opiates and opiate antagonists: A review of their mechanisms of action in relation to clinical problems. Public Health Monograph No. 52, U.S. Dept. of Health, Education & Welfare, Washington, D.C.
5. JUDD, L. L., D. S. JANOWSKY, D. S. SEGAL, et al. 1981. Behavioral effects of methadone in schizophrenic patients. Am. J. Psychiatry **138(2):** 243–245.
6. LIPMAN, R. S., K. RICKELS, E. H. ULENHUTH, L. C. PARK & S. FISHER. 1965. Neurotics who fail to take their drugs. Br. J. Psychiatry **111:** 1043–1049.
7. McCLELLAN, T. A. & G. COWAN. 1970. Use of antipsychotic and antidepressant drugs by chronically ill patients. Am. J. Psychiatry **126(12):** 1771.
8. SALZMAN, B., M. KURIAN, A. DEMIRJIAN, et al. 1973. The paranoid schizophrenic in a methadone maintenance program. 5th Natl. Conf. on Methadone Treatment, Wash., D.C., Natl. Assoc. for Prevention of Addiction to Narcotics.
9. ROUNSAVILLE, B. J., M. M. WEISSMAN, H. D. KLEBER & C. WILBER. 1981. The heterogeneity of psychiatric diagnosis in treatment of opiate addicts. Arch. Gen. Psychiatry. In press.

THE PROVISION OF OPIOID THERAPY
TO THE MENTALLY ILL:
CONCEPTUAL AND PRACTICAL CONSIDERATIONS

Robert B. Millman

Departments of Public Health and Psychiatry
Cornell University Medical College
New York, New York 10021

INTRODUCTION

A controlled study is presently being developed in the Department of Psychiatry of the Cornell University Medical College-Payne Whitney Clinic to assess the efficacy of opioids in selected schizophrenic patients. Provocative data from a number of similar and dissimilar studies have been published; additional data are being presented in this volume.[1] A number of important conceptual and organizational issues arise in considering this mode of therapy. These include who should be tried on opiates, how these should be given, particularly on an outpatient basis, and what constitute the potential risks of the medication or the system of delivery. This discussion will focus on some of the issues integral to the development of further studies and demonstration treatment programs.

The need for new treatments is clear. Whereas the major tranquilizers have proven to be of immense value in the treatment of the chronically mentally ill, patients are often loath to take them. Although these drugs may be tolerated when patients are acutely ill and in relapse, they are often unpalatable when patients are feeling better or leave the hospital milieu. It has been well documented that a major factor in the relapse of psychotic patients and over 50% of psychiatric hospital readmissions, is the reluctance and subsequent failure of these patients to adhere to their prescribed posthospital medication schedules.[3, 4]

There is a dearth of systematically obtained information available as to what sort of patients will respond to opiates. There is good evidence that opiates are useful in certain patients with acute psychotic illness. This information is derived from ancedotal reports made for several hundred years, as well as clinical observations made more recently. The normalizing effects of heroin on street addicts, the use of illicit opiates in treating the acute psychotic episodes induced by psychedelic drugs, and reports from methadone maintenance treatment programs are quite persuasive.[1, 2, 5, 6] It is probable that an important element in some acute psychotic episodes is anxiety; perhaps the anxiety precipitates or fuels the disordered thinking. There is some evidence that benzodiazepines may be useful in these episodes, though this class of drugs is also in disfavor in psychiatric hospitals. It is suggested that opioids or perhaps benzodiazepines should be given a careful trial in these patients. Manic or depressed patients may also under certain circumstances be candidates for opioid therapy.

At the same time, since drugs in conventional usage, particularly major tranquilizers, are reasonably effective in these acute states, it is difficult to justify the use of opiates as a first-line medication in such situations. The administration of opioid drugs is fraught with significant dangers. Continued or prolonged use will induce tolerance and physical dependence and may lead to craving and

178

0077-8923/82/0398-0178 $1.75/0 © 1982, NYAS

drug-seeking behavior. The risk of opiate overdose is ever present. The media and lay public including family and friends, have an extremely jaundiced view of opioid drugs. They may view as addicts opioid-maintained people with no history of drug abuse. Then too, physicians are not familiar with these drugs and may not handle them with competence and restraint. Diversion of the drugs for illicit purposes is likely to occur unless careful regulation is insured. These problems may well be answerable. For example, there is good evidence that patients who change settings or others who are not drug abusers will experience abstinence syndromes when they are withdrawn, but will not continue or initiate drug-seeking behavior. Viet Nam veterans who were able to cease opiate use when they returned home, or the pain patients who had no continued drug craving when their pain defervesced, have been so described.[7, 8] Given these very real problems, however, it is not likely that committees on human experimentation or public narcotic regulatory agencies will be sanguine about encouraging the investigations or use of these drugs in this new patient population who already have acceptable treatments available.

PSYCHIATRIC PERSPECTIVES AND NOSOLOGY

It is probable that in most early studies chronically ill patients who are quite disorganized, who have well-defined psychotic symptoms, and who have not responded to other modes of therapy will be allowed a therapeutic trial of opiates. These will include patients with persistent symptomatology and disability or those whose assaultive or belligerent behavior is difficult to control. There are good data from existing studies that suggest that some of these difficult chronic patients do respond to opiates, but also that many do not. Others respond to narcotic antagonists.[1, 9] A major problem in these studies may relate to psychiatric nosology. It is likely that a number of different illnesses are presently subsumed under the diagnosis of psychotic thinking disorders or affective disorders. The Diagnostic Statistical Manual (DSMIII) attempts to refine diagnostic discriminative decisions, though for the most part it remains descriptive and quite primitive. It is likely that presenting signs and symptoms may be quite similar in some of these states though the psychobiology and characteristics of neurotransmitters or receptors may be quite different. Perhaps comprehensive discussions of a small number of cases will be more useful than the present mode of collecting superficial data on a large number of cases. For example, a patient who presents with paranoid psychotic signs and symptoms with anxiety may be quite different from one without anxiety; it is probable that the former would be more likely to respond to opiates. Perhaps a careful analysis of the opiate responders and nonresponders may result in more precise diagnostic formulations.

Many workers in the field have come to appreciate these diagnostic difficulties. Despite the admonitions of our teachers who have borrowed phrases from other branches of medicine, accurate diagnosis is often not the key to selection of appropriate therapies in psychotic patients. The severity of the disorder may be more important than the diagnostic formulation. Parenthetically, I might mention that in an hour-long psychiatric case conference, 50 minutes are traditionally devoted to diagnostic formulation with input from a wide variety of people including psychiatrists, social workers, and recreational therapists. Routinely, 10 minutes are devoted to therapy, and the selection of the therapeutic strategy often derives little from the interminable discussion.

Despite the presumed therapeutic efficacy, there are significant conceptual difficulties that are likely to compromise the success of opioid pharmacotherapy. The first of these arises from the understandable eagerness of psychiatry to emulate medicine and the other heretofore more biologically oriented clinical disciplines. In medicine or surgery we were taught to compare the medical management of gallbladder disease with cholecystectomy; results were measured in morbidity and mortality. The technology was what was being compared, and that is what biologically oriented psychiatric workers also are doing. There seems to be undue reliance on the search for specific technological solutions to cure mentally ill people. Even if schizophreniform or affective illness is biologically or genetically determined, social and dynamic factors may also be important determinants of the illness. Etiology is often complex, and nonbiological factors may be necessary modifiers of biological predisposition. Then too, given a particular psychiatric illness, whatever the cause, it is likely that social and psychodynamic adjustment will be importantly influenced.

CHRONIC MENTAL PATIENTS

An additional conceptual difficulty derives from the idea that if replacement or corrective medication can be found, mental illness will become like pneumococcal pneumonia, an acute illness and liable to complete cure. This seems to be an unrealistic assumption. Even if a biochemical deficit or derangement such as inadequate endorphins or abnormal receptors is corrected, it is probable that many of these people will remain disabled to some extent. Perhaps only because they have lived for some years with disease and have not mastered some of the social and economic tasks that remain a trial for healthy people.

Most mental illness is likely to remain chronic just as most physical illness is. The pneumonia model is extremely limited in medicine. For example, most internists devote their time to treating diabetes or congestive heart failure. They have excellent tools to do this, of course—insulin and digitalis, for example—but these merely control the disease or slow deterioration. Treatment in these diseases, as in most forms of mental illness even with better pharmacotherapies, must be seen as long-term in nature and requiring a diverse array of therapeutic tools in addition to pharmacological agents.

To belabor a point, during the last 20 to 30 years, remarkable pharmacological strides have been made in the treatment of mental illness, but the clear impression remains that the chronically ill are receiving inadequate treatment and will continue to do so even if opiates prove to be effective and are widely accepted. This inadequacy derives from economic and procedural issues in addition to the serious and chronic nature of the illnesses being treated.[10]

Practicing psychiatrists do not often treat the chronically mentally ill, particularly psychotics or others whose function is severely impaired. A primary reason for this is that many of these people are not wealthy enough to afford the onerous costs of private psychiatric care. These chronic patients come disproportionately from the poorer classes; the evidence suggests that many patients started poor and, in fact, poverty may be a determinant of the expression of their illness. In other cases, chronically ill patients drift downward because they lose their jobs or become separated from their families.[11] They are thus dependent on institutions and the public system, where they are generally given infrequent and superficial care. The so-called medication clinics of a university hospital reflects this reliance on pharmacotherapy with almost no resources available to provide any other sort of support. Patients are seen monthly or less, for 5 to 15 minutes; they are asked some desultory questions and their prescriptions are refilled. When they deteriorate, and they often do, they drop out of outpatient care and are eventually readmitted to the hospital.

This is not to say that the therapists are inexpert or inhumane; they are doing the best they can given the economics and organization of the system. Then too, anyone who has cared for these chronically ill people understands that it is grindingly difficult work.

It may be useful to translate the idea of the chronically mentally ill into clinical terms. These people do not change much. There might be some improvement; more often there is some deterioration. Clinic treatment staff must see the same patients day after day, year after year. Crises do occur and staff must be able to handle these episodes. But these merely punctuate the essentially unchanging nature of the patient care experience. It is not surprising that staff become depleted or "burnt out" in this endeavor. There is often little to talk about and interactions become routine and boring. It is no wonder that when private therapists are able to afford to, they transfer these patients to other younger, less-experienced therapists or to clinic situations.

It is interesting to conjecture why other sorts of psychiatric chronic-care givers—for example, psychoanalysts or some private psychotherapists in contrast to clinic personnel—are able to retain their enthusiasm. It may in part be related to the fact that the population they treat is often not very disabled and lead reasonably interesting lives, with change and even improvement to be expected. In addition, the jargon, dogma, and perspectives of dynamic and biological psychiatry insulate therapists from the failures and chronicity of their patients. Therapists are able to talk about the intricacies of diagnosis and transference and not be so sensitive to the defeats of caring for chronically ill people. Research is also a useful way to insulate the therapist from the patient; interest in failure as well as success may be maintained. This is considerably more difficult in medication clinics, charged with the care of psychotic and impoverished patients. The patients are more disabled and the staff are often less well trained, less professional, and so less able to protect themselves from the experience of the patient.

METHADONE MAINTENANCE

The existing model for delivering opioids to patients, methadone maintenance for narcotic addicts, reflects these same procedural and conceptual difficulties. Patients are in essence chronic mental patients, though even less appreciated. The determinants of addiction are chronic, including psychological, social, and pharmacological factors. Programs are organized to safeguard the methadone, deliver it in a controlled fashion, and provide some psychosocial supports, all in as inexpensive a manner as possible. They are subject to a complicated and confusing array of regulations and inspections to insure that the possibility of narcotic diversion is minimized and that minimum levels of care, or at least paper work, are provided. Of necessity, most of the programs deliver methadone efficiently but are unable to provide the extensive psychosocial supports necessary, even to the most severely disturbed patients. Counselor-patient ratios may be one to 50 or 75 and there is generally little psychiatric backup.

Although many of these patients are helped significantly, in other cases the treatment merely stabilizes the situation or perhaps slows the deteriorative processes.[6, 12] In the face of these conditions, and similar to what happens to front-line therapists for the nonaddicted chronically ill, staff become depleted and are unable to extend themselves for the care of these patients. It is likely that the problems inherent to the present care systems for chronic mental patients as well as for heroin addicts maintained on methadone, will be compounded should opioid therapy be provided for psychiatric patients.

TREATMENT OF NONDISEASE

Opioids may well prove to be useful in the treatment of a variety of psychiatric disease states. This is well within the medical model, and the responsibility for diagnosis and treatment remains firmly in the hands of physicians and other certified practitioners. Prescribing euphoriants to make people feel or do better is more problematic. Pain, grief, insomnia, and anxiety may all occur in the absence of disease or pathology and are often treated with drugs by physicians. Athletes, astronauts, and entertainers are also treated by physicians to improve their performance. Propranolol, for example, has received some acceptance as a treatment of "stage fright." Physicians and others also employ nonpharmacological means to enhance the sense of well-being, pleasure, or performance of "normal" or "healthy" people. Examples would include cosmetic surgery, sex therapy, sports medicine, and perhaps some psychoanalysis. Opioids are a powerful tool, and the implications of treating simple unhappiness, prolonged grief or situational depression, or "normal" senile dementia must be carefully considered. It is questionable whether physicians or biomedical scientists have the necessary perspective or wisdom to make these decisions. Perhaps some of these decisions should be left in the hands of the "patients," though it will then be difficult to distinguish these people from drug abusers.[13]

OUTPATIENT TREATMENT MODEL

The provision of opioids to patients with psychiatric illness while they are inpatients may be effected within existing medical care structures. Certainly patients with severe pain are routinely treated with opiates within the hospital, albeit often inadequately. It is when psychiatric patients leave the hospital that difficulties arise. The criteria for an acceptable outpatient treatment model should include the following:

1. provision for effective pharmacotherapy;
2. provision for a positive therapeutic milieu, psychosocial supports, and psychotherapy;
3. manageable costs;
4. reduced risk of diversion of the medication; and
5. acceptability to patients.

There are four possible models under consideration. They are the private psychiatrist, the hospital-based psychiatric clinic, inclusion of these patients in existing methadone maintenance treatment programs for opiate addicts, and development of a new generation of maintenance programs for psychiatric patients. These are compared in TABLE 1. The traditional model for delivering

TABLE 1

DELIVERY OF OPIOID THERAPY TO PSYCHIATRIC PATIENTS

Treatment Modality	Effective Psychotherapy and Pharmacotherapy	Positive Therapeutic Milieu	Cost	Risk of Diversion	Patient Acceptability
Private psychiatrist-psychotherapist	High	Low	High	High	High
Hospital-based psychiatric clinic	Variable, low	Low	Variable	High	Low
Existing methadone program for addicts	Low	Variable, low	Low	Low	Low
New generation of maintenance program for psychiatric patients	Variable, potentially high	Variable, potentially high	Variable, potentially high	Low	Variable, potentially high

medical care, including psychiatric services, is that of the private physician on a fee-for-service basis. This model might be appropriate for opioid maintenance of certain patients provided they have the money to pay for private care and do not require extensive psychosocial supports. Private care is generally limited to one or two sessions per week. Psychotherapy is supportive in nature, but issues of residential or vocational placement and economic support are often not well considered. In this model the risk of diversion of the medication is high.

A subcommittee of The New York Academy of Medicine is presently considering the development of a system whereby private practitioners might provide methadone treatment for selected narcotic addicts. It was recognized that some well-functioning patients would be less inconvenienced and would do better in a more traditional medical care system. The issue is particularly pressing in the current era of waiting lists for overcrowded programs, where the quality of the therapeutic milieu is questionable. This proposal would also be applicable to psychiatric patients.

It is likely that at the outset of these studies, opioid outpatient treatment will be provided in hospital-based outpatient programs in modified medication clinics. These have the many liabilities described earlier. Provision of effective psychotherapy or a positive therapeutic milieu will be difficult in this model, the risk of diversion will be high, though it will not be difficult to develop this capability. Inclusion of these patients in existing methadone maintenance programs would also not be difficult to effect and costs would be low. At the same time, there are many liabilities in this system, as well. Of primary concern is that psychiatric patients in this environment would not be comfortable for social and cultural reasons. Many of them would be harassed. In addition, these programs are unable to provide sufficient psychiatric services to this population.

Perhaps the most promising model for delivering opioid therapy to chronic mental patients would be the development of a new generation of programs related to the methadone maintenance model but focused on psychiatric patients. The major development would be the application of day-hospital or milieu therapy techniques to the existing maintenance model. Caseloads could be reduced to 10 or 20 patients per counselor and comprehensive psychiatric backup would be available. Liaison with an inpatient unit of a psychiatric hospital would be necessary so that easy transition could be made between the inpatient and the outpatient phase, or vice versa. The physical facility would be sufficiently large and attractive so that patients might spend significant portions of time in the facility on a daily basis. Comprehensive services including legal, vocational, and educational services might be available in this program. This is an expensive undertaking, to be sure. It is likely that the effectiveness of existing methadone maintenance programs could be enhanced by development of this model, as well.[6]

CONCLUSION

Psychobiological and clinical data suggest that opioids may prove to be useful in the treatment of psychiatric disorders. A great deal of work must be done to determine which patients will benefit from this pharmacotherapy and how treatment might best be delivered. Consideration of this therapeutic modality also raises important conceptual and ethical issues.

REFERENCES

1. VEREBEY, K. 1981. Opioids and psychological disorders. Adv. Alcohol Substance Abuse **4**(1): 99–121.
2. COMFORT, A. 1977. Morphine as an antipsychotic. Lancet 448, 449, August 27.
3. SACKETT, D. L. 1976. The magnitude of compliance and noncompliance. *In* Compliance with Therapeutic Regimes. D. L. Sackett & R. G. Haynes, Eds. Johns Hopkins University Press. Baltimore, MD.
4. VAN PATTEN, T., E. CRUMPTON & C. YALE. Drug refusal in schizophrenia and the wish to be crazy. 1976. Arch. Gen. Psychiatry **33**: 1443–1446.
5. KHANTZIAN, E. J., J. E. MACK & E. F. SCHATZBERG. Heroin use as an attempt to cope: Clinical observations. 1974. Am. J. Psychiatry **131**: 160–164.
6. MILLMAN, R. B., E. T. KHURI & M. E. NYSWANDER. Therapeutic detoxification of adolescent heroin addicts. 1978. Ann. NY Acad. Sci. **311**: 153–164.
7. ROBINS, L. W., J. E. HELZER & D. H. DAVIS. Narcotic use in Southeast Asia and afterward. 1975. Arch. Gen. Psychiatry **32**: 955–972.
8. KANNER, R. M. & K. M. FOLEY. Patterns of narcotic drug use in a cancer pain clinic. 1981. Ann. NY Acad. Sci. **362**: 161–172.
9. PICKAR, D. *et al.* Short term naloxone administration in schizophrenic and manic patients. 1982. Arch. Gen. Psychiatry **39**: 313–319.
10. TALBOTT, J. A. (Editorial) Care of the chronically mentally ill—still a national disgrace. 1979. Am. J. Psychiatry **136**(5): 688, 689.
11. DOHRENWEND, B. P. 1975. Sociocultural and socio-psychological factors in the genesis of mental disorder. J. Health Soc. Behavior **16**: 365–392.
12. DOLE, V. P., M. E. NYSWANDER, D. DES JARLAIS & H. JOSEPH. Performance based rating of methadone maintenance programs. 1982. N. Engl. J. Med. **306**(3): 169–172.
13. MICHELS, R. Doctors, drugs used for pleasure and performance and the medical model. *In* Feeling Good and Doing Better. Hastings Center, Institute of Society, Ethics and the Life Sciences. In preparation.

PART VI.   THERAPEUTIC AND SOCIOPOLITICAL CONSIDERATIONS: GENERAL DISCUSSION

R. B. RESNICK (*Department of Psychiatry, New York Medical College, New York*): One prospective on the problems that both Dr. Millman and Dr. Kleber raised is the likelihood that should opioid agonists prove efficacious in treating mental illness it will serve to stimulate the pharmaceutical industry to develop drugs that have opioid-like effects without the dependence liability that the current ones do, drugs such as buprenorphine, for example, and probably the greater utilization of existing technology for decreased dosing. The techniques are available today to dose patients on a once per month basis and obtain constant and sustained blood levels of the drug.

They are not being utilized now because of the lack of financial incentive to do so.

R. B. MILLMAN (*Cornell University Medical College, New York*): I agree there will be increased incentives for the pharmaceutical industry to develop a new class of drugs. Buprenorphine is particularly interesting in this regard in that it is reported to have opioid agonist effects but supposedly will not induce dependence or a severe withdrawal syndrome.

RESNICK: Of course, much needs to be learned about its particular effects in the mentally ill population. The floor is open for comments or questions for the papers by Drs. Kleber and Millman.

A. CORBASCIO (*Oakland, CA*): I believe that the most pertinent objection to the last two papers is the fact that, at least in California, severely ill psychotics are treated in State institutions. In this setting the safe administration of controlled dose of opiates is easily feasible. The danger of addiction has to be weighed against the well-known toxicity of neuroleptics and antidepressants. One further point I would like to make about opiates. Neuroleptics are dysphoric drugs; they are the main cause of the unpopularity of psychiatrists on the part of mental patients. The mentally ill are forced to live in semidetention and subject to a relentless and unpleasant pharmacological siege. It is possible that opiates may constitute a more humane therapeutic alternative for a more compliant and less resistant population of patients.

MILLMAN: I certainly agree; the point is even more vividly made in psychiatric patients with a history of drug abuse who are treated with major tranquilizers. Their choice is, in essence, whether to take their drugs, feel good for a while, and be dysfunctional or take our drugs (major tranquilizers), feel terrible, but be somewhat functional. When they leave the hospital or escape our purview, they frequently choose the drugs of abuse.

QUESTION: Is it ethical or even proper to make the psychiatrist responsible as primary physician or would the medical physician in the methadone program be responsible for the total care of a psychotic, violent patient?

H. D. KLEBER (*Yale Medical School, New Haven, CT*): The most appropriate person to treat these psychotic patients has to do with the area of expertise. Certainly, if we are dealing with drugs where the major problems are cardiotoxic, you would want someone with an internal medicine background having primary care or someone with that kind of experience readily available.

In our methadone program, for example, we have both counsellors who deal with the everyday reality and our patients lives and, then, we use our psychiatric residents and our psychiatrists to deal with the more severely psychologically disturbed. So, we have that division of responsibility. I would see the same thing holding with the new model.

E. NYGREN (*Metropolitan Hospital, New York*): This question is for Dr. Zinberg. Anybody who treats drug addicts very quickly learns that they are not very reliable. They are adept at concealing their drug abuse by substituting somebody else's urine or liquid soap. What makes you convinced that you can believe what your group of drug users say?

N. ZINBERG (*Harvard Medical School at Cambridge Hospital, Cambridge MA*): We certainly know that we cannot get into their heads. I do think, that certain kinds of interviews are pretty reliable, and we have done follow up interviews now over 8 years with a huge percentage of our sample. So, we have probably seen them, five to seven times—it varies. We also interviewed others who confirmed our interviews.

The interviews last about 2 hours and we have lots of ways of going back and forth to pick up discrepancies in the interview. One can tell a great deal by how people are dressed, by their addresses and telephone numbers and by the consistency of their stories. I can only tell you that all of that has been taken into account. I think there is little doubt that we are getting, if not exactly a straight story, awfully close to it.

KLEBER: I think there is also evidence in the literature and we have done some studies looking at opiate addicts in the community who have never come in for treatment. In an APA paper that I presented last May we discussed a hundred opium addicts who never applied for treatment and our results have certain similarities to Dr. Zinberg's. Telling the truth has often to do with what the consequences of lying are. Patients in methadone programs may try to give false urines not out of any particular enjoyment of beating the system, although there are some that do that, but, more because there is a good reason for it. If you come up with an illicit drug in your urine certain consequences follow. You have to say, what are the bad consequences that would come from telling Dr. Zinberg that you used this. Is he going to report you to the police or not pay you his 10 dollars or something? If there are no adverse consequences, then people, as has been shown with studies of alcoholics and a number of other follow-up studies, are likely to tell you at least a version of the truth.

R. CHIPKIN (*Schering Corp., Bloomfield, NJ*): My question is, perhaps, a general one. We know a fair amount of the reinforcing properties of opiates, and we know that drugs that are euphorogenic reinforce behavior. It seems to me that if you are giving euphorogenic drugs to patients with the idea of causing a cessation of some sort of behavior you may end up in a bind that will not work. You may be just increasing the likelihood of schizophrenic behavior because the patient says, "Well, if I am schizophrenic, I get opiates. I will feel better. I will be more schizophrenic." Do you see the possibility of the cycle you are getting into? You are reinforcing by the very nature of the drug the behavior that you are supposed to be eliminating.

RESNICK: I think that one can provide many, many speculations about what will happen under a variety of unknown circumstances. We really need to wait until the experiments have been done and the data are in.

Well, you know, opiates are not always that reinforcing. Even in animal models it is not easy to get a rodent to self-administer opiates. One has got to go through a lot of work to get an animal to do that, and it has been shown recently in Vancouver that when animals who are made physically dependent on opiates are put in a social environment, that is, they have a rat park where they can run free and engage in the normal interactions that rats engage in with other rats and are not isolated in cages, not only will they not take an opiate to start with, but, if they have been made physically dependent they will give it up. They cannot addict these animals under those circumstances.

The animals that are addicted and for whom opiates are reinforcing are animals that are in restricted environments and one might speculate from the human experience that not all people like them, not all people find them reinforcing, and it may only be certain individuals in certain circumstances. One of the things for which we have to thank Dr. Zinberg for constantly reminding us is that the problem is not the drug, but it is the person who uses the drug and that the circumstances and the setting all contribute equally to the consequences of the drug use in addition to the particular pharmacology of the drug.

I would also like to thank Dr. Kleber and Dr. Millman for raising the questions that they did. I hope that we do someday come to a point where we have to really confront those issues in reality.

INTRODUCTORY REMARKS

Yasuko Jacquet

Center for Neurochemistry
Rockland Research Institute
Wards Island, New York 10035

As chairman, I would like to welcome you to this session on animal studies relevant to the topic of opiates and mental illness. As a quick background, I would like to show one slide (FIG. 1) demonstrating the behavioral effects of β-endorphin following microinjection into rat brain. In 1976, we published this in *Science,* showing that nanomolar amounts of β-endorphin administered in a critical region of the brain resulted in profound analgesia, sedation and passive immobility during which state the rat could be molded into any position (as shown in this slide) that would be maintained for long periods. We proposed that such a behaviorally potent neuropeptide may be an endogenous neuroleptic-antipsychotogen, and that some forms of psychopathology may be due to a deficiency of the enzyme that cleaves β-endorphin from its prohormone, β-

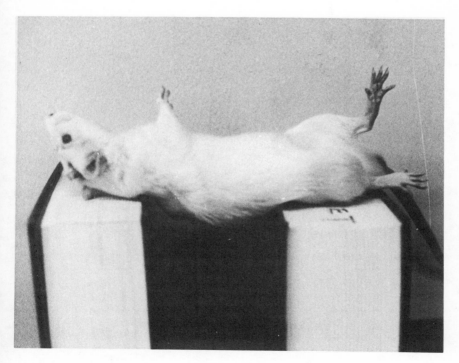

FIGURE 1.

189

lipotropin. Today, 5 years later, there are other peptide candidates for this role of endogenous antipsychotogen. However, a simple test is not possible because β-endorphin, as well as many of these other neuropeptides, does not penetrate the blood-brain barrier readily, and significant amounts do not reach the brain by the peripheral route. In the case of human patients, it is not possible to inject these neuropeptides directly into brain sites as we do with rats. Therefore, alternate strategies have to be devised. One possibility is to return to animal studies and to analyze the various actions of these peptides from different perspectives. The papers in this section will provide this perspective.

THE INFLUENCE OF A CENTRALLY ACTIVE PEPTIDE ON RECEPTOR MACROMOLECULAR DYNAMICS: TOWARD A NEUROPSYCHOPHARMACOLOGY OF PHASE *

Arnold J. Mandell

Department of Psychiatry
University of California, San Diego
La Jolla, California 92093

In addressing the relationship between neurobiological and behavioral phenomena as it may involve centrally active polypeptides, I shall examine the potential nonspecific and distributed (as contrasted to stereospecific and local) influences of thyrotropin-releasing hormone (TRH) on macromolecular dynamics, with particular reference to the temporal phasing of autonomous statistical motions in dopaminergic receptor binding activity and the observation of the same (entropic) property at several scales of time and space in other measures of neurobiological function.[1]

In contrast to the sensitivity of pituitary cell cultures to 10^{-8} M TRH for specific hormone release, micromolecular concentration of TRH induces a change in the pattern of fluctuations in crude rat brain striatal membrane dopaminergic ligand binding activity and has a similar effect on the statistical mechanical description of electrophysiological events. Those phenomena, considered with the behavioral changes induced by the peptide in animals and humans, suggest that TRH can alter macromolecular cooperativity (coherence) by randomizing the pattern of intermodulations of frequency, amplitude, and phase among the system's participants. This state of higher phase variance is manifested across levels as fast variational behavior in time, a lowered threshold for activation of neural systems by a multiplicity of neurotransmitters, and disruption of the rhythms of such phase-dependent phenomena as sleep cycles and some pathological affective states. A general corollary to our examination of distributed pharmacological influences on patterns of macromolecular dynamics that ramify across neurobiological levels is that descriptive properties derived from more abstract dimensions of central nervous system data may serve to relate to one another the effects seen at the basic and clinical levels.[2, 3]

MACROMOLECULAR SYSTEM STABILITY

Two current lines of biophysical research suggest that time- and space-dependent instabilities in the motions of and cooperativity among macromolecules may play an elementary role in the dynamics of larger biological systems. The first involves the finding that as a function of their innate structural instabilities,[4] intrinsic structural energy,[5] and low energy barriers between multiple quasi-stable states,[6] globular proteins in solution manifest spontaneous and vertically cooperative motions across scales of time.[7] Linderstrøm-Lang

* This work was supported by the National Institute on Drug Abuse (Grant DA–00265–09).

0077–8923/82/0398–0191 $1.75/0 © 1982, NYAS

concluded that small fast rotational, vibrational, and translational motions within proteins gather to produce slow larger semicoherent movements.[51] For example, the relaxation times of structural protein fluctuations range from 10^{-2} to 10^4 seconds,[7, 30] depending on the method of measurement and the size of the moiety under observation. The large motions reflect the amplitude and frequency of conformational transitions, and even such nonspecific influences as solvent viscosity have been shown to alter patterns of binding—for instance, those of CO binding to protoheme or O_2 and CO binding to myoglobin.[8] Moreover, as charged macro-ions in an ensemble, proteins in solution are interdependent; they manifest considerable short-range order (coherence) in their motions.[52]

FIGURE 1 illustrates characteristic fluctuations over time in the behavior of representative globular proteins with respect to immunoreactivity, binding, and catalysis. (A) reflects the multiphasic renaturation of porcine pancreatic elastase over time in both immunological and enzymatic measures; [18] (B) illustrates quasi-periodic deviations from linearity in quinacrine-bound cholinergic receptor fluorescence-difference measures in metabolically poisoned T. marmorata microsacs, suggesting physical, not metabolic instability; [10, 11] (C) demonstrates oscillatory binding of ^{3}H-cyclic adenosine monophosphate to purified plasma membrane (with no diesterase activity as a feedback mechanism to terminate the action) from cells of D. discoideum, showing an average period of two minutes; [19] (D) graphs oscillations around the mean velocity of ^{3}H-spiroperidol binding to an enriched membrane preparation from rat corpus striatum; [3] (E) shows quasi-regular fluctuations in initial rates of striatal tyrosine hydroxylase activity from rat brain in the presence of 5 μM propranolol; [20] and (F) shows fluctuations in rat raphé tryptophan hydroxylase activity as examined by repeated sampling over time in a preparation that was mechanically phased with a one-second burst of sonication.[21]

In the second relevant line of research, the motions of a particular class of globular proteins, membrane receptor molecules, have been inferred from studies of ionic conductance noise,[9] of fluctuations in fluorescence-difference measures,[10, 11] and, with respect to lateral diffusion, of the rate of recovery after photobleaching of the fluorescence of specifically labeled receptor proteins.[12, 13] Recent applications of the bleaching technique have demonstrated that polypeptide hormones (insulin, epidermal growth factor, nerve growth factor, and pituitary gonadotropins) alter the spatial-temporal patterns of lateral movement in the membrane by receptor molecules as well as their cooperativity.[14-16] The results of linear changes in coupling between elements in complex dissipative systems are nonlinear, so whereas a critical range of polypeptide hormone concentration (as a parameter in such a system) may induce functional order among receptor proteins, lower or higher levels are as likely to disorganize the system in space and/or time.[17]

STOCHASTIC DESCRIPTORS OF THE BEHAVIOR OF NONLINEAR
COOPERATIVE DETERMINISTIC SYSTEMS

Systems of partial differential equations with low dimension representing the dynamics of interdependent elements may evolve over time into unpredictable behavior. The classic example is the Saltzman–Lorenz equations, which repre-

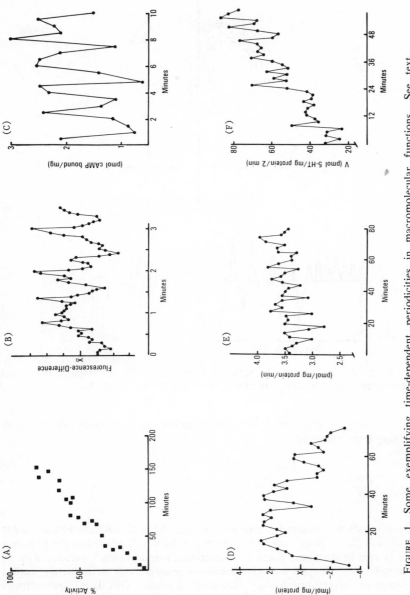

FIGURE 1. Some exemplifying time-dependent periodicities in macromolecular functions. See text.

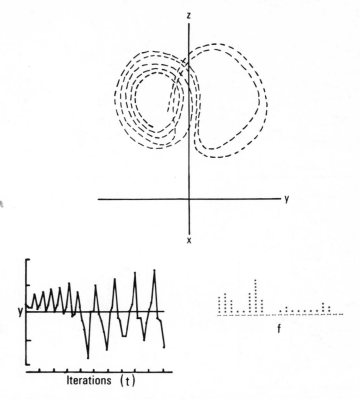

FIGURE 2. The behavior of the Saltzman-Lorenz attractor in the phase plane and the frequency spectrum across its orbital transition to the second basin.

sent the emergent convective order in a model hydrodynamic system with increasing Rayleigh number:

$$\dot{x} = g(y - x)$$
$$\dot{y} = x(r - z) - y$$
$$\dot{z} = xy - bz,$$

where x stands for material convection; y, for thermal convection; and z, for variations in the vertical temperature profile.[22] FIGURE 2 illustrates the behavior of the system in the phase plane (y/z over time) and graphs y versus t with its power spectrum. Several hundred iterations generate one y frequency until a "spontaneous" bifurcation leads to two spectral peaks. This figure demonstrates that a deterministic harmonic oscillator (pacemaker) is not required for quasi-ordered oscillations in a dissipative system and that statistical averages rather than predicted coefficients are necessary to characterize the dynamical behavior of a cooperative system. Indeed, we find in such a scheme a very apt model for the microdomain/microdomain; polypeptide ligand/microdomain; protein/protein; protein/polypeptide ligand interactions manifested in the binding kinetics of an interdependent macromolecular system.[6, 8, 47] Recent mathematical research in nonlinear dynamics attests to the usefulness of the descriptors usually applied to random systems for characterizing such nonlinear behavior, i.e., moments,[23] spectra,[24] and dimensional exponents.[25] We have approached the analysis of variational kinetics of brain enzyme systems by these means with some success.[20, 21]

FIGURE 3 is a diagram representing the probability density distribution of an ensemble of measures of the behavior of a dynamical system in which the average time-dependent amplitude is seen as the variance and the higher moments (skew, kurtosis) describe its symmetry and shape. The frequency of variations is seen in the power spectrum; the dominant wavelength, in the autocorrelation function. Systems of interdependent differential equations that do not evolve to a stable equilibrium point, to equally dense ergodicity over the energy surface (Boltzmann), to a simple limit cycle (Poincaré–Bendixon theorem [26]), or as invariant tori (KAM surface [27]) may manifest the dynamical structure of a strange attractor.[28] Strange attractors (FIGURE 2) have exponential dependence on initial conditions; a small change at t_0 is magnified many-fold over iterations, a behavior known as the mixing property. That is, in one or more dimensions, adjacent points move away from one another over time. Partially compromised order emerges because in other dimensions the orbits come together as a function of the system's phase condensation.[55] Thus autocorrelation and frequency spectra manifest increased replicability over specific orbital trajectories,[24] and indices of stability such as the spectrum of Lyapounov characteristic exponents (LCE) and measures of dimension may be even more reliable.[25, 53, 55] In the stochastic context, the Hausdorff–Besicovitch

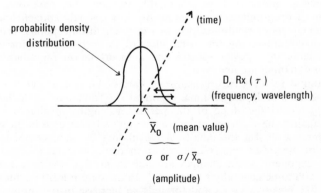

PARAMETERS OF STOCHASTIC PERIODICITY

FIGURE 3. Diagram representing a probability density distribution around the mean of an ensemble of determinations in which the ordinate indicates the percentage of the total number of data points at each value along the abscissa. The standard deviation, σ, or the coefficient of variation, σ/X_0, represents the average amplitude of the time-dependent variations. The autocorrelation function, $Rx(\tau)$, and the dimensional exponent, D, indicate the frequency with which the variations are changing along the time axis.

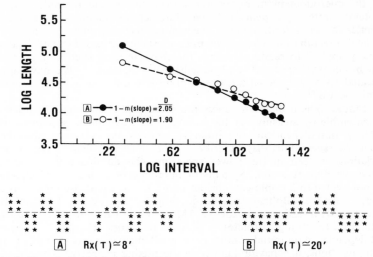

FIGURE 4. Two indices of variational frequency, the autocorrelation length, $Rx(\tau)$, and the dimensional exponent, D, in quickly (A) and slowly (B) changing periodic processes. See text.

dimension D characterizes frequency of variation in terms of the "roughness" of the surface of the random function, $f(A)$.[54] In our work this describes the frequency aspect of the dynamics of A, which equals the deviation of the observed from the calculated value established by linear or exponential regression analysis, normalized for slope and intercept. We have observed that the direction of drug-induced changes in this dimensional exponent may sometimes resist the effects of randomization of the order in data points, thus affording a means of circumventing the instabilities of the orbital behavior of the system more reliably than power spectra and autocorrelation functions when strange attractor dynamics are involved.

FIGURE 4 features two measures of variational frequency: the auto-correlation function and the dimensional exponent D. The latter is calculated as $1 - m$, where m equals the slope of the perimeter lengths of the random function plotted against the sequence of increasing interval sizes used in the measurement. See Reference 20 for the details of calculating D. A decrease in D indicates slowing of the variational frequency; an increase indicates quickening. Because D is an exponent, small changes are important, and we have found shifts of 0.04 to 0.06 to be generally replicable.[20] In the deterministic context, a decrease in D is like negative LCEs and foretells an increase in the predictability of the final state of a system with variations in the initial conditions.[25, 53, 55] The amplitude term we use in conjunction with $D(A)$ is $RMS(A)$, the square root of the sum of the squared differences from the mean regression line. Assuming N to be conserved, we view slowing as a sign of increased cooperativity (coupling, phasing, synchronization) and a higher D as indicating either greater independence among the contributing elements of the system or a post-bifurcational interference pattern of multiple frequencies. The assumption in the first case is that increased cooperativity accompanies phase condensation and that, through randomization of phase, loss of cooperativity destabilizes the system, leading to more diffuse occupancy of state as well as probability space. Dimension, D, appears to be closely related to LCEs, which describe a system's stability in critical zones.[25, 53, 55] As noted above, high phase variance makes small inputs declarative, so an increase in D reflecting that state would be predicted to accompany manifestations of both faster (random) variation and increased sensitivity to perturbation.[1] An increase in D due to spectral bifurcation and the interference pattern of two or more incommensurate frequencies would predict less sensitivity to perturbation because of decreased capacity for coherent action.[11]

POLYPEPTIDE EFFECTS ON ^{3}H-SPIROPERIDOL BINDING FLUCTUATIONS

Methods for these experiments were adapted from those described by Burt *et al.*[29] Striate regions from rat brain were homogenized in ice cold sodium–potassium phosphate buffer, 0.02 M, 10:1, pH 7.4 (with a Brinkmann Polytron PT-10, 10 sec at No. 6). The homogenate was centrifuged twice at 20,000 × g for 10 min (Sorvall RC2-B) with rehomogenization of the intermediate pellet in fresh buffer. The final pellet was homogenized in cold buffer (5:1 wt/vol) containing 0.1% ascorbic acid, 120 nM NaCl, 5 mM KCl, 2 mM $CaCl_2$, and 1 mM $MgCl_2$; final pH was 7.1 at 37° C. ^{3}H-Spiroperidol, 25.64 Ci/mmol, was diluted so that 0.22 nM equaled approximately 5000 cpm, which in 100 μl (including 1% ascorbic acid) was added to 0.1 ml of tissue suspension. Tissue suspensions with or without polypeptide ligand were allowed to stabilize on ice until sampled by incubations with ^{3}H-spiroperidol. For time courses, duplicate samples were drawn every two min across 80 to 100 min and incubated for one min to yield 40 to 50-point functions. Alternatively, duplicate samples were incubated for one minute with increasing concentrations of ^{3}H-spiroperidol (0 to 0.70 nM in increments of 0.01 nM). After incubation, tubes were quickly filtered under vacuum (Whatman GF/B filters), and the filters were rinsed three times with 5 ml ice cold phosphate buffer. Radioactivity on the filters was counted by liquid scintillation spectrometry in a 10 ml solution (BioCount Fluid). Duplicate blanks contained 10^{-6} M cold spiroperidol.

A time-dependent ^{3}H-spiroperidol binding curve, showing means of duplicate determinations, appears in FIGURE 1(D). FIGURE 5 (left) shows the usual wide-band noise of the ill-defined spectral character in the ligand binding fluctuations, which is characteristic of many strange attractors.[24] The spectrum is almost Lorentzian, with 10 to 20 min as the half-width in time and a $1/f$-like pattern over increasing ligand concentration. Incubation of membrane preparations that were kept on ice in the presence of 10^{-6} M TRH tended to induce flatter spectra or ones with faster average frequencies (FIGURE 5, center and right). These and other experiments under control conditions failed to demonstrate the degree of spectral order in time observed in our studies of rat brain tyrosine hydroxylase[20] or tryptophan hydroxylase.[21] With the ^{3}H-spiroperidol binding, autocorrelational and spectral evidence of periodicity (one region of broad or narrow band noise) appeared more often in fluctuations over increasing ligand concentration than in those over time, but not consistently. Those experiments also showed considerably less replicable spectral morphology than our enzyme substrate–velocity curves.[48] Nevertheless, $D(A)$, which is sensitive

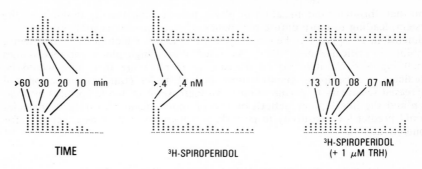

FIGURE 5. Spectral representation of TRH effects on ³H-spiroperidol binding fluctuations across ligand and time. See text.

to the finer texture of the random functions, showed small but consistent changes in the presence of TRH.

TABLE 1 summarizes the results of analyzing kinetic fluctuations in ³H-spiroperidol binding over increasing ligand. In the presence of 10^{-6} M TRH (but not at 10^{-7} M or below) variational frequency as seen in $D(A)$ was increased; RMS(A) as an indicator of variational amplitude (variance) did not change. TABLE 2 lists results from studies of ³H-spiroperidol binding fluctuations over time in the presence of various polypeptide ligands. Note a similar small increase in stochastic frequency of fluctuations in the presence of either the 1-methyl or 3-methyl TRH analog, which, along with the requirement of 10^{-6} M levels of TRH (those that elicit nonspecific release of hormones from cultured pituitary cell preparations), suggests that the polypeptide has a nonspecific effect. The frequency-increasing effect of somatostatin in the same concentration was more marked and contrasted with the "phasing" (slowing) action of the guanine nucleotide (GTP) at a concentration of 10^{-5} M. GTP is a ligand known to decrease the affinity of crude striatal membrane preparations for binding dopaminergic agonists.[49]

TABLE 1

THYROTROPIN RELEASING HORMONE (TRH) INFLUENCE ON ³H-SPIROPERIDOL BINDING FLUCTUATIONS OVER INCREASING ³H-SPIROPERIDOL CONCENTRATIONS *

Condition	RMS(A) (fmol/mg protein/min)	$D(A)$
Control	5.19	1.88
	4.72	1.94
	4.65	1.94
	5.51	1.93
10^{-6} M TRH	3.49	1.98
	6.80	2.08
	5.42	2.01
	3.37	2.04

* RMS$_A$ = index of variational amplitude; D$_A$ = index of variational frequency.

Fast motions and high affinity binding have been related to one another by Colquhoun in the dynamics of cholinergic drug receptor binding.[50] The inverse, decreased sensitivity with increased systems coherence, is consonant with response characteristics related to phase dynamics in complex cooperative systems.[1] Contrasting with the actions of GTP, the TRH effect in the preparations may be consistent with nonspecific potentiating actions on cholinergic, dopaminergic, serotonergic, and noradrenergic receptor-mediated functions (TABLE 3).

TABLE 2

POLYPEPTIDE INFLUENCES ON ^{3}H-SPRIOPERIDOL BINDING FLUCTUATIONS OVER TIME

Condition	RMS(A) (fmol/mg protein)	$D(A)$
Control	1.65	2.01
	1.44	1.97
	1.49	2.03
TRH (10^{-6} M, 1-CH$_3$)	1.42	2.05
	1.55	2.08
	1.36	2.06
TRH (10^{-6} M, 3-CH$_3$)	0.67	2.04
	0.94	2.04
	0.73	2.02
Somatostatin (10^{-6} M)	0.93	2.10
	1.31	2.17
	0.83	2.07
GTP (10^{-5} M)	0.47	1.89
	0.81	1.92
	1.51	1.92

DISCUSSION

We present preliminary evidence suggesting that TRH in concentrations above that required for high affinity binding to pituitary membranes and specific release of thyroid stimulating hormone from pituitary cell cultures [60] increases the frequency of variations in ^{3}H-spiroperidol binding to crude striatal membrane preparations from rat brain. FIGURE 6 diagrams two dynamical routes to such an effect in a population of partially coupled dissipative oscillators: (a) a randomization of phase, represented on the far left by a wide distribution of oscillators over a single cycle, a nearly equiprobable density distribution, a flat spectrum, a fast relaxation of the autocorrelation function, and (not shown) a high D; (b) a post-coherence bifurcation of frequency-phase, seen in the progression of the four descriptors to the right, resulting in fluctuations that manifest fast frequencies due to the interference patterns of two or more dominant frequencies.[11] This second mechanism has been speculated by Landau to constitute a common bifurcational route to randomness.[56]

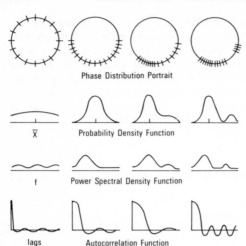

FIGURE 6. Phasing and bifurcational dynamics as seen in four statistical representations. See text.

These two kinds of statistical mechanical mechanisms can be differentiated by the system's sensitivity to perturbation. Whereas the bifurcated system loses sensitivity, having lost capacity for concerted action,[1, 11] the system with random phase would manifest increased sensitivity. TABLE 3 refers to several studies indicating that TRH increases neuronal membrane and receptor sensitivity to a variety of neurotransmitter and electrical input. The higher frequencies generated by somatostatin suggested to us that it might bifurcate the system because we had seldom observed a flat or single-peaked specrtum associated with a D

TABLE 3

REPRESENTATIVE EFFECTS OF TRH ACROSS NEUROBIOLOGICAL LEVELS

Preparation	Finding
Rat striatal ³H-spiroperidol binding	Fast fluctuations without dominant phase [30]
Frog motoneuron	Facilitation of spontaneous discharge [31]
Mammalian cortical neurons	Facilitation of spontaneous discharge [31]
EEG (rabbit)	Low voltage, fast activity [32, 33]
Sleep (cat)	Increased awakeness, decreased REM and SWS [34]
Exploratory behavior (rat)	Behavioral excitation;[43] hyperactivity [35, 46]
Neuronal, turnover, behavioral measures	Facilitated ACh, DA, 5-HT, NE actions [36-39]
Behavior, EEG measures in many species	Antagonism of sedatives [40, 41]; Potentiation of stimulants [42]
Clinical studies	Some reports of antidepressive and antimanic effects [44, 45]

greater than 2.06. FIGURE 7 contains three spectra from studies of ^{3}H-spiro-peridol binding in the presence of 10^{-6} M somatostatin. The two regions of narrow band noise are consistent with our suspicion of bifurcation (compare FIGURE 5). A bifurcated spectrum with its attendant decrease in responsivity could explain inhibition of specific pituitary hormone release and the decrease in exploratory behavior observed after intraventricular administration of somato-statin to rats,[35] both of which contrast to the influence of TRH. We have demonstrated a relationship between response inhibition and bifurcation in several neurobiological systems.[11]

That such a TRH-induced "dephasing" mechanism with respect to molecular cooperativity may be a distributed property across temporal-spatial scales is indicated by the fast, more random fluctuations in multiple measures, increased sensitivity to perturbation by agonists, and loss of coherence in cyclic phase functions listed in TABLE 3. As has been reported for the psychotropic changes

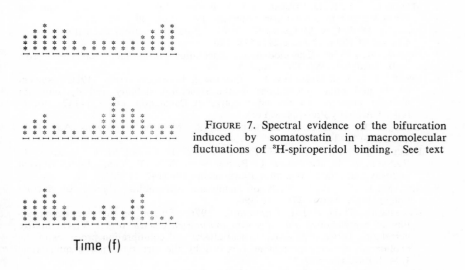

FIGURE 7. Spectral evidence of the bifurcation induced by somatostatin in macromolecular fluctuations of ^{3}H-spiroperidol binding. See text

Time (f)

induced in humans by β-endorphins,[57] the clinical effects of TRH are evident hours to days after administration.[58] Such latencies to action are more con-sistent with an influence on macromolecular population dynamics than they are with a lock and key receptor-mediated trigger.

The high concentrations and lack of stereospecificity required for this TRH effect in molecular dynamics suggest that, aside from pharmacological studies of TRH in animals and human subjects, it may be relevant to psychobiology only when circulating peptides are pathologically elevated. For example, during times of end organ failure, as in the involutional period, high circulating levels of neurally active peptides (of a variety of sorts) may create a distributed condition of molecular desynchronization in the central nervous system. The anxiety, tension, increased sensitivity, irritability, hyperarousal with increased sleep cycle disturbances, and agitated depression characteristic of some post-menopausal syndromes may represent such an entity.[59]

ACKNOWLEDGMENTS

Appreciation is expressed to Kim D. Stewart for technical assistance; to Drs. Jean Rivier, Nicholas Ling, and Roger Burgus for the generous gifts of 1- and 3-methyl TRH; and to Dr. Roger Guillemin for enlightening discussions.

REFERENCES

1. WINFREE, A. T. 1980. The Geometry of Biological Time. pp. 205–230, 258–276. Springer-Verlag. New York.
2. MANDELL, A. J. 1980. Vertical integration of levels of brain function through parametric symmetries within self-similar stochastic fields. *In* Information Processing in the Nervous System. H. Pinsker & W. Willis, Eds. pp. 177–197. Raven Press. New York.
3. MANDELL, A. J., K. D. STEWART & P. V. RUSSO. 1981. The Sunday syndrome: From kinetics to altered consciousness. Fed. Proc. **40:** 2693–2698.
4. KARPLUS, M. & J. A. MCCAMMON. 1971. Protein structural fluctuations during a period of 100 ps. Nature **277:** 578–580.
5. COOPER, A. 1976. Thermodynamic fluctuations in protein molecules. Proc. Natl. Acad. Sci. USA **73:** 2740–2741.
6. FINNEY, J. L., B. J. GELLATLY, J. C. GOLTON & J. GOODFELLOW. 1980. Solvent effects and polar interactions in the structural stability and dynamics of globular proteins. *In* Second Biophysical Discussion. pp. 131–142. Rockefeller University Press. New York.
7. GURD, F. R. N. & T. M. ROTHGEB. 1979. Motions in proteins. Adv. Prot. Chem. **33:** 73–165.
8. BEECE, D., L. EISENSTEIN, H. FRAUENFELDER, D. GOOD, M. C. MARDEN, L. REINSCH, A. H. REYNOLDS, L. B. SORENSEN & K. T. YUE. 1980. Solvent viscosity and protein dynamics. Biochemistry **19:** 5147–5157.
9. STEVENS, C. F. 1977. Study of membrane permeability changes by fluctuation analysis. Nature **270:** 391–396.
10. GRUNHAGEN, H.-H. & J.-P. CHANGEUX. 1976. Studies on the electrogenic action of acetylcholine with *Torpedo marmorata* electric organ. V. Qualitative correlation between pharmacological effects and equilibration processes of the cholinergic receptor protein as revealed by the structural probe quinacrine. J. Mol. Biol. **106:** 517–535.
11. MANDELL A. J. & P. V. RUSSO. 1983. Toward a neuropsychopharmacology of habituation: A vertical integration. Pharmacol. Rev. In press.
12. ELSON, E. L. & J. A. REIDLER. 1979. Analysis of cell surface interactions by measurements of lateral mobility. J. Supramol. Struct. **12:** 481–489.
13. TAYLOR, D. L. & Y.-L. WANG. 1980. Fluorescently labelled molecules as probes of the structure and function of living cells. Nature **284:** 405–410.
14. SCHECHTER, Y., J. SCHLESSINGER, S. JACOBS, K.-J. CHANG & P. CUATRECASAS. 1978. Fluorescent labeling of hormone receptors in viable cells: Preparation and properties of highly fluorescent derivatives of epidermal growth factor and insulin. Proc. Natl. Acad. Sci. USA **75:** 2135–2139.
15. SCHLESSINGER, J., Y. SHECHTER, M. C. WILLINGHAM & J. PASTAN. 1978. Direct visualization of binding, aggregation, and internalization of insulin and epidermal growth factor on living fibroblastic cells. Proc. Natl. Acad. Sci. USA **75:** 2659–2663.
16. HAZUM, E., P. CUATRECASAS, J. MARIAN & P. M. CONN. 1980. Receptor-mediated internalization of fluorescent gonadotropin-releasing hormone by pituitary gonadotropes. Proc. Natl. Acad. Sci. USA **77:** 6692–6695.

17. GUCKENHEIMER, J. M. 1981. Instabilities and chaos in nonhydrodynamic systems. *In* Hydrodynamic Instabilities and the Transition to Turbulence. H. L. Swinney & J. P. Gollub, Eds. pp. 271–288. Springer-Verlag. New York.

18. GHELIS, C. 1980. Transient conformational states in proteins followed by differential labeling. *In* Second Biophysical Discussion. pp. 401–408. Rockefeller University Press. New York.

19. KING, A. C. & W. A. FRAZIER. 1979. Properties of the oscillatory cAMP binding component of *Dictyostelium discoideum* cells and isolated plasma membrane. J. Biol. Chem. **254:** 7168–7176.

20. MANDELL, A. J. & P. V. RUSSO. 1981. Striatal typrosine hydroxylase activity: Multiple conformational kinetic oscillators and product concentration frequencies. J. Neurosci. **1:** 380–389.

21. KNAPP, S. & A. J. MANDELL. 1981. Calcium, cofactor, and propranolol-induced changes in the kinetic variations of rat raphe tryptophan hydroxylase activity. *In* Function and Regulation of Monoamine Enzymes: Basic and Clinical Aspects. E. Usdin, N. Weiner & M. Youdim, Eds. pp. 215–222. Macmillan. London.

22. LORENZ, E. N. 1963. Deterministic nonperiodic flow. J. Atmos. Sci. **20:** 130–141.

23. KRAICHNAN, R. H. 1980. Realizability, in equalities and closed moment equations. Ann. N.Y. Acad. Sci. **357:** 37–46.

24. FARMER, D., J. CRUTCHFIELD, H. FROEHLING, N. PACKARD & R. SHAW. 1980. Power spectra and mixing properties of strange attractors. Ann. N.Y. Acad. Sci. **357:** 453–472.

25. MORI, H. 1980. Fractal dimensions of chaotic flows of autonomous dissipative systems. Prog. Theor. Phys. **63:** 1044–1047.

26. HIRSCH, M. W. & S. SMALE. 1974. Differential Equations, Dynamical Systems, and Linear Algebra. pp. 239–254. Academic Press. New York.

27. GREEN, J. M. 1980. The calculation of KAM surfaces. Ann. N.Y. Acad. Sci. **357:** 80–89.

28. RUELLE, D. 1980. Strange attractors. Math. Intellig. **2:** 126–137.

29. BURT, D. R., I. CREESE & S. H. SNYDER. 1976. Properties of [³H]haloperidol and [³H]dopamine binding associated with dopamine receptors in calf brain membranes. Mol. Pharmacol. **12:** 800–812.

30. MANDELL, A. J. 1981. Statistical stability in random brain systems: Possible implications for polydrug abuse in the borderline syndrome. Adv. Subst. Abuse **2:** 299–341.

31. RENAUD, L. P. & A. PADJEN. 1978. Electrophysiological analysis of peptide action in neutral tissue. *In* Centrally Acting Peptides. J. Hughes, Ed. pp. 59–84. University Park Press. Baltimore, MD.

32. ANDRY, D. K. & A. HORITA. 1977. Thyrotropin-releasing hormone: Physiological concomitants of behavioral excitation. Pharmacol. Biochem. Behav. **6:** 58–59.

33. WHITE, R. P. & J. S. BEALE. 1975. Electroencephalographic (EEG) effects of thyrotropin releasing hormone on rabbits. Neurosci. Abst. **1:** 727.

34. KIND, C. D. 1975. Inhibition of slow wave sleep and rapid eye movement sleep by thyrotropin releasing hormone in cats. Pharmacologist **17:** 211.

35. SEGAL, D. S. & A. J. MANDELL. 1974. Differential behavioral effects of hypothalamic polypeptides. *In* Thyroid Axis, Drugs, and Behavior. A. J. Prange, Ed. pp. 129–124. Raven Press. New York.

36. GREEN, A. R. & D. G. GRAHAME-SMITH. 1974. TRH potentiates behavioral changes following increased brain 5-hydroxytryptamine accumulation in rats. Nature **251:** 524–526.

37. YARBROUGH, G. G. 1976. TRH potentiates excitatory actions of acetylcholine on cerebral cortical neurones. Nature **263:** 523–524.

38. KELLER, H. H., G. BARTHOLINI & A. PLETSCHER. 1974. Enhancement of cerebral noradrenaline turnover by thyrotropin-releasing hormone. Nature 248: 528–529.

39. PLOTNIKOFF, N. P., A. J. PRANGE, G. R. BREESE, M. A. ANDERSON & I. C. WILSON. 1972. Thyrotropin releasing hormone: Enhancement of DOPA activity by a hypothalamic hormone. Science 178: 417–418.

40. BROWN, M. & W. VALE. 1975. Central nervous system effects of hypothalamic peptides. Endocrinology 96: 1333–1336.

41. BREESE, G. R., J. M. COTT, B. R. COOPER, A. J. PRANGE, M. A. LIPTON & N. P. PLOTNIKOFF. 1975. Effects of thyrotropin-releasing hormone (TRH) on the actions of pentobarbital and other centrally acting drugs. J. Pharmacol. Exp. Ther. 193: 11–22.

42. GREEN, A. J., D. J. HEAL, D. G. GRAHAME-SMITH & P. H. KELLEY. 1976. The contrasting actions of TRH and cycloheximide in altering the effects of centrally acting drugs: Evidence for the noninvolvement of dopamine sensitive adenylate cyclase. Neuropharmacology 15: 591–599.

43. CARINO, M. A., J. R. SMITH, B. C. WEICK & H. HORITA. 1976. Effects of thyrotropin-releasing hormone (TRH) microinjected into various brain areas of conscious and pentobarbital-treated rabbits. Life Sci. 19: 1687–1692.

44. PRANGE, A. J., J. C. WILSON, P. P. LARA, L. B. ALLTOP & G. R. BREESE. 1972. Effects of thyrotropin-releasing hormone in depression. Lancet (2): 999–1002.

45. HUEY, L. Y., D. S. JANOWSKY, A. J. MANDELL, L. L. JUDD & M. PENDERY. 1975. Preliminary studies on the use of thyrotropin-releasing hormone in manic states, depression, and the dysphoria of alcohol withdrawal. Psychopharmacol. Bull. 11: 24–27.

46. VOGEL, R. A., B. R. COOPER, T. S. BARLOW, A. J. PRANGE, R. A. MUELLER & G. R. BREESE. 1979. Effects of thyrotropin-releasing hormone on locomotor activity, operant performance and ingestive behavior. J. Pharmacol. Exp. Ther. 208: 161–168.

47. KARPLUS, M. & D. L. WEAVER. 1976. Protein-folding dynamics. Nature 260: 404–406.

48. MANDELL, A. J. & P. V. RUSSO. 1981. Striatal tyrosine hydroxylase: The role of cofactor concentration in the scaling of enzyme periodicity and behavioral stereotypy. In Function and Regulation of Monoamine Enzymes: Basic and Clinical Aspects. E. Usdin, N. Weiner & M. Youdim, Eds. pp. 271–280. Macmillan. London.

49. CREESE, I. & S. H. SNYDER. 1979. Multiple dopamine receptors. In Catecholamines: Basic and Clinical Frontiers. Vol. 1: 601–603. E. Usdin, I. Kopin & J. Barchas, Eds. Pergamon Press. New York.

50. COLQUHOUN, D. 1980. The link between drug binding and response: Theories and observations. In The Receptors. Vol 1: 93–142. R. D. O'Brien, Ed. Plenum Press. New York.

51. LINDERSTRØM-LANG, K. J. & J. A. SCHELLMAN. 1959. Protein structure and enzyme activity. In The Enzymes. 2nd edit. Vol. 1: 443–480. P. D. Boyer, H. Lardy & K. Myrback, Eds. Academic Press. New York.

52. BROWN, J. C., P. N. PUSEY, J. W. GOODWIN & R. H. OTTEWILL. 1975. Light scattering study of dynamic and time-averaged correlations in dispersions of charged particles. Phys. A: Math. Gen. 8: 664–682.

53. LADRAPPIER, F. 1981. Some relations between dimension and Lyapounov exponents. Commun. Math. Phys. 81: 229–238.

54. MANDELBROT, B. B. 1977. Fractals: Form, Chance, and Dimension. W. H. Freeman, San Francisco, CA.

55. FROEHLING, H., J. CRUTCHFIELD, D. FARMER, N. H. PACKARD & R. SHAW. 1981. On determining the dimension of chaotic flows. Physica 3D: 601–617.

56. LANFORD, O. E. 1981. Strange attractors and turbulence. *In* Hydrodynamic Instabilities and the Transition to Turbulence. H. L. Swinney & J. P. Gollub, Eds. pp. 7–26. Springer-Verlag. New York.
57. KLINE, N. S. & H. E. LEHMANN. 1979. β-Endorphin therapy in psychiatric patients. *In* Endorphins in Mental Health Research. E. Usdin, W. E. Bunney & N. S. Kline, Eds. pp. 500–517. Oxford University Press. New York.
58. PRANGE, A. J., C. B. NEMEROFF, P. T. LOOSEN, G. BISSETTE, A. J. OSBAHR, I. C. WILSON & M. A. LIPTON. 1979. Behavioral effects of thyrotropin-releasing hormone in animals and man: A review. *In* Central Nervous System Effects of Hypothalamic Hormones and Other Peptides. R. Collu, A. Barbeau, I. R. Ducharme & J.-G. Rochfort, Eds. pp. 75–96. Raven Press. New York.
59. REISER, M. F. & L. WHISNANT. 1980. Endocrine disorders. *In* Comprehensive Textbook of Psychiatry III. H. Kaplan, A. Freedman & B. Sadock, Eds. pp. 1917–1929. Williams & Wilkins. Baltimore, MD.
60. GRANT, G., W. VALE & R. GUILLEMIN. 1973. Characteristics of the pituitary binding sites for thyrotropin-releasing factor. Endocrinology **92:** 1629–1633.

DISCUSSION OF THE PAPER

J. V. VOLAVKA (*New York University School of Medicine, New York*) What is the signal-to-noise ratio in these events that you showed?

A. J. MANDELL (*University of California at San Diego, La Jolla*): Between 1:1 and 3:1. I would like to mention the signal-to-noise ratio with respect to either stochastic or Fourier analysis. You can pick up 0.5 signal to 1.0 noise if there are consistent statistical wave properties. In other words, I can send noise over the telephone to the extent of 1.0 and send my signal on top of that to the extent of 0.5 and the pattern will be received on the other end using the analytic methods we are talking about. Usually we work in these systems from about 1:1 to 3:1. In some systems it is even higher, but it does not have to be; it can be less than 1:2.

G. C. DAVIS (*Case Western Reserve School of Medicine, Cleveland, OH*): Dr. Mandell, I did not fully comprehend the concentrations. These are still at pharmacological concentrations as opposed to physiological concentrations, are they not?

MANDELL: Absolutely, and that is important. We are working at about 10^{-6} M; 10^{-7} or 10^{-8} M will not give it to us.

Except for subcellular compartments with higher, but quite local concentrations, we suspect that these phenomena may be relevant only to pharmacological or pathophysiological effects. For example, in post-menopausal syndromes, when target organs are withering despite large amounts of various polypeptides, perhaps a nonspecific effect would involve a diffuse action on a macromolecular phase. That could be relevant in some clinical conditions. Remember, I reported that 1-methyl and 3-methyl analogues of TRH had the same effect as physiological TRH, a finding consistent with a distributed and nonspecific effect.

H. M. EMRICH (*Max Planck Institute for Psychiatry, Munich, FRG*): How do you really measure the fluctuation in enzyme protein activity?

MANDELL: We examine the activity in three ways. We assay across very small increments in pterin cofactor (0.5 μM) to obtain fluctuations over the mean saturation function in the linear range with cofactor less than K_m. Then, in our long residence time courses, all the samples are incubated simultaneously in the presence or absence of ligand or drug and duplicates or triplicates are removed every minute for 60 minutes and the product concentrations are determined. Finally, in our short residence time experiments, where we are looking at initial rates, duplicate samples are removed from iced homogenate with or without ion or drug every 1.5 minutes and incubated with 20 μM cofactor and 10 μM substrate for two minutes; then we determine the product concentrations. The deviations of those concentrations from the mean velocity as determined by least squares regression and normalized for slope and intercept are then analyzed as time series as I described.

OPIOID PEPTIDES IN THE HIPPOCAMPUS: ANATOMICAL AND PHYSIOLOGICAL CONSIDERATIONS *

Steven J. Henriksen,† Guy Chouvet,‡ Jacqueline McGinty, and Floyd E. Bloom

The Salk Institute
San Diego, California 92138
‡ INSERM U171
Claude Bernard University
Lyons, France

The recent explosive growth in knowledge concerning the possible functions of newly identified neuroactive peptides is reminiscent of the period from the early to mid 1960s when biogenic amines were the subject of intensified investigation as possible substrates for various neuropsychiatric disorders. Presently, several neuroactive peptides, including the endorphins, somatostatin, vasoactive intestinal peptide (VIP), and cholecystokinin (CCK) are under scrutiny as possible participants in psychiatric pathology. This situation, in part, derives from the recent localization of these neuropeptides in mammalian limbic system structures.[1-8] Significantly, preclinical and clinical investigations of one class of neuropeptide, the endorphins, have suggested a correlation between certain neuropsychiatric conditions and the central function of these peptides (as outlined by Verebey, this volume). Albeit tempered by the experience with biogenic amines, there seems to be a growing optimism that the investigation of neuropeptides, and the endorphins in particular, may shed light on neuropsychiatric dysfunction.

Although early pharmaco-behavioral laboratory studies suggested a possible link between endogenous opioid mechanisms and schizophrenia,[9] there was neither physiological nor anatomical evidence to support these behavioral observations. However, more recent neurochemical and cellular physiological studies have suggested an important role for endogenous opioid peptides in limbic system function, particularly in the hippocampus (HPC).[5, 10-12]

IMMUNOCHEMICAL STUDIES

Early immunohistochemical investigations of endogenous opioids demonstrated their broad distribution in most limbic structures, but very sparse labeling of cells in the hippocampus.[8, 12-15] This histochemical evidence was compatible with parallel radioimmunoassay data suggesting little, if any, endorphin immunoreactivity (IR) in whole rat hippocampus. Regional studies in rodents also indicated low levels of enkephalin (ENK) immunoreactivity

* This work supported by the National Institutes of Health (Grants DA 01785 and AA 03504), The Klingenstein Foundation, and the Fondation de l'Industrie Pharmaceutique pour la Recherche.
† Address for correspondence: The Salk Institute, P.O. Box 85800, San Diego, CA 92138.

0077–8923/82/0398–0207 $01.75/0 © 1982 NYAS

(IR) (using an antibody to Leu[5]-enkephalin) in the CA1 pyramidal cell field.[2] However, more recent immunochemical studies have revealed that the highest concentration of ENK-IR resides in the dentate-CA4-CA3 cell fields with only half as much ENK-IR in CA1 and the subiculum.[1, 16] FIGURE 1 illustrates the correlation between ENK-like immunohistochemical staining of rat dorsal hippocampus, and enkephalin radioimmunoassay data from regionally dissected rat hippocampi.

However, recent immunohistochemical studies in our laboratory, in conjunction with collaborative immunochemical studies (performed by A. Goldstein at Stanford University), have suggested to us that the major opioid peptide found in the hippocampus is not a "classical" endorphin, but *dynorphin*. This 17-amino-acid residue neuropeptide is one member of a growing class of neuropeptides containing the Leu[5]-enkephalin sequence at its N-terminus.[17] Antisera raised against dynorphin 1-17 and antisera raised against leucine-enkephalin both demonstrate immunoreactivity in rat, squirrel monkey, and cat hippocampal mossy fibers and dentate granule cells. In addition, the rat CA1 hippocampal field demonstrated scattered dynorphin IR and enkephalin IR in cells and fibers.

Enkephalin IR is also observed in cells of the entorhinal cortex. These cells give rise to fibers which innervate rat hippocampus and dentate gyrus. However, this group of cells is *not* dynorphin immunoreactive. Moreover, we have observed that the dynorphin IR in the rat hippocampus is qualitatively denser in immunocytochemical preparations and quantitatively greater in radioimmunoassay preparations than is enkephlin IR. Furthermore, dynorphin IR staining throughout the hippocampus is eliminated *only* by adsorption with

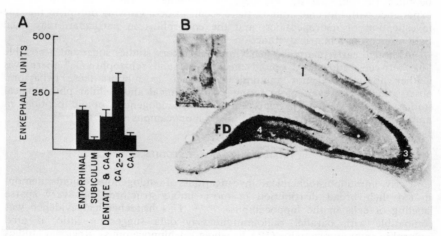

FIGURE 1. (A) Immunochemical analysis of enkephalin immunoreactivity (ENK-IR) from regional dissection of rat hippocampal gyrus. Note relative differences in ENK-IR in various cell fields illustrated in (B).

(B) Enkephalin immunoreactivity in mossy fibers of hippocampus (HPC) from a rat treated 2 days previously with 1 μg/μl kainic acid, i.c.v. Coronal section. Numbers 1 through 4 refer to CA fields of HPC. FD = fascia dentata. Calibration bar = 500 μm.

1–100 μM dynorphin 1-17, whereas enkephalin IR staining is eliminated by adsorption with 10 μM Leu-enkephalin, 1 μM dynorphin 1-17, 1-13, or α-neo-endorphin (J. McGinty *et al.*, in press). Intrahippocampal injections of colchicine, which selectively destroys dentate granule cells, significantly reduces the dynorphin IR and enkephalin IR in rat hippocampal mossy fibers. Intra-ventricular kainic acid, which selectively destroys the CA3-4 pyramidal cells, results in an increase of both dynorphin IR and enkephalin IR in rat hippo-campus. Therefore, our data suggest that, throughout the hippocampus, enkephalin IR is likely to be due to cross-reactivity with dynorphin or α-neo-endorphin. Conversely, enkephalin IR fibers afferent to the hippocampus, arising from the lateral entorhinal/perirhinal cortex,[5] are *not* dynorphin IR containing. Thus, the endorphin IR in two major opioid peptidergic pathways of the hippocampal formation may represent the presence of two entirely different prohormonal systems.

Physiological Studies

Early investigations of the role of endogenous opioid peptides in the central nervous system suggested a role for this class of peptides in the regulation of brain excitability. Intraventricular administration of nanomolar amounts of several opioid peptides elicits in rodents a variety of electrographic signs in the subcortical and cortical electroencephalogram (EEG), suggesting epileptogenic properties of these peptides.[18, 19] A major aspect of these opioid-induced electrographic abnormalities is the development of repetitive paroxysmal sharp EEG waveforms primarily confined to limbic brain areas, and particularly observable in the hippocampus (FIGURE 2).[19]

This suggests that one of the major pharmacological sites of action of this naloxone-reversible epileptogenic effect could be the rat limbic system; and a major role of opioid peptides could be the regulation of limbic excitability.[19] In addition, ^{14}C-2-deoxy-glucose autoradiographs of rats administered the potent endogenous opioid peptide, β-endorphin, demonstrate that the hippocampus is particularly sensitive to this epileptogenic action (FIGURE 3).[20]

These early encephalographic studies are compatible with more recent microelectrophoretic cellular investigations suggesting a *unique* excitatory effect of opioid peptides in the rat hippocampus.[22, 23, 26] The role of endorphins in limbic activity has been further clarified by evidence suggesting that this unique excitatory (epileptogenic) action of endorphins may be the result of a disinhibitory process within the microcircuitry of the hippocampus.[23] Although controversy still exists with respect to the exact mechanism of this excitatory effect,[10, 24, 25] it now appears probable that opioid peptides play a significant role in regulating limbic excitability.

Preliminary studies in rats injected intraventricularly with microgram amounts of dynorphin 1-13 demonstrated a variety of behavioral effects but no epileptogenic response, thus pharmacologically differentiating dynorphin from other epileptogenic opioids. Prompted by our recent observations of the apparent predominance of dynorphin in the rat hippocampus (J. McGinty *et al.*, in press), we have recently investigated the response of hippocampal neurons to electrophoretically administered dynorphin. To date, we have studied more than 180 hippocampal neurons *in vivo* and assessed the response of each neuron to electrophoretically (or pneumatically) applied dynorphin. We have com-

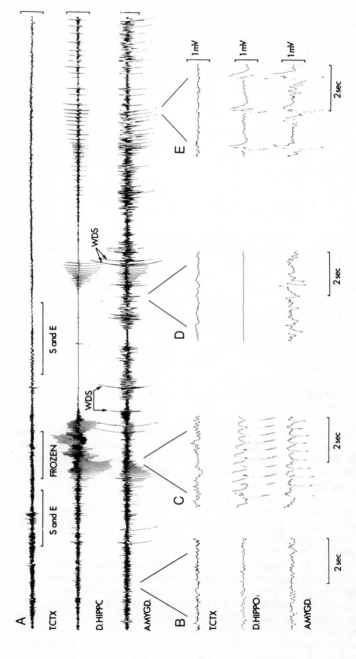

FIGURE 2. Multitrace EEG record of β-endorphin-induced epileptiform activity in rats (3 nM i.c.v.). (A) Slow time-base record showing onset and subsequent postictal epileptiform events. β-endorphin injected at start of trace. Note high voltage (1–2 mV) paroxysmal spikes (ictal episode) followed by prolonged isoelectric period prominent in the hippocampal trace. (B) Baseline EEG prior to onset of seizural activity, fast time-base. (C) Ictal paraoxysmal waves, fast-base. (D) Postictal period of hippocampal depressing and complex spiking in amygdala. (E) Postictal period of prolonged isolated paroxysmal waves. T.CTX — bipolar transcortical electrode EEG trace; D.HIPPO = bipolar dorsal hippocampal electrode trace; AMYGD. = bipolar amygdala electrode trace; S and E = sniffing and exploring; WDC = wet dog shakes.

pared the difference in cellular responses to dynorphin (1-13 and 1-17), Leu⁵-enkephalin, morphine sulfate, and the excitatory amino acids acetylcholine and glutamic acid. We have also investigated the ability of the opiate antagonist naloxone to antagonize hippocampal responses to the above peptides and morphine.

Male rats (Sprague-Dawley, $n = 41$) were prepared for electrophoretic tests by conventional surgical techniques. Following halothane anesthesia and tracheotomy, rats were fixed in a stereotaxic head-holder and maintained at

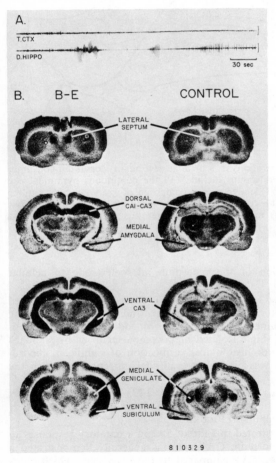

FIGURE 3. EEG traces and ¹⁴C—2-deoxyglucose (2DG) autoradiographic illustrations of the response to intraventricularly administered β-endorphin (B-E, 3 nM) in a representative rat. (A) Electrographic tracing of ictal seizure episode elicited by B-E. (B) ¹⁴C-2DG autoradiographs of representative sections of control rat brain and a brain of a rat exhibiting seizure shown in FIGURE 2A following B-E. Visual inspection of the autoradiographs reveal marked uptake of DG, bilaterally, in the dorsal and ventral hippocampus, posterior and ventral subiculum, dentate gyrus, lateral septum, and the posterior part of the medial nucleus of the amygdala (amygdala-hippocampal area). There was also a marked decrease of uptake bilaterally in the medial geniculate body.

low anesthetic levels (1.0–1.5% halothane) and constant temperature (37° C). A craniotomy was performed in order to allow placement of a bipolar stimulating electrode as well as standard 5-barrel electrophoretic/recording electrodes aimed in a vertical plane to allow each penetration to pass through both CA1 and CA3 cellular fields (FIGURE 4). The bipolar stimulating electrode was aimed toward the dentate gyrus within the laminar confluence of the granule cell mossy fibers, allowing field-potential laminar analysis of the hippocampus. This greatly

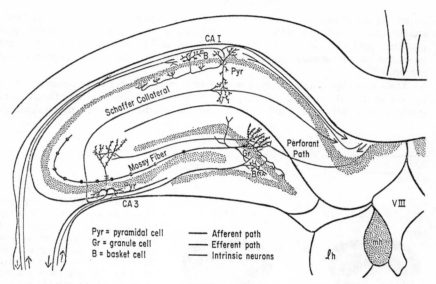

FIGURE 4. Diagrammatic illustration of a frontal section of dorsal hippocampus (septal pole). The major cellular groups include (1) the continuous pyramidal cell field CA1 through CA4; and the dentate gyrus, composed of granular cells sending primary axons to the pyramidal cells in CA3–4 by way of the so-called mossy fibers. Schaffer collateral axons arise from CA3–4 neurons and innervate CA1–2 cell fields.

facilitated "on-line" localization of the recording microelectrode to cellular targets.

Each 5-barrel micropipette (4–7 μm diameter) consisted of 3 drug-filled barrels, a 3 M NaCl current compensation barrel, and a central recording barrel containing 2% pontamine sky blue in 0.5 M sodium acetate. Drugs were ejected in the vicinity of single isolated hippocampal neurons by standard electrophoretic techniques.[11] For histological verification of significant recording sites, pontamine sky blue was ejected by cathodal current applied to the recording barrel.

Most hippocampal neurons tested (67%, $n = 122$) exhibited excitatory responses to dynorphin in a manner similar to that reported by ourselves [11, 21] and others [22] for other opioid peptides (FIGURE 5).

Although both neurons illustrated in FIGURE 5 show excitatory responses to electrophoretically applied dynorphin, CA1 neurons generally demonstrated a short lasting excitation (FIGURE 5A) compared to CA3 neurons, which characteristically demonstrated very long periods of excitation (FIGURE 5B). However, *both* CA1 and CA3/4 neurons generally responded with short-latency and short-lasting excitatory responses to electrophoretically applied Leu[5]-enkephalin, and to a lesser extent, morphine sulfate. Iontophoretically applied naloxone, a potent opiate antagonist, successfully antagonized 84% of all induced excitatory responses of hippocampal neurons tested ($n = 25$) (FIGURE 6).

Dynorphin elicited long-lasting excitations (up to 4 min) in CA3-4 neurons whether applied by short (usually 3–15 sec) electrophoretic or micropressure pulses, indicating that the dynorphin-induced effects were not attributable to nonspecific mechanisms (i.e., current stimulation) (FIGURE 7).

Although the majority of cells studied in all hippocampal cell fields exhibited naloxone-reversible excitatory responses to dynorphin, a significant number of neurons (10%, $n = 18$) demonstrated a clear inhibitory response to the peptide. Even though we have not attempted to classify these neurons further, many of these hippocampal neurons appeared to have a more rapid spontaneous discharge rate than those neurons excited by dynorphin, and thus could presumably constitute a separate class of hippocampal cell. In addition, for all cells inhibited by dynorphin, iontophoretically applied naloxone was unable to antagonize this inhibitory effect (FIGURE 8).

Previous studies in our laboratory [23, 24] and work by others [26] have suggested an indirect, disinhibitory, synaptic mechanism underlying the excitatory responses of hippocampal cells to opiates and opioid peptides. Magnesium ions have previously been used to demonstrate the possibility of such an indirect

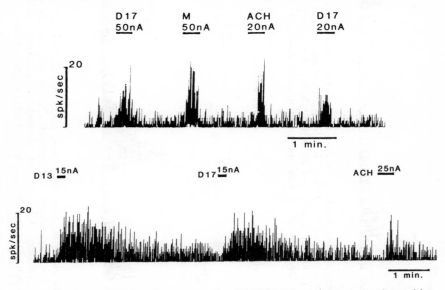

FIGURE 5. (*Top*) Excitatory responses of a CA1 hippocampal neuron to dynorphin, morphine, and acetylcholine. Rate meter records of the effect of electrophoretically applied dynorphin (D17, 3 mM in saline), morphine sulfate (M, 10 mM in distilled water [DH$_2$O], and acetylcholine (ACh, 1 M in DH$_2$O), of single neuron action potentials recorded from a CA1-hippocampal neuron. Note the relatively similar and short lasting effect of electrophoretically applied D17, morphine and ACH. (*Bottom*) Excitatory responses of a CA3 hippocampal neuron to dynorphin and ACH. Note similar but much longer lasting excitatory action of dynorphin (both dynorphin 1–13 [D13] and dynorphin 1–17 [D17]) on a CA3 hippocampal neuron compared to the response to dynorphin seen for CA1 neurons. However, ACH exhibits a similar short lasting response in CA3 and CA1. Abbreviations: nA = nanoamperes of ejection current; spk/sec = number of individual action potentials observed in 1 sec bins; bar (1 min.) = length of electrophoretically applied drug.

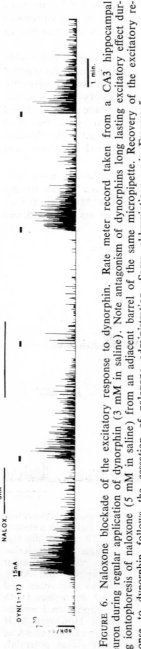

FIGURE 6. Naloxone blockade of the excitatory response to dynorphin. Rate meter record taken from a CA3 hippocampal neuron during regular application of dynorphin (3 mM in saline). Note antagonism of dynorphins long lasting excitatory effect during iontophoresis of naloxone (5 mM in saline) from an adjacent barrel of the same micropipette. Recovery of the excitatory response to dynorphin follows the cessation of naloxone administration. Same abbreviations as in FIGURE 5.

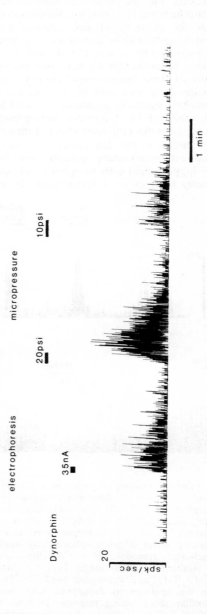

FIGURE 7. Comparison of the effects of dynorphin applied electrophoretically or by micropressure to a CA3 hippocampal neuron. Rate meter illustration of the similarity between electrophoretically and pneumatically (micropressure) applied dynorphin [3 mM in saline]. Note the long periods excitation elicited by both administration-paradigms. Abbreviation: nA = nanoamperes of current applied; psi = pounds per square inch of air applied to the sealed head of the microelectrode barrel.

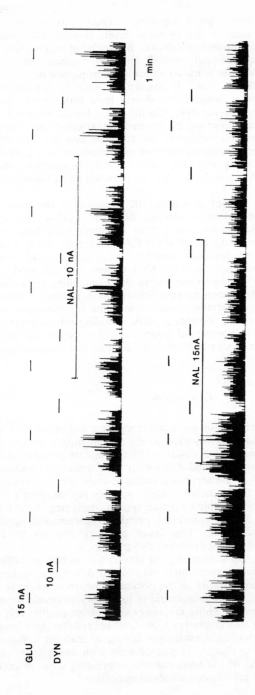

FIGURE 8. Inhibitory response to dynorphin and lack of antagonist by naloxone. Rate meter records taken from a CA3 hippocampal neuron during electrophoretic administration of dynorphin (3 mM in saline) and glutamate (0.5 M in DH₂O). Even with an iontophoresis current of naloxone (5 mM in H₂O) sufficient to suppress glutamate-induced excitation of the neuron, naloxone failed to suppress the dynorphin-induced inhibition of spontaneous activity. Abbreviations: NHC = no holding current: diffusion of dynorphin, no cathodal current applied; Glut = glutamic acid (0.5 M in DH₂O).

mechanism of action for other opioid peptides.[24] These ions are believed to interfere with calcium uptake at the synaptic level, thereby disrupting the calcium-coupled process of transmitter release. By applying magnesium to the microenvironment of a hippocampal neuron, one can examine the effect of subsequently delivered dynorphin from an adjacent micropipette barrel, on that neuron's spontaneous discharge rate. If dynorphin were to act directly on somatic or dendritic receptors, magnesium should have little or no effect on the peptide-induced response of the cell. On the other hand, observed alterations in the peptide-induced response by magnesium suggest that dynorphin may affect the recorded neuron indirectly via adjacent neurons (FIGURE 9). Moreover, as naloxone alters dynorphin-induced excitations in both CA1 as well as CA3-4 cell fields, it is likely that dynorphin containing neurons, observed by immunochemistry in CA1 as well as CA3, are presynaptic to these presumed inhibitory interneurons.

More confusing is the role of dynorphin IR obesrved in the mossy fiber system—the acknowledged primary intrinsic input to CA3-4 hippocampal pyramidal neurons. Classically, the mossy fiber terminals have been thought to synapse directly on the proximal dendrites of CA3-4 neurons and to release an excitatory amino acid, as yet uncharacterized.[27] It remains unclear what role dynorphin may have in this major intrinsic fiber system, yet it is intriguing to speculate that it may play a role in regulating the excitability pyramidal cell activity. It is possible that the non-naloxone-reversible inhibitory responses to electrophoretically applied dynorphin observed in some hippocampal neurons may be a reflection of this effect. Further studies, including intracellular investigation of the response of hippocampal neurons to dynorphin (in progress) are necessary to clarify the precise role of dynorphin in this hippocampal fiber system.

DISCUSSION

Immunohistochemical studies in our laboratory have suggested that at least three possible opioid peptide systems exist in the rodent hippocampus. Potentially, the most significant pathway is described by the dentate granule cell-mossy fiber system where we have identified dynorphin both immunohistochemically and radioimmunochemically. Dynorphin-containing cells are also found scattered throughout CA1 and CA3-4 cellular fields, possibly representing a subclass of hippocampal interneuron. A third peptide system impinging on the hippocampus derives from the lateral entorhinal/perirhinal cortex and appears to synapse on dentate granule cells. This latter pathway appears to contain enkephalin immunoreactivity but is devoid of dynorphin.

Parallel neurophysiological studies suggest similarities as well as differences in the response of identified hippocampal neurons to dynorphin, enkephalin, and morphine sulfate. The majority of hippocampal neurons we have tested elicit a naloxone-reversible, Mg^{2+} antagonizable excitatory response to electrophoretically applied dynorphin. Those responses are similar qualitatively to the effects observed following electrophoresis of Leu[5]-enkephalin and morphine sulfate. However, dynorphin induces longer lasting excitations compared to the rapid onset and short excitatory responses seen with enkephalin. In fact 80% of the neurons in CA3 of the hippocampus responding with an excitatory response to dynorphin, had prolonged periods of excitation.

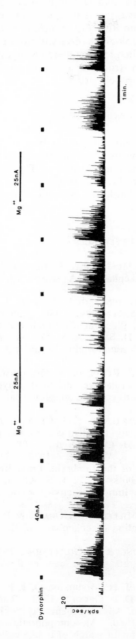

FIGURE 9. Mg^{2+} antagonism of dynorphin-induced excitation of a CA3 hippocampal neuron. Note the typical long-lasting excitatory response of this CA3 neuron to electrophoretically applied dynorphin (3 mM in saline). When Mg^{2+} (1 M in DH_2O) is concurrently applied to the environment of the cell from an adjacent barrel of the same microelectrode used for recording the spontaneous activity of the cell, Mg^{2+} is capable of suppressing the normal excitation seen following pulses of dynorphin. Note recovery of the normal excitatory response following the cessation of Mg^{2+} iontophoresis.

We have utilized the hippocampus of the *in vivo* anesthesized rat to assess cellular responses to an endogenous neuroactive peptide, dynorphin. Immuno-histochemical studies have demonstrated a unique distribution of this peptide in the hippocampus separate from the distribution of Leu-enkephalin. We feel that such microneuropharmacological observations in the hippocampus in conjunction with this new histochemical evidence suggest an important role for dynorphin in this limbic system structure, and may provide insights as to the role of endorphin peptides in neuropsychiatry.

ACKNOWLEDGMENTS

We thank Drs. Avram Goldstein, Alejandro Bayon, George Siggins, and Walter Zieglgansberger for allowing us to summarize portions of our collaborative research. We acknowledge the contribution of Drs. Nicholas Ling, Roger Guillemin, and Lars Terenius for the availability of the opioid peptides and antisera used in these studies. We thank Ms. Nancy Callahan for the preparation of the manuscript.

REFERENCES

1. BAYON, A., W. SHOEMAKER, J. McGINTY & F. BLOOM. 1982. Immunodetection of endorphins and enkephalins—A search for reliability. Int. Rev. Neurobiol. In press.
2. BLOOM, F. E., A. BAYON, E. BATTENBERG, E. FRENCH, L. KODA, G. KOOB, M. LEMOAL, J. ROSSIER & W. SHOEMAKER, 1980. Endorphins: Developmental and Behavioral Aspects. Adv. Biochem. Psychopharmacol. **22:** 619–632.
3. BROWNSTEIN, M., A. ARIMURA, H. SATO, A. V. SCHALLY & J. S. KIZER. 1975. The regional distribution of somatostatin in the rat brain. Endocrinology **96:** 1456–1461.
4. EMSON, P. C., S. P. HUNT, J. F. REHFELD, N. GOLTERMAN & J. FAHRENKRUG. 1980. Cholecystokinin and vasoactive intestinal polypeptide on the mammalian CNS: Distribution and possible physiological roles. Adv. Biochem. Psychopharmacol. **22:** 63–74.
5. GALL, C., N. BRECHA, H. J. KARTEN & K.-J. CHANG. 1981. Localization of enkephalin-like immunoreactivity to identified axonal and neuronal populations of the rat hippocampus. J. Comp. Neurol. **198:** 335–350.
6. KOBAYASHI, R. M., M. BROWN & W. VALE. 1977. Regional distribution of neurotensin and somatostatin of the rat brain. Brain Res. **126:** 584-588.
7. PETRUSZ, P., M. SAR, G. H. GROSSMAN & J. S. KIZER. 1977. Synaptic terminals with somatostatin-like immunoreactivity in the rat brain. Brain Res. **137:** 181–187.
8. SAR, M., W. E. STUMPF, R. J. MILLER, K.-J. CHANG & P. CUATRACASAS. 1978. Immunohistochemical localization of enkephalin in the rat brain spinal cord. J. Comp. Neurol. **187:** 17–38.
9. BLOOM, F. E., D. SEGAL, N. LING & R. GUILLEMIN. 1976. Endorphins: Profound behavioral effects in rats suggest new etiological factors in mental illness. Science **194:** 630–632.
10. SIGGINS, G. R., J. F. McGINTY, J. H. MORRISON, Q. J. PITTMAN, W. ZIEGLGANSBERGER, P. J. MAGISTRETTI & D. L. GRUOL. 1982. The role of neuropeptides in the hippocampal formation. Adv. Biochem. Psychopharmacol. In press.
11. FRENCH, E. D. & G. SIGGINS. 1980. An iontophoretic survey of opioid peptide actions in the rat limbic system: In search of opiate epileptogenic mechanisms. Reg. Peptides **1:** 127–146.

12. BLOOM, F. E. & J. MCGINTY. 1981. Cellular distribution and functions of endorphins. *In* Endogenous Peptides and Learning and Memory Processers. Academic Press, pp. 199–229. New York.
13. HÖKFELT, T., R. ELDC, O. JOHANSSON, L. TERENIUS & L. STEIN. 1977. The distribution of enkephalin-immunoreactive cell bodies in rat central nervous system. Neurosci. Lett. **5:** 25–31.
14. UHL, G., R. GOODMAN, S. CHILDERS & S. SNYDER. 1978. Immunohistochemical mapping of enkephalin containing cell bodies and nerve terminals in the brain stem of the rat brain. Brain Res. **166:** 75–94.
15. WAMSLEY, J., W. YOUNG & M. KUHAR. 1980. Immunohistochemical localization of enkephalin in rat forebrain. Brain Res. **190:** 153–174.
16. HONG, J. S. & R. SCHMID. 1981. Intrahippocampal distribution of Met-enkephalin. Brain Res. **205:** 415–418.
17. GOLDSTEIN, A. & R. GHAZAROSSIAN. 1980. Immunoreactive dynorphin in pituitary and brain. Proc. Natl. Acad. Sci. USA **77:** 6207–6210.
18. URCA, G., H. FRENK, J. C. LIEBESKIND & A. N. TAYLOR. 1977. Morphine and enkephalin: Analgesic and epileptic properties. Science **197:** 83–86.
19. HENRIKSEN, S. J., F. E. BLOOM, F. MCCOY, N. LING & R. GUILLEMIN. 1978. β-endorphin induces nonconvulsive limbic seizures. Proc. Natl. Acad. Sci. USA **75:** 5221–5225.
20. HENRIKSEN, S. J., F. MORRISON & F. E. BLOOM. 1979. β-endorphin induced epileptiform activity increases local cerebral metabolism in hippocampus. Soc. Neurosci. Abstracts **5:** 528.
21. NICOLL, R. M., G. R. SIGGINS, N. LING, F. E. BLOOM & R. GUILLEMIN. 1977. Neuronal actions of endorphins and enkephalins among brain regions: A comparative microiontophoretic study. Proc. Natl. Acad. Sci. USA **74:** 2584–2588.
22. HILL, R. G., J. F. MITCHELL & C. M. PEPPER. 1977. The excitation and depression of hippocampal neurons by iontophoretically applied enkephalins. J. Physiol. **272:** 50–51P.
23. ZIEGLGANSBERGER, W., E. D. FRENCH, G. R. SIGGINS & F. E. BLOOM. 1979. Opioid peptides may excite hippocampal pyramidal neurons by inhibiting adjacent inhibitory interneurons. Science **205:** 415–417.
24. SIGGINS, G. R. & W. ZIEGLGANSBERGER. 1981. Morphine and opioid peptides reduce inhibitory synaptic potentials in hippocampal pyramidal cells *in vitro* without alterations of membrane potential. Proc. Natl. Acad. Sci. USA **78:** 5935–5239.
25. DINGLEDINE, R. 1981. Possible mechanism of enkephalin action on hippocampal CA1 pyramidal neurons. J. Neuroscience **9:** 1022–1035.
26. NICOLL, R. A., B. E. ALGER & C. E. JAHR. 1980. Enkephalin blocks inhibitory pathways in the vertebrate CNS. Nature **287:** 22–25.
27. COTMAN, C. 1981. Acidic amino acid as excitatory transmitters. *In* Regulatory Mechanisms of Synaptic Transmission, R. Tapia and C. Cotman, Eds. Plenum Press. New York.

DISCUSSION OF THE PAPER

QUESTION: Don't you have difficulty with the stability of dynorphin, because it is a rather unstable compound?

Second, have you tried any antagonists in your experiments?

S. J. HENRIKSEN (*The Salk Institute, La Jolla, CA*): Before I answer the question, I have to add that the dynorphin we have been using is 1–13 rather than 1–17, although it has been demonstrated that there is very little or no significant physiological difference between the two. At the time we did not have the 1–17. The stability of dynorphin is an important issue biochemically. We put 10 mM dynorphin in the pipettes that we fill just prior to the experiment. The fact that we are getting the proportional effect suggests to us that it has not broken down.

If we left the dynorphin in the pipette overnight and tried it later in a couple of experiments, we were not able to see anything, so there may be a breakdown on standing.

To answer the second question, we have not done any experiments with antagonists yet, but we are planning to use the κ antagonist in studies very soon. The problem, of course, is that there are no very specific κ antagonists, but we have some Winthrop Laboratory compounds that we are planning to administer to see whether they won't block the effects, although I do not think that this is a real critical issue. Whether one describes a particular peptide as being opioid or not on the basis of naloxone is becoming more and more suspect. This is an important peptide in the hippocampus and it is our job to find the antagonists that work.

BRAIN ENDORPHINS:
POSSIBLE ROLE IN LONG-TERM MEMORY

James D. Belluzzi and Larry Stein

Department of Pharmacology
College of Medicine
University of California
Irvine, California 92717

A role for endorphins in the mediation of behavioral reinforcement is suggested by several lines of evidence: (1) injections of Met- or Leu-enkephalin or a degradation-resistant analog may serve as reinforcement for self-administration behavior; [1, 2] (2) electrical stimulation of many enkephalin-rich regions supports high rates of self-stimulation; [1, 3] and (3) such brain stimulation reinforcement may be antagonized in a dose-related fashion by naloxone. [1, 4-7] Thus, results both from self-administration testing (which demonstrates reinforcement from exogenously administered endorphins) and from self-stimulation testing (which demonstrates reinforcement from endogenously released endorphins) are consistent with the hypothesis that brain endorphins may regulate or mediate behavioral reinforcement.

The self-administration and self-stimulation tests, while providing convenient analysis of reinforcement mechanisms, nevertheless have certain limitations. Administration of pure peptides in the self-administration experiments strictly controls the chemical nature of the reinforcing injection, but because the distribution of injected peptide to active sites cannot exactly duplicate that of naturally released endorphins, the ensuing pattern of receptor activation could be artifactual or misleading. On the other hand, while electrical activation of peptide pathways during self-stimulation presumably releases the chemical messenger in a relatively natural distribution at appropriate postsynaptic sites, the electrical stimulus must also cause the simultaneous release of many different transmitters and neurohormones, including some that are still unknown. Furthermore, since both self-stimulation and self-administration typically allow the animal subjects to respond freely on schedules of continuous or densely spaced reinforcement, direct carry-over effects of drug injections and electrical brain stimulation on closely following responses pose serious problems. These drug–behavior and stimulation–behavior interactions may be avoided by use of the single-trial learning test described below.

Here we report that enkephalins and morphine enhance retention of a learned response when given immediately after training in a one-trial passive avoidance test. [8] Other workers also have investigated the role of endorphins in memory formation, but no consensus has been reached since opiates have been found both to facilitate and to inhibit retention. We attempt here to resolve the apparent contradictions.

The subjects were male albino Charles River rats (Sprague-Dawley–derived) weighing 300–400 g and individually housed with food and water available *ad libitum*. Some rats had permanently indwelling 27-gauge stainless steel cannulas stereotaxically implanted in the lateral ventricle to permit administration of drugs directly into the brain. All rats were gentled by frequent handling

0077–8923/82/0398–0221 $1.75/0 © 1982 NYAS

for 7–10 days prior to avoidance training. Animals were trained in an acrylic (Plexiglas) chamber with a grid floor for delivery of electric shock from a constant current shock source; an electrically insulated aluminum shelf extended along the back wall of the apparatus 9.4 cm above the grid floor. On the training day each rat was placed on the shelf and the time to step completely off the shelf (step-down latency) was recorded automatically within 0.1 sec by the operation of a microswitch under the shelf.[9] Trial 1 was an habituation trial; no shock was given after the step-down response and the rat was permitted to explore the box for 3 min. Trial 2 was the learning trial; the rat received a mildly painful foot shock immediately after stepping off the shelf. Mild intensities of footshock were used to produce moderate levels of avoidance learning and thus provide a sensitive baseline for measurement of memory enhancement by drugs. The rat was removed from the apparatus 10 sec after the shock, injected either intraventricularly or subcutaneously with test compound or vehicle, and returned to its home cage. Three days later, long-term memory was evaluated in a retention test by placing the rat on the shelf, exactly as before, and recording the step-down latency. If no response occurred within 180 sec, the trial was terminated and a score of 180 sec was recorded.

In the first experiment, different groups of rats received intraventricular injections of morphine, enkephalins, or Ringer's solution either immediately or 15 minutes after the shock, as indicated in TABLE 1. The Ringer's controls exhibited moderate learning and stayed on the shelf in the retention test for an average of 36.2 sec as compared to their preshock latency of 8.2 sec (FIGURE 1). Significantly increased step-down times (an average of 78.2 sec) were observed in the group treated immediately after the shock with morphine. This morphine-induced increase in retention latency could be due to an enhanced memory of the shock, but other explanations are possible. First, one must rule out direct inhibitory effects of morphine on performance in the retention test. Since the retention test occurred 3 days after the drug injection, such carry-over effects seem unlikely and, indeed, are ruled out by the results of a "morphine delayed" group. These rats received the same training as the morphine group, but the

TABLE 1

EFFECTS OF POSTTRAINING INJECTIONS OF MORPHINE AND ENKEPHALIN ON
STEP-DOWN PASSIVE AVOIDANCE

Treatment	Dose (μg)	No. of Rats	Step-Down Latency (sec) Mean ± SE
Ringer's	—	17	36.2 ± 9.4
Morphine	20	19	78.2 ± 12.1 *
Morphine (shock withheld)	20	8	5.8 ± 0.9 **
Morphine (15 min delay)	20	7	39.5 ± 23.7
Leu-Enkephalin	100	10	49.2 ± 22.0
	200	8	47.0 ± 19.7
Met-Enkephalin	100	5	8.8 ± 1.8
	200	10	114.2 ± 27.7 *

* p < 0.02 vs Ringer's.
** p < 0.001 vs Morphine.

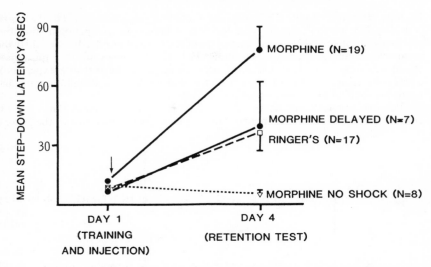

FIGURE 1. Intraventricular administration of morphine (20 μg) immediately after step-down passive avoidance training (arrow) facilitates (p < 0.02) retention measured three days later. Morphine had no effect on retention scores if the injections were delayed for 15 min after training or if the shock was omitted during training. Bars indicate standard errors.

injection was delayed for 15 min after the shock. In this case, the same carry-over effects should occur, but the retention latencies did not differ from those of the Ringer's group (FIGURE 1).

Direct effects on retention performance seem unlikely to explain the increased retention latencies, but other direct effects of the morphine injections could possibly have produced these results. For example, the morphine injection might have produced a rewarding or euphoric state in the animal. However, if morphine reinforced the step-down response, one would expect animals to step off the shelf more quickly in the retention test. Evidence also exists that a first injection of morphine can be punishing.[10] In such a case, the step-down latency in the retention test would be increased and could erroneously be interpreted as memory facilitation. To test for such direct punishing effects of morphine an additional group of rats was trained and injected with morphine immediately after the step-down response, but these rats were not shocked. If the morphine injection was punishing, then these animals also should exhibit long retention latencies. On the other hand, if morphine acts to strengthen the memory of the shock, then animals in this group should step down quickly in the retention test since there was no shock to remember. FIGURE 1 shows such quick step-down latencies in the morphine no-shock group, suggesting that the morphine injection had little or no punishing effects under the conditions of these experiments, and that the long latencies in the morphine group may be attributed to memory enhancement.

Since temporal contiguity between the response and the reinforcement is crucial for memory formation, another group of rats was trained and received the shock in a normal manner, but the morphine injection was delayed for

15 min after the shock. Delaying the morphine injection beyond the usual consolidation period should demonstrate whether time-dependent memory processes are involved.[11] This delayed administration completely abolished the memory-enhancing effects of morphine (FIGURE 1), suggesting that the opiate effects are time-dependent and must occur soon after the learning experience. These results are consistent with the idea that memory consolidation mechanisms are facilitated by opiate receptor activation.

Possible memory-enhancing effects of Met- and Leu-enkephalin were examined in the same experiment. The peptides were injected in the lateral

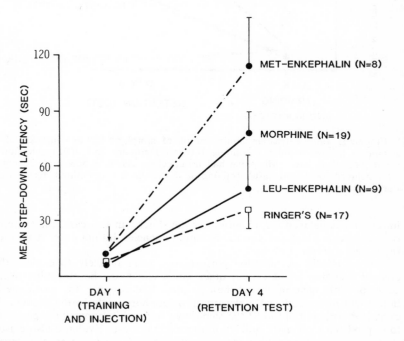

FIGURE 2. Intraventricular administration of Methionine-enkephalin (200 µg) immediately after step-down passive avoidance training (*arrow*) facilitates (p < 0.02) retention measured three days later. Identical administration of Leucine-enkephalin had no significant effects. Bars indicate standard errors.

ventricle at doses of 100 or 200 µg per injection in different groups of rats. The 200 µg-dose of Met-enkephalin significantly facilitated retention of the learned response as compared to the Ringer's control (FIGURE 2, TABLE 1). No significant effect on retention was observed following either dose of Leu-enkephalin (TABLE 1). Interestingly, 100 µg of Met-enkephalin produced an apparent amnesia, which, however, failed to achieve statistical significance.

The memory-enhancement induced by Met-enkephaline is consistent with the results produced by morphine. The failure of Leu-enkephalin to share this effect is unexpected, especially since Leu-enkephalin is a more potent reinforcer than Met-enkephalin in the self-administration test.[1] The present result may simply reflect differences in the dose–response curves for the two pentapeptides. On the other hand, it is possible that functional differences exist between Met- and Leu-enkephalin systems, and that the present findings reflect the possible separation of reinforcing and memory-facilitatory effects.

The second experiment examined the effects of naloxone on memory facilitation induced by morphine and Met-enkephalin. Demonstration of naloxone blockade would further suggest involvement of opiate receptors. Animals received avoidance training and administration of morphine (20 μg) or Met-enkephalin (200 μg) immediately after training as before. Two additional groups were given morphine or Met-enkephalin in a solution also containing naloxone (10 μg). Naloxone was delivered in the same solution as the opiates so that all groups would be injected only once following training. Naloxone completely blocked the memory-enhancing effects of morphine ($p < 0.05$), but had no significant effect on the facilitation induced by Met-enkephalin (TABLE 2). We do not know whether a higher dose of naloxone will antagonize the action of Met-enkephalin or whether this effect of the peptide cannot be reversed by naloxone.

In a final experiment the memory-enhancing effects of a peripherally active enkephalin analog (Wy–42,896; N(Me)Tyr-D-Ser-Gly-N(Me)Phe-D-Ser-NH$_2$) were examined. Again, experimental procedures were identical to the previous tests except that the peptide was administered subcutaneously. Potent analgesic activity by this route has been demonstrated for this compound in our laboratory. Different groups of rats received injections of either the enkephalin analog (Wy–42,896) or the saline vehicle. Control rats, injected subcutaneously with saline immediately after the shock, exhibited moderate learning and stayed on the shelf in the retention test on the average for 49.8 sec. Significant facilitation ($p < 0.02$) of the learned response was observed with 5–10 mg/kg of Wy–42,896 (TABLE 3, FIGURE 3). If the drug injection was delayed for 15 minutes after the shock trial (15′ Delay group), or if the shock was omitted (No Shock group) the memory-enhancing effect of Wy–42,896 was abolished. These results replicate our findings following central injections of morphine. Similar subcutaneous

TABLE 2

EFFECTS OF NALOXONE ON MORPHINE- AND ENKEPHALIN-INDUCED
MEMORY FORMATION

Treatment	Dose (μg)	No. of Rats	Step-Down Latency (sec) Mean ± SE
Ringer's	—	18	7.1 ± 2.2
Morphine	20	14	38.3 ± 9.0 **
Morphine + Naloxone	20 10	8	5.5 ± 2.3
Met-Enkephalin	200	18	31.0 ± 13.1 *
Met-Enkephalin + Naloxone	200 10	6	28.6 ± 12.9 *

* Significantly different from Ringer's, $p < 0.05$.
** $p < 0.02$.

TABLE 3

EFFECTS OF POSTTRAINING INJECTIONS OF ENKEPHALIN ANALOGS
ON STEP-DOWN PASSIVE AVOIDANCE

Treatment	Dose (mg/kg, s.c.)	No. of Rats	Step-Down Latency (sec) Mean ± SE	
			Training (Pre-Shock)	Retention (72 hr)
Vehicle	—	25	4.4 ± 0.8	49.8 ± 11.0
Wy–42,896 †	2.5	6	10.6 ± 2.0	63.2 ± 31.6
	5.0	12	9.7 ± 3.5	100.8 ± 16.8 *
	10.0	5	13.8 ± 6.6 **	139.5 ± 19.2 **
Wy–42,896 (No shock)	5.0	8	8.1 ± 3.0	5.6 ± 1.7
Wy–42,896 (15' delay)	5.0	5	5.1 ± 1.8	57.1 ± 34.8
Morphine	2.5	10	9.6 ± 3.0	43.6 ± 22.9
	5.0	13	9.3 ± 3.7	42.9 ± 17.6
	10.0	11	13.0 ± 4.5 *	46.7 ± 20.8
Wy–42,186 ‡	5.0	11	3.4 ± 0.6	63.0 ± 23.1
	10.0	11	7.8 ± 3.4	25.1 ± 6.8

* Significantly different from vehicle, $p < 0.02$, ** $p < 0.01$.
† N(Me)Tyr-D-Ser-Gly-N(Me)Phe-D-Ser-NH$_2$.
‡ Tyr-D-Ala-Gly-Phe-D-Pro-NH$_2$.

treatments with equianalgesic doses of morphine (2.5–10 mg/kg) or a related analog (Wy–42,186; Tyr-D-Ala-Gly-Phe-D-Pro-NH$_2$, 5–10 mg/kg), failed to alter retention performance. The 2.5 mg/kg dose of Wy–42,896 also failed to enhance memory formation, although this dose of drug produces analgesia.

The present observations that morphine, Met-enkephalin, and a potent analog of enkephalin facilitate retention in one-trial avoidance learning supports the idea that opiate receptor activation is involved in memory formation. A number of other laboratories have also studied the effects of opiates and opioid peptides in memory and learning tests, but no consensus has emerged regarding their role in memory formation; in fact, contradictory conclusions have been reported. However, it may be possible to reconcile these findings by giving consideration to differences in training methods and drug administration procedures, as discussed below.

As we report here, administration of morphine or enkephalins in high doses immediately after a single training trial consistently enhances memory formation.[8, 12–14] Especially noteworthy is a study [15] demonstrating memory facilitation by morphine in appetitive learning: 100 μg of morphine administered intraventricularly immediately following a single training trial facilitated retention of a water-finding response. In this case, punishing and memory-enhancing effects of morphine cannot be confused, since drug-induced punishment would increase retention latencies while drug-induced memory enhancement would decrease retention latencies. However, problems of interpretation would arise if the morphine treatment had rewarding effects, since reinforcement of the water-finding response by morphine also would decrease retention latencies. This possibility seems to be ruled out by parallel experiments in rats that learned that water was not present in the familiar water tubes. In these rats, the morphine treatment produced increased retention latencies. This result is consistent with morphine-induced memory enhancement but not with morphine-induced reward, since rewarding effects of the drug should have caused the rats to approach the empty water tube.

In the positive experiments described above, high doses of opiates were used to facilitate learning. On the other hand, deficits in retention are reported when low doses of opiates are administered immediately after training in a one-trial inhibitory avoidance task.[12, 16, 17] Thus, Jensen et al.[12] found retention deficits after intraventricular administration of 3 μg of morphine, although 40 μg facilitated retention performance. Using peripheral administration, the same authors found that 1–3 mg/kg of morphine induced amnesia, whereas 10–30 mg/kg had no inhibitory or facilitatory effect. Martinez and Rigter[16] similarly report that 0.1 mg/kg of β-endorphin administered immediately after training produces a retention deficit, whereas 100 μg/kg of β-endorphin did not alter retention.

The studies reviewed above present a complicated picture of the role of endogenous opiate systems in memory formation. On the one hand, five laboratories report that high doses of enkephalin or morphine cause memory facilitation.[8, 12–15] On theoretical grounds, this result is pleasing since it is consistent with the well-established facilitatory relationship between natural rewards and learning. In apparent contradiction, a number of studies demonstrate amnesia following administration of low doses of opiates.[12, 16, 17] Dose-dependent opposite actions are also found with opiates in other behavioral

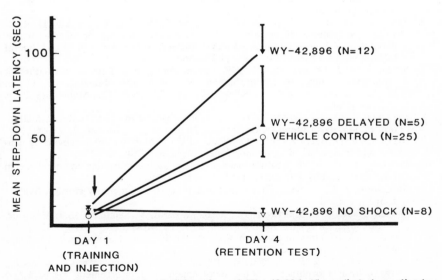

FIGURE 3. Intraperitoneal administration of Wy–42,896 (5 mg/kg) immediately after step-down passive avoidance training (arrow) facilitates (p < 0.02) retention measured three days later. Wy–42,896 had no effect on retention scores if the injections were delayed for 15 min after training or if the shock was omitted during training. Bars indicate standard errors.

tests.[18-20] One possibility is that the opposite effects of high and low opiate doses are due to differences in the relative activation of presynaptic and post-synaptic receptor sites. Low opiate doses could actually reduce postsynaptic receptor activity by presynaptic inhibition of endogenous endorphin release; such reduction in net opiate activity might produce amnesia. On the other hand, high opiate doses could override their presynaptic effects by direct activation of the postsynaptic receptor; such increase in net opiate activity might facilitate memory formation. However, it is also possible that differential interactions with other neurotransmitter systems (such as catecholamines) or differences in effective concentration at different brain sites is involved in the dual actions of opiates.

REFERENCES

1. BELLUZZI, J. D. & L. STEIN. 1977. Enkephalin may mediate euphoria and drive-reduction reward. Nature **266:** 556–558.
2. MELLO, N. K. & J. H. MENDELSON. 1978. Self-administration of an enkephalin analog by rhesus monkey. Pharmacol. Biochem. Behav. **9:** 579–586.
3. STEIN, L. & J. D. BELLUZZI. 1978. Brain endorphins and the sense of well-being: a psychobiological hypothesis. In C. Costa & M. Trabucchi, Eds. Adv. Biochem. Psychopharmacol. **18:** 299–311.
4. CHILDRESS, A. R. 1979. Naloxone suppression of brain self-stimulation: Evidence for endorphin-mediated reward. Doctoral dissertation, Bryn Mawr College.
5. KELSEY, J. E., J. D. BELLUZZI & L. STEIN. 1979. Does naloxone suppress self-stimulation by decreasing reward or increasing aversion? Society for Neuroscience Abstracts **5:** 530.
6. STAPELTON, J. M., V. J. MERRIMAN, C. L. COOGLE, S. D. GELBARD & L. D. REID. 1979. Naloxone reduces pressing for intracranial stimulation of sites in the periaqueductal gray area, accumbens nucleus, substantia nigra, and lateral hypothalamus. Physiol. Psychol. **7:** 427–436.
7. STEIN, L. & J. D. BELLUZZI. 1979. Brain endorphins: Possible mediators of pleasurable states. In Endorphins in Mental Health Research. E. Usdin, W. E. Bunney, Jr. & N. S. Kline, Eds. pp. 375–389. The Macmillan Press Ltd., London.
8. BELLUZZI, J. D. & L. STEIN. 1977. Enkephalin- and morphine-induced facilitation of long-term memory. Society for Neuroscience Abstracts **3:** 230.
9. STEIN, L., J. D. BELLUZZI & C. D. WISE. 1975. Memory enhancement by central administration of norepinephrine. Brain Res. **84:** 329–335.
10. JACQUET, Y. F. 1973. Conditioned aversion during morphine maintenance in mice and rats. Physiol. Behav. **11:** 527–541.
11. McGAUGH, J. L. 1966. Time dependent processes in memory storage. Science **153:** 1351–1358.
12. JENSEN, R. A., J. L. MARTINEZ, JR., R. B. MESSING, V. SPIEHLER, B. J. VASQUEZ, B. SOUMIREU-MOURAT, K. D. LIANG & J. L. McGAUGH. 1978. Morphine and naloxone alter memory in the rat. Society for Neuroscience Abstracts **4:** 260.
13. MONDADORI, C. & P. G. WASER. 1979. Facilitation of memory processing by posttrial morphine: Possible involvement of reinforcement mechanisms? Psychopharmacology **63:** 297–300.
14. STAUBLI, U., & J. P. HUSTON. 1980. Avoidance learning enhanced by post-trial morphine injection. Behav. Neural Biol. **28:** 487–490.
15. WHITE, N., R. MAJOR & J. SIEGEL. 1978. Effects of morphine on one-trial appetitive learning. Life Sci. **23:** 1967–1972.

16. MARTINEZ, J. L. & H. RIGTER. 1980. Endorphins alter acquisition and consolidation of an inhibitory avoidance response in rats. Neurosci. Lett. **19:** 197–201.

17. MESSING, R. B., R. A. JENSEN, B. J. VASQUEZ, J. L. MARTINEZ, JR., V. R. SPIEHLER & J. L. McGAUGH. 1981. Opiate modulation of memory. *In* Endogenous Peptides and Learning and Memory Processes. J. L. Martinez, Jr., R. A. Jensen, R. B. Messing, H. Rigter & J. L. McGaugh, Eds.: 431–443. Academic Press. New York.

18. BELLUZZI, J. D. & L. STEIN. 1978. Do enkephalin systems mediate drive reduction? Society for Neuroscience Abstracts **4:** 405.

19. HOLTZMAN, S. G. 1975. Effects of narcotic antagonists on fluid intake in the rat. Life Sci. **16:** 1465–1470.

20. LORENS, S. A. & C. L. MITCHELL. 1973. Influence of morphine on lateral hypothalamic self-stimulation in the rat. Psychopharmacologia **32:** 271–277.

PHENCYCLIDINE-LIKE DISCRIMINATIVE STIMULUS PROPERTIES OF PSYCHOTOMIMETIC OPIOIDS *

Stephen G. Holtzman

Department of Pharmacology
Emory University School of Medicine
Atlanta, Georgia 30322

The opioids comprise a heterogeneous mixture of compounds that include among their number the following: morphine and related classical agonists; naloxone and naltrexone, antagonists that are essentially devoid of intrinsic activity; and numerous drugs, such as cyclazocine, that display various combinations of agonist and antagonist properties. Tests of opioids in human subjects sophisticated in the use of narcotics and other drugs have revealed two distinct syndromes of subjective symptomology.[1] Morphine and drugs with morphine-like agonist activity produce subjective effects that are often described as pleasurable, including feelings of "coasting" and well-being (i.e., "euphoria"). In contrast, cyclazocine and certain other mixed agonist-antagonists produce a largely unpleasant dysphoric syndrome of subjective changes that range from tiredness and drunkenness to disorientation and psychotomimetic symptomology.

Differences in the spectra of activity among opioids suggest that the effects of these drugs are mediated by more than one type of neuronal substrate. Martin and co-workers [2, 3] have proposed a three-receptor model for opioids based upon the results of physiological experiments in the chronic spinal dog preparation. According to this model, effects of the various opioids are mediated at receptors designated *mu, kappa,* and *sigma,* after the proposed prototype agonists morphine, ketocyclazocine (or ethylketocyclazocine), and SKF 10,047 (*N*-allylnormetazocine). Opioids may interact with more than one receptor subtype. For example, SKF 10,047 was suggested to be an antagonist at the mu receptor in addition to being an agonist at the sigma receptor, and cyclazocine, an antagonist at the mu receptor and an agonist at both the kappa and sigma receptors. Naloxone and naltrexone are antagonists at all of the receptors, but have the highest affinity for the mu site. According to this model, the dysphoric and psychotomimetic effects of opioids are subserved by the sigma receptor. Like cyclazocine, SKF 10,047 is psychotomimetic in man.[4]

Drug discrimination techniques appear to afford an animal model for studying components of action of the opioids that reflect the different neuronal substrates with which these drugs have been proposed to interact. In a typical discrimination paradigm, an animal is trained to emit one response when injected with a certain drug and a different response when injected with saline. Under these circumstances the drug serves as an interoceptive discriminative stimulus to occasion the differential behavioral responses. A well-trained animal

* This work was supported in part by U. S. Public Health Service Grants DA 00541 and DA 02208 and Research Scientist Development Award K02 DA 00008 from the National Institute on Drug Abuse.

0077–8923/82/0398–0230 $01.75/0 © 1982 NYAS

will emit the drug-appropriate response when injected with a novel drug that has discriminative stimulus properties similar to those of the training drug; that is, stimulus control of behavior will generalize to the novel compound being tested.

MORPHINE-LIKE DISCRIMINATIVE STIMULUS EFFECTS

Rats and squirrel monkeys were trained to discriminate between saline and 3.0 mg/kg of morphine in two-choice discrete-trial avoidance procedures. The rats were trained until they reliably completed at least 18 trials of a 20-trial session on the choice lever appropriate for the substance that they had been injected with 30 min prior to the session (i.e., saline or morphine, s.c.).[5] The monkeys were trained in a 25-trial session with the criterion performance being at least 22 trials on the appropriate choice lever following the i.m. injection of saline or morphine 15 min before the session.[6]

The results of stimulus generalization tests were consistent across species and indicate that the stimulus effects of morphine are mediated by the same receptors that subserve other well-known actions of the drug such as analgesia. The stimulus effects of morphine are: (1) produced by all other drugs traditionally classified as narcotic analgesics with an order of potency similar to that seen in other procedures involving interactions with the morphine receptor; (2) stereoselective for the levorotatory isomer; (3) blocked by low doses of naloxone and naltrexone (0.1 mg/kg or less); and (4) centrally mediated.[5-10] Stimulus generalization is characterized by a high degree of pharmacologic specificity; the animals respond predominantly on the saline-appropriate choice lever when tested with a variety of nonopioid psychoactive drugs, including pentobarbital, chlorpromazine, diazepam, mescaline, ketamine, and phencyclidine (PCP).

Results such as these have been consistently obtained regardless of whether the training drug was morphine or another morphine-like agonist, such as fentanyl,[11] heroin,[12] or etorphine.[13] On the strength of these types of data, we[14] and others[15, 16] have postulated that there is an analogy between discriminative stimulus effects of opioids in animals and subjective drug effects in man.

Rats and monkeys trained to discriminate saline from morphine generalize partially to cyclazocine.[5, 17] Conversely, rats trained to discriminate saline from 0.3 mg/kg of cyclazocine[18] and squirrel monkeys trained to discriminate saline from 0.1 mg/kg of cyclazocine[19] generalize partially to morphine. These partial cross-generalizations between morphine and cyclazocine in the rat are illustrated in the left and middle panels of FIGURE 1. Although interpretation of partial generalizations can be troublesome, it is most probable that levels of drug-appropriate responding intermediate to those engendered by saline and the training drug reflect commonalities in the stimulus properties of the training and test drugs.[20]

CYCLAZOCINE-LIKE DISCRIMINATIVE STIMULUS EFFECTS

If the extent to which morphine and cyclazocine cross-generalize to each other is a reflection of their shared stimulus properties, it follows that the extent to which the drugs fail to be generalized completely to each other is an indication of the differences in their stimulus properties. In fact, the overlap in the stimulus effects of morphine and cyclazocine can be almost entirely eliminated by training animals to discriminate concurrently among morphine, saline, and cyclazocine.[21] Under these conditions it is presumably the differences between the two drugs that serve as the salient cues to occasion differential behavioral responses.

In order to develop a fuller profile of the stimulus properties of cyclazocine, rats and squirrel monkeys trained to discriminate between saline and cyclazocine were tested for stimulus generalization to a variety of opioid and nonopioid compounds. Both species generalized completely to the postulated kappa-receptor agonists ketocyclazocine and ethylketocyclazocine, and to the postu-lated sigma-receptor agonist SKF 10,047.[18, 19, 22] Consistent with these observa-tions is the recent demonstration that rhesus monkeys trained to discriminate saline from ethylketocyclazocine generalize completely to cyclazocine.[23]

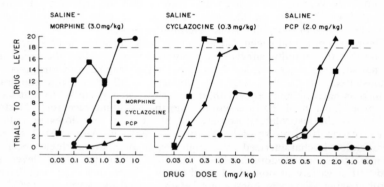

FIGURE 1. Discriminative stimulus effects of graded doses of morphine, cyclazo-cine, and PCP in rats trained to discriminate between saline and one of the following: 3.0 mg/kg of morphine (Left); 0.3 mg/kg of cyclazocine (Center); or 2.0 mg/kg of PCP (Right). Each point is the mean number of trials resulting in the choice of the drug-appropriate lever in a 20-trial session; the remaining trials were completed on the saline-appropriate lever. The upper and lower horizontal dashed lines indicate the minimum levels at which the discrimination performance was maintained with the training drug and saline, respectively. Means are based upon one observation in at least four rats.

The stimulus effects of cyclazocine in the monkey are blocked completely by naltrexone, but at a dose 10–30 times higher than the dose needed to block the stimulus effects of morphine-like agonists in monkeys trained with morphine and saline.[24] These results accord well with those of other studies showing that mixed agonist-antagonists of the benzomorphan family are less sensitive to antagonism by naloxone than are pure morphine-like agonists,[25, 26] and pro-vide further support for the view that the stimulus effects of morphine and cyclazocine are mediated by different neuronal substrates.

In the rat, the stimulus effects of cyclazocine are only partially attenuated by naltrexone, even at doses up to 30 mg/kg.[18] The relative efficacy of naltrexone for antagonizing the stimulus effects of morphine and cyclazocine in the rat can be seen in FIGURE 2. These results suggest that the stimulus effects of cyclazocine are composed of both a naltrexone-sensitive "opiate" com-ponent and a naltrexone-insensitive "nonopiate" component. It is the former component that is presumably responsible for the partial cross-generalizations

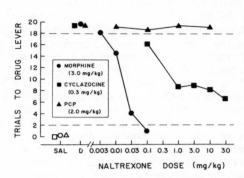

FIGURE 2. Comparison of the sensitivity of the discriminative stimulus effects of morphine (3.0 mg/kg), cyclazocine (0.3 mg/kg), and PCP (2.0 mg/kg) to antagonism by graded doses of naltrexone in different groups of rats trained to discriminate between saline and one of those three drugs. The mean number of trials completed with the animal choosing the drug-appropriate lever in test sessions with saline or with one of the training drugs alone is indicated by the points above SAL and D, respectively. Other details as in FIGURE 1.

between morphine and cyclazocine and for the complete generalization of cyclazocine with kappa-receptor agonists. The stimulus control of behavior by cyclazocine in the squirrel monkey [24] and by ethylketocyclazocine in the rhesus monkey [23] are stereoselective for the levorotatory isomer, concordant with other receptor-mediated effects of mixed-acting opioids.

Whereas the discriminative stimulus properties of mu-receptor agonists appear to be relatively consistent across species,[27] there are considerable interspecies differences in the stimulus properties of opioids believed to interact with the kappa receptor. Examples of the species dependence of the discriminative stimulus properties of ethylketocyclazocine are shown in TABLE 1. Differences among species are manifested both in pattern of stimulus generalization and in sensitivity to antagonism by naloxone or naltrexone. If pharmacokinetic variables can be ruled out, such interspecies differences may be a reflection of differences in the ratios of the various neuronal substrates that subserve the stimulus effects of some opioids. Regardless of the reason for these interspecies differences, their existence points out the need for caution in drawing conclusions from data derived from a single animal species.

TABLE 1

SPECIES DEPENDENCE OF THE DISCRIMINATIVE STIMULUS PROPERTIES OF
ETHYLKETOCYCLAZOCINE

Species	Stimulus Effects Resemble:	Antagonism By Naltrexone	Reference
Rat	Cyclazocine	Yes	Teal & Holtzman [18] and unpublished observation
Monkey	Cyclazocine	No	Teal & Holtzman [22]
Pigeon	Morphine	Yes	Herling et al.[28]

PHENCYCLIDINE-LIKE DISCRIMINATIVE STIMULUS EFFECTS

The results of stimulus generalization tests with nonopioid psychoactive drugs provide a clue to the nature of the naltrexone-insensitive component of the discriminative stimulus effects of cyclazocine. Rats trained to discriminate saline from cyclazocine generalize completely to PCP, a dissociative anesthetic with prominent psychotomimetic effects in man,[29] and to ketamine, another dissociative anesthetic and structural analog of PCP.[30] The significance of this outcome derives from the pharmacologic specificity of the drug discrimination paradigm. Cyclazocine-trained rats respond primarily on the saline-appropriate choice lever when tested with other nonopioid psychoactive drugs, such as mescaline, LSD, and d-amphetamine.[18] Hence, generalization to PCP and ketamine is based upon the stimulus effects that these drugs have in common with cyclazocine rather than being the mere consequence of the simple presence

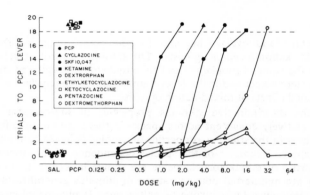

FIGURE 3. Discriminative stimulus effects of graded doses of PCP, ketamine, and various opioids in rats trained to discriminate between saline and 2.0 mg/kg of PCP. The mean number of trials completed on the drug (PCP)—appropriate lever in test sessions with saline or the training dose of PCP, which were interspersed among each of the dose-response curves, is indicated by the points above SAL and PCP, respectively. Other details as in FIGURE 1. (From Holtzman,[31] by permission of Williams & Wilkins.)

of a drug. As can be seen in FIGURE 1, PCP elicits no drug-appropriate responding in animals trained with morphine (left panel) over the same dose range that engenders prominent drug-appropriate responding in animals trained with cyclazocine (middle panel). The cyclazocine-like stimulus effects of PCP and ketamine are unaffected by up to 10 mg/kg of naloxone.[18]

The apparent similarities in the discriminative stimulus properties of PCP and certain opioids were evaluated further in animals trained to discriminate between saline and PCP. Rats were trained with intraperitoneal injections of saline and 2.0 mg/kg of PCP given 30 min before a session; squirrel monkeys were injected intramuscularly with saline and 0.25 mg/kg of PCP 10 min before a session.

FIGURE 3 shows that rats trained with PCP generalize completely to cyclazocine and SKF 10,047, but respond only on the saline-appropriate choice lever

TABLE 2

SUMMARY OF THE RESULTS OF TESTS OF STIMULUS GENERALIZATION TO OPIOIDS IN
SQUIRREL MONKEYS TRAINED TO DISCRIMINATE BETWEEN SALINE AND PCP
(0.25 MG/KG)*

	Drug	Highest Dose Tested, mg/kg
Opioids that are generalized completely to PCP:	Cyclazocine	1.0
	d-Cyclazocine	2.0
	SKF 10,047	2.0
	Dextrorphan	5.7
	Normetazocine	22.6
Opioids that are not generalized to PCP:	Ethylketocyclazocine	0.25
	Ketocyclazocine	0.5
	Levorphanol	1.0
	Levallorphan	4.0
	Pentazocine	4.0
	Naltrexone	16.0

* Tests were conducted with 4 squirrel monkeys.

in generalization tests with ketocyclazocine and ethylketocyclazocine. The latter two drugs were tested up to the highest doses at which the rats could still complete the 20 trials of the test session, which are several times higher than the doses that engender cyclazocine-like stimulus control of behavior in rats trained to discriminate saline from cyclazocine.[18] In another study, Shannon[32] has also demonstrated similarities in the stimulus effects of PCP and SKF 10,047 in the rat. Neither the PCP-like stimulus effects of cyclazocine[31] nor the stimulus effects of PCP itself (FIGURE 2) are blocked by naltrexone.

In addition to opioids proposed as agonists at the sigma opiate receptor, rats trained with PCP also generalize completely to dextrorphan (FIGURE 3), the dextrorotary isomer of the classical narcotic analgesic, levorphanol. This finding is particularly interesting in view of our earlier observation that the stimulus effects of dextrorphan as well as those of several other dextrorotatory isomers of narcotic analgesics overlap to a notable extent with the stimulus effects of cyclazocine in the squirrel monkey.[24] Commonalities in the discriminative stimulus effects of PCP, cyclazocine, and dextrorphan have also been observed in the pigeon.[33] On the other hand, dextromethorphan, the dextrorotatory isomer of levomethorphan, engenders little or no PCP-appropriate responding in the rat (FIGURE 3).

Squirrel monkeys trained with PCP display a pattern of stimulus generalization to opioids that is very similar to that seen in the rat (TABLE 2). However, the potency of the opioids relative to PCP in the squirrel monkey is less than that in the rat by a factor of approximately 2. The association between PCP-like stimulus effects and dextrorotatory opioid isomers is strengthened by the finding that d-cyclazocine is as efficacious and one-half as potent as racemic cyclazocine in engendering PCP-like stimulus control of behavior. A report that d-N-allylnormetazocine is more efficacious than its levorotatory counterpart as a PCP-like discriminative stimulus in the squirrel monkey [34] suggests a stereoselectivity for PCP-like stimulus control of behavior that favors the dextrorotatory isomer, the converse of the steric requirement for stimulus control of behavior by mu- and kappa-receptor agonists.

However, the generality of these observations remains to be established. Dextromethorphan, which is almost inactive as a PCP-like stimulus in the rat, is generalized to only partially by PCP-trained monkeys. An average of 13 out of 25 trials were completed on the PCP-appropriate choice lever after the administration of 16 mg/kg of dextromethorphan, the highest dose that could be tested safely. Thus, PCP-like stimulus effects may not be a universal property of the dextrorotatory isomers of opioids, and, by extension, the opioid structure may simply be coincidental to the PCP-like stimulus effects of these compounds.

SUMMARY AND CONCLUSIONS

The discriminative stimulus properties of opioids are heterogeneous and reflect the differences in the spectra of activity of the various opioids that have been seen in other procedures. The diverseness of stimulus properties supports the concept that the effects of opioids are mediated by multiple populations of receptors.

Opioids can be partitioned into three broad groupings on the basis of: (1) the extent to which their stimulus effects in the rat and squirrel monkey resemble those of morphine, cyclazocine, and PCP (e.g., FIGURE 1); and (2) the sensitivity of their stimulus effects to antagonism by naloxone or naltrexone (e.g., FIGURE 2). The three groups are shown in TABLE 3. Group I includes those drugs that have traditionally been classified as morphine-like narcotic analgesics. They are generalized completely to morphine and their stimulus effects are easily and completely blocked by pure antagonists. Drugs that are generalized completely to cyclazocine, but not to morphine or PCP (Group II) appear to be those compounds that have been proposed to act at the kappa opiate receptor. Their stimulus effects can be blocked at least partially by high doses of naltrexone; sensitivity to antagonism may vary between species. Drugs that are generalized completely to both cyclazocine and PCP but not to morphine comprise Group III. Included among these are opioid mixed agonist-antagonists, dextrorotatory isomers of narcotic analgesics, and nonopioid psychoactive drugs such as ketamine. The stimulus effects of drugs in Group III are relatively insensitive to antagonism by naltrexone in both cyclazocine- and PCP-trained animals.

This categorization of opioids is based on a composite of data obtained in both the rat and squirrel monkey and ignores minor inconsistencies between the species. Such inconsistencies as well as other interspecies differences in the stimulus effects of opioids [27] (i.e., TABLE 1) remain to be reconciled.

It is no accident that the examples presented in TABLE 3 are the prototype mu, kappa, and sigma opiate receptor agonists proposed by Martin et al.[2] The discriminative stimulus effects of the opioids seem to fit within the construct of this three-receptor model with one important difference. The stimulus effects of drugs in Group III do not appear to be mediated by neuronal sites that have usually been associated with the activity of opiates: the effects are not blocked by specific antagonists, show the "wrong" stereoselectivity, and are mimicked by nonopioid compounds.

Specific [³H]PCP binding sites have recently been identified in rat brain homogenates.[35, 36] [³H]PCP binding is displaced by micromolar concentrations of cyclazocine and SKF 10,047; ketocyclazocine and ethylketocyclazocine have a relatively low order of potency in this assay, and naloxone and morphine are essentially inactive.[37] The evidence suggests that the stimulus effects of opioids in Group III are mediated, in part, by neuronal substrates associated with actions of PCP rather than by sites traditionally associated with opiate activity. The neuronal sites of action common to PCP and opioids such as SKF 10,047 and cyclazocine may account for the psychotomimetic effects of these opioids in man.

TABLE 3

CLASSIFICATION OF OPIOIDS ON THE BASIS OF THEIR DISCRIMINATIVE
STIMULUS PROPERTIES IN THE RAT AND SQUIRREL MONKEY

Group	Complete Stimulus Generalization to:	Antagonism by Naltrexone	Example
I	Morphine	Complete ($\leq$ 0.1 mg/kg)	Morphine
II	Cyclazocine	Complete ($\geq$ 1.0 mg/kg) or Partial	Ketocyclazocine
III	Cyclazocine and PCP	Partial or None	SKF 10,047

REFERENCES

1. JASINSKI, D. R. 1977. Assessment of the abuse potentiality of morphine-like drugs (methods used in man). *In* Handbook of Experimental Pharmacology. W. R. Martin, Ed. Vol. 45: 197–258. Springer-Verlag, Berlin.
2. MARTIN, W. R., C. G. EADES, J. A. THOMPSON, R. E. HUPPLER & P. E. GILBERT. 1976. The effects of morphine- and nalorphine-like drugs in the nondependent and morphine-dependent chronic spinal dog. J. Pharmacol. Exp. Ther. **197**: 517–532.
3. GILBERT, P. E. & W. R. MARTIN. 1976. The effects of morphine- and nalorphine-like drugs in the nondependent, morphine-dependent and cyclazocine-dependent chronic spinal dog. J. Pharmacol. Exp. Ther. **198**: 66–82.
4. KEATS, A. S. & J. TELFORD. 1964. Narcotic antagonists as analgesics: Clinical aspects. *In* Molecular Modification in Drug Design [Advances in Chemistry Series 45]. R. F. Gould, Ed. pp. 170–176, American Chemical Society, Washington, D.C.
5. SHANNON, H. E. & S. G. HOLTZMAN. 1976. Evaluation of the discriminative effects of morphine in the rat. J. Pharmacol. Exp. Ther. **198**: 54–65.
6. SCHAEFER, G. J. & S. G. HOLTZMAN. 1977. Discriminative effects of morphine in the squirrel monkey. J. Pharmacol. Exp. Ther. **201**: 67–75.
7. SHANNON, H. E. & S. G. HOLTZMAN. 1976. Blockade of the discriminative effects of morphine in the rat by naltrexone and naloxone. Psychopharmacologia **50**: 119–124.
8. SHANNON, H. E. & S. G. HOLTZMAN. 1977. Further evaluation of the discriminative effects of morphine in the rat. J. Pharmacol. Exp. Ther. **201**: 55–66.

9. SHANNON, H. E. & S. G. HOLTZMAN. 1977. Discriminative effects of morphine administered intracerebrally in the rat. Life Sci. **21**: 585–594.
10. TEAL, J. J. & S. G. HOLTZMAN. 1980. Stimulus effects of morphine in the monkey: Quantitative analysis of antagonism. Pharmacol. Biochem. Behav. **12**: 587–593.
11. COLPAERT, F. C., H. LAL, C. J. E. NIEMEGEERS & P. A. J. JANSSEN. 1975. Investigations on drug produced and subjectively experienced discriminative stimuli. 1. The fentanyl cue, a tool to investigate subjectively experienced narcotic drug actions. Life Sci. **16**: 705–715.
12. OVERTON, D. A. & S. K. BATTA. 1979. Investigation of narcotics and antitussives using drug discrimination techniques. J. Pharmacol. Exp. Ther. **211**: 401–408.
13. HERLING, S. & J. H. WOODS. 1981. Discriminative stimulus effects of etorphine in rhesus monkeys. Psychopharmacology **72**: 256–267.
14. HOLTZMAN, S. G., H. E. SHANNON & G. J. SCHAEFER. 1977. Discriminative properties of narcotic antagonists. *In* Discriminative Stimulus Properties of Drugs, H. Lal, Ed. pp. 47–72. Plenum Publishing Corp. New York.
15. LAL, H., G. GIANUTSOS & S. MIKSIC. 1977. Discriminable stimuli produced by analgesics. *In* Discriminative Stimulus Properties of Drugs, ed. by H. Lal, pp. 23–45, Plenum Press. New York.
16. COLPAERT, F. C. 1978. Discriminative stimulus properties of narcotic analgesic drugs. Pharmacol. Biochem. Behav. **9**: 863–889.
17. SCHAEFER, G. J. & S. G. HOLTZMAN. 1981. Morphine-like stimulus effects in the monkey: Opioids with antagonist properties. Pharmacol. Biochem. Behav. **14**: 241–245.
18. TEAL, J. J. & S. G. HOLTZMAN. 1980. Discriminative stimulus effects of cyclazocine in the rat. J. Pharmacol. Exp. Ther. **212**: 368–376.
19. SCHAEFER, G. J. & S. G. HOLTZMAN. 1978. Discriminative effects of cyclazocine in the squirrel monkey. J. Pharmacol. Exp. Ther. **205**: 291–301.
20. SHANNON, H. E. & S. G. HOLTZMAN. 1979. Morphine training dose: A determinant of stimulus generalization to narcotic antagonists in the rat. Psychopharmacology **61**: 239–244.
21. WHITE, J. M. & S. G. HOLTZMAN. 1981. Three-choice drug discrimination in the rat: Morphine, cyclazocine and saline. J. Pharmacol. Exp. Ther. **217**: 254–262.
22. TEAL, J. J. & S. G. HOLTZMAN. 1980. Discriminative stimulus effects of prototype opiate receptor agonists in monkeys. Europ. J. Pharmacol. **68**: 1–10.
23. HEIN, D. W., A. M. YOUNG, S. HERLING & J. H. WOODS. 1981. Pharmacological analysis of the discriminative stimulus characteristics of ethylketazocine in the rhesus monkey. J. Pharmacol. Ther. **218**: 7–15.
24. TEAL, J. J. & S. G. HOLTZMAN. 1980. Stereoselectivity of the stimulus effects of morphine and cyclazocine in the squirrel monkey. J. Pharmacol. Exp. Ther. **215**: 369–376.
25. HUTCHINSON, M., H. W. KOSTERLITZ, F. M. LESLIE, A. A. WATERFIELD & L. TERENIUS. 1975. Assessment in the guinea-pig ileum and mouse vas deferens of benzomorphans which have strong antinociceptive activity but do not substitute for morphine in the dependent monkey. Brit. J. Pharmacol. **55**: 541–546.
26. HOLTZMAN, S. G. 1976. Comparison of the effects of morphine, pentazocine, cyclazocine and amphetamine on intracranial self-stimulation in the rat. Psychopharmacologia **46**: 223–227.
27. HERLING, S. & J. H. WOODS. 1981. Discriminative stimulus effects of narcotics: Evidence for multiple receptor-mediated actions. Life Sci. **28**: 1571–1584.
28. HERLING, S., E. H. COALE, R. J. VALENTINO, D. W. HEIN & J. H. WOODS. 1980. Narcotic discrimination in pigeons. J. Pharmacol. Exp. Ther. **214**: 139–146.

29. DOMINO, E. F. 1964. Neurobiology of phencyclidine (Sernyl), a drug with an unusual spectrum of pharmacological activity. Int. Rev. Neurobiol. **6:** 303–347.
30. DOMINO, E. F., P. CHODOFF & G. CORSSEN. 1965. Pharmacologic effects of CI-581, a new dissociative anesthetic in man. Clin. Pharmacol. Ther. **6:** 279–291.
31. HOLTZMAN, S. G. 1980. Phencyclidine-like discriminative effects of opioids in the rat. J. Pharmacol. Exp. Ther. **214:** 614–619.
32. SHANNON, H. E. 1981. Evaluation of phencyclidine analogs on the basis of their discriminative stimulus properties in the rat. J. Pharmacol. Exp. Ther. **216:** 543–551.
33. HERLING, S., E. H. COALE, JR., D. W. HEIN, G. WINGER & J. H. WOODS. 1981. Similarity of the discriminative stimulus effects of ketamine, cyclazocine, and dextrorphan in the pigeon. Psychopharmacology **73:** 286–291.
34. BRADY, K. T., R. L. BALSTER & E. L. MAY. 1982. Stereoisomers of N-allylnormetazocine: Phencyclidine-like behavioral effects in squirrel monkeys and rats. Science **215:** 178–180.
35. VINCENT, J. P., B. KARTALOVSKI, P. GENESTE, J. M. KAMENKA & M. LAZDUNSKI. 1979. Interaction of phencyclidine ("angel dust") with a specific receptor in rat brain membranes. Proc. Natl. Acad. Sci. USA **76:** 4678–4682.
36. ZUKIN, S. R. & R. S. ZUKIN. 1979. Specific [^{3}H]phencyclidine binding in rat central nervous system. Proc. Natl. Acad. Sci. USA **76:** 5342–5376.
37. ZUKIN, R. S. & S. R. ZUKIN. 1981. Demonstration of [^{3}H]cyclazocine binding to multiple opiate receptor sites. Mol. Pharmacol. **20:** 246–254.

DISCUSSION OF THE PAPER

H. M. EMRICH (*Max Planck Institute for Psychiatry, Munich, FRG*): For the theory that endorphins may play a role in schizophrenia Terenius, quoting the work of Jasinski and Martin, made an important observation that cyclazocine produces hallucinations which can be blocked by naloxone. How do you look on this from your work? Do you think the psychotogenic parts of cyclazocine can be blocked by naloxone or not?

S. G. HOLTZMAN (*Emory University School of Medicine, Atlanta, GA*): The discriminative stimulus effects of cyclazocine that we believe reflect the psychotomimetic component of action of the drug are not blocked by either naloxone or naltrexone. Therefore, the prediction from our results would be that the psychotomimetic effects of cyclazocine in man cannot be reliably blocked by naloxone. The study by Jasinski and his colleagues that you referred to may have been misinterpreted. In that particular study, cyclazocine did not produce psychotomimetic effects; its subjective effects were primarily morphine- and barbiturate-like. Cyclazocine also has a morphine-like component of action in our animal model. The morphine-like discriminative effects of cyclazocine are blocked by the pure antagonists.

Y. JACQUET (*Rockland Research Institute, Wards Island, NY*): Do you think you might get different results with naloxone instead of naltrexone?

HOLTZMAN: No, we have used naloxone as well as naltrexone in our experiments, and have obtained results with the two drugs that are entirely comparable. Naltrexone is more convenient to use than naloxone because of its longer duration of action: we don't have to worry about loss of antagonist activity during behavioral test sessions.

G. KING (*Pointe Claire, Que., Canada*): Can PCP effects be reversed by any other antagonists? Have you tried atropine or propranolol?

HOLTZMAN: The approach that you mentioned has not proven to be very productive in drug discrimination research. Thus, we have tended to avoid those types of experiments. The only drug other than the pure opiate antagonists that we have tested was haloperidol which did not block the phencyclidine cue.

UNIDENTIFIED SPEAKER: Have you tried to determine whether anesthetic drugs would generalize in your PCP- or cyclazocine-trained animals?

HOLTZMAN: There is one other drug that I am aware of: etoxadrol, a drug that was being developed as an intravenous anesthetic by Upjohn, is generalized to phencyclidine. The drug was withdrawn from clinical trials because of a high incidence of psychotomimetic side effects during emergence from anesthesia. In contrast, barbiturates, which have no psychotomimetic activity, are not generalized to either cyclazocine or to phencyclidine.

UNIDENTIFIED SPEAKER: Is there any evidence that the *d*-isomers of the opiates that generalize to the PCP- and cyclazocine-trained animals might have psychotomimetic effects?

HOLTZMAN: Yes, there is. In the early 1950s, Isbell and Fraser reported that both dextrorphan and dextromethorphan produced dysphoric subjective effects in postaddict volunteers in tests at the Addiction Research Center in Lexington. These observations were confirmed and extended in the early 1970s by Jasinski and his colleagues, also at the Addiction Research Center. They reported that high doses of dextromethorphan produced dysphoric and actual psychotomimetic symptoms that resembled the effects of high doses of nalorphine, a narcotic mixed agonist–antagonist with well-documented psychotomimetic activity.

R. S. ZUKIN (*Albert Einstein College of Medicine, Bronx, NY*): One of your illustrations points to another very interesting conclusion: that a number of the prototypic opiate ligands, which were predicted to target κ or σ opiate receptors selectively, actually crossreact with multiple receptor subclasses. Thus, your data are consistent with the idea that cyclazocine, for example, interacts with μ, κ and σ opiate receptors, if we can call the σ receptor an opiate receptor. I also wanted to point out that our binding data concur with the altered stereoselectivity pattern you observe at the sigma/PCP binding site.

BIOBEHAVIORAL BASES OF THE REINFORCING
PROPERTIES OF OPIATE DRUGS *

Conan Kornetsky and George Bain

Laboratory of Behavioral Pharmacology
Division of Psychiatry
Boston University School of Medicine
Boston, Massachusetts 02118

INTRODUCTION

One thing that is certainly not in short supply in the field of drug abuse is theories. A recent NIDA monograph edited by Lettieri *et al.*[1] gives 43 theories presented by 43 different researchers and commentators. Each of the theories is classified into one of four types of theories: self, others, society, and nature. The editors of the monograph point out that many theories could be classified into more than one category. What the monograph clearly indicates is that there are multiple contributions to initiation, continuation, cessation, and relapse to substance abuse. Despite these multiple factors, the focus of the present essay is that there exists a commonality of central nervous system action of many substances of abuse that for the user is translated into some pleasurable feelings that have been described as the "high." At the level of the CNS it is translated into an activation of those areas of the brain for which electrical stimulation is rewarding. At a behavioral level in an animal it is translated into abuse substances causing a lowering of the threshold for rewarding brain stimulation. Of interest for the main focus of this meeting, opioids in mental illness, is that the experiments described implicate an important interaction between the catecholaminergic and the endorphinergic systems.

ABUSE

As mentioned, there are multiple reasons why opioids are abused, and many of these reasons are unrelated to the pharmacological action of the drugs. Certainly peer pressure, psychopathology, and, most important, availability of drugs contribute to nonmedical use. However, none of these reasons or the reasons expressed in the NIDA monograph would have any causative factor in drug use if the drugs were not in some way reinforcing. It could be argued that this is a tautology. If the taking of the drugs leads to drug-seeking behavior, then by definition the taking of the drug is reinforcing. However, the question is not really whether the drug is reinforcing, but why and how it is reinforcing? This question may be looked at in various ways. The effects of two aspirin tablets can be reinforcing if we find that as a result of taking these two tablets our headache is relieved. Even though the aspirin-taking

* Much of the research and preparation of this paper was supported by Grant DA 02326 from the National Institute of Drug Abuse (NIDA).

241

behavior is reinforcing, and even if the aspirin is taken every four hours around the clock, it is not considered drug abuse. The person who continually takes a benzodiazepine for the relief of anxiety, fear or tension is also not usually considered a drug abuser.

What is unique in the aspirin or benzodiazepine example is that the drug is used to relieve some discomfort, be it physical or psychological. Both psychological as well as biological theories have emphasized the restorative nature of drug use as the reinforcement of drug use. For example, Beckett [2] poetically stated, "that heroin addiction in some is symptomatic of an underlying chronic depression in a wounded personality . . ." and that drug use is adaptive. This position is not different from that of Chein et al. 10 years earlier [3] or Wikler 12 years earlier.[4] Many writers have argued that the use of opiates protects the user from feelings of "unmitigated aggression." [5] Even the more biological theories have studied the adaptive nature of the opiate use. For example, Dole and Nyswander [6] have argued that there is a metabolic deficiency in the narcotic addict, and opiate use is restorative.

These theories have emphasized the negative aspects of the user to explain the reinforcement properties of narcotic use. However, the need to relieve the withdrawal symptoms is also an example of the adaptive nature of drug taking that makes no statement regarding a predisposing psychopathology.

Mello [7] has argued that the major effects of opiates and most other abuse substances is unpleasant or negatively reinforcing, and, if this be so, then these aversive effects become positively reinforcing. This hypothesis is based on the finding that electric shock that can maintain escape and avoidance behavior, may under certain conditions be self-administered by the same monkey.[8, 9] Although response-produced shock in animals may be a reasonable model for the reinforcing properties of abuse substances for a few individuals, it is not particularly parsimonious, and it makes the assumption that the prepotent effect of the drug is unpleasant even in initial use. This model ignores the fact that abuse substances differ from the non-abuse substances in that all of the former cause some euphoria and well-being in the subject, even in the presence of aversive actions, while none of the latter cause such euphoriant effects. If this were not the case, all substances that had aversive properties would be abused by a significant number of people.

In the NIDA monograph on theories, only 7 of the 43 proffered theories have euphoria as a key variable. For the most part theories have ignored the euphoriant-producing aspects of opiate use. Margaret Mead more than a decade ago at a Congressional hearing on drug abuse characterized society's attitude toward drug use when she defined the difference between virtue and vice: "Virtue is when you have pain followed by pleasure, while vice is when you have pleasure followed by pain." Thus, despite the fact that drug use has pharmacologically as well as societally caused pain, it also has a pharmacologically caused pleasure that we believe accounts for much of the reinforcing properties of drug use. Further, a model for this euphoric action is suggested by the effects of opioids, as well as of other abuse substances, on brain-stimulation reward (also referred to as intracranial self-stimulation.) [10, 11]

BRAIN STIMULATION

Although the phenomenon of intracranial self-stimulation was first described by Olds and Milner in 1954,[12] it was not until 1960 [13] that the effects of opiates on self-stimulation was first described. Although Olds and Travis found that morphine (7.0 mg/kg i.p.) caused significant decrease in response rate in most of their preparations, some facilitation in rate was seen in some animals.

Of interest is that after the 1960 paper by Olds and Travis there was, as far as we could find, not a single publication on the effects of any opiate on intracranial self-stimulation until a paper by Adams et al. in 1972.[14] Although Adams and coworkers found that morphine facilitated self-stimulation behavior, the increase in response rate was not seen until three hours after drug administration. The immediate effect was inhibitory. The lack of interest in intracranial self-stimulation as a method for the study of the reinforcing properties of opioids for over 10 years after the Olds and Travis paper in 1960 was probably due to the growth and interest in the intravenous self-administration of drugs by animals first described by Weeks in 1962 [15] as a model for the study of reinforcing properties, and secondly to the fact that the major effect of morphine reported by Olds and Travis [13] was to inhibit self-stimulation behavior.

In addition to the 1972 Adams et al. paper,[14] we reported in 1972 [16] on the effects of morphine on the EEG recorded from depth electrodes implanted in areas of the brain that elicit self-stimulation behavior. This work was, in part, based on a 1970 dissertation by Nelsen.[17] In the late 1960s Nelsen became interested in determining if the phenomenon of single dose tolerance to morphine [18, 19] could be demonstrated in the EEG recorded from intracranial sites. As it was wished to emphasize the possible difference between the effects of morphine as an analgesic and as a euphoriant, each animal was prepared with two electrodes, one in a negatively reinforcing site and one in a positively reinforcing site. Since epochs of EEG were simultaneously recorded from the two sites in each animal, the results indicated that morphine could simultaneously cause both depression (increased amplitude) in those areas of the brain for which stimulation is aversive and stimulation (decreased amplitude) in the EEG in those areas of the brain for which stimulation is rewarding.

THRESHOLD MEASURES

The Nelsen findings raised the obvious question of whether or not the results could be functionally demonstrated. That is, is the intensity of stimulation to positively reinforcing sites enhanced by morphine while the intensity of stimulation to negatively reinforcing sites decreased? Since we were primarily interested in whether or not the rewarding value of the stimulation was increased or decreased after morphine, we believed that a direct approach would be to determine the effect of the drug on the threshold for the stimulation rather than the effect on rate of response. There has been sufficient evidence from experiments by Hodos and Valenstein [20] and a review by Valenstein [21] that rate of response does not necessarily reflect the rewarding value of the stimulation. Also, current work in our laboratory by Payton [22] indicates that rate of response for intracranial stimulation does not correlate with the absolute threshold for rewarding brain stimulation. The product moment correlation between rate of response and threshold was 0.02. It is highly possible that a change in rate of response after a drug could be affecting nonspecific depressant or stimulating effects without altering the value of the reinforcer. Although an individual animal's response rate will be, within limits, proportional to the intensity of stimulation, a change in response rate after drug taking does not necessarily reflect a change in the reinforcement value.

The first experiment in which we looked at the functional manifestation of the Nelsen findings was reported in a 1973 Ph.D. thesis by Marcus [23] and published in 1974.[24] This was the first published experiment indicating (1) that the effect of morphine on facilitating brain-stimulation reward occurred within the first 30 minutes after an injection of morphine, and (2) that the drug actually increased the sensitivity of the animal to rewarding brain-stimulation.

In the Marcus experiment, animals were prepared with electrodes in either positive or negative reinforcement sites. FIGURE 1 shows the percent change in threshold after morphine for each of three animals with electrodes in positive sites and three animals with electrodes in negative sites. As can be seen,

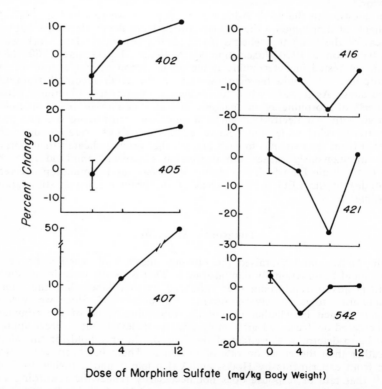

Dose of Morphine Sulfate (mg/kg Body Weight)

FIGURE 1. Mean percent change in threshold after morphine from three animals stimulated in "negative" reinforcement sites (on the left) and three animals stimulated in "positive" reinforcement sites (on the right). The standard error for approximately 10 threshold determinations after saline (0 dose) is indicated for each animal. (After Marcus & Kornetsky.[24])

the threshold for rewarding brain-stimulation is lowered by morphine while the threshold for negatively reinforcing brain-stimulation is raised by morphine. These results gave clear functional confirmation to the results obtained by Nelsen.

The double staircase psychophysical method [25] was used in the Marcus experiment. And in subsequent experiments we have used a modification of the psychophysical method of limits.[26] With both psychophysical methods a rate-free discrete trial procedure is used. Also a cylindrical wheel manipulandum, mounted in one wall of the experimental chamber, is used rather than the usual lever. This is shown in FIGURE 2 from Kornetsky and Bain [27] along with a schematic of a single trial in which the animal did not respond (labeled I) and one in which the animal did respond (labeled II).

Generally we find that the absolute threshold in the CDF rat (Charles River, Fisher-derived rat) usually is between 65 and 125 μA at 160 Hz. Morphine at doses from 2–8 mg/kg s.c. lowers the threshold approximately 20 μA. Details of the procedure have been published by Esposito and Kornetsky.[28]

FIGURE 3 summarizes the mean effects of morphine from a number of our experiments on the threshold for brain-stimulation reward.[27] These are percentage changes based on post-pre difference. Thus negative scores indicate a lowering of the threshold. Of interest is that although 12 mg/kg seems to bring the threshold change back to that seen after saline, higher doses did not cause a raising of the threshold. At higher doses, and for some animals at doses as low as 6 mg/kg, we could not measure the threshold since the animal is incapable of performing the task.

TOLERANCE

Of interest is the failure to find tolerance to either the rate facilitating effect [14, 29, 30] or threshold lowering effect [28] of opioids on brain-stimulation reward. In the Adams et al. experiment,[14] the effects of five consecutive days of morphine injections were studied. As with most studies they found a significant decrease in rate of response for the first two hours after drug administration on day 1 with significant increases subsequently. However, by day 3 there was complete tolerance to the inhibitory effect on rate with no tolerance to the facilitatory action of the morphine. However, after chronic administration the facilitatory effect appeared earlier after treatment. Other investigators also found that there was no tolerance to the facilitatory effect, only tolerance to the inhibitory effects.[30, 31] Contrary results have been reported by Glick and Rapaport.[32] They found tolerance to both the facilitatory and inhibitory effects of morphine on self-stimulation to animals with electrodes in the medial forebrain bundle. This report of tolerance to the facilitatory effect, contrary to the findings of most investigators, is difficult to explain and may, as suggested by Esposito and Kornetsky,[33] be due to subtle differences in training or baseline rates of response which were not reported in the Glick and Rapaport study. Using a threshold measure we have found that a relatively high dose, which previously had no effect on threshold, lowered the threshold after a number of days of daily drug administration. FIGURE 4 shows the results of animals from a number of our experiments in which the same animals were studied after single doses of morphine and after 14–38 days of daily administration. Of interest is that not only do these results indicate that

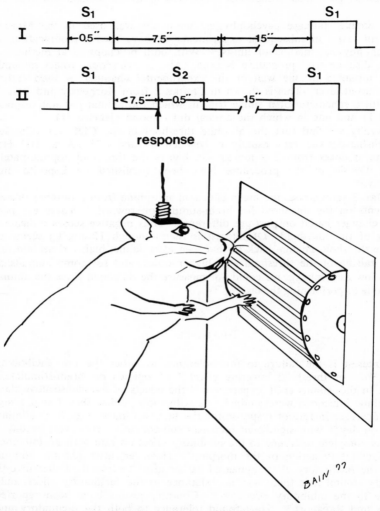

FIGURE 2. A schematic representation of the method for determining brain-stimulation reward thresholds. (I) A sequence of a single trial when an animal does not respond. (II) The sequence when the animal makes a response. A trial begins with the delivery of a noncontingent stimulus train (S_1), if the animal fails to respond by turning the wheel within 7.5 sec from the onset of the S_1 the trial is terminated and 15 sec later the next trial is begun. If the wheel is turned as indicated in example II, the rat receives a contingent stimulus (S_2). Intensity of stimulation is varied according to a modification of the method of limits.[26] A response after the 7.5-sec available response time postpones the presentation of the next stimulus for 15 sec.

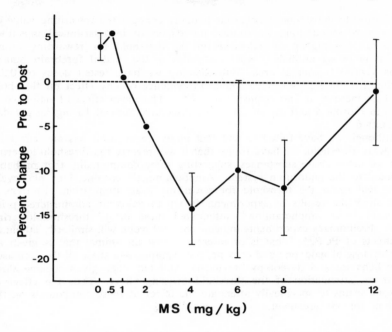

FIGURE 3. Mean effect of various doses of morphine on the threshold for brain-stimulation reward. Data summarized from a number of experiments in our laboratory (References 24, 28, 29, and some unpublished data). Standard errors are only indicated at doses in which five or more animals were tested. The large standard errors are primarily the result of individual animals obtaining maximum threshold lowering effect at different doses. The curve was U-shaped for all animals.

there is no tolerance to the reward threshold lowering effect of morphine, but that there is an increased effect of morphine. This suggests either a supersensitivity whose functional significance is not evident or that tolerance to the depressant effects allows for a greater manifestation of the threshold lowering effect.

NALOXONE

The facilitation of self-stimulation by opioids has suggested that the critical neurochemical basis for rewarding brain-stimulation may indicate a role for the endorphins or enkephalins.[34, 35] Not only does electrical stimulation of enkephalin-rich regions of the brain serve as a reinforcer, but enkephalins as well, have been reported to serve as reinforcers in self-administration behavior. Belluzzi and Stein [34] have also reported that naloxone will decrease self-stimulation behavior in animals with electrodes in the central gray. Although some investigators have also reported inhibition of self-stimulation rate after naloxone,[36] other investigators have found no effect on rate of response.[37–41]

In order to determine if naloxone actually changes the rewarding value of the electrical stimulation, we studied the effects of intraperitoneal injections of 2.0 to 16.0 mg/kg of naloxone on the threshold for rewarding brain-stimulation in six animals [42] with electrodes in the medial forebrain bundle or the ventral tegmental area. Subsequently we have tested doses of 0.25, 0.5, and 1.0 mg/kg. We have found no evidence of any effect on threshold except an increase in intrasubject variability. The mean effect of naloxone is shown in FIGURE 5 and the effects of 5 consecutive days of 16 mg/kg per day in FIGURE 6.[43]

Although we have failed to find that naloxone by itself has any effect on the reward threshold, we have found that it will reverse the threshold-lowering effects of other abuse substances, suggesting some commonality that probably is related to the endorphin system. Amphetamine,[42] cocaine,[44] or phencyclidine [10] will lower the threshold for rewarding brain-stimulation. FIGURES 7 and 8 show the results of experiments in which naloxone administered prior to cocaine [45] or amphetamine [42] attenuated these drugs' threshold-lowering action. Preliminary experiments indicate that naloxone will similarly attenuate the effects of PCP.[46] What is of interest is that an animal that is given an effective dose of naloxone and cocaine, for example, will show all the increased motor behavior and stereotypy previously exhibited when given cocaine alone despite an attenuation of the threshold-lowering effect. Thus the effect of naloxone seems to specifically attenuate the effect of these compounds on the threshold for reinforcement.

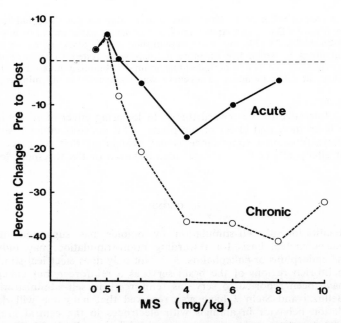

FIGURE 4. Mean effect of various doses of morphine reward threshold before and after chronic treatment (14–38 days) in the same animals ($N = 9$, not all animals tested at all doses).

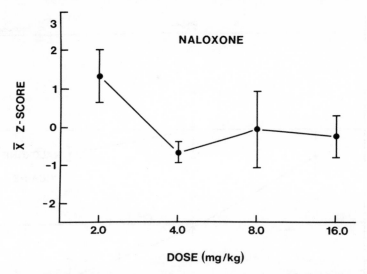

FIGURE 5. Mean effect of various doses of naloxone on brain-stimulation reward. Data are presented as Z-scores based on the mean and standard deviation of saline treatments. Vertical bars indicate standard errors. (After Esposito *et al.*[42])

German and Bowden,[47] Crow,[48] Wise,[49] and Fibiger [50] have all implicated catecholamines in self-stimulation behavior with particular emphasis on a dopaminergic substrate. Our failure to find a direct effect of naloxone on the absolute threshold for self-stimulation and the reported attenuation of

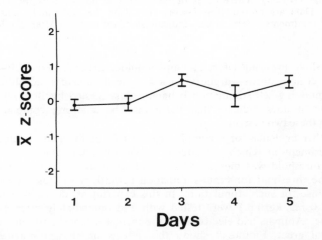

FIGURE 6. Mean effect of daily intraperitoneal administration (5 days) of 16 mg/kg of naloxone. Data are expressed by Z-scores as previously described. (After Perry *et al.*[43])

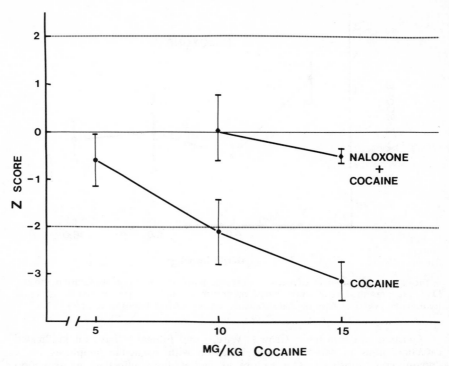

FIGURE 7. Mean effect of various doses of cocaine and cocaine and naloxone on the reward threshold. The dose of naloxone was either 2 or 4 mg/kg depending on the animal ($N = 4$). These doses of naloxone had no effect by themselves in these animals. Data are presented as Z-scores based on the mean and standard deviation of saline treatments. Vertical bars indicate standard errors. (After Kornetsky et al.[45])

the threshold-lowering effect of amphetamine, cocaine, and PCP—all indirect dopaminergic agonists—argue against a tonically active endorphinergic system for maintaining self-stimulation behavior as suggested by Belluzzi and Stein.[34] However, it does indicate that there may be a strong complementary role between these two systems.

Further evidence for a complementing role of the two systems is given in an experiment in which the effects of naloxone and chlorpromazine on the reward threshold was measured.[51, 52] Chlorpromazine, like other neuroleptics, raises the threshold for brain-stimulation reward as well as increases the rate of response for such stimulation. In this experiment, doses of chlorpromazine (0.25–2.0 mg/kg, i.p.) were tested with and immediately after 4.0 mg/kg of naloxone. Animals had electrodes in the medial forebrain bundle or the ventral tegmental area. FIGURE 9 shows that effects of chlorpromazine alone and after naloxone. As can be seen, the naloxone potentiated the threshold-raising effect. This effect was seen in each of the four animals represented in the mean effects in the figure. Also, it has been reported that naloxone will

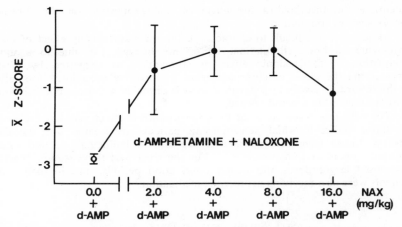

FIGURE 8. Mean effect of various doses of naloxone and the maximum threshold lowering dose of *d*-amphetamine for the individual animals ($N = 6$). These doses varied from 1–2 mg/kg. The effect of this dose of *d*-amphetamine is shown on the left. Data are presented as Z-scores as previously described. (After Esposito *et al.*[42])

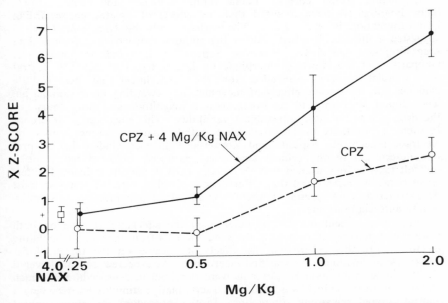

FIGURE 9. Mean effects of various doses of chlorpromazine and chlorpromazine plus 4 mg/kg naloxone of the threshold for rewarding brain stimulation. Effects of naloxone alone are shown on the left. Results are expressed as Z-scores as previously described. Vertical bars indicate standard scores ($N = 4$). (After Esposito *et al.*[51])

potentiate the threshold-raising effect of chlorpromazine on the threshold for nociceptive stimulation.[53, 54]

Although it is difficult to characterize the threshold-raising effect of chlorpromazine on brain stimulation, we do not believe it is due to a simple attenuation of the hedonic effect of stimulation as suggested by Wise.[55] Considering the effect of chlorpromazine on attentive behavior,[56] the raising of the reward threshold by chlorpromazine is probably a more subtle behavioral disruption on attention and reward.

The naloxone potentiation of the chlorpromazine effect may have relevance for those studies in which schizophrenic patients are treated with naloxone. Several studies have demonstrated a decrease in hallucinations and bizarre thought content after naloxone.[57–60] For the most part these studies generally have used larger doses and longer observation periods, and in many cases patients were also receiving neuroleptic medication.

SITE SPECIFICITY OF DRUG ACTION

Since a number of sites within the brain will support brain-stimulation reward, the technique seemed ideally suited for site specificity studies. Morphine will facilitate self-stimulation from a variety of brain sites.[33] These areas include the lateral hypothalamus,[30, 61] locus coeruleus,[62] ventral tegmental area,[63] medial frontal cortex,[61] dorsal raphe nucleus,[64] and central gray.[65] Some investigators have reported that the effects of opiates on rewarding brain-stimulation is site specific. The earliest study by Olds and Travis[13] suggested a site-specific effect. All of the authors above have presented data suggesting site specificity. However, Schenk et al.[65] did an intrasubject comparison of the effects of morphine on lateral hypothalamic and central gray stimulation. They concluded from their experiment that there is little evidence for site-specific effects of morphine on rewarding brain-stimulation. They found large intersubject differences in magnitude and time course of the drug effects but little intrasubject variability. This suggested a difference in subjects' sensitivity to the drug's effect rather than a difference caused by electrode placement. Esposito and Kornetsky[33] also concluded that a "precise description of the critical anatomical pathways involved would be a difficult task." They argued that there may exist important individual differences between animals and that differences in baseline rates of response must be considered in interpreting differences in the effect of morphine on stimulation to different brain sites.

In a more recent study,[66] we determined the effects of cocaine on both reward and detection threshold in the same animals from the same stimulating electrodes. In this experiment the effects of cocaine on the threshold for rewarding brain-stimulation was first determined. As expected, cocaine lowered the threshold in all animals. Animals were retrained in a procedure in which stimulation to the animal was used as a discriminative stimulus for receiving a supra-threshold rewarding stimulation. In this procedure the noncontingent stimulation was varied as described (FIGURE 2) for determination of the reward threshold. However, a response by the animal within 7.5 sec after the discriminative stimulus was followed always by a supra-threshold reinforcing brain stimulation. The intensity of noncontingent stimulus was varied according to the psychophysical method of limits. In this experiment the absolute threshold for rewarding stimulation was 65–125 μA while in the same animals the detection threshold was 7–22 μA. FIGURE 10 shows the results of this experiment and what can easily be seen is the clear dissociation in effect between detection and rewarding thresholds. This dissociation was evident in every animal. If we assume that the detection threshold represents a functionally significant measure of sensitivity at the site of stimulation, as suggested by Phillips and LePiane [67] and Swett and Bourassa,[68] then these findings suggest that the action of drugs on reinforcement levels may be mediated at a site(s) other than the locus of stimulation.

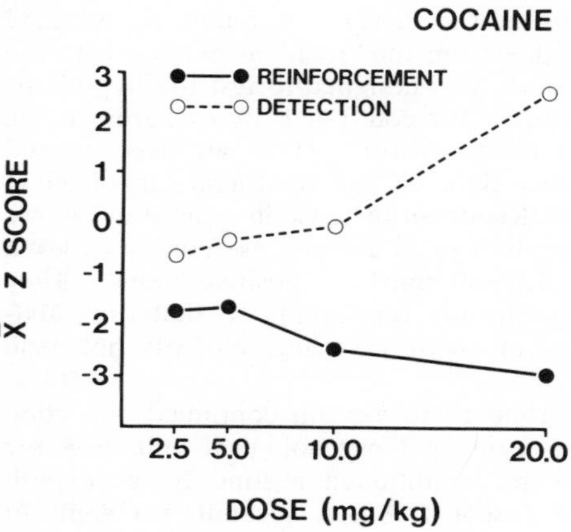

FIGURE 10. Mean effect of various doses of cocaine on the threshold for brain-stimulation reward (reinforcement) and on the threshold for brain-stimulation detection. Data are expressed as Z-scores based on the respective mean and standard deviation of the effects of saline ($N = 4$). (After Marcus & Kornetsky.[66])

HUMAN DRUG USE

Although it is well established that opioids facilitate intracranial self-stimulation, the question of whether or not this increase in rate of response and the lowering of threshold for self-stimulation is related to the euphoria-producing effect of these drugs is not proven. Human subjects who have received electrical stimulation to areas of the brain that are homologous to those for which animals will self-stimulate, report pleasurable sensation.[69, 70] Nelsen [17] pointed out the similarity between these reports and the reports of narcotic users describing their opiate-induced euphoria. Implicit, if not explicit, in most of the experiments in which there is facilitation of responding for rewarding brain-stimulation is the hypothesis that continued opiate-seeking behavior in many may be due to the drug causing an increase in the activity of central reward pathways.

This hypothesis implicating the reward system in opiate abuse was explicitly made by Marcus and Kornetsky [24] based on the results of their experiments showing that morphine lowered the threshold for rewarding brain-stimulation. Earlier, Collier [71] in a theoretical paper suggested that activation of the "reward or depression of the punishment system would have comparable results—a lessening of drives, accompanied by a sense of gratification and the reinforcement of the behavior leading to these effects." Kumar et al.[72] also evoked the hypothalamic reward system in attempting to explain drug-seeking behavior. However, these investigators did not look directly at opiate effects on intracranial self-stimulation. Subsequently the hypothesis that the "high" or euphoriant effects of morphine are related to activation of the reward system has been made by a number of investigators.[73–75]

The lack of tolerance to the threshold lowering effect of morphine suggests that the narcotic user may be continuing to use the drug not simply to avoid withdrawal signs. If there was tolerance to the euphoric effect, avoidance of withdrawal would be the major pharmacological reinforcer unless one subscribed to the previously mentioned theory that the aversiveness of the drug effect becomes positively reinforcing. Studies of street users of heroin by McAuliffe and Gordon[76] report that physically dependent subjects (and most likely tolerant to many of the actions of the drug) still report a sustained euphoria or high that can be differentiable from the "rush" associated with the intravenous injection of heroin. This study was designed to test the hypothesis of Lindesmith[77] that the primary reinforcer for continued use of heroin is the avoidance of withdrawal signs. Meyer and Mirin[78, 79] in an experimental study of heroin use in man shed further light on the reinforcers involved in continued drug use. They reported that despite an increase in a more dysphoric mood state and an increase in psychopathology as chronic use continues, each drug injection caused a brief period (30–60 min) of positive mood. They stated that "these acute effects are significantly reinforcing so that drug self-administration is perpetrated in the face of measurable degree of psychological and social deterioration."

A number of theories have been proposed to explain continued and compulsive opiate use, and it is clear that social and psychological influences are most important. Certainly there may be conditioned abstinence, as experimentally demonstrated by Wikler and Pescor,[80, 81] that accounts for some of the continued use; however, there seems to be a primary unconditioned effect of opioids that is reinforcing.

CONCLUSIONS

These experiments clearly indicate that morphine increases the sensitivity of animals to rewarding brain stimulation and suggest that brain-stimulation reward may be a useful model for understanding the rewarding effects of the opiate drugs. Naloxone's ability to attentuate the threshold-lowering effect of ampetamine, cocaine, and PCP and to potentiate the threshold-raising effect of chlorpromazine suggests that there is an important interaction between the catecholiminergic and endorphinergic systems. Finally, this interaction may have relevance for the clinical use of naloxone with neuroleptics in the treatment of schizophrenic patients.

REFERENCES

1. LETTIERI, D. J., M. SAYERS & H. W. PEARSON, Eds. 1980. Theories on Drug Abuse: Selected Contemporary Perspectives. NIDA Research Monograph 30. U.S. Government Printing Office, Washington, D.C.

2. BECKETT, H. D. 1974. Hypotheses concerning the etiology of heroin addiction. *In* Addiction. P. G. Bourne, Ed. pp. 38–54. Academic Press. New York.
3. CHEIN, I., D. L. GERARD, R. E. LEE & E. ROSENFELD, Eds. 1964. The Road to H. Basic Books. New York.
4. WIKLER, A. 1952. A psychodynamic study of patients during experimental self-regulated readdiction to morphine. Psychiat. Quart. **26:** 270–293.
5. KHANTZIAN, E. J. 1974. Opiate Addiction: A critique of theory and some implications for treatment. Am. J. Psychother. **28:** 59–70.
6. DOLE, V. P. & M. E. NYSWANDER. 1967. Addiction—A metabolic disease. Arch. Int. Med. **120:** 19–24.
7. MELLO, N. K. 1978. Control of drug self-administration: The role of aversive consequences. *In* Phencyclidine (PCP) Abuse: An Appraisal. R. C. Peterson & R. C. Stillman, Eds. pp. 289–308. NIDA Research Monograph 21. U.S. Government Printing Office, Washington, D.C.
8. KELLEHER, R. T., W. C. RIDDLE & L. COOK. 1963. Persistent behavior maintained by unavoidable shocks. J. Exp. Anal. Behav. **6**(4): 507–517.
9. KELLEHER, R. T. & W. H. MORSE. 1968. Schedules using noxious stimuli III. Responding maintained with response-produced electrical shocks. J. Exp. Anal. Behav. **11**(6): 819–838.
10. KORNETSKY, C., R. U. ESPOSITO, S. McLEAN & J. O. JACOBSON. 1979. Intracranial self-stimulation thresholds: A model for the hedonic effects of drugs of abuse. Arch. Gen. Psychiat. **36:** 289–292.
11. KORNETSKY, C. & R. U. ESPOSITO. 1979. Euphorigenic drugs: Effects on the reward pathways of the brain. Fed. Proc. **38:** 2473–2476.
12. OLDS, J. & P. MILNER. 1954. Positive reinforcement produced by electrical stimulation of septal area and other regions of rat brain. J. Comp. Physiol. Psychol. **47:** 419–427.
13. OLDS, J. & R. P. TRAVIS. 1960. Effects of chlorpromazine, meprobamate, pentobarbital and morphine on self-stimulation. J. Pharmacol. Exp. Ther. **128:** 397–404.
14. ADAMS, W. J., S. A. LORENS & C. L. MITCHELL. 1972. Morphine enhances lateral hypothalamic self-stimulation in the rat. Proc. Soc. Exp. Biol. **140:** 770–771.
15. WEEKS, J. 1962. Experimental morphine addiction: method for automatic intravenous injections in unrestrained rats. Science **138:** 143–144.
16. NELSEN, J. M. & C. KORNETSKY. 1972. Morphine induced EEG changes in central motivational systems: evidence for single dose tolerance. Fifth Int. Cong. Pharmacol. 166.
17. NELSEN, J. M. 1970. Single dose tolerance to morphine sulfate: Electroencephalographic correlates in central motivational systems. Doctoral Dissertation, Boston University. No. 70–22425. University Microfilms, Ann Arbor, MI.
18. COCHIN, J. & C. KORNETSKY. 1964. Development and loss of tolerance to morphine in the rat after single and multiple injections. J. Pharmacol. Exp. Ther. **145:** 1–10.
19. KORNETSKY, C. & G. BAIN. 1968. Morphine: Single-dose tolerance. Science **162:** 1011–1012.
20. HODOS, W. & E. VALENSTEIN. 1962. A evaluation of response rate as a measure of rewarding intracranial stimulation. J. Comp. Physiol. Psychol. **55:** 80–84.
21. VALENSTEIN, E. S. 1964. Problems of measurement and interpretation with reinforcing brain stimulation. Psychol. Rev. **71:** 415–437.
22. PAYTON, M. The relationship between absolute threshold and rate of response for brain-stimulation reward. Manuscript in preparation.

23. MARCUS, R. A. 1973. Morphine: Effects on positive and negative intracranial reinforcement thresholds. Doctoral dissertation, Boston University. University Microfilms. Ann Arbor, MI.
24. MARCUS, R. & C. KORNETSKY. 1974. Negative and positive intracranial reinforcement thresholds: Effects of morphine. Psychopharmacologia **38:** 1–13.
25. CORNSWEET, T. N. 1962. The staircase method in psychophysics. Am. J. Psychol. **75:** 485–491.
26. STEVENS, S. S. 1951. Mathematics, measurement, and psychophysics. *In* Handbook of Experimental Psychology. S. S. Stevens, Ed. pp. 1–49. John Wiley and Sons. New York.
27. KORNETSKY, C. & G. T. BAIN. 1982. Effects of opiates on rewarding electrical brain stimulation. *In* Neurobiology of Opiate Reward Mechanisms. J. E. Smith & J. D. Lane, Eds. Elsevier/North Holland Biomedical Press. In press.
28. ESPOSITO, R. & C. KORNETSKY. 1977. Morphine lowering of self-stimulation thresholds: Lack of tolerance with long term administration. Science **195:** 189–191.
29. ESPOSITO, R. U., S. MCLEAN & C. KORNETSKY. 1979. Effects of morphine on intracranial self-stimulation to various brain stem loci. Brain Res. **168:** 425–429.
30. LORENS, S. A. & C. L. MITCHELL. 1973. Influence of morphine on lateral hypothalamic self-stimulation in the rat. Psychopharmacologia **32:** 271–277.
31. BUSH, H. D., M. F. BUSH, M. A. MILLER & L. D. REID. 1976. Addictive agents and intracranial stimulation: Daily morphine and lateral hypothalamic self-stimulation. Physiol. Psychiat. **4:** 79–85.
32. GLICK, S. D. & G. RAPAPORT. 1974. Tolerance to the facilitatory effect of morphine on self-stimulation of the medial forebrain bundle of rats. Res. Commun. Chem. Pathol. Pharmacol. **9:** 647–652.
33. ESPOSITO, R. U. & C. KORNETSKY. 1978. Opioids and rewarding brain stimulation. Neurosci Biobehav. Rev. **2:** 115–122.
34. BELLUZZI, J. D. & L. STEIN. 1977. Enkephalin may mediate euphoria and drive reduction reward. Nature **266:** 556–558.
35. STEIN, L. & J. D. BELLUZZI. 1979. Brain endorphins: possible role in reward and memory formation. Fed. Proc. **38:** 2468–2472.
36. STAPELTON, J. M., V. J. MERRIMAN, C. L. COOGLE, S. D. GELBARD AND L. D. REID. 1979. Naloxone reduces pressing for intracranial stimulation of sites in the periaqueductal gray area, accumbens nucleus, substantia nigra, and lateral hypothalamus. Physiol. Psychol. **7**(4): 427–436.
37. WAUQUIER, A., C. J. E. NIEMEGEERS & H. LAL. 1974. Differential antagonism by naloxone of inhibitory effects of haloperidol and morphine on brain self-stimulation. Psychopharmacologia **37:** 303–310.
38. HOLTZMAN, S. G. 1976. Comparison of the effects of morphine, pentazocine, cyclazocine, and amphetamine on intracranial self-stimulation in the rat. Psychopharmacologia **46:** 223–227.
39. VAN DER KOOY, D., F. G. LEPIANE & A. G. PHILLIPS. 1977. Apparent independence of opiate reinforcement and electrical self-stimulation systems in rat brain. Life Sci. **20:** 981–986.
40. LORENS, S. A. & S. M. SAINATI. 1978. Naloxone blocks the excitatory effect of ethanol and chlordiazepoxide on lateral hypothalamic self-stimulation behavior. Life Sci. **23:** 1359–1364.
41. STILWELL, D. J., R. A. LEVITT, C. A. HORN, M. D. IRVIN, K. GROSS, D. S. PARSONS, R. H. SCOTT & E. L. BRADLEY. 1980. Naloxone and shuttlebox self-stimulation in the rat. Pharmacol. Biochem. Behav. **13:** 739–742.
42. ESPOSITO, R. U., W. PERRY & C. KORNETSKY. 1980. Effects of d-amphetamine and naloxone on brain stimulation reward. Psychopharmacology **69:** 187–191.

43. PERRY, W., R. U. ESPOSITO & C. KORNETSKY. 1981. Effects of chronic naloxone treatment on brain-stimulation reward. Pharmacol. Biochem. Behav. **14:** 247–249.
44. ESPOSITO, R. U., A. H. D. MOTOLA & C. KORNETSKY. 1978. Cocaine: Acute effects on reinforcement thresholds for self-stimulation behavior to the medial forebrain bundle. Pharmacol. Biochem. Behav. **8:** 437–439.
45. KORNETSKY, C., G. BAIN & M. RIEDL. 1981. Effects of cocaine and naloxone on brain-stimulation reward. Pharmacologist **23:** 192.
46. KORNETSKY, C., R. A. MARKOWITZ & R. U. ESPOSITO. 1981. Phencyclidine and naloxone: Effects on sensitivity to aversive and rewarding stimulation in the rat. In PCP (Phencyclidine): Historical and Current Perspectives. F. Domino, Ed. pp. 321–330. NPP Books. Ann Arbor, MI.
47. GERMAN, D. C. & D. M. BOWDEN. 1974. Catecholamine systems as the neural substrate for intracranial self-stimulation: A hypothesis. Brain Res. **73:** 381–419.
48. CROW, T. J. 1976. Specific monoamine systems as reward pathways: Evidence for the hypothesis that activation of the ventral mesencephalic dopaminergic neurones and noradrenergic neurones of the locus coeruleus complex will support self-stimulation responding. In Brain-Stimulation Reward. A. Wauquier and E. T. Rolls, Eds. pp. 211–238. American Elsevier Publishing Co. New York.
49. WISE, R. A. 1978. Catecholamine theories of reward: A critical review. Brain Res. **152:** 215–247.
50. FIBIGER, H. C. 1978. Drugs and reinforcement mechanisms: A critical review of the catecholamine theory. In Annual Review of Pharmacology and Toxicology. R. George, R. Okun & A. K. Cho, Eds. pp. 37–56. Annual Reviews, Inc. Palo Alto, CA.
51. ESPOSITO, R. U., W. PERRY & C. KORNETSKY. 1980. Chlorpromazine and brain-stimulation reward: Potentiation of effects by naloxone. Society for Neuroscience Abstracts **6:** 700.
52. ESPOSITO, R. U., W. PERRY & C. KORNETSKY. 1981. Chlorpromazine and brain-stimulation reward: Potentiation of effects by naloxone. Pharmacol. Biochem. Behav. **15:** 903–905.
53. KELLY, D. D., R. J. BODNAR, M. BRUTUS, C. F. WOODS & M. GLUSMAN. 1978. Differential effects upon liminal-escape pain thresholds of neuroleptic, antidepressant, and anxiolytic agents. Fed. Proc. **37:** 470.
54. KELLY, D. D., M. BRUTUS & R. J. BODNAR. 1978. Differential effects of naloxone upon elevation of liminal escape pain thresholds induced by psychotropic drugs: Reversal of chlordiazepoxide but enhancement of neuroleptic "analgesia." 7th Int. Con. Pharmacol. (Abstract) 119 (No. 270).
55. WISE, R. A. 1982. Neuroleptics and operant behavior: The anhedonia hypothesis. Behav. Brain Sci. In press.
56. MIRSKY, A. F. & C. KORNETSKY. 1964. On the dissimilar effects of drugs on the Digit Symbol Substitution and Continuous Performance Tests. Psychopharmacologia **5:** 161–177.
57. DAVIS, G. C., W. E. BUNNEY, E. G. DEFRAITES, J. E. KLEINMAN, D. P. VAN KAMMEN, R. M. POST & R. J. WYATT. 1977. Intravenous naloxone administration in schizophrenia and affective illness. Science **197:** 74–77.
58. EMRICH, H. M., C. CORDING, S. PIRCE, A. KNOLLING, D. VZERSSEN & A. HERZ. 1977. Indication of an antipsychotic action of the opiate antagonist naloxone. Pharmakopsychiat. Neuropharmakol. **10:** 265–270.
59. GUNNE, L.-M., L. LINDSTROM & L. TERENIUS. Naloxone-induced reversal of schizophrenic hallucinations. J. Neural Trans. **40:** 13–19.
60. WATSON, S., P. A. BERGER, H. AKIL, M. J. MILLS & J. D. BARCHAS. 1978. Effects of naloxone in schizophrenia: Reduction in hallucinations in a subpopulation of subjects. Science **201:** 73–76.

61. LORENS, S. A.   1976.   Comparison of the effects of morphine on hypothalamic and medial frontal cortex self-stimulation in the rat. Psychopharmacology **48:** 217–224.

62. JACKLER, F., S. S. STEINER, R. J. BODNAR, R. F. ARKERMANN, W. T. NELSON & S. J. ELLMAN.   1979.   Morphine and intracranial self-stimulation in the hypothalamus and dorsal brainstem: Differential effects of dose, time, and site. Int. J. Neurosci. **9:** 21–35.

63. BROEKKAMP, C. L., J. H. VAN DEN BOGGARD, H. J. HEIJNEN, R. H. ROPS, A. R. COOLS & J. M. VAN ROSSUM.   1976.   Separation of inhibiting and stimulating effects of morphine on self-stimulation behavior by intracerebral microinjections. Eur. J. Pharmacol. **4:** 443–446.

64. LIEBMAN, J. & S. D. SEGAL.   1977.   Differential effects of morphine and *d*-amphetamine on self-stimulation from closely adjacent regions in rat midbrain. Brain Res. **136:** 103–117.

65. SCHENK, S. T. WILLIAMS, A. COUPAL & P. SHIZGAL.   1980.   A comparison between the effects of morphine on the rewarding and aversive properties of lateral hypothalamic and central gray stimulation. Physiolog. Psychol. **8:** 372–378.

66. KORNETSKY, C. & R. U. ESPOSITO.   1981.   Reward and detection thresholds for brain stimulation: Dissociative effects of cocaine. Brain Res. **209:** 496–500.

67. PHILLIPS, A. G. & F. G. LEPAINE.   1978.   Electrical stimulation of the amygdala as a conditioned stimulus in a bait-shyness paradigm. Science **201:** 536–538.

68. SWETT, J. E. & C. M. BOURASSA.   1980.   Detection thresholds to stimulation of ventrobasal complex in cats. Brain Res. **183:** 313–328.

69. SEM-JACOBSEN, C. W. & A. TORKILDSEN.   1960.   Depth recording and electrical stimulation in the human brain. *In* Electrical Studies on the Unanesthetized Brain. E. R. Ramey & D. S. O'Doherty, Eds. pp. 275–290. Paul S. Hoeber. New York.

70. HEATH, R. G. & W. A. MICKLE.   1960.   Evaluation of seven years experience with depth electrode studies in human patients. *In* Electrical Studies on the Unanesthetized Brain. E. R. Ramey & D. S. O'Doherty, Eds. pp. 214–242. Paul S. Hoeber. New York.

71. COLLIER, H. O. J.   1968.   Supersensitivity and dependence. Nature **20:** 228–231.

72. KUMAR, R., E. MITCHELL & I. P. STOLERMAN.   1971.   Disturbed patterns of behavior in morphine tolerant and abstinent rats. Brit. J. Pharmacol. **42:** 473–484.

73. LEVITT, R. A., J. H. BALTZER, T. M. EVERS, D. J. STILWELL & J. E. FURBY.   1977.   Morphine and shuttle-box self-stimulation in the rat: A model for euphoria. Psychopharmacology **54:** 307–311.

74. FARBER, P. D. & L. D. REID.   1976.   Addictive agents and intracranial stimulation (ICS): Daily morphine and pressing for combinations of positive and negative ICS. Physiol. Psychol. **4:** 262–268.

75. WISE, R.   1980.   Actions of drugs of abuse on brain reward systems. Pharmacol. Biochem. Behav. **13** (Suppl. 1): 213–224.

76. McAULIFFE, W. E. & R. A. GORDON.   1974.   A test of Lindesmith's theory of addiction: The frequency of euphoria among long term addicts. Am. J. Soc. **79:** 795–840.

77. LINDESMITH, A. R.   1965.   Problems in the social psychology of addiction. *In* Narcotics. D. M. Wilner & G. G. Kassebaum, Eds. pp. 118–139. McGraw-Hill. New York.

78. MEYER, R. E. & S. M. MIRIN.   1979.   The Heroin Stimulus. Plenum Press. New York.

79. MIRIN, S. M., R. E. MEYER & H. B. McNAMEE.   1976.   Psychopathology and mood during heroin use. Arch. Gen. Psychiat. **33:** 1503–1508.

80. WIKLER, A. & F. T. PESCOR. 1967. Classical conditioning of a morphine abstinence phenomenon, reinforcement of opioid-drinking behavior and "relapse" in morphine addicted rats. Psychopharmacologia **10**: 255–284.
81. WIKLER, A. & F. T. PESCOR. 1970. Persistence of "relapse-tendencies" of rats previously made physically dependent on morphine. Psychopharmacologia **16**: 375–384.

◆

DISCUSSION OF THE PAPER

UNIDENTIFIED SPEAKER: Would naloxone change the threshold for the adversive, punishing stimuli?

C. KORNETSKY (*Boston University School of Medicine, Boston, MA*): Yes, we have actually done that, and if electrodes are put into areas of the brain that are aversive, that is, not rewarding at any intensity, you find a very systematic dose–effect increase in sensitivity in those areas. In other words, the threshold is lowered.

UNIDENTIFIED SPEAKER: At what dose of naloxone?

KORNETSKY: Doses of 2 and 4 mg/kg.

A. L. STEIN (*University of California at Irvine*): Your last experiment is a particularly interesting one and gave me the following idea—an idea that may resolve both our findings and explain some of the effects you have shown.

In the last experiment naloxone demonstrated a profound effect in the presence of chlorpromazine. It made me wonder whether most self-stimulation sites involve the action of opioids and catecholamines jointly. In certain sites, such as the substantia nigra and the medial forebrain bundle, where we show naloxone insensitivity, the opiate effect may be largely masked by massive release of catecholamines. If you block those catecholamine effects with chlorpromazine, then you may see a residual opiate effect which can be nicely blocked by naloxone.

So this method of using the two kinds of antagonists may, in fact, reflect that at many self-stimulation sites there are simultaneously both endorphin- and catecholamine-reversed actions. This idea may be particularly inviting because Hökfelt has shown that many catecholamine-containing neurons also may contain endorphins. Conceivably, both transmitters may be simultaneously released from the same neuron and may interact to produce behavioral reinforcement.

KORNETSKY: If you are correct, Dr. Stein, it would explain the discrepancy between our results, or at least one aspect of the discrepancy.

THE ROLE OF ENDORPHINS IN
STRESS-INDUCED ANALGESIA

Dennis D. Kelly

New York State Psychiatric Institute
and
Department of Psychiatry
College of Physicians & Surgeons of Columbia University
New York, New York 10032

The scientific study of pain, apart from clinical observations, is only decades old. Nevertheless, during the past decade this area of research has produced one of the major advances in our understanding of the brain, one that introduces the possibility of altering dramatically the methods by which patients suffering pain will be treated in the future. This discovery is the existence in the human brain of systems whose specific function is to modulate or inhibit sensitivity to painful stimuli. The endogenous neural inhibitory system contains both opiate and serotonergic links,[1, 2] and it appears to be composed of a set of phylogenetically primitive areas of the brain, structures that line the medial and caudal portions of the ventricular system.[3] This phylogenetic perspective suggests two things. First, we share this capability for pain inhibition with many living species. Hence the properties of the system can be studied experimentally in animals. Second, the pain inhibitory system most likely evolved before the earliest hominids, and we may assume that it did so, and survived to be represented in the human brain, because it offered a significant selective advantage to its possessors. However, we do not yet know how to characterize that presumed advantage.

Although we normally strive to avoid pain or to relieve it when it occurs, pain also represents a primitive, protective sensory experience that warns of danger. It is not immediately clear under what environmental circumstances it would be advantageous for an organism to be denied information about pain.[4] Therefore, although we have witnessed a rapid expansion of knowledge concerning the anatomical, biochemical and physiological properties of the pain inhibitory system, we still know relatively little about its biological significance or its adaptive value. It was in this context that the initial reports of the phenomenon of stress-induced analgesia (SIA) appeared to be so important.[5, 6]

When an experimental animal was exposed to a novel and severe stressor, such as inescapable footshock or a brief, forced swim in cold water, its sensitivity to other painful stimuli was reduced for a measurable period afterwards. Repeated exposures to the same environmental stressor resulted in a progressive decline of the analgesic response, in much the same manner that the pituitary-adrenal responses to stress show adaptation.

If an important part of an organism's response to emergency situations was reduced sensitivity to pain, then it seemed reasonable that the newly discovered pain inhibitory system might be involved, and, thereby, so might endogenous opioids. Stress-induced analgesia was a simple empirical finding, yet it represented the only experimental clue that addressed the possible be-

0077-8923/82/0398-0260 $01.75/ © 1982 NYAS

havioral utility of endogenous pain inhibition. The extended version of this theory suggested that it is in meeting the behavioral demands prompted by exposure to stressful situations, such as those involving predation, defense, dominance, or adaptation to an extreme environmental demand, that an organism's normal reactions to pain could prove disadvantageous. Pain normally promotes a profile of reflex withdrawals, escape, rest and other recuperative behaviors. During the stressful encounter these reactions to pain might be suppressed automatically in favor of more adaptive behavior.

There also appeared to be strong intuitive support for the existence of SIA in humans. Soldiers wounded in battle and athletes injured in sports sometimes report that they do not feel pain.[7] However, it is still not clear whether these instances represent examples of a natural response of the body to a novel stressor, or rather some isolated and complicated exceptions to the more common rule that people feel pain when injured. In fact, most athletes and most soldiers do feel pain, and perhaps the latter represents the more adaptive response. Pain as a warning of serious physical damage can represent vital information that in normal, even stressful, circumstances ought not to be ignored. Patients who are congenitally insensitive to pain develop serious, often lethal, medical problems in the absence of such signals.[8] Therefore, whether normal pain sensitivity or analgesia should be the more adaptive property of a stressed nervous system is not intuitively obvious. Perhaps both would be, at different times.

Because of its theoretical importance, it may be valuable to examine some of the properties of the laboratory phenomenon of SIA. The focus will be upon the paradigm that we have studied most extensively in our own laboratory, the exposure of a rat to a brief (3.5 min) swim in cold water (2°C). We will try to relate these findings to the hypothesis that stress may induce analgesia by activating endogenous opioids. Finally, in light of the conflicting data that will be reviewed, we will also consider the possibility that some examples of diminished pain reflexes following exposure to a stressor may not reflect analgesia *per se*, but rather a more generalized behavioral deficit.

THE PSYCHOPHYSICS OF ANALGESIA IN ANIMALS

As we will see, when an animal's responsivity to pain is tested following an experimental procedure, the method selected to measure pain is a major determinant of the results obtained and the conclusions drawn. Since there is no individual pain test that currently offers sufficient psychophysical precision to be used alone, we normally employ a pain test battery, which combines two standard reflex tests with an operant escape procedure.

In the tail-flick test, a collimated light is focused upon a rat's tail and the latency to withdrawal is recorded. The response is a reflex and can be elicited even in a spinal transected animal.[9] We have found it essential to test the tail-flick reflex at different light intensities (and thereby plot a psychophysical function for tail-flick, instead of a simple point-estimate threshold) for we have found that short and long tail-flick latencies are differentially responsive to drugs, as have others.[10] For instance, naloxone shortens long tail-withdrawal latencies to low-intensity noxious stimuli, but has no effect upon rapid flicks to high-intensity stimuli.

The flinch-jump test is also a reflex test, which differs from the tail-flick in terms of the response measured and the aversive stimulus employed. A rat is presented with a series of brief, but successively more intense shocks. Using an ascending method of limits, the lowest shock intensities are determined that elicit first a flinch in any limb and, subsequently, a jump off of the grid floor.

The third method employed in our laboratory to measure pain sensitivity is a trained operant psychophysical procedure called liminal escape. As its name implies, this is not a reflex test, even though it employs the same aversive shock stimuli as does the flinch-jump test. Unlike the two preceding reflex tests, the liminal escape procedure incorporates both an animal's evaluation of the relative aversiveness of a given shock stimulus and its motivation to terminate its presence. As outlined schematically in FIGURE 1, shock is presented on each trial for 10 secs, unless the rat responds three times by pressing a lever. The third response immediately terminates shock, as illustrated in the right hand trial in FIGURE 1. Fewer than three responses, as in the left-hand trial, have no effect upon shock, and the response requirement is reset for the next trial. The intertrial interval is fixed at 20 secs and responses during this period, though recorded, are also ineffective. Sessions consist of 100 trials distributed evenly over five shock intensities. The sequence of intensities on successive trials is varied in a Latin square design. They range from a shock intensity from which the rat rarely escapes within the 10 sec interval, to one from which it always escapes rapidly.

A psychophysical analysis based upon a profile of results from these three pain tests administered as a battery offers greater inferential strength than can be drawn from any individual test, for the three tests can be paired in two important ways. The first two, tail-flick and flinch-jump, are reflex tests, though they differ in the type and location of the noxious stimulus. The second two, flinch-jump and liminal escape, employ the same aversive stimulus, but they differ in that one is a reflex test and the other a trained operant performance. The value of these comparisons will be illustrated in the next section, in which the first property of SIA will be discussed.

The Time Course of Stress-Induced Analgesia

Stress-induced analgesia refers to a phenomenon that outlasts the exposure to stress. A post-stress time course for analgesia is important to distinguish the phenomenon from the attentional variables that are known to alter reactions to pain. A number of laboratories, including our own, have attempted to

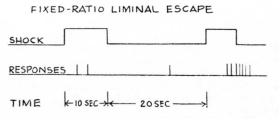

FIGURE 1. Schematic diagram of the liminal escape procedure.

correlate various physiological changes with the time course of SIA. However, estimates of the duration of SIA have ranged from minutes to hours depending upon the stressor employed, its severity, and, as will be shown here, the method used to measure pain thresholds. For example, Akil *et al.*[5] and Madden *et al.*[11] reported that following acute exposure to inescapable foot shock there were parallel changes in the tail-flick latencies of rats and in the inhibition of stereospecific opiate binding in brain tissue. On the strength of this temporal correlation, they proposed that the analgesia induced by stress was an opiate-dependent process. However, a major question of interpretation posed by such studies is: If stress-induced analgesia can display many different time courses, with which one should the physiological variable be correlated?

In the experiment shown in FIGURE 2, each subject was exposed to a cold-water swim and then, after a given delay, administered a battery of three tests in the order: flinch-jump, liminal escape, and tail-flick. This particular sequence produces no interactions among the tests, with threshold values equal to those determined when each test is administered alone. Following stress the test sequence was begun either 15, 30, 60, 120, or 180 minutes later, as indicated in the middle panel for the first test in the battery, flinch-jump. All six subjects were exposed to all five delay conditions. The order of exposure was balanced in a Latin square design.

When the sequence was begun either 15 or 30 minutes following the cold-water swim, pain thresholds measured by all three tests were significantly elevated relative to the no stress condition. Liminal escape thresholds were the first to return to normal by 70 minutes after the stress, whereas flinch-jump thresholds did not return to normal until 120 minutes later, and tail-flick thresholds remained elevated for over 3 hours. Thus, for example, on

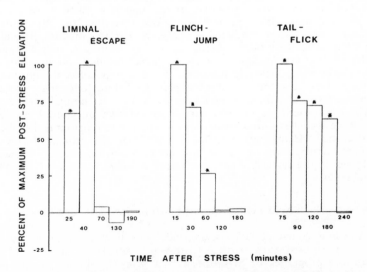

FIGURE 2. Time course of analgesia following cold-water stress depends upon the method employed to measure pain thresholds. N = 6 rats. * = statistically significant elevation relative to no-stress baseline. (p < .05)

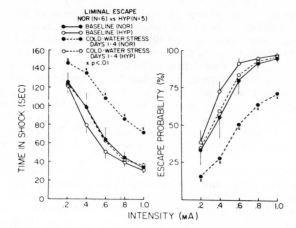

FIGURE 3. Adaptation of stress-induced analgesia. Liminal escape threshold functions (± SEM) are more elevated 30 minutes following the first 4 daily cold water swims than following the last 4 of 14 daily swims.

the day when the test sequence was started 60 minutes after exposure to stress, the same animal would be judged analgesic by the flinch-jump test, normal by the liminal escape test, and analgesic by the tail-flick test.

These results argue that there is no single time course of analgesia induced by stress. The effective duration of analgesia is clearly dependent upon the selection of the pain test. A second implication of these results is that there appears to be no unitary analgesic process that is initiated by stress and that decays over time. It is particularly informative that the procedure which produced the shortest estimate of analgesia was the operant liminal escape task. This schedule reflects, among other parameters, the subject's perception of the relative aversiveness of a given shock stimulus and its willingness to make the effort necessary to terminate it. So it is possible, though not proven by these data, that for a prolonged period of time following exposure to a severe stressor, an animal may report by way of its liminal escape response that it can experience noxious stimuli as aversive or painful, while at the same time its reflex withdrawal responses to the same stimuli may be slowed or weakened. If this interpretation is true, then the prolonged elevations in tail-flick latencies, which last several hours following stress, may not reflect analgesia in the normal sense, but rather a slow recovery of function in a spinal reflex arc.

ADAPTATION OF STRESS-INDUCED ANALGESIA

The time course of SIA also depends upon how many times the organism has been exposed to a particular stressor. Adaptation is one of the most interesting properties of SIA, for it is a property shared by the hormonal responses of the pituitary-adrenal system. FIGURE 3 shows the progressive decline in analgesia induced by 14 daily cold swims as tested by the liminal escape method 30 minutes following stress. The left panel of FIGURE 3 plots the total time cumulated by the subjects during the last 16 trials at each intensity. (Since the trial duration was 10 seconds, the maximum possible score is 160 seconds.) This measure represents a blend of escape probability, shown in the right panel, and escape latency. Adaptation is such an important property of SIA that it is tempting to argue that any putative example of SIA that does not show adaptation is probably an artifact of direct exposure to the stressor and not the organism's reaction to the stressor.

Nonanalgesic Stressors

Not all stressors result in analgesia. Although stress may be a necessary condition for SIA (by definition SIA excludes other nonstressful, environmentally produced, analgesic states such as hypnosis), it is clearly not a sufficient condition. For there are many quite severe environmental stressors that do not induce analgesia. For this reason we collaborated with Dr. Murray Glusman of this Institute and Drs. Dorothy T. Krieger and Gloria Colurso, Mt. Sinai School of Medicine, to examine the peripheral endocrine consequences of analgesic and nonanalgesic stressors.[12]

Forty-two male albino rats were exposed to one of seven stressful conditions or to a no-stress condition. Flinch-jump and tail-flick tests were used to assess analgesia. At varying times following separate exposures to the same stress conditions, the rats were sacrificed by swift decapitation and trunk blood collected. Plasma corticosterone was determined by a competitive protein binding assay, and ACTH and β-endorphin by radioimmunoassay.

Exposure to ether stress for 1, 2.5, or 10 minutes produced a graded series of significant elevations in all three hormones 20 minutes after the stress, but analgesia was induced only by the longest two durations of prior anesthesia. A cold-water swim induced near maximal elevations in plasma levels of all three hormones, when measured at 30 minutes after the stress, and also elevated thresholds. However, an identical swim in warm water (28°) produced statistically similar hormonal responses unaccompanied by analgesia. Finally, both a 3.5 min exposure to loud noise and exposure to the pain test battery by itself significantly elevated ACTH and corticosterone. β-Endorphin showed a nonsignificant trend in the same direction.

We concluded that neither the blood level of corticosterone, ACTH, or β-endorphin was able to predict whether a stressor would induce analgesia or not. Therefore, whereas analgesic stressors tend to be severe both in terms of the hormonal responses and the range of behavioral deficits they induce, many other stressors can prompt similar plasma elevations in stress hormones without inducing analgesia or other behavioral deficits. This finding is in agreement with other data that suggest that the maximal β-endorphin response induced by the most extreme stress (limb fracture) [13] is manifold lower than levels required to induce analgesia via systemic injections.[14]

Hypophysectomy and Stress-Induced Analgesia

This is an area fraught with many conflicting results. Some examples of SIA are attenuated by removal of the pituitary,[15–19] others are enhanced,[17, 20] and many are simply unaffected by the operation.[21, 22] In our own laboratory we have found that an important variable determining the direction of the effects of hypophysectomy upon SIA may be the postoperative schedule of hormone replacement therapy. Cold water swim analgesia was attenuated by removal of the pituitary when the rats were supported by daily injections of corticosterone and thyroxin [16]; however, when the paradigm was repeated in unsupplemented subjects, hypophysectomy enhanced SIA.[20] It is surprising that removal of the pituitary does not interact more consistently with SIA as there is such a wide variety of ways in which the operation might alter the body's response to stress and, thereby, stress's analgesic properties.

THE INTERACTION OF OPIATE AGONISTS AND ANTAGONISTS WITH STRESS-INDUCED ANALGESIA

Because SIA and the endogenous opioids were discovered at approximately the same time, a question of repeated concern in the literature is whether SIA is an opiate-mediated phenomenon. There are at least two forms of this hypothesis: the first involving systemic endorphins, as discussed in the preceding sections; the second involving CNS opioid neurons. The most common experimental tests of the latter have been the sensitivity of SIA to opiate receptor blockade by naloxone and to the development of cross tolerance with morphine. Again the data present a highly inconsistent pattern across analgesias induced by different stressors.[23] These two methods of testing opioid involvment in SIA may also diverge with respect to the same stressor, as in our laboratory.

Richard J. Bodnar [24] showed that there was no cross tolerance in either direction between cold swim analgesia and systemic morphine analgesia. The analgesic properties of this stressor developed with equal facility in both naïve and morphine-tolerant rats. One might expect, therefore, that naloxone would be similarly without effect upon cold-swim analgesia. Instead Bodnar [25] found an orderly, dose-dependent attenuation of analgesia by naloxone, albeit at rather high doses (up to 20 mg/kg), and then only to a moderate extent. These findings are not startling if we recall that naloxone is a drug with many CNS effects. They do not argue with any strength, however, that cold-swim analgesia is an opiate-dependent phenomenon. In this respect, these pharmacological data concur with the neuroendocrine experiments above.

A seminal development in this area occurred when several laboratories showed that a single stressor could elicit either a naloxone-sensitive or a naloxone-insensitive form of analgesia at different experimental parameters. For example, Lewis, Cannon and Liebeskind [26] showed that inescapable footshock will interact with naloxone only at certain temporal parameters of the shock. Unlike the effects of cold-water swims or of morphine, the analgesia induced by this procedure is mild and lasts only several minutes. With repeated exposure to the footshock stressors, tolerance developed to the naloxone-sensitive, but not the naloxone-insensitive stressor.[27] On this basis, they have argued for the probable existence of two neurochemically discrete pain-inhibitory systems, opioid and nonopioid.

In a similar manner, Cobelli et al.[28] and Watkins and Mayer [21] have shown that inescapable shock applied to the forepaws of a rat produces a brief tail-flick analgesia that is antagonized by systemic and spinal naloxone and by morphine tolerance, whereas hindpaw shock results in a naloxone-insensitive analgesia with a similar time course. Moreover, Maier *et al.*[29] have found that acute exposure to an extended series of inescapable shocks (80 5-second shocks at an average interval of 1 minute) produces a naloxone-insensitive analgesia that dissipates quickly. However, 24 hours later a more prolonged and naloxone-reversible analgesia can be reinstated by a brief reexposure to mild shock, which by itself is insufficient to induce analgesia.

One difficulty in interpreting naloxone's diverse interactions with different examples of SIA is that there are multiple opiate receptors [30] and that naloxone is not an equally effective antagonist of them all. At the δ receptor preferred by enkephalins, the affinity of naloxone is 10 times less than at the μ receptor preferred by morphine. The affinity of naloxone is even lower at the κ receptor.[31] From the distribution of receptor types within the CNS, and the structure-activity relationships of opioids, Chang, Hazum and Cuatrecasas [32] have concluded that the μ receptors are those most likely involved in pain inhibition and that where endogenous analgesic mechanisms are opioid-operated they should be naloxone-sensitive.

	Tail-flick	Flinch-Jump
Normal and Sham	↑	↓
Hypophysectomized	↑↑	↓↓

FIGURE 4. Differential effects of inescapable footshock stress upon two reflex tests of pain. Both effects are exaggerated following removal of the pituitary.

HYPERALGESIA AND ANALGESIA INDUCED BY THE SAME STRESSOR

Earlier we noted that the method selected to measure an animal's responsiveness to pain was a major determinant of the time course of analgesia induced by a cold-water swim. The analgesia ranged from minutes to hours depending upon whether thresholds were measured by liminal escape, flinch-jump or tail-flick. Perhaps more importantly, we have recently found that a single stressor, inescapable footshock, produced both analgesia and hyperalgesia in the same subject depending upon how pain thresholds were measured. Moreover, both effects were enhanced by hypophysectomy.

In the first experiment, five rats were exposed to inescapable footshock stress (IFS) consisting of 300-msec shocks of 3.5 ma repeated at 2-sec intervals for 5 minutes, the same parameters reported by Millan *et al.*[15] to induce tail-flick analgesia. Each rat was exposed four times to IFS, and combined flinch-jump and tail-flick testing occurred either 0, 15, 30, or 60 minutes later. Three no-stress baseline test days separated the IFS sessions. The sequence of exposure to the IFS conditions was counterbalanced across rats in an incomplete Latin square design. As shown schematically in the top row of FIGURE 4, flinch-jump thresholds were decreased for 30 minutes following IFS, while tail-flick thresholds were increased. These paired results demonstrated that the method employed to assess pain thresholds can determine the very direction of threshold shifts induced by stress.

In a second experiment, 16 hypophysectomized and 16 sham-operated adult rats were exposed to IFS followed by pain testing 10 minutes later. The animals were stressed twice during the 2nd post-operative week and twice again in the 14th week following regeneration of the neurohypophysis (and recovery of water balance). The animals did not differ in normal pain thresholds. However, when stressed, hypophysectomized rats displayed both potentiated tail-flick analgesia and potentiated flinch-jump hyperalgesia. This is a particularly valuable pair of findings, for the greater responsivity to flinch-jump shocks argues that the potentiation of tail-flick analgesia induced by the same stressor in the same rats was not due to a motor deficit.

SPECIFICITY OF SENSORY CHANGES IN STRESS-INDUCED ANALGESIA

It has never been proven that the sensory deficit induced by stress is limited to the modality of pain. This is an extremely important issue, and it represents a significant lacuna in our understanding of the phenomenon. If stress were found to induce not only changes in pain sensitivity but in other sensory modalities as well, then the adaptive value of such a response to the organism would be much less clear, as would its potential relevance to endogenous pain inhibitory mechanisms. For this phenomenon to be of maximum teleological benefit to the organism, stress should induce only analgesia, and not other sensory changes, which might prove a hindrance to adaptive behavior. Were we to find a generalized sensory deficit following stress, we would not look toward a specific pain inhibitory system as an explanation of the phenomenon, but toward a more general mechanism for sensory disruption. In turn, this would reopen the question, considered at the beginning of this article, of the biological significance of the intrinsic CNS capability to modulate pain.

SUMMARY

We have seen that exposure of an organism to any of a wide range of stressful situations can induce alterations in sensitivity to pain that outlast the exposure. Not all stressors induce analgesia; among those that do not are some that produce maximal elevations in plasma beta-endorphin, ACTH, and adrenal corticosteroids. Some examples of SIA are sensitive to opiate receptor blockade by naloxone, but others are not. Hypophysectomy produces a similarly uneven profile of effects across different stressors. This diversity has often been interpreted as evidence for the existence of an array of pain inhibitory systems, with differing physiological properties and activated by different stressors. However, it might also suggest that stressors can prompt a variety of behavioral changes, many of which can be interpreted as analgesia if a pain reflex test is employed as the dependent measure.

REFERENCES

1. BASBAUM, A. I. & H. L. FIELDS. 1978. Endogenous pain control mechanisms: Review and hypothesis. Ann. Rev. Neurobiol. 4: 451–462.
2. SNYDER, S. H. & S. CHILDERS. 1979. Opiate receptors and opioid peptides. Ann. Rev. Neurosci. 2: 35–64.

3. BOWSHER, D. 1976. Role of the reticular formation in responses to noxious stimulation. Pain **2:** 361–378.
4. KELLY, D. 1981. Somatic sensory system IV: Central representations of pain and analgesia. Chapter 18 *In* Principles of Neural Science. E. R. Kandel & J. H. Schwartz, Eds.: 199–212. Elsevier/North-Holland. New York.
5. AKIL, H., J. MADDEN, R. L. PATRICK & J. D. BARCHAS. 1976. Stress-induced increase in endogenous opiate peptides: Concurrent analgesia and its partial reversal by naloxone. *In* Opiates and Endogenous Opioid Peptides. H. W. Kosterlitz Ed.: 63–70. Elsevier/North-Holland. Amsterdam.
6. HAYES, R. L., G. J. BENNETT, P. G. NEWLON & D. J. MAYER. 1978. Behavioral and physiological studies of non-narcotic analgesia in the rat elicited by certain environmental stimuli. Brain Res. **155:** 69–90.
7. BEECHER, H. K. 1956. Relationship of significance of wound to pain experienced. J. Am. Med. Assn. **161:** 1609–1613.
8. STERNBACH, R. 1963. Congenital insensitivity to pain: A critique. Psychol. Bull. **60:** 252–264.
9. DEWEY, W. L., J. W. SNYDER, L. S. HARRIS & J. F. HOWES. 1969. The effect of narcotics and narcotic antagonists on the tail-flick response in spinal mice. J. Pharm. Pharmacol. **21:** 548–550.
10. DEWEY, W. L. & L. S. HARRIS. 1975. The tail-flick test. *In* Methods in Narcotics Research. S. Ehrenpreis & A. Neidle, Eds.: 101–109. Marcel Dekker. New York.
11. MADDEN, J., H. AKIL, R. L. PATRICK & J. D. BARCHAS. 1977. Stress-induced parallel changes in central opioid levels and pain responsiveness in the rat. Nature **265:** 358–360.
12. KELLY, D. D., G. COLURSO, D. T. KRIEGER & M. GLUSMAN. 1981. Pituitary-adrenal correlates of analgesic and non-analgesic stressors. Bull. Psychonomic Soc. **18:** 70. (#270).
13. GUILLEMIN, R., T. VARGO, J. ROSSIER, S. MINICK, N. LING, C. RIVIER, W. VALE & F. BLOOM. 1977. β-endorphin and adrenocorticotropin are secreted concomitantly by the pituitary gland. Science **197:** 1367–1369.
14. TSENG, L. F., H. LOH & C. H. LI. 1976. Beta-endorphin as a potent analgesic by intravenous injection. Nature **263:** 239–240.
15. MILLAN, M. J., R. PRZEWLOCKI & A. HERZ. 1980. A non-beta-endorphinergic adenohypophyseal mechanism is essential for an analgesic response to stress. Pain **8:** 343–353.
16. BODNAR, R. J., M. GLUSMAN, M. BRUTUS, A. SPIAGGIA & D. D. KELLY. 1979. Analgesia induced by cold-water stress: Attenuation following hypophysectomy. Physiol. Behav. **23:** 53–62.
17. BODNAR, R. J., D. D. KELLY, A. MANSOUR & M. GLUSMAN. 1979. Differential effects of hypophysectomy upon analgesia induced by two glucoprivic stressors and morphine. Pharmacol. Biochem. Behav. **11:** 303–308.
18. AMIR, S. & Z. AMIT. 1979. The pituitary gland mediates acute and chronic pain responsiveness in stressed and non-stressed rats. Life Sci. **24:** 439–448.
19. GLUSMAN, M., R. J. BODNAR, D. D. KELLY, C. SIRIO, J. STERN & E. A. ZIMMERMAN. 1979. Attenuation of stress-induced analgesia by anterior hypophysectomy in the rat. Neurosci. Abstr. **5:** 609.
20. Unpublished observations.
21. WATKINS, L. R. & D. J. MAYER. The neural organization of endogenous opiate and non-opiate pain control systems. Science. In press.
22. LEWIS, J. W., J. T. CANNON, E. H. CHUDLER & J. C. LIEBESKIND. 1981. Effects of naloxone and hypophysectomy on electroconvulsive shock-induced analgesia. Brain Res. **208:** 230–233.
23. BODNAR, R. J., D. D. KELLY, M. BRUTUS & M. GLUSMAN. 1980. Stress-induced analgesia: Neural and hormonal determinants. Neurosci. Biobehav. Rev. **4:** 87–100.

24. BODNAR, R. J., D. D. KELLY, S. S. STEINER & M. GLUSMAN. 1978. Stress-produced analgesia and morphine-produced analgesia: Lack of cross-tolerance. Pharmac. Biochem. Behav. **8:** 661–668.
25. BODNAR, R. J., D. D. KELLY, A. SPIAGGIA, C. EHRENBERG & M. GLUSMAN. 1978. Dose-dependent reductions by naloxone of analgesia induced by cold-water stress. Pharmacol. Biochem. Behav. **8:** 667–672.
26. LEWIS, J. W., J. T. CANNON & J. C. LIEBESKIND. 1981. Opioid and non-opioid mechanisms of stress analgesia. Science **208:** 623–625.
27. LEWIS, J. W., J. E. SHERMAN & J. C. LIEBESKIND. 1981. Opioid and non-opioid stress analgesia: Assessment of tolerance and cross-tolerance with morphine. J. Neurosci. **1:** 358–363.
28. COBELLI, D. A., L. R. WATKINS & D. J. MAYER. 1980. Dissociation of opiate and non-opiate foot-shock produced analgesia. Soc. Neurosci. Abstr. **6:** 247. No. 92.11.
29. MAIER, S. F., R. C. DRUGAN, J. W. GRAU, R. HYSON, A. J. MacLENNAN, J. MADDEN IV & J. D. BARCHAS. 1981. Opioid and non-opioid mechanisms of long-term analgesia. Soc. Neurosci. Abstr. **7:** 166. (#57.7).
30. LORD, J. A. H., A. A. WATERFIELD, J. HUGHES & H. W. KOSTERLITZ. 1977. Endogenous opioid peptides: multiple agonists and receptors. Nature **267:** 495–499.
31. HILL, R. G. 1981. The status of naloxone in the identification of pain control mechanisms operated by endogenous opioids. Neurosci. Lett. **21:** 217–222.
32. CHANG, K.-J., E. HASUM & P. CUATRECASAS. 1980. Multiple opiate receptors. Trends Neurosci. **3:** 160–162.

DISCUSSION OF THE PAPER

C. KORNETSKY (*Boston University School of Medicine, Boston, MA*): I am glad to hear you say that there have as yet been no studies in other sensory modalities. That is something that I have been inquiring about over and over again. Why hasn't any investigator really looked at stress-induced changes in other modalities?

Another group of people have been doing similar work that is rarely mentioned. This other line of research is related more directly to mental illness. I refer to the so-called learned helplessness phenomenon in which animals do not seem to be responsive to a lot of various phenomena.

I would like to make a couple of additional points. Would you say that when you are describing stress-induced analgesia it is related to the sort of thing that Hardy, Wolff and Goodell did in the 1940s? They measured pain thresholds using the thermal radiation technique in women during labor, and found an elevated threshold to experimental pain during labor.

A bit of evidence that is contrary to the analgesic properties of stress is a study by Hill and Wickler back in the early 1950s or late 1940s, in which they found that they could raise the theshold of pain in humans by decreasing the stress. As they decreased stress directly related to the painful stimulus, the threshold was actually raised.

D. D. KELLY (*College of Physicians and Surgeons of Columbia University, New York*): In many scientific contexts the word stress is used more as a metaphor than as an operational term. Clearly we are dealing with as many different types of stressors as we are behavioral consequences of exposure to stress. Although they may both involve stress, it does not seem reasonable to attempt to compare the behavioral correlates of a woman in labor to those of a rat swimming in ice water.

I would also like to emphasize the distinction between stress-induced analgesia and threshold shifts that are due to attentional variables. If you rivet your attention on a potential pain-producing situation, such as some screams emanating from dentist's office during drilling, then your pain threshold is likely to be lower when it is your turn to be drilled. On the other hand, if you focus on anything other than the potential pain-producing situation, it is likely that you threshold will be elevated.

In order for stress to induce analgesia in experimental paradigms we attempt to rule out such concurrent variables by insisting that the analgesia outlast the stressor. In other words, SIA should be a defined time-dependent, post-stress effect.

DUAL ACTIONS OF MORPHINE ON THE
CENTRAL NERVOUS SYSTEM: PARALLEL
ACTIONS OF β-ENDORPHIN AND ACTH

Yasuko F. Jacquet

Center for Neurochemistry
Rockland Research Institute
Ward's Island, New York 10035

The 1973 demonstration [1-3] of a stereospecific receptor that binds selectively to opiates spurred the search for endogenous ligands that mimic opiate action,[4] culminating in the discovery of β-endorphin.[5] The demonstration of β-endorphin's potent sedative and analgesic actions in brain,[6, 7] and its biosynthetic link to the potent neurohormone, ACTH,[8-10] have raised the possibility that, apart from its opiate action, this new class of neuromodulators may have profound importance in the functional regulation of the brain. Clinical studies on the therapeutic efficacy of β-endorphin to treat mental illness, however, have been hampered not only by its high cost, but also by its demonstrated inability to cross the blood-brain barrier and reach the brain to produce pharmacological actions.[11] This has prompted a renewed examination of opiates, not just as an analgesic to be used in the therapeutic management of pain, but as an inexpensive alternative (with proven ability to effectively cross the blood-brain barrier) to be used as a possible tool in the therapy of functional disorders of the brain. In this connection, it may be of some relevance to review our studies in experimental animals of the CNS actions of morphine (the prototypic opiate), and of the correlated actions of endogenously occurring neuropeptides that mimic morphine's actions.

The intracerebral microinjection technique (the method used in the studies reported here), whereby a drug can be administered directly into CNS sites in the rat brain and thus bypass the blood-brain barrier, provides an important means of investigating drug actions at specific sites in the living brain of the unanesthetized experimental animal. This method is especially appropriate for investigating the CNS actions of compounds that have poor penetration of the blood-brain barrier. A drawback of the intracerebral microinjection method, however, is the need to limit the injection volume to 0.5 μg/site since larger volumes may lesion the injection site. Therefore, a highly concentrated solution is administered, and this diffuses within a small radius representing 0.1% or less of the total brain. (In contrast, numerous sites are activated by more moderate concentrations of circulating drug following a peripheral injection.) Only those drugs that can be solubilized in physiological saline at high concentrations are used. In this sense, the intracerebral microinjection method is suitable for revealing pharmacological, rather than physiological, actions of the microinjected drug. On the other hand, the advantages of this method are its ability to correlate a drug's action with mediation by a discrete CNS site, and to reveal drug action at a specific CNS site that may otherwise be masked or modified following a peripheral administration due to modulatory interactions with other CNS sites that are simultaneously activated.

0077–8923/82/0398–0272 $01.75/0 © 1982 NYAS

Morphine, a naturally occurring plant alkaloid, exerts potent pharmacological actions mediated by the CNS, yet very little of the peripherally administered dose penetrates the blood-brain barrier and reaches the CNS . (It has been estimated that less than 1% of the peripherally administered dose penetrates into brain.[12]) Once at CNS sites, morphine exerts potent opiate action. In the present studies, the intracerebral microinjection technique was used to identify CNS sites in the rat brain that are sensitive to morphine. At these sites, the microinjection method revealed pharmacological actions of morphine that are normally masked following peripheral administration. In the periaqueductal gray (PAG), morphine exerted dual actions: inhibitory and excitatory. The former was mediated by a stereospecific receptor that was antagonized by naloxone, the latter by a nonstereospecific receptor that was not antagonized by naloxone. β-endorphin mimicked the former, suggesting that it may be the endogenous ligand for the inhibitory receptor, while adrenocorticotropic hormone (ACTH) mimicked the latter, indicating that it may be the endogenous ligand for the excitatory receptor. Thus, the CNS actions of morphine paralleled those of the biosynthetically linked neuropeptides, β-endorphin and ACTH.

METHOD

The details of the intracerebral microinjection technique used in these studies have been described elsewhere.[13]

Adult male Wistar rats, weight approximately 300–350 g, under chloral hydrate (360 mg/kg) anesthesia were stereotaxically implanted with bilateral intracerebral cannulas made of 30-gauge stainless steel tubing (outer diameter $= 0.30$ mm), the tips of which were aimed at sites 3 mm dorsal to the intended sites. Injection needles were prepared from 35-gauge stainless steel tubing (outer diameter $= 0.13$ mm) and calibrated to extend precisely 3 mm beyond the tip of the guide cannula. The stereotaxic coordinates for the PAG were (with head position of lamda $=$ bregma at the horizontal plane): 6.00 mm below the skull surface, 0.50–0.75 mm lateral to the midline, and A-P ranged from 0.50 mm posterior to 1.00 mm anterior to lamda. The coordinates for the midbrain reticular formation (MRF) were (with incisor bar at 5.00 mm above interaural zero): 9.25 mm below skull surface, and 1.00–1.50 mm lateral to, and 0.20 mm posterior to the interaural zero. Each rat was allowed one week for postsurgical recovery. For the intracerebral microinjection, the rat was wrapped in a soft towel covering the entire head and body, leaving only the cannula exposed to view. Injection volume was 0.5 μl/site, infused at the rate of 0.1 μl/15 sec. (All drugs and peptides were dissolved in physiological saline, with solutions made up fresh on each day of use.) Immediately following the microinjection, the rat was placed in a transparent plastic bin (30 cm wide, 60 cm high) to allow observation of its behavior for a predetermined interval. At the end of each study, the subjects were perfused with formalin under chloral hydrate anesthesia, the brains removed, and alternate 100–μm sections (containing cannula tracks) stained with cresylviolet and mounted permanently on glass slides.

Drugs and peptides were obtained from the following sources: morphine sulfate, Mallinckrodt, St. Louis, MO [1]; naloxone hydrochloride, Endo Labs, Garden City NY; β-endorphin, Peninsula Labs Inc., San Carlos, CA; and ACTH, a kind gift from Organon, NJ.

RESULTS AND DISCUSSION

Morphine

Following microinjection of morphine (2.6×10^{-8} mol) into bilateral sites in the PAG, two concurrent behavioral syndromes were observed: (a) fearful hyperreactivity to mild auditory and visual stimuli that are normally neutral to the rat (with the rat responding with shrill shrieks and repetitive jumping when presented with a waving towel or a mild tapping sound), and (b) profound analgesia, as indicated by analgesiometric tests (e.g., the tail-flick, hotplate, and paw-pinch tests). These dual actions of morphine were dose-dependent, as seen in FIGURE 1.[14] The hyperreactivity had an onset latency of 5 min and a duration of 20–40 min, while the analgesic action had an onset latency of 10 min and a duration of 1–2 hr.

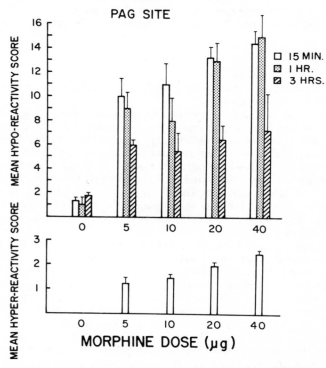

FIGURE 1. Dose-dependent scores of hyperreactivity and hyporeactivity (i.e., analgesia) of rats after intracerebral (IC) microinjections of morphine in periaqueductal gray (PAG). The hyperreactivity was measured at 5, 10, and 15 min after IC administration, and the highest score achieved (1, 2, or 3) during this interval was assigned to the rat. The analgesia at 15, 60, and 180 min after IC administration was measured by a battery of tests including pinches, pinpricks, and thermal stimuli (as described in Reference 14). Separate groups, consisting of 4–6 rats, are shown at each morphine dose. (The injection volume was invariably 0.5 µl for each bilateral site.) (From Jacquet & Lajtha.[14] By permission of *Science*.)

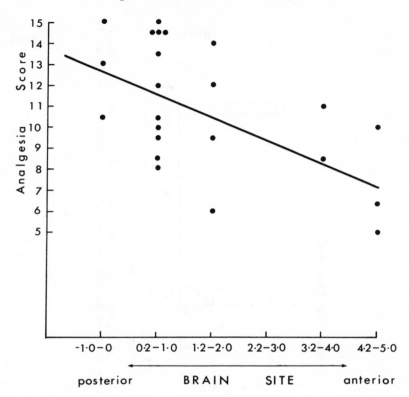

FIGURE 2. Analgesia scores of rats as a function of anterior-posterior (AP) placements of the bilateral intracerebral cannulae ranging from AP −1.0 to +5.0 within the periventricular-periaqueductal gray. The line, drawn free-style through the points, indicates an increase in analgesia with more posterior placements. (Pellegrino and Cushman atlas.) (From Jacquet & Lajtha.[15] By permission of *Brain Research*).

A neuroanatomical mapping of the PAG showed that these dual actions were correlated with rostro-caudal variations in cannula placement within the PAG; both effects increased as placements were more caudal (FIGURES 2 & 3).

Two-way analgesic cross tolerance between peripheral (intraperitoneal) and PAG administration of morphine was found, confirming that the PAG is an important component of the analgesic action of morphine following peripheral administration (FIGURES 4 & 5).[15] (However, this is not to say that the PAG is the only CNS site that mediates morphine analgesia.) (The fearful hyperreactivity syndrome is never seen following a peripheral injection of morphine no matter how high the dose; therefore, it was not possible to demonstrate two-way cross tolerance for this action of morphine.)

These dual actions of morphine were also observed following morphine infusion (6.6×10^{-7} mol) into the lateral ventricle—possibly because of diffusion of morphine into the PAG. Naloxone not only failed to block, but, on

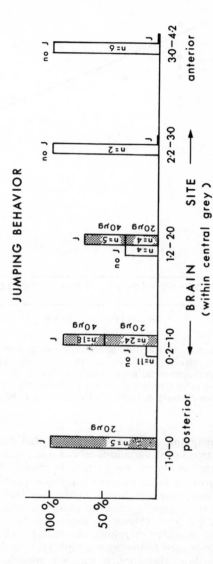

FIGURE 3. Occurrence (*stipled bars*) or absence (*open bars*) of hyperreactivity (jumping behavior) in rats as a function of anterior-posterior cannula placements within the PAG (*central gray*). The hyperreactivity was associated with more posterior placements. (Pellegrino and Cushman atlas.)

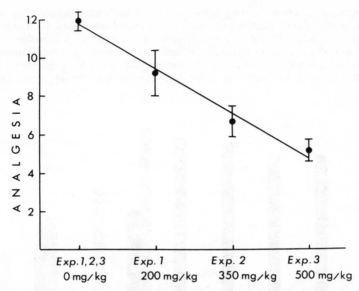

FIGURE 4. Dose-dependent decreases of analgesia in rats following a constant test dose of IC morphine (20 μg) in the PAG as a function of the pretreatment with systemically administered morphine (i.p.) of either 200, 350, or 500 mg/kg. The point at 0 indicates the mean analgesia scores of three saline-pretreated control groups combined. The decrease indicates dose-dependent analgesic cross-tolerance due to the pretreatment. (From Jacquet & Lajtha.[15] By permission of *Brain Research*.)

the contrary, *increased* the incidence of hyperreactivity (from 38% in saline-pretreated control to 64% in naloxone (1 mg/kg) pretreated rats).

A unilateral microinjection of morphine (5.2×10^{-8} mol) into another CNS site, the midbrain reticular formation (MRF), resulted in bouts of rapid ipsilateral rotation (similar to an ice skater's spin) elicited by mild auditory and visual stimuli.[16] This hyperreactivity had an onset latency of 15 min and a duration of 2–8 hr (FIGURE 6). Naloxone (20 mg/kg) given intraperitoneally potentiated, while pretreatment with the dopamine blocker, pimozide (1 or 3 mg–kg), failed to block this behavior. The rate of rotation (greater than 2/sec) was at least severalfold higher than that reported to follow administration of dopamine agonists and antagonists in animals with unilateral nigrostriatal lesions. Thus, morphine was considerably more potent in inducing rotation than the latter. No analgesic action of morphine at this site was observed.

These effects of morphine in the PAG and MRF indicated that the dual actions of morphine—hyperreactivity following mild stimulation, and analgesia to painful stimuli—are dissociable effects of morphine, and site specific.

The unnatural (+)-enantiomer of morphine was assayed in parallel in 3 *in vitro* and 2 *in vivo* assays (FIGURE 7).[17] In the *in vitro* assays, the following was found: (1) the unnatural (+)-morphine, compared with its natural (−)-enantiomer, was found to be 10,000-fold weaker in its ability to displace ³H-dihydromorphine from binding sites in rat brain homogenates; (2) in the electrically stimulated guinea pig ileum, (+)-morphine failed to inhibit contractions at a dose 100 times greater than the dose of (−)-morphine, or of (−)-normorphine that is normally effective in inhibiting contractions, and failed to antagonize the action of (−)-morphine or of (−)-normorphine in this assay; (3) in the assay of adenylate cyclase activity in neuroblastoma

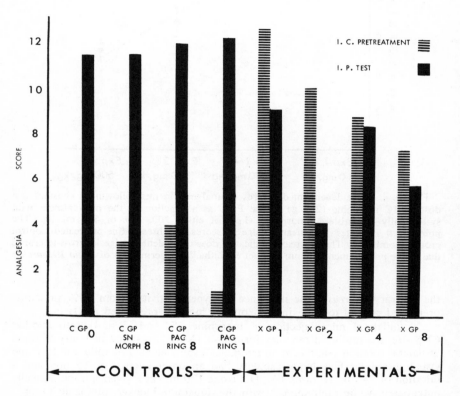

FIGURE 5. Analgesia scores of control groups (at left) and experimental groups (at right) pretreated with IC morphine and tested for analgesic cross tolerance following systemically administered morphine (i.p.) 2 days later. Controls were: 0 = no pretreatment; SN Morph 8 = pretreatment 8 times (at 2–day intervals) with IC morphine injected into the substantia nigra; PAG Ring 8 = pretreatment 8 times with Ringers solution (vehicle) in PAG; PAG Ring 1 = pretreatment once with Ringers in PAG. Experimental groups were pretreated with IC morphine given 1,2,4, or 8 times (at 2-day intervals) as indicated. All groups were tested for analgesic cross tolerance following a constant dose (20 mg/kg) of systemically administered (i.p.) morphine 2 days after the last IC pretreatment. Stipled bars indicate analgesia scores on last day of pretreatment. Solid black bars indicate analgesia scores on test day. An analysis of variance for test day analgesia scores was significant ($F = 6.35$; df 4/12; $p < 0.01$. For details, see Reference 15), indicating the occurrence of analgesic cross tolerance in experimental groups pretreated with IC morphine in the PAG, but not in control groups not pretreated with IC morphine in the PAG.

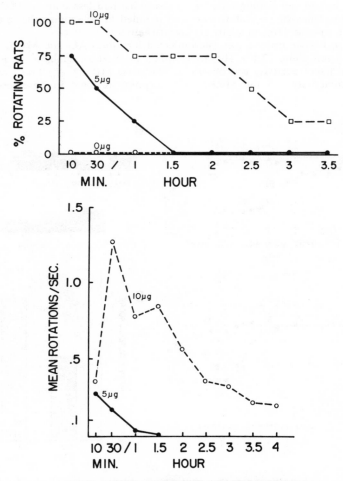

FIGURE 6. Morphine-induced rotations as a function of morphine dose. Rats were tested at 10 and 30 min, and every 30 min thereafter following IC morphine in the midbrain reticular formation (MRF). The test was a white cloth waved over the rat's head for 1 min during which 360° rotations were counted. Half of the rats were injected in the left MRF, the other half in the right MRF; all rotations were ipsilateral to the side of injection. Upper graph depicts incidence of rotators as a function of morphine dose. The 0-μg group, injected with vehicle (Ringers solution) alone, showed no rotation; the 5-μg group showed a moderate, and the 10-μg group a 100%, incidence of rotation. All rats were subsequently tested with a standard dose of 20 μg in the MRF and ascertained to be vigorous rotators. Lower graph depicts rotation speed as a function of morphine dose. The 0-μg group showed no rotations, while the 5-μg group showed moderate, and the 10-μg group robust, speeds. (From Jacquet et al.[16] By permission of Science.)

X glioma hybrid cell homogenates, (+)-morphine had less than 1/1000 of the inhibitory potency of (−)-morphine, and it failed to antagonize the inhibitory action of (−)-morphine on adenylate cyclase activity.

In vivo, (+)-morphine was microinjected into the PAG and MRF. In the PAG, (+)-morphine (2.1×10^{-7} mol) failed to exert an analgesic action, but the fearful hyperreactivity was observed. Naloxone (10 mg/kg) failed to block the hyperreactivity. In the MRF, (+)-morphine resulted in dose-dependent

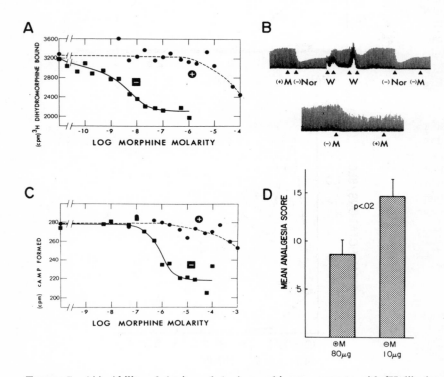

Figure 7. (A) Ability of (+)- and (−)-morphine to compete with ^{3}H-dihydromorphine for binding to receptors in rat brain membrane preparations. (B) Effects of (+)- and (−)-morphine and (−)normorphine on the electrically stimulated contractions of the guinea pig ileum. Note the lack of inhibition following additions of (+)-morphine to the bath, and its lack of antagonism to the inhibitory effects of (−)-morphine and (−)-normorphine. The doses were (upper tracing): 10^{-5} M (+)-morphine, and 4×10^{-7} M (−)-normorphine; (lower tracing): 2×10^{-7} M (−)-morphine and 2×10^{-5} M (+)-morphine. (C) Adenylate cyclase activity of neuroblastoma X glioma hybrid cell homogenates measured in the presence of the indicated concentrations of (+)- or (−)-morphine. (D) Mean analgesia scores and standard errors of rats ($N = 8$) microinjected with 2.1×10^{-7} mol of (+)-morphine into the PAG, and 2 days later, with 2.6×10^{-8} mol of (−)-morphine into the same site. Analgesia was measured by a battery of tests, including pinches, pinpricks, and thermal stimuli (as described in Reference 14). A t-test of the difference between paired scores was significant at p < 0.02. (From Jacquet *et al.*[17] By permission of *Science*.)

bursts of ipsilateral rotation following mild stimulation. Again, these were not blocked by naloxone (10 mg/kg). No analgesia was observed following (+)-morphine microinjection at this site.

These results suggested that there are at least two classes of opiate receptors, one stereospecific and blocked by naloxone, the other not stereo-specific and not blocked by naloxone. The former mediated the inhibitory actions of morphine observed in standard *in vitro* opiate assays, as well as the morphine-induced analgesia observed in the *in vivo* assay. The latter mediated the hyperreactivity observed following microinjection into CNS sites. Significantly, these latter behaviors, i.e., repetitive jumping or bursts of rapid rotation elicited by mild stimuli following morphine microinjection into the PAG or MRF, have never been observed following a peripheral injection of morphine. Even following high peripheral doses, rats typically remain stuporous, occasionally showing spurts of abrupt running, but never violent jumping or rotation. These discrepancies may be attributed to different morphine distributions in the CNS. An intracerebral microinjection delivers the intended morphine dose to a single discrete CNS site. Peripherally administered morphine, on the other hand, must pass through the blood-brain barrier, resulting in a lower concentration that activates multiple systems throughout the CNS, of which some may exert an inhibitory action that masks its excitatory action in the PAG or MRF. Such a "silent" function may explain why there is a puzzling lack of correlation between those CNS sites found to be rich in stereospecific opiate binding, and those CNS sites found to mediate morphine analgesia.

However, other species readily exhibit both inhibitory and excitatory effects of morphine. In the cat, both analgesia and fearful hyperreactivity are observed following peripherally administered morphine. Other species that exhibit the excitatory action of peripherally administered morphine are: pigs, cows, sheep, goats, lions, tigers, bears, and horses.[18] An excitatory action of morphine in man, although rare, has also been reported.[19] In these cases, the ratio of excitatory receptors to inhibitory receptors are probably more favorable for the expression of the excitatory action of morphine.

In the electrically stimulated contractions of the rat vas deferens, both natural (−)-morphine and its unnatural enantiomer, (+)-morphine, exerted excitatory actions, while β-endorphin exerted an inhibitory action. Pre-exposure to (−)-morphine, but not to (+)-morphine, however, resulted in an attenuation of β-endorphin's inhibitory action, indicating the development of cross-tolerance. (−)-Naloxone, but not (+)-naloxone, blocked the inhibitory action of β-endorphin. These results indicated that morphine exerted a dual action in this peripheral tissue: one an inhibitory action mediated by the stereospecific receptor that is blocked stereospecifically by naloxone, the other an excitatory action mediated by the nonstereospecific receptor not blocked by naloxone. The lack of inhibitory action by morphine in the rat vas deferens was explicable when viewed as a reverse example of morphine's dual actions: The masking of the inhibitory action of morphine by its concomitant and more potent excitatory action (FIGURES 8 & 9).[20]

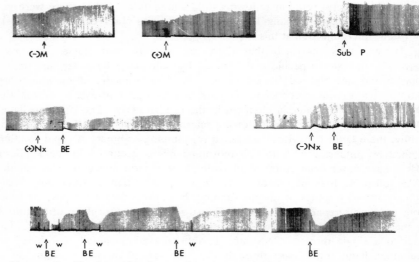

FIGURE 8. Tracings showing excitatory and inhibitory actions of opiates and peptides on the electrically stimulated contractions of rat vas deferens. (A) Left, excitation after addition of $(-)$-morphine (M) (final dilution $= 1 \times 10^{-4}$ M); center, after $(+)$-morphine (1×10^{-4} M); right, after substance P (SP) (2.5×10^{-6} M). (B) Left, excitation after addition of $(+)$-naloxone (Nal) (1×10^{-4} M) followed by inhibition (no blockade) when β-endorphin (B-E) (1.4×10^{-6} M) was added in its presence; right, excitation after addition of $(-)$-naloxone (1×10^{-4} M); no inhibition (blockade) followed when β-endorphin (1.4×10^{-6} M) was added in its presence. (C) Inhibition in a vas deferens preexposed to $(+)$-morphine (1×10^{-4} M) when β-endorphin (1.4×10^{-7} M) was added 1, 10, 30, and 60 min later (i.e., no cross tolerance). Three minutes after each of the first three additions, the strips were washed (w). (From Jacquet.[20] By permission of *Science*.)

Other Opiates: Etorphine, Levorphanol, Methadone, and Heroin

The analgesic potencies of etorphine, levorphanol, and methadone following intracerebral microinjections failed to parallel their analgesic potencies following systemic administration.[14] It had been previously reported by Kutter, et al.,[21] that by the intravenous route, etorphine, levorphanol, and methadone required 1/5,000, 1/11, and 1/5, respectively, of the morphine dose to achieve comparable analgesic action, whereas by the intracerebroventricular route, the ratio was reduced or *reversed* to 1/34, 7, and 30 times the morphine dose, respectively. This was attributed to the lipophilicity of these opiates that enabled them to penetrate the blood-brain barrier and reach receptor sites more rapidly before being metabolized than the more hydrophilic opiate, morphine. Moreover, lipophilic drugs can traverse the blood-brain barrier readily in both directions, and therefore may be rapidly eliminated from receptor sites and redistributed elsewhere by the circulation. These factors may explain why only moderate levels of analgesia, and never any hyperreactivity, was observed following microinjections of levorphanol (2–4 times the morphine dose) and methadone (4 times the morphine dose). (Higher concentrations of these opiates were not tested since it was not possible to achieve solubilization without precipitation in physiological saline.) Intracerebrally administered etorphine, on the other hand, exerted analgesic action (without hyperreactivity) but only after a relatively high dose (2 μg) equivalent to the systemically effective dose. This suggests that etorphine was rapidly absorbed and redistributed by the circulation, thereby activating those CNS sites that exerted an inhibitory action that masked its excitatory action. Intracerebral microinjecion of heroin (at the same dose as morphine) resulted in the same dual actions seen with morphine, i.e., potent analgesia and fearful hyperreactivity (with perhaps a faster onset of action than morphine). Although lipophilic, heroin (diacetylmorphine) is hydrolyzed to 6-monoacetylmorphine and morphine in the brain, and its pharmacological actions have been attributed to these hydrolysis products. These may resist rapid uptake and redistribution by the circulatory system, and may explain heroin's potent actions following intracerebral microinjection in the PAG in contrast to the other lipophilic opiates. Thus, the behavioral effects of an opiate differ depending not only on route of administration (whether peripheral, intracerebroventricular, or intracerebral), but also as a function of its ability to traverse the blood-brain barrier (in both directions), as well as factors regulating its peripheral and central metabolism and elimination, and specific drug–receptor interaction.

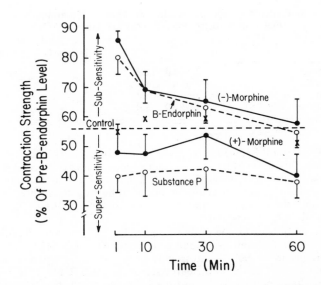

FIGURE 9. Mean contraction strength ($\pm$ standard error) of vasa deferentia (6 per group) after β-endorphin (1.4×10^{-7} M) was added 1, 10, 30, and 60 min after a 30-min pre-exposure to either ($-$)-morphine (1×10^{-4} M), ($+$)-morphine (1×10^{-4} M), β-endorphin (1.4×10^{-6} M), substance P (SP) (2.5×10^{-6} M), or no drug (X). The smallest contraction during the 3-min exposure to β-endorphin was measured and expressed as a percentage of the contraction height before β-endorphin was added. Note cross tolerance after ($-$)-morphine, but not ($+$)-morphine. (From Jacquet.[20] By permission of *Science*.)

NALOXONE

A high naloxone dose ($1.6–3.0 \times 10^{-7}$ mol) microinjected in the rat PAG resulted in fearful hyperreactivity, similar to morphine-induced fearful hyperreactivity.[22] In contrast, a high dose of naloxone given systemically in mice [23] and rats [22] resulted in lethargic immobility similar to the lethargy reported in human subjects.[24] Thus, different behaviors occurred depending on the route of administration, whether systemic or intracerebral. The lethargy following systemic naloxone was attributed to interactions with a nonopiate receptor,[25] whereas the fearful hyperreactivity following microinjection into the PAG may be due to an agonist interaction with the same excitatory receptor stimulated by morphine. Multiple lines of evidence [26] now indicate that naloxone is not a "pure" opiate antagonist, especially at high doses.

β-Endorphin and ACTH

Only β-endorphin, of the naturally occurring putative "opiate" peptides, was found to exert an analgesic action following microinjection into the PAG

TABLE 1

ANALGESIA AND CATATONIA FOLLOWING INTRACEREBRAL MICROINJECTION OF OPIATE
PEPTIDES INTO THE PERIAQUEDUCTAL GRAY (PAG)

		analgesia	catatonia
Met-enkephalin	2×10^{-7} mol	—	—
Leu-enkephalin	2×10^{-7} mol	—	—
α-endorphin	3×10^{-8} mol	—	—
β-endorphin	1×10^{-9} mol	+	+

(TABLE 1).[6] Fearful hyperreactivity was never observed. Methionine enkephalin (Tyr, Gly, Gly, Phe, Met), with a homologous sequence to β-LPH (61–65), leucine enkephalin (Tyr, Gly, Gly, Phe, Leu), and alpha-endorphin (β-LPH (61–76)) failed to exert an analgesic action following microinjection into the PAG. Raising the dose of β-endorphin, even to toxic levels (1.7×10^{-7} mol) failed to result in hyperreactivity.

Pro-opiomelanocortin, the prohormone of B-LPH, contains the full sequence of ACTH(1–39) (as well as homologous sequences of MSH.[10] This common biosynthetic origin of ACTH and β-endorphin suggests a potential relationship between the actions of the two neurohormones. ACTH has long been known for its potent hormonal actions, but little is known about its CNS actions. Terenius et al.[27] reported that ACTH displaced ^{3}H-dihydromorphine (as well as ^{3}H-naloxone) from binding sites in rat brain homogenates (although with low affinity). Potent behavioral effects in various avoidance paradigms following peripheral administrations of ACTH and its fragments were reported by DeWied and his associates.[28] Gispen [29] observed that naloxone antagonized grooming behavior induced by intraventricular injections of ACTH(4–10) and ACTH (1–24). Krivoy and Zimmermann [30] reported that ACTH(1–24) and related

TABLE 2

CORRELATED OCCURRENCE OF HYPERREACTIVITY FOLLOWING PAG MICROINJECTION
OF MORPHINE (5.2×10^{-8} MOL) AND ACTH (1.7 OR 3.4×10^{-8} MOL)

| | | Morphine | |
		yes	no
ACTH	yes	75.9%	10.3%
	no	3.5%	10.3%

* Half of the rats were given morphine first, the others ACTH first, in a counter-balanced design. The two intracerebral microinjections were given at 2-day intervals.

fragments antagonized morphine's depressant actions in the cat spinal cord. These studies suggested that ACTH and/or its fragments may have a central site of action related to opiate action.

Microinjection of ACTH(1–24) in the PAG (1.7 or 3.4×10^{-8} mol) resulted in fearful hyperreactivity similar to morphine-induced fearful hyperreactivity, but no analgesia.[31] The onset latency of the hyperreactivity was 10 min, and duration of action was approximately 20–40 min. When identical rats were micro-injected with morphine and ACTH separately (at 2-day intervals in a counterbalanced design), a significant correlation was obtained between morphine-induced, and ACTH-induced hyperreactivity (TABLE 2), suggesting that the same neuronal substrates mediated the two behaviors.[32] Histological examination of the brains of these rats indicated that the occurrence of this behavioral syndrome was critically dependent on accurate bilateral placements of the cannulas within caudal PAG, with minimal damage inflicted on this structure by the cannulas and injection procedure (FIGURE 10).[32]

Thus, ACTH and β-endorphin each duplicated one of the dual actions of morphine in the PAG. β-endorphin microinjected in the PAG resulted in potent analgesia and sedation, while ACTH microinjected in the same site resulted in fearful hyperreactivity. These results suggest that in the mammalian

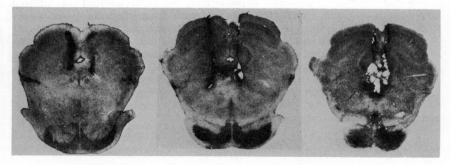

FIGURE 10. Photomicrographs of rat brain sections (middlemost of cannula tracks): left with injection sites within PAG; middle with injection sites ventral to PAG; right with extensive lesions throughout the PAG. (From Jacquet & Wolfe.[32] By permission of *Brain Research*.)

CNS, the exogenous plant alkaloid, morphine, exerts its dual actions by stimulating receptors for the two biosynthetically related endogenous neuropeptides, β-endorphin and ACTH.

Temporal Aspects of the CNS Actions of β-Endorphin and ACTH

Acute analgesic tolerance following a single microinjection of β-endorphin in the PAG was observed 7 days later (FIGURE 11). At the same time, acute sensitization to the hyperthermic action of a single microinjection of β-endorphin in the PAG was also observed (FIGURE 11). These opposite temporal effects, tolerance (i.e., habituation) to the analgesic action, but reverse tolerance (sensitization) to the hyperthermic action of β-endorphin microinjected into the same site (PAG), raise the possibility that two separate receptors may mediate these effects.

TABLE 3

POTENTIATION (+) OR ATTENUATION (−) OF β-ENDORPHIN EFFECTS FOLLOWING
INTRACEREBRAL MICROINJECTION INTO THE PAG

	Analgesia	Catatonia	Body Temp Changes
Hypophysectomy	+ +	+ +	− −
Adrenalectomy	+	+	−
Dexamethasone pretreatment	−	?	+

Modulation by the Pituitary-Adrenal Axis of the CNS Actions of β-Endorphin

The analgesic and catatonic effects of β-endorphin following microinjection in the PAG were potentiated in hypophysectomized rats, while the hyperthermic action was reversed to profound hypothermia. Adrenalectomized rats showed similar, but less potent effects. Pretreatment with dexamethasone (1 mg/kg 24 hr previous to, and 100 μg/kg 1 hr previous to, the β-endorphin microinjection) of normal rats resulted in an attenuation of the analgesic action of β-endorphin in the PAG, while the hyperthermic action was potentiated (TABLE 3). The potentiation of the analgesic and catatonic actions of β-endorphin in hypophysectomized and adrenalectomized rats may indicate the absence of an antagonist that normally modulates some of β-endorphin's actions. We previously reported [33] that crude rat brain homogenates contained an antagonist of β-endorphin's actions in the guinea pig ileum assay.

SUMMARY

In the studies described above, the intracerebral microinjection technique was used to study the actions of morphine at morphine-sensitive sites, the periacqueductal gray (PAG) and the midbrain reticular formation (MRF). In

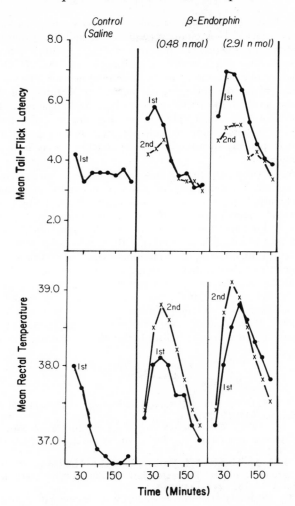

FIGURE 11. *Mean tail-flick latencies (upper half)*. The two curves in each of the middle and right panels represent mean tail-flick latencies during the two sessions separated by a 7-day interval. Testing was conducted at 2–5 min after the micro-injection, followed by testing every 30 min thereafter for eight determinations (210 min). The middle panel shows results of the 0.48 nmol β-endorphin group, the right panel those of the 2.9 nmol group. The "2nd" session was conducted 7 days after the "1st." Note the significant ($p < 0.05$) elevation of mean tail-flick latencies of both β-endorphin groups during the 1st session over the control saline session (left panel), and the significant decrease in the mean tail-flick latencies from the 1st to the 2nd session for both groups. (* indicates $p < 0.05$, t-test for paired measures, one-tail.)

Mean rectal temperatures (lower half). Rectal temperatures were determined immediately following the tail-flick test for each rat over the 210 min of the experiment. Note the significant increase from the 1st to the 2nd sessions in the hyperthermia of both groups. (* indicates $p < 0.05$, t-test for paired measures, one-tail.)

the PAG, morphine exerted dual actions: inhibitory and excitatory. In the MRF, morphine exerted an excitatory action only, indicating that the dual actions of morphine are dissociable and site specific. Following microinjection into the PAG, β-endorphin exerted an inhibitory, and ACTH an excitatory, action, i.e., each duplicated one of morphine's dual actions. These results indicated that receptors for the endogenously occurring peptides, β-endorphin and ACTH, may play a role in morphine's potent pharmacological actions. Although these studies do not shed direct light on the physiological role of these neuropeptides and their receptors, nor on their potential roles in the functional regulation of brain (especially in diseased mental states), it may be permissible to offer some speculations.

We previously proposed that β-endorphin may be an endogenous antipsychotogen, and that a deficiency in brain β-endorphin may underlie some forms of psychopathology. In view of β-endorphin's biosynthetic link to ACTH, and the behavioral effects of β-endorphin (sedated immobility) that was found to be opposite in kind to those of ACTH (fearful hyperreactivity) following administration into brain, it is possible that these two neuropeptides may have regulatory roles in maintaining a functional balance in brain. (It may be speculated that these biosynthetically linked neuropeptides served survival functions of "flight" and "freeze" in our evolutionary ancestors.) An imbalance in the bioavailability of either of the two neuropeptides, e.g., a deficiency of β-endorphin or an excess of ACTH (perhaps due to the lack of the specific enzymes that cleave these peptides from their parent prohormone) may be an etiological factor in some forms of chronic functional disorders of the brain.

REFERENCES

1. PERT, C. B. & S. H. SNYDER. 1973. Opiate receptor: Demonstration in nervous tissue. Science **179:** 1011–1014.
2. TERENIUS, L. 1973. Characteristics of the receptor for narcotic analgesics in synaptic plasma membrane fraction from rat brain. Acta Pharmacol. Toxicol. **33:** 377–384.
3. SIMON, E. J., J. M. HILLER & I. EDELMAN. 1973. Stereospecific binding of the potent narcotic analgesic (^{3}H) etorphine to rat-brain homogenate. Proc. Natl. Acad. Sci. USA **70:** 1947–1949.
4. HUGHES, J. 1975. Isolation of an endogenous compound from the brain with pharmacological properties similar to morphine. Brain Res. **88:** 295–308.
5. BRADBURY, A. F., D. G. SMYTH, C. R. SNELL, N. J. M. BIRDSALL & E. C. HULME. 1976. C-fragment of lipotropin has a high affinity for brain opiate receptors. Nature (Lond.) **260:** 793–795.
6. JACQUET, Y. F. & N. MARKS. 1976. The C-fragment of B-lipotropin: An endogenous neuroleptic or antipsychotogen? Science **194:** 632–635.
7. BLOOM, F., D. SEGAL, N. LING & R. GUILLEMIN. 1976. Endorphins: Profound behavioral effects in rats suggest new etiological factors in mental illness. Science **194:** 630–632.
8. MAINS, R. E., B. A. EIPPER & N. LING. 1977. Common precursor to corticotropins and endorphins. Proc. Natl. Acad. Sci. USA **74:** 3014–3018.
9. ROBERTS, J. L. & C. HERBERT. 1977. Characterization of a common precursor to corticotropin and b-lipotropin: Cell-free synthesis of the precursor and identification of corticotropin peptides in the molecule. Proc. Natl. Acad. Sci. USA **74:** 4826–4830.

10. NAKANISHI, S., A. INOUE, T. KITA, M. NAKAMURA, A. C. Y. CHANG, S. N. COHEN & S. NUMA. 1979. Nucleotide sequence of cloned cDNA for bovine corticotropin-B-lipotropin precursor. Nature **278:** 423–427.
11. JACQUET, Y. F. 1980. B-endorphin, blood-brain barrier, and schizophrenia. Lancet: 831–832.
12. MULÉ, S. J. 1971. Physiological disposition of narcotic agonists and antagonists. In Narcotic Drugs: Biochemical Pharmacology, D. H. Clouet, Ed. pp. 99–121. Plenum Press. New York.
13. JACQUET, Y. F. 1975. Intracerebral administration of opiates. In Methods of Narcotics Research, S. Ehrenpries & A. Neidle, Eds. pp. 33–57. Dekker. New York.
14. JACQUET, Y. F. & A. LAJTHA. 1974. Paradoxical effects after microinjection of morphine in the periaqueductal gray matter in the rat. Science **185:** 1055–1057.
15. JACQUET, Y. F. & A. LAJTHA. 1976. The periaqueductal gray: Site of morphine analgesia and tolerance as shown by 2-way cross tolerance between systemic and intracerebral injections. Brain Res. **103:** 501–513.
16. JACQUET, Y. F., M. CAROL & I. S. RUSSELL. 1976. Morphine-induced rotation in naive, nonlesioned rats. Science **192:** 261–263.
17. JACQUET, Y. F., W. A. KLEE, K. C. RICE, I. IIJIMA & J. MINAMIKAWA. 1977. Stereospecific and nonstereospecific effects of (+)- and (−)-morphine: Evidence for a new class of receptors? Science **198:** 842–845.
18. JAFFE, J. H. & W. R. MARTIN. 1980. Opioid analgesics and antagonists, In The Pharmacological Basis of Therapeutics. L. S. Goodman & A. Gilman, Eds., 6th edit. pp. 494–534. Macmillan Publishing Co. New York.
19. BERRYHILL, R. E., J. L. BENUMOF & D. S. JANOWSKY. 1979. Morphine-induced hyperexcitability in man. Anesthesiology **50:** 65–66.
20. JACQUET, Y. F. 1980. Excitatory and inhibitory effects of opiates in the rat vas deferens: A dual mechanism of opiate action. Science **210:** 95–97.
21. KUTTER, E., A. HERZ, H. J. TESCHEMACHER & R. HESS. 1970. Structure-activity correlations of morphine-like analgetics based on efficiencies following intravenous and intraventricular application. J. Med. Chem. **13:** 801–805.
22. JACQUET, Y. F. 1980. Different behavioral effects following intracerebral, intracerebroventricular or intraperitoneal injections of naloxone in the rat. Behav. Brain Res. **1:** 543–546.
23. JACQUET, Y. F. 1980. Stereospecific, dose-dependent antagonism by naloxone of non-opiate behavior in mice. Pharmacol. Biochem. Behav. **13:** 585–587.
24. JUDD, L. L., D. S. JANOWSKY, D. S. SEGAL & L. Y. HUEY. 1980. Naloxone-induced behavioral and physiological effects in normal and manic subjects. Arch. Gen. Psychiat. **37:** 583–586.
25. VOLAVKA, J. & Y. F. JACQUET. 1981. Naloxone-induced lethargy. Arch. Gen. Psychiat. **38:** 844.
26. SAWYNOK, J., C. PINSKY & F. S. LABELLA. 1979. On the specificity of naloxone as an opiate antagonist. Life Sci. **25:** 1621–1632.
27. TERENIUS, L., W. H. GISPEN & D. DE WIED. 1975. ACTH-like peptides and opiate receptors in the rat brain: structure activity studies. Eur. J. Pharmacol. **33:** 395–399.
28. DE WIED, D., A. WITTER & H. M. GREVEN. 1975. Behaviorally active ACTH analogues. Biochem. Pharmacol. **24:** 1463–1468.
29. GISPEN, W. H. & W. M. WIEGANT. 1976. Opiate antagonists suppress ACTH 1–24–induced excessive grooming in the rat. Neurosci. Lett. **2:** 159–164.
30. KRIVOY, W. A. & E. ZIMMERMANN. 1977. An effect of B-melanocyte stimulating hormone (B-MSH) on α-motoneurons of cat spinal cord. Eur. J. Pharmac. **46:** 315–322.
31. JACQUET, Y. F. 1978. Opiate effects after adrenocorticotropin or B-endorphin injection in the periaqueductal gray matter of rats. Science **201:** 1032–1034.

32. JACQUET, Y. F. & G. WOLF. 1981. Morphine and ACTH(1–24): Correlative behavioral excitations following microinjections in rat periaqueductal gray. Brain Res. **219:** 214–218.
33. JACQUET, Y. F., W. A. KLEE & D. G. SMYTH. 1978. B-endorphin: Modulation of acute tolerance and antagonism by endogenous brain systems. Brain Res. **156:** 396–401.

DISCUSSION OF THE PAPER

E. L. WAY (*University of California, San Francisco*): Is the excitatory effect just peculiar for morphine or does it hold for all opiate agonists?

Y. JACQUET: I have only experimented with a limited number of opiates. Heroin will definitely produce this action, but etorphine and levorphanol will not.

D. GMEREK (*Temple University School of Medicine, Philadelphia*): Have you tried unilateral injection? Do you have to inject bilaterally to find this response?

JACQUET: I tried unilateral injections, and the same effect is produced, but it is somewhat weaker. The best effects occur when bilateral injection is used, probably because more tissue is being stimulated.

MORPHINE- AND ENDORPHIN-INDUCED BEHAVIORAL ACTIVATION IN THE MOUSE: IMPLICATIONS FOR MANIA AND SOME RECENT PHARMACOGENETIC STUDIES *

R. J. Katz

Department of Psychology
The Johns Hopkins University
Baltimore, Maryland 21218

Because systemic injections of morphine and related endogenous and exogenous opiates are behaviorally depressant for most laboratory species (e.g., rats, rabbits, guinea pigs, dogs, and primates), their stimulating effects in other species, including mice [1] and cats [2] as well as such less commonly employed animals as asses,[2] lions,[3] panthers,[3] bears,[4] and hedgehogs (however, only in the summer [5]) are often overlooked. Nonetheless, highly stereotyped behavioral activation to morphine consisting of the Straub tail response [6] and continuous, exclusively horizontal, hyperkinesis were described for the mouse well over a century ago,[1] and strain differences in murine responses to opiates were noted as early as 1912.[7]

We (Drs. B. J. Carroll, P. T. Sharp, R. Moreines, and I) were interested in further characterizing the murine opiate activation syndrome for several reasons. For one thing, murine running represented an easily replicated and highly quantifiable index of opiate activity, which could be obtained without causing any obvious pain to the animal. In addition, when account was taken of different routes of administration and catabolism, the running response (as defined by horizontal hyperkinesis and Straub tail) was as sensitive to endorphins as it was to plant alkaloids. More immediate to our own interests, however, was the fact that, upon several critical grounds, it offered an interesting preclinical analog of human mania.[8] Finally, because the mouse is an excellent species for behavior-genetic analysis, it subsequently enabled us to examine the influences of genotype upon the morphine response. Indeed, as we will demonstrate, in several cases it was possible to isolate and analyze the effects of a single gene upon the opiate response.

In the following sections we review three aspects of our research: the relationship of muroid running to human mania, the influence of opioid peptides in producing the running syndrome, and the influence of genetic factors in determining the quality and degree of behavioral response to morphine.

OPIOID RUNNING AS A MODEL FOR MANIA

Although several acceptable preclinical screening procedures are available for the identification of compounds with antidepressant potential,[9] few are suitable for the specific detection of antimanic activity.[9] Given the paucity of

* This work was supported in part by an Alfred P. Sloan Foundation Research Fellowship in Neuroscience and Grant MH 31588 from the National Institutes of Health.

0077-8923/82/0397-0291 $1.75/0 © 1982, NYAS

drugs beyond lithium for the specific treatment of mania, the need for accurate and specific preclinical procedures of this last class is acute.

Clearly, mice are not human, and behavioral parallels can be taken only so far. However, it might be noted that murine activation and human mania do share a number of basic behavioral similarities. Both are characterized by an impulsive, driven quality, present in each to a pathological degree. Moreover, in both cases some few activities occur to the exclusion of normal adaptive behavior. Clinically, mania is characterized by a narrowing of behaviors to that class which is directed towards immediate gratification (especially for the grandiose subtypes) or (in more atypical and hostile cases), to responding to paranoid ideation. In both cases the lability of manic ideation results in a general dropping out of actual goal attainment.[10, 11] Likewise in the case of the murine model, treatment with a compound with highly reinforcing properties narrows behavior to an extreme stereotype lacking any immediate significance or apparent goal.

In a series of elegant studies, Carroll and Sharp demonstrated that virtually all clinical or experimental therapeutic interventions that reduced mania also reduced the running response. Lithium,[12] reserpine, acetylcholinesterase inhibitors such as physostigmine, and antiserotonergic drugs such as methysergide all produced parallel clinical and experimental reductions in mania and the running response.[13] The only failure we know of in the model is the tricyclic antiepileptic drug, carbamazepine, which may have antimanic properties clinically, but which actually increased the running response.[14] We have argued elsewhere that this may reflect intrinsic anticonvulsant properties of the latter, since anticonvulsants generally increase the running response to morphine or d-Ala^2-Leu enkephalinamide.[14, 15]

As an opiate-mediated syndrome, the running response is subject to receptor blockade by naloxone. Thus a strong prediction emerging from these initial studies nearly a decade ago was that, at a clinical level, naloxone might possess antimanic activity. Although naloxone is not universally effective in this regard, it has recently been demonstrated to possess a therapeutic effect in a subpopulation of manics.[16] It might be predicted that more potent or long-lasting antagonists would be yet more effective. At the very least, at present, the opiate running response offers one of the few acceptable procedures for identifying compounds with therapeutic profiles similar to the lithium ion. Thus in the future the running model might lead to an improved understanding of the substrates of mania and to such practical developments as novel classes of antimanic drugs.

ENDORPHINERGIC NATURE OF THE ACTIVATION RESPONSE

The discovery in 1975 by Hughes and Kosterlitz [17] of endogenous opioid neuropeptides prompted us to examine central injections of Leu and Met enkephalins in the running model. Following intraventricular injections of 10–200 μg, mice typically displayed a brief (10–20 min) period of activity that was quantitatively and qualitatively similar to vehicle injection in all respects. In a few exceptional cases (perhaps 5%) at higher doses some stereotyped running was observed. This was uncommon, however, and represented a highly variable response.

Reasoning that the peptides might normally have been broken down prior to their having produced any biological or behavioral effects, we next examined the d-Ala^2-substituted amides of Leu and Met enkephalin. Central injections of both compounds (6–50 μg) produced profound dose-related stereotyped running behaviorally identical to that seen after systemic morphine.[18] Of the two peptides, the Leu form was more potent, possibly pointing to a δ-like peptide effect at a receptor level. It might be noted that Wei and co-workers independently have found similar behavioral effects, and additionally have reported that β-endorphin lacks activity-enhancing properties of the enkephalins.[19]

In more recent experiments we have examined *kyotorphin,* an endogenous dipeptide isolated by Takagi and co-workers.[20] This peptide, although devoid of direct receptor-stimulating properties, potentiates endogenous enkephalin activity by inhibiting the catabolic enzyme enkephalinase. Typical results, based upon intracerebroventricular injections of the neuropeptide approximately 5 minutes prior to the onset of recording, may be seen in FIGURE 1. As was the

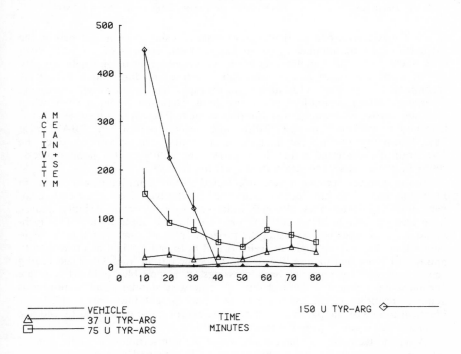

FIGURE 1. Effects of the dipeptide Tyr-Arg (kyotorphin) upon behavioral activation in the HA/ICR mouse. Adult male mice at 30 g were prepared by the method of Katz *et al.*[18] and injected intracerebroventricularly with 0.9% vehicle, or peptide in vehicle into the lateral ventricle. 5 μl injections were used with infusion times of < 30 sec. Recording based upon capacitance sensing [14, 15, 18] began 5 min after injection and continued for 30 min. All data as means $\pm$ SE. Main effects for dose ($F_{3, 24} = 5.1$), time ($F_{7, 168} = 19.7$), and their interaction ($F_{21, 108} = 10.1$) are all significant beyond $p < 0.01$. Note that the highest dose was toxic for all mice by min 30.

case with the degradation-resistant pentapeptides, kyotorphin produced unambiguous increases in activity. It should be noted that lower doses of kyotorphin produced increases in general activity without a pronounced stereotyped quality. Rearing, horizontal translation, and other aspects of the normal repertoire were all increased. At doses above 150 μg mice showed the stereotyped response, generally for 10–20 min. This was invariably succeeded by convulsions and death. Thus, although enkephalinase inhibitors can mimic the actions of endogenous and exogenous opiates, their actions possibly on other endorphinergic systems render them less specific than the former compounds.

Given the above evidence from degradation-resistant analogs of endogenous opioid peptides and also from enkephalinase inhibitors that prolong the action of endogenous opiates, it is apparent that endogenous opioid peptides may play a functionally significant role in the activation syndrome.

A PHARMACOGENETIC ANALYSIS OF THE RUNNING SYNDROME

As noted above, one particular advantage of using mice as subjects is the existence of a large number of genetically well-defined lines of subjects. Such lines allow both initial molar ascriptions of genetic control and subsequently permit a more detailed analysis through selective breeding and a variety of recombinant techniques. Goldstein,[21] for example, has demonstrated increasing divergence across generations with mice bred from one common stock when selection across generations was for opiate-elicited activity. Likewise, Castellano and co-workers [22] using C57BL6J mice in comparison with DBA2J mice have shown that the loci for analgesia and running are orthogonal, since the first strain demonstrated a high level of running activity but a poor analgesic response while the second strain shows just the reverse.

In our own research we have concentrated on the definition of effects due to individual loci. This has been accomplished by the use of congenic and coisogenic lines. Congenic lines, although widely used for histocompatability studies, have seen only slight behavioral and pharmacological applications. This technique involves repeatedly crossing the progeny from two lines back to a single parent line. For example, given strains A and B, their F1 might be crossed to B, and the F1 from that mating likewise, to the same parent line. Over succeeding generations and by repeated back crossings, it is possible to insert a single chromosomal segment of interest onto an otherwise standard and homogenous genome, resulting in the existence of two pure parent lines and a third line identical to one of the parents in all respects except those controlled by the one chromosomal segment from the second parent line.

A second technique we have made use of is the insertion of a single gene of interest onto a constant genetic background. This second technique (of coisogenic lines) involves breeding a point-mutation from a given parent stock and comparing it to the latter. It should be evident that this second technique results in the production of an essentially limitless number of identical siblings and a second group of identical siblings differing from the first by a single locus. Using both the above techniques in concert, we are able to identify and independently validate the role of a given locus in controlling a pharmacological response. We review below our efforts involving the c locus, the gene controlling albinism, and the pallid (pa) locus. Finally, we present recent studies on the effects of inserting a novel locus (the gene for audiogenic seizure susceptibility, the locus *ep*) upon a *randomly* outbred (rather than a constantly inbred) genetic background, using the deer mouse, *Peromyscus maniculatus*.

The c Locus

We began studying the locus for albinism using both congenic and coisogenic lines. The *c* locus was chosen for initial study because of its established pleiotropic effects both upon behavior and upon drug responses. Using either of two genetic techniques and either of two dependent measures [a behavioral measure (the running response), or a physiological measure (core temperature reduction)], we found significant losses in opiate sensitivity to be due to the presence of the gene. These findings for single gene insertions are presented in FIGURES 2 and 3 for running and hypothermia, respectively. Results for congenic lines were essentially similar (i.e., a chromosomal segment for albinism significantly reduced both the behavioral and physiological response) and have been published elsewhere.[23]

The Pallid Locus

We next examined the locus *pa* (pallid), again using the single gene insertion technique. The pallid mouse (57BL6Jpapa) and its parent line (C57BL6JPaPa) were of interest because of the established effects of the gene upon reduced

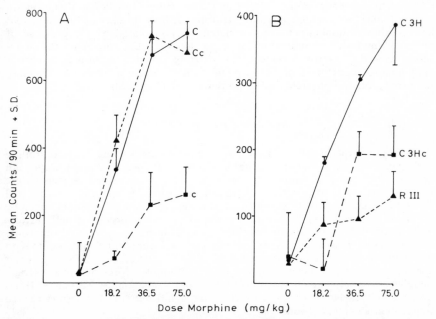

FIGURE 2. Effects of systemic morphine or vehicle upon stereotyped behavioral activation in the C57BL6J mouse and a coisogenic albino line. All data as means ± SE.

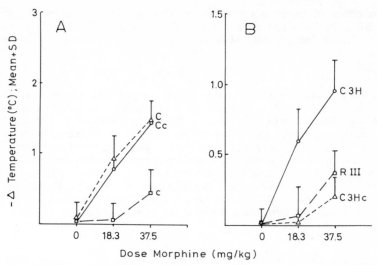

FIGURE 3. Effects of systemic morphine or vehicle upon core temperature elevation in the C57BL6J mouse and a coisogenic albino line. All data as means ±SE.

transport of aromatic amino acids,[24] and concomitant functional alterations in
catechol- and indolamine-containing neurons. It may be seen in FIGURE 4 that
opiate-induced running activity was significantly increased by the presence of
the pallid mutation. Similar findings were noted for the core temperature response as well.[25] Thus it is evident that changing a single gene of a given genetically homogeneous strain of mouse is sufficient to radically increase or decrease
the behavioral and physiological responses to opiate agonists.

Studies on Epileptic Mice

In recent experiments we have also begun to examine the gene controlling
audiogenic seizure sensitivity in the deer mouse, *Peromyscus maniculatus*. In
contrast with previous studies in which genes or chromosomal segments were
inserted upon a fixed genetic background, the gene for epilepsy was inserted
upon a genetically random background, since epileptic mice were maintained by
outbreeding to wild stock. Thus, in previous cases background genetic factors
were controlled by the highly specified and stable nature of the strain; while
in the present case all genes except the gene *ep* were sufficiently random to
allow statistical rather than experimental control. The choice of this particular
species was partially dictated by the limited amount of previous pharmacogenetic work and also by observations by Bloom,[26] Liebeskind,[27] Tortella,[28] Holaday,[29] and ourselves [14, 15] for a functionally significant role for seizure-related
phenomena in opiate actions.

Our findings are summarized in FIGURE 5. Particularly at higher doses epileptic mice were behaviorally more sensitive to morphine. Indeed they appeared
to run at twice the normal levels of their genetic controls. This confirms that

seizure susceptibility is a sufficient condition to modify opiate sensitivity. It must be emphasized that these changes are not a result of convulsions *per se.* None of the mice were convulsed at any time prior to testing, although at the close of testing litter mates of convulsive and convulsion-resistant mice were tested for seizure susceptibility. All homozygous epileptic mice did seize, while neither heterozygotes nor homozygous dominant (i.e., resistant) mice did.

Final evidence that convulsions are not the basis of the above effect are found in the observation that immediately (< 30 sec) post-ictal mice showed no behavioral activation to any dose of morphine. Finally, in a recent series of experiments, Mansour (personal communication) has repeatedly convulsed *ep* mice and then tested them for behavioral activation. He reports that mice given

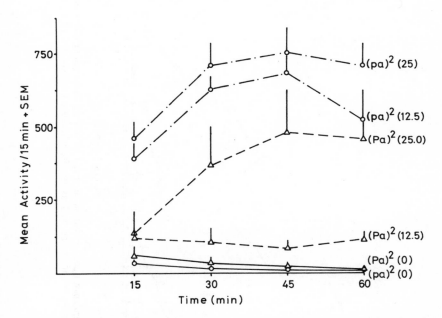

FIGURE 4. Effects of morphine upon behavioral activation in the C57BL6J mouse and a coisogenic (pallid) line. All data as means ± SE.

a series of convulsions are behaviorally supersensitive to morphine. This may point to a kindling-like process, since we have seen a similar effect when C57BL mice were repeatedly kindled.[36]

We feel the results with epileptic mice point to the existence of two factors in seizure-behavioral interactions. One immediate result of seizures is behavioral inhibition; a second, opioid-related process may increase long-term behavioral responsiveness. This model is consistent with a recent hypothesis of Engel,[31] attributing behaviorally facilitatory properties to interictal spikes, possibly through the mediation of endogenous opiates.

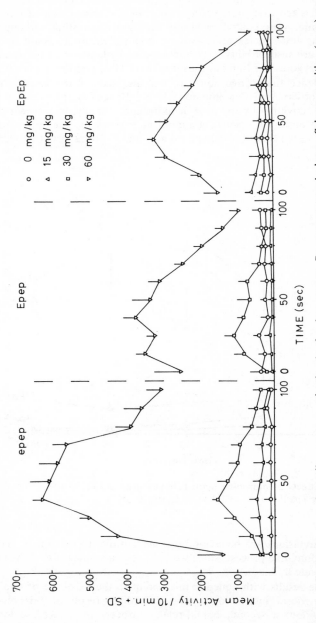

FIGURE 5. Effects of a gene for epilepsy upon activation in the deer mouse, *Peromyscus maniculatus*. Seizure sensitive (*epep*) and seizure resistant (*EpEp*) homozygotes are shown, as well as the heterozygous resistant line (*Epep*). All data as means ± SE.

CONCLUSION

We have attempted to describe three interrelated aspects of behavioral and other responses of mice to opiates. First, the response has clinical relevance since it may speak to certain behavioral and motivational abnormalities also found in mania. At the preclinical level it represents one of the few acceptable models of manic disorders. Additionally, the response appears to be mediated by enkephalins or enkephalin-like neuropeptides. Thus, the response also is psychobiologically relevant as a model of peptide-induced activation. Finally, because of the particular choice of subjects, the model has a further advantage of allowing extensive genetic studies of a pharmacological syndrome. It is neither apparent nor necessary that all the above three aspects reflect the same common neurobiological substrate. It is not clear, for example, that genetic manipulations of the running response reflect identical genetic patterns in human manics. They may speak to homologous processes, however.

Given the above studies and their implications, it is possible to frame novel hypotheses upon mania and the action of neuropeptides. We close by re-emphasizing the clinical complexity of mania and the psychobiological complexity of opiate-induced activation. It is our hope that with continued investigation perhaps in the future the twain will meet.

ACKNOWLEDGMENTS

The technical assistance of Giulio Baldrighi and the statistical assistance of W. Robert Shea are gratefully acknowledged.

REFERENCES

1. HARLEY, J. 1868. The old vegetable neurotics, hemlock, opium, belladonna, and henbane; their physiological action and therapeutical use alone and in combination; being the Gulstonian Lectures of 1868, extended and including a complete examination of the active constituents of opium. Brit. Med. J. **1:** 293–295, 319–321, 343–345.
2. GUINARD, L. 1898. La Morphine et L'apomorphine Etude Experimentale de Pharmacodynamie Compare. Paris.
3. MILNE-EDWARDS. 1890. Note in discussion of paper by Guinard. Compt. Rend. Acad. Sci. **111:** 983.
4. MACHT, D. I. & M. E. DAVIS. 1936. Responses to drugs of *Ursus americanus*. Am. J. Physiol. **116:** 105.
5. NOE, J. 1903. Variabilite et specificite de effets des substances toxiques. Arch. Int. Pharmacodyn. Therap. **12:** 153.
6. STRAUB, H. 1911. Eine empfindliche biologische reaktion auf morphin. Deuts. Med. Bedschr. **37:** 1462.
7. HERRMANN, O. 1912. Eine biologische nachweismethode des morphins. Biochem. Z. **39:** 216–231.
8. CARROLL, B. J. & P. T. SHARP. 1972. An animal model of mania. Psychopharmacologia **26** (suppl.): 10.
9. KATZ, R. J. 1981. Animal models and human depressive disorders. Neurosci. Biobehav. Res. (In press.)
10. CARLSON, G. A. & I. GOODWIN. 1973. The stages of mania. Arch. Gen. Psychol. **18:** 221–228.

11. TAYLOR, M. A. & R. ABRAMS. 1973. The phenomenology of mania. Arch. Gen. Psychol. **29:** 520–522.
12. CARROLL, B. J. & P. T. SHARP. 1971. Rubidium and lithium: Opposite effects on amine-mediated excitement. Science **172:** 1355–1357.
13. CARROLL, B. J. & P. T. SHARP. 1972. Monoamine mediation of the morphine induced activation of mice. Brit. J. Pharmacol. **46:** 124–139.
14. KATZ, R. J. & K. SCHMALTZ. 1981. Behavioral interactions between opiate and antiepileptic drugs. Neuropharmacology **20:** 375–379.
15. KATZ, R. J. & K. SCHMALTZ. 1979. Facilitation of opiate and enkephalin induced motor activity in the mouse by phenytoin sodium and carbamazepine. Psychopharmacology **65:** 65–69.
16. JUDD, L. L., D. S. JANOWSKY, D. S. SEGAL & L. Y. HUEY. 1980. Naloxone induced behavioral and physiological effects in normal and manic subjects. Arch. Gen. Psychol. **37:** 583–586.
17. HUGHES, J. 1975. Isolation of an endogenous compound with pharmacological properties similar to morphine. Brain Res. **88:** 295–308.
18. KATZ, R. J., B. J. CARROLL & G. BALDRIGHI. 1978. Behavioral activation by enkephalins in mice. Pharmacol. Biochem. Behav. **8:** 493–496.
19. WEI, E. T., L. F. TSENG, H. H. LOH & C. H. LI. 1977. Comparisons of the behavioral effects of β-endorphin and enkephalin analogs. Life Sci. **21:** 321–328.
20. TAKAGI, H., H. SHIOMI, H. SHIOMI, H. UEDA & H. AMANO. 1979. Morphine-like analgesic by a new dipeptide l-tyrosyl-l-arginine (kyotophin) and its analogue. Eur. J. Pharmacol. **55:** 109–111.
21. JUDSON, B. A. & A. GOLDSTEIN. 1978. Genetic control of opiate induced locomotor activity in mice. J. Pharmacol. Exp. Ther. **206:** 56–60.
22. CASTELLANO, C. & A. OLIVERIO. 1975. A genetic analysis of morphine induced running and analgesia in the mouse. Psychopharmacologia **41:** 197–200.
23. KATZ, R. J. 1980. The albino locus produces abnormal responses to opiates in the mouse. Eur. J. Pharmacol. **68:** 229–232.
24. COTZIAS, G. C., L. C. TANG, S. T. MILLER, D. SLADIC-SIMIC & L. S. HURLEY. 1972. A mutation influencing the transportation of manganese, l-dopa, and l-tryptophan. Science **176:** 410–412.
25. KATZ, R. J. & R. DOYLE. 1980. Enhanced responses to opiate produced by a single gene substitution in the mouse. Eur. J. Pharmacol. **67:** 301–303.
26. BLOOM, F., D. SEGAL, N. LING & R. GUILLEMIN. 1976. Endorphins: Profound behavioral effects in rats suggest new etiological factors in mental illness. Science **194:** 630.
27. URCA, G., H. FRENK, J. C. LIEBESKIND & A. N. TAYLOR. 1977. Morphine and enkephalin: Analgesic and epileptic properties. Science **197:** 83–86.
28. TORTELLA, F. C., J. E. MORETON & N. KHAZAN. 1978. Electroencephalographic and behavioral effects of d-Ala^2-methionine-enkephalinamide and morphine in the rat. J. Pharmacol. Exp. Ther. **206:** 636–642.
29. BELENKY, G. L. & J. W. HOLADAY. 1980. Electroconvulsive shock (ECS) in rats: Naloxone modification of post ECS behaviors provides evidence for functional endorphin release. In Endogenous and Exogenous Opiate Agonists and Antagonists. E. L. Way, Ed. pp. 487–490. Pergamon. New York.
30. MANSOUR, A., R. DOYLE, R. KATZ & E. S. VALENSTEIN. 1980. Altered morphine sensitivity following amygdaloid kindling in C57B1/6J mice. Soc. Neurosci. Abstr.
31. ENGEL, J. R., J. ACKERMAN, R. F. CALDECOTT, S. HAZARD & D. E. KUHL. 1981. Epileptic activation of antagonistic systems may explain paradoxical features of experimental and human epilepsy: A review and hypothesis. In Kindling. J. A. Wada, Ed. Academic Press. New York. In press.

DISCUSSION OF THE PAPER

G. KING (*Pointe Claire, Quebec*): What is the possibility in your genetically different mice that the uptake of morphine into the central nervous system is less than it is in the C57 black mice?

R. J. KATZ (*Johns Hopkins University, Baltimore, MD*): I cannot exclude that possibility. I do not have direct measurements of morphine in the brain.

KING: Have you injected morphine directly into the CNS?

KATZ: We have done that in other cases and can exclude disposition as a factor in those, but not in the present case. I doubt that it is true, but I cannot give you hard evidence for that.

M. ADLER (*Temple University School of Medicine, Phildelphia, PA*): I am concerned about the conclusions that you are drawing in your paper. We do not know what happens to these compounds once they are injected. The differences you find may be pharmacokinetic ones between various strains.

The problem is that we do not know what happens to these compounds once they are given intracerebroventricularly. They may not be getting to the same sites at the same time or they may not be handled in the same way. Unless one determines by measurement where a compound goes after intracerebroventricular administration, conclusions as to receptors or mechanisms can be very prone to error.

KATZ: You are right, in essence. On the other hand, there is no general problem of drug disposition with other drugs. In the pallid animals, particularly, drugs evoke a greater response. Amphetamines do, for example, as do dopamine and 5-HT agonists. Thus, pharmacokinetic differences may be restricted to opiates or some small class of drugs.

Regarding the point about the receptors, there are at least four different receptor classifications, and I am not sure where all the ligands fit at this point.

Taking a conservative point of view, we have shown, as our title suggests, strain-selective effects of opioids. I would be willing to leave it at that, rather than to try to defend a weak case, especially given the confusion about receptors at this point.

C. O'BRIEN (*University of Pennsylvania, Philadelphia*): I was fascinated by this genetic *tour de force*. It reminds me of a comment that Dr. Costa made off the cuff at a recent Gordon conference about how the tremendous differences found in opiate receptors in the guinea pig ileum depended upon which strain was used. He felt that the tremendous genetic heterogeneity made clinical research more difficult.

I have just one question. What is the duration of the post-ictal depressant effect that you showed? [refers to inhibition after audiogenic seizures]

KATZ: We can test up to 15 minutes but have not tested past that. The effect may be longer; however, at least it is intact for that first quarter of an hour.

L. STEIN (*University of California, Irvine*): [Suggests the flatness of dose response curves as an argument against dispositional effects.]

KATZ: Possibly that is one piece of evidence. I might add, we drew our lines to zero.

ACTIVATION OF OPIOID-CONTAINING SYSTEMS DURING GESTATION

Alan R. Gintzler

Departments of Biochemistry and Psychiatry
State University of New York
Downstate Medical Center
Brooklyn, New York 11203

The biochemical demonstration of specific opiate [1-3] receptors and the discovery of endogenous ligands (endorphins) for these receptors [4-7] suggest that in addition to mediating the pharmacologic effects of alkaloids these receptors are also involved in mediating certain physiological processes. Consequently, considerable attention has been focused on trying to determine the various physiological states in which there is an activation of endogenous opioid systems.

Considerable evidence indicates that endorphins may play an important role in modulating responsiveness to aversive stimuli. For example, pain thresholds were found to be considerably higher in patients with elevated endorphin levels in the cerebrospinal fluid (CSF) than in patients with low endorphin levels.[8] In addition, it has been demonstrated that electrical stimulation of the medial thalamus results in the release of β-endorphin into the ventricular system.[9] Since periventricular stimulation often causes pain blockade,[10, 11] it could be inferred that the release of β-endorphin may participate in such relief. In this regard, it is interesting to note that naloxone, a pure opiate antagonist, has been reported to alter pain perception as well as somatosensory evoked potentials in normal subjects.[12] On the other hand, it should be realized that it has also been reported that rats treated with doses of naloxone sufficient to block morphine analgesia showed no change in the threshold for escape from shock.[13] Thus, the role of endorphins in modulating the perception of pain is by no means clear.

Evidence is accumulating that indicates that opioid-containing systems may be quiescent under normal basal conditions, that is, they do not appear to be tonically active.[13, 14] There are, however, a variety of external and internal stimuli, known collectively as stressors, that cause significant activation of endorphin systems; examples of such stimuli would be chronic, inescapable foot shock and insulin-induced hypoglycemia.[15, 16] Thus, it appears that there must be a perturbation of an animal's system in order for opioid pathways to be activated. The responsiveness of the endorphin system(s) to stressful events coupled with their potent analgesic activity [17-19] suggests that the endorphins may play a role in the adaptation of the organism to such stresses.

Since pregnancy, labor, and parturition are states that require adaptation to stress, considerable attention has been focused on the possible involvement of endorphins in the physiological sequelae of pregnancy. Data obtained from several laboratories independently have shown that during the latter stages of pregnancy and, in particular, during labor, there are substantial increases in the plasma concentration of opioids.[20, 21] However, despite these biochemical data

302

0077–8923/82/0398–0302 $01.75/0 © 1982, NYAS

indicating the activation of opioid systems during pregnancy and labor, the specific behavioral and physiological consequences of this activation have not yet been elucidated. In addition, it should be realized that despite the substantial magnitude of the increase in plasma β-endorphin during labor and delivery, the levels that are achieved are still well below the analgesic effective concentration of the peptide that is indicated by the potency of intravenously administered β-endorphin.[22] Accordingly, this report describes experiments that were designed to obtain physiological evidence indicating a natural role for endorphins in the processes underlying gestation and labor.

Jump (pain) thresholds were determined by subjecting the animals to successively more intense shocks. The jump threshold was defined as the lower of two consecutive intensities that elicited simultaneous withdrawal of both front paws from the grids.[23] Tests were conducted in a standard chamber with a 30- by 24-cm floor grid composed of 14 bars spaced 1.8 cm apart. Scrambled electric shock was delivered to the grids by a constant-current shock generator. Each trial was begun by giving the animal a 300-msec foot shock at a current intensity of 0.1 mA. Subsequent shocks were increased in 0.05-mA steps at 20-sec intervals. After each trial, the current intensity was reset to 0.1 mA for the next trial until eight determinations of jump threshold were completed for each animal (intertrial intervals, 30 seconds). The mean jump threshold for each animal was then calculated.

Two groups of eight pregnant rats and two groups of eight nonpregnant rats were housed individually and given free access to food and water. Pain thresholds were determined for one group of pregnant animals beginning 16 days before parturition and continuing until 41 days afterward. One group of nonpregnant rats was tested in parallel with the pregnant group an equal number of times with the same interval between tests. To determine whether endorphins are involved in modulating responsiveness to aversive stimuli during pregnancy, the remaining pregnant and nonpregnant groups were implanted with long-acting naltrexone pellets [24] and tested in the same way, except that testing was discontinued after parturition. Also, before pellet implantation and testing, five baseline pain thresholds were determined for the nonpregnant group.

FIGURE 1 shows the alterations in pain threshold during pregnancy and parturition for the unimplanted pregnant group and thresholds for the unimplanted nonpregnant group during repeated testing over the same time span. Two-way analysis of variance indicates that before parturition the jump thresholds were significantly different between groups [$F(1, 13) = 29.36$, $p < 0.001$] and over days [$F(6, 78) = 5.65$, $p < 0.001$]. There was also a significant interaction between treatment and days [$F(6, 78) = 4.13$, $p < 0.001$]. Scheffe post hoc comparisons showed that while none of the thresholds for the nonpregnant animals differed significantly from those of the first test day ($p > 0.01$), all of the thresholds for the pregnant animals prior to parturition were significantly different ($p < 0.01$) from those of the first test day. The thresholds for the pregnant and nonpregnant animals on the first day of testing were not significantly different [$t(13) = 1.35$, $p > 0.05$]. However, there was a gradual increase in jump threshold between 16 and 4 days before parturition and a more abrupt increase 1 to 2 days before that event. The mean threshold increased to 0.51 mA 2 days and 0.59 mA 1 day before birth, compared with 0.35 mA on the first day of testing.

Analysis of variance of jump thresholds after parturition indicates that there was no significant difference in threshold between the pregnant and nonpregnant

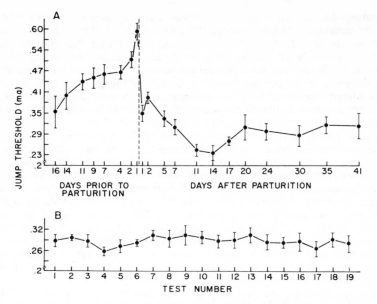

FIGURE 1. (A) Mean jump threshold in pregnant rats as a function of days before and after parturition (*dashed line*). Each point represents the mean threshold of eight rats ± standard error (SE). (B) Mean jump threshold in nonpregnant females as a function of repeated test. These determinations were made in parallel with the schedule shown in (A). Each point represents the mean threshold of seven rats ± SE.

groups [$F(1, 13) = 1.06$, $p < 0.05$], while there was a significant change in threshold over days [$F(11, 143) = 36.32$, $p < 0.001$] and a significant interaction between days and groups [$F(11, 143) = 13.09$, $p < .001$]. One day after parturition there was an abrupt decrease in jump threshold followed by a more gradual decline over the next 13 days (the mean jump threshold 14 days postpartum was 0.24 mA, compared to 0.59 mA 1 day before parturition).

In seven of eight animals, the jump thresholds 11 days postpartum were actually less than the thresholds measured on day 7; this was also observed on day 14 for all but two of the eight animals. Moreover, on days 11 and 14, six of the eight animals had lower thresholds than on day 17. After day 17 there did not appear to be any systematic changes in jump threshold. Essentially the same pattern of change was demonstrated when five additional pregnant rats were tested 15, 13, 11, 8, 6, and 2 days before parturition and 2, 6, 8, 10, 13, 15, 17, and 21 days afterward. In all, jump thresholds for 13 of 13 pregnant rats were higher during pregnancy than in the period after they gave birth.

Subcutaneously implanted naltrexone pellets markedly reduced the increase in jump threshold observed during pregnancy (FIG. 2A) without altering either the length of gestation or the average litter size (10.3 pups for naltrexone-implanted mothers, 9.8 pups for unimplanted mothers). Naltrexone pellets did not induce significant alteration in the jump threshold of any of the seven nonpregnant females (FIG. 2B). The mean jump threshold, determined over five baseline trials (35 determinations), was 0.29 ± 0.009 mA, and was unchanged over a 15-day period after pellet implantation (0.29 ± 0.007 mA; 56 determinations).

The results presented in this study indicate that intrinsic mechanisms that modulate responsiveness to aversive stimuli are activated concomitantly with pregnancy and parturition. Different stages of pregnancy are associated with different degrees of attenuation of pain responsiveness; the highest threshold was observed 1 to 2 days before parturition. Moreover, during the postpartum period maternal rats apparently go through transient hyperalgesia before the pain threshold returns to baseline levels. This transient hyperalgesia observed in postpartum rats might have some relationship to postpartum depression observed in humans. Additional studies are obviously necessary to confirm or disprove this speculation.

The failure of naltrexone to alter jump threshold in nonpregnant female rats indicates that the opioid system(s) that modulates responsiveness to aversive stimuli in this animal is not tonically active. Furthermore, it illustrates that the ability of naltrexone to markedly reduce the increase in pain threshold observed during pregnancy is due to a pharmacologic and not physiological antagonism of endogenous pain-attenuating processes.

Thus, during pregnancy there is an activation of an opioid system(s) that is apparently quiescent in nonpregnant female rats treated in identical fashion. Opioids therefore appear to be an important component of intrinsic mechanisms that modulate responsiveness to aversive stimuli during pregnancy. Various deficiencies or abnormalities in the controlled activation of this system(s) could conceivably result in a myriad of maternal as well as fetal complications during the gestational and postpartum periods.

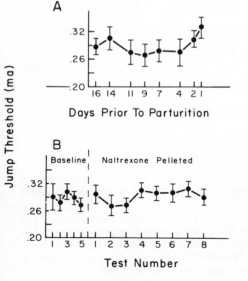

FIGURE 2. (**A**) Mean jump thresholds of pregnant rats implanted with two naltrexone pellets, presented as a function of days before parturition. Testing was begun 1 day after implantation. Each point represents the mean threshold of seven rats $\pm$ SE. (**B**) Jump thresholds in nonpregnant females before and after implantation. Thereafter, determinations were made in parallel with the schedule shown in (**A**). Each point is the mean threshold of seven rats $\pm$ SE.

REFERENCES

1. SIMON, E. J., J. M. HILLER & I. EDELMAN. 1973. Proc. Natl. Acad. Sci. USA 70: 1947–1949.
2. PERT, C. & S. SNYDER. 1973. Science 179: 1011–1014.
3. TERENIUS, L. 1973. Acta Pharmacol. Toxicol. 33: 377–384.
4. HUGES, J. 1975. Brain Res. 88: 295–308.
5. PASTERNAK, G. W., R. GOODMAN & S. SNYDER. 1975. Life Sci. 16: 1765–1769.
6. TERENIUS, L. & A. WAHLSTRÖM. 1975. Life Sci. 16: 1759–1764.
7. GOLDSTEIN, A., S. TACHIBANA, L. I. LOWNEY, M. HUNKAPILLER & L. HOOD. 1979. Proc. Natl. Acad. Sci. USA 76(N012): 6666–6670.
8. VONKNORRING, L., B. G. L. ALMAY, F. JOHANSSON & L. TERENIUS. 1978. Pain 5: 359–365.
9. AKIL, H., D. E. RICHARDSON, J. D. BARCHAS & C. H. LI. 1978. Proc. Natl. Acad. Sci. USA 75: 5170–5172.
10. D. G. MAYER, T. L. WOLFLE, B. CARDER, H. AKIL & J. C. LIEBESKIND. 1971. Science 174: 1351–1354.
11. MAYER, D. J. & R. L. HAYNES. 1975. Science 188: 941–943.
12. BUCHSBAUM, M. S., G. C. DAVIS & W. E. BUNNEY. 1977. Nature 270: 620–622.
13. GOLDSTEIN, A., G. T. PRYOR, L. S. OTIS & F. LARSEN. 1976. Life Sci. 18: 599–604.
14. EL-SOBKY, A., J. O. DOSTROVSKY & P. D. WALL. 1976. Nature 263: 783–784.
15. ROSSIER, J., E. D. FRENCH, C. RIVIER, N. LING, R. GUILLEMIN & F. BLOOM. 1977. Nature 720: 618–620.
16. KRIEGER, D. T., A. LIOTTA & C. H. LI. 1977. Life Sci. 21: 1771–1777.
17. TSENG, L. F., H. H. LOH & C. H. LI. 1976. Nature 263: 239–240.
18. BELLUZZI, J. D., N. GRANT, V. GARSKY, V. D. SARANTAKIS, C. D. WISE & L. STEIN. 1976. Nature 260: 625–626.
19. GROF, L., J. I. SZEKELY, A. Z. RONAI, Z. DUNAI-KORRACS & S. BAJUSZ. 1976. Nature 263: 240–241.
20. AKIL, H., S. J. WATSON, J. D. BARCHAS & C. H. LI. 1979. Life Sci. 24: 1659–1665.
21. CSONTOS, K., M. RUST, V. HOLT, W. MAHR, U. KROMER & H. J. TESCHEMACHER. 1979. Life Sci. 25: 835–844.
22. LOH, H. H., L. F. TSENG, E. NEI & C. H. LI. 1976. Proc. Natl. Acad. Sci. USA 73: 2895–2898.
23. EVANS, W. O. P. 1961. Psychopharmacologia 2: 318–325.
24. MISRA, A. L., R. B. PONTANAI & N. L. VADLAMANI. 1973. Res. Commun. Chem. Pathol. Pharmacol 20: 43–50.

DISCUSSION OF THE PAPER

UNIDENTIFIED SPEAKER: In view of the very low levels of β-endorphin in plasma, have you considered the possibility that the levels in the cerebrospinal fluid may be more relevant?

A. R. GINTZLER: Yes, absolutely. I referred to the plasma level because it is one variable of endorphin function that has been measured and seems to change with pregnancy. However, opioid levels in the CNS could certainly be more relevant to changes in maternal pain threshold. Alternatively, there might be enhanced activity of endorphinergic neuronal activity in the CNS.

R. CHIPKIN (*Schering Corporation, Bloomfield, NJ*): Did the naltrexone experiments last for a couple of weeks?

GINTZLER: Yes.

CHIPKIN: Did you challenge any of the animals with morphine to make sure that the naltrexone was exerting a pharmacologic blockade?

GINTZLER: No, I did not, but similar studies were performed by Dr. Misra. In his studies similar pellets continued to release naltrexone in excess of the time period that was used in the present study. The duration of action of the naltrexone pellets was determined in both rats and cats.

R. S. ZUKIN (*Albert Einstein College of Medicine, Bronx, NY*): In the case of the animals with long-term treatment with naltrexone pellets, did you also test nonpregnant female rats to see whether they exhibit any changes in pain threshold?

GINTZLER: Yes; we obtained five pain thresholds in nonpregnant female rats prior to pellet implantation. When we obtained what looked like stable baseline values, we placed pellets in those same animals and continued to determine flinch–jump threshold. Flinch–jump thresholds obtained subsequent to pellet implantation were not significantly different from those obtained prior to naltrexone administration. Thus, naltrexone only affected pain threshold in rats that were pregnant. This was shown in FIGURE 2.

P. C. GOLDSMITH (*University of California School of Medicine, San Francisco*): Have you considered the endorphin contribution from the fetuses present in the mother? Or do you consider that this is all a maternal system?

GINTZLER: It certainly does not have to be an all-maternal system. At this point, I do not mean to make any inference about the relative contribution of maternal versus fetal systems. Right now the question is still open.

METABOLISM OF ENKEPHALIN ANALOGUES AND SURROGATES HAVING ENHANCED PHARMACOLOGIC ACTIVITIES *

Neville Marks, Myron Benuck,
Martin J. Berg, and Len Sachs

*Center for Neurochemistry
Rockland Research Institute
Ward's Island, New York 10035*

INTRODUCTION

The promise of opiate peptides as psychoactive agents arose in part from observations made in this Institute by Jacquet and Marks [1] and at the Salk Institute by Bloom *et al.*[2] in 1976 on the central effects of endorphin $_{1-31}$ when microinjected into rat brain. These observations led to clinical trials in man, but such studies were limited by the scarcity and cost of endorphins or their analogues. Although pentapeptidyl enkephalins (E_5) gave poor response relative to endorphins or morphine,[1,2] the enhanced effects of enkephalin surrogates having C-terminal extensions,[3-6] or of biostable E_5 analogues,[7-9] have revived interest in the use of the simpler enkephalin forms. From a clinical point of view two strategies appear to be of promise for the enhancement of E_5 *in vivo*: (1) synthesis of analogues resistant to digestion by tissue enzymes when administered orally or systemically or (2) interference with E_5 degradation by the use of specific enzyme inhibitors. As will be seen, progress in these two areas has been predicated upon knowledge of enkephalin metabolism reviewed briefly below.

That tissues contain a variety of peptidases degrading E_5 is now well established, but the relevance of each is still a matter of debate. Candidate enzymes acting as enkephalinases include soluble and particulate bound aminopeptidases [1,10-14] and others acting at the Gly^3-Phe^4 site such as peptidyl dipeptidases or metalloendopeptidases [15-20] (FIG. 1). Pentapeptide enkephalins, by virtue of their structure, are substrates for monocarboxypeptidases, but, surprisingly, those present in brain do not appear to be of significance for inactivation, although they may play a role in the conversion of putative precursors [21] (FIG. 1).

The existence of multiple pathways poses problems in assigning importance to any one hydrolase. Despite observations that homogenates or their fractions contain aminopeptidases rapidly acting on the Tyr-Gly bond, there is a body of opinion that favors the action of a metalloendopeptidase as the key enkephalinase, as recounted later. This situation contrasts with that of the biogenic amines, where a single enzyme is largely responsible for inactivation at the target site, making the task for the synthesis of stable analogues, or enzyme inhibitors, far simpler. For E_5, a neurotransmitter candidate, several chemical

* This work was supported by Grant NS–12578 from the National Institute of Neurological and Communicative Disorders and Stroke (NM) and by Grant HRC–II–029 from the Health Research Council of New York State (MB).

0077–8923/82/0398–0308 $01.75/0 © 1982 NYAS

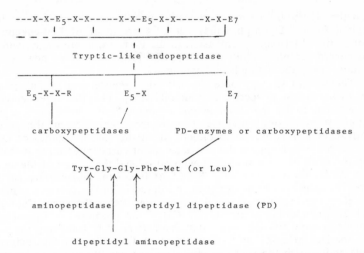

FIGURE 1. Scheme for the production of enkephalin surrogates and of E_5 enkephalins from an original gene product. The one indicated is based on the 27,000-dalton unit isolated from adrenal medullary (chromaffin) cells.[41] Note that PD enzymes can play dual roles in the conversion of E_7 (Met-enkephalin-Arg-Phe). Inactivation of the Gly-Phe site is mediated by a metalloendopeptidase.

modifications are required to block degradation by tissue enzymes. These include either modification of N-terminal Tyr (F-Tyr; *N*-methyl; *N',N*-dimethyl) [25] or presence of a D-amino acid in position 2 to block action of aminopeptidases, along with the modification or presence of a D-amino acid in positions 3–5 to block action of peptidyl dipeptidases or other enzymes acting at the Gly-Phe bond. Scores of such analogues have been synthesized, far too many to review in this article, but those that are active *in vivo* demonstrate the need for a minimum of two substitutions, as illustrated later in this study. Enhanced potencies arise not only from reduced rates of degradation, but also from alteration of biological properties (receptor affinities, stability in serum or tissue en route to the target sites, altered transport across the blood-brain barrier system). Many of the stable analogs, for example, interact with μ receptors as compared to δ ones of E_5, and their actions may be mediated by an independent pathway. Examples include D-Ala-enkephalinamide and FK 33–824 as μ agonists; enkephalin surrogates such as enkephalin-Arg-Phe (E_7), which is a δ agonist, and dynorphins 1–13 or 1–17, which are κ-agonists.[22-24] Indeed, synthesis of E_5 analogs or its surrogates may provide new avenues for the rational design of stable peptides targeted for a specific receptor subpopulation, as illustrated by recent studies of Gacel *et al.*[26] This is likely to have an impact on clinical use since some agonists, κ ones for example, have fewer side effects compared with those of morphine and are more suited for use as drugs. Dynorphin, a CNS component, although without marked activity *in vivo,* is reported to antagonize morphine actions [24]; E_7, another surrogate, is active *in vivo* as an analgesic agent and is sevenfold more potent than E_5.[3] Since metabolism of these forms may be of equal interest to that of pentapeptides, the metabolism of E_7 used as a model is covered in this report. A question of importance is whether E_5 itself in some instances is merely an end-product of more active opioid forms. Dynorphin may act as a precursor of Leu-enkephalin, which forms the N-terminus; conversion to the E_5 form, interestingly, will then result in altered receptor affinity (κ to δ), illustrating a possible new regulatory role for enzymes modulating ligand expression.

The second strategy noted earlier for enhancement of enkephalin actions *in vivo* is the use of specific enzyme inhibitors. That this approach is of promise is attested to by the development of angiotensin-converting enzyme (ACE) inhibitors active orally and useful for the treatment of essential hypertension.[27-29] Advances in this area stem directly from the elegant studies of Quiocho and Lipscomb [30] in mapping the active center of carboxypeptidase A, followed later by the work of Ondetti *et al.*,[28] who postulated the nature of the active subsites for ACE. Carboxypeptidase A and ACE are metalloenzymes for which site-specific reagents can be designed to interact with the catalytic centers: Ondetti *et al.*,[28] starting from succinyl proline, developed the agent Captopril (or SQ 14225), containing groups (-SH, -CH$_3$) that promoted its interaction with the major enzyme subsites; and later Patchett *et al.*,[29] following the same theme, synthesized MK-421, an *N*-carboxymethyl dipeptide. These structures and their interaction with the subsites of the enzyme are illustrated in FIGURE 2. Such inhibitors are of interest to E_5 metabolism since purified brain ACE acts also on the Gly^3-Phe^4 bond with the release of the C-terminal dipeptide.[19] Since there is some evidence that enkephalins play a role in mediating homeostatic mechanisms related to blood pressure regulation, it is possible that some of the *in vivo* effects of ACE inhibitors are mediated via an opioid–peptidergic system. Another possible role for brain ACE is for conversion of enkephalin precursors to form E_5. This will be illustrated later by actions of purified brain ACE and enzyme(s) present in synaptosomal plasma membranes (SPM) acting on E_7 (see also FIG. 1). In the presence of an aminopeptidase inhibitor, SPM can be shown to contain a second enkephalinase, unaffected by ACE inhibitors, cleaving E_5 at the Gly^3-Phe^4 bond, but not acting on typical angiotensin substrates.[17] Roques *et al.*,[31] using SPM as a model, have synthesized an inhibitor for this enkephalinase on the basis of differences between its active center and that of ACE. The inhibitor, Thiorphan, closely resembles the C-terminal of E_5 (Phe-Met or Phe-Leu) with an aromatic residue in the penultimate position (FIG. 2); like Captopril, it contains a -SH group on the N-terminus for promoting interaction with the metallo subsite. Aside from the fact that this SPM enzyme is masked by aminopeptidases *in vitro* (it requires addition of puromycin or bestatin), there is evidence supporting the notion that this is a relevant enkephalinase. Recent data show that one of the SPM enzymes acting at the Gly-Phe bond of E_5 is a Thiorphan-sensitive endopeptidase.[16] It is known that membranes cleave E_5 with release of Tyr-Gly-Gly and C-terminal dipeptide by a mechanism that is insensitive to ACE inhibitors. Other evidence suggesting a relevant role for such an enzyme is based on kinetic data (higher substrate affinity for E_5 than aminopeptidases), a correlation between enzyme distribution in brain and that of opiate receptors, or changes that result during development, effects of chronic morphine treatment or other pharmacologic treatments on enzyme levels in brain striatum, and on the recovery of enkephalin from K$^+$-stimulated slices *in vitro* bathed in media containing Thiorphan, but not other peptidase inhibitors.[17, 18, 31-33] Impressive as this evidence appears, it must be stressed that studies *in vitro* generally require manipulation (presence of aminopeptidase inhibitor) and they take little account of possible aminopeptidase heterogeneity. One of the aminopeptidases may be highly specific and present at or near the receptor. It can be noted that the striatum used in studies by Schwartz *et al.*[17] and rich in opiate receptors is also ranked among the highest containing ACE together with appreciable levels of aminopeptidase.[19] The existence of these multiple pathways for E_5 inactivation *in vitro* indicates that new strategies are required in order to pinpoint the key enzyme(s) associated with inactivation *in situ*. The SPM used under the conditions stated enabled

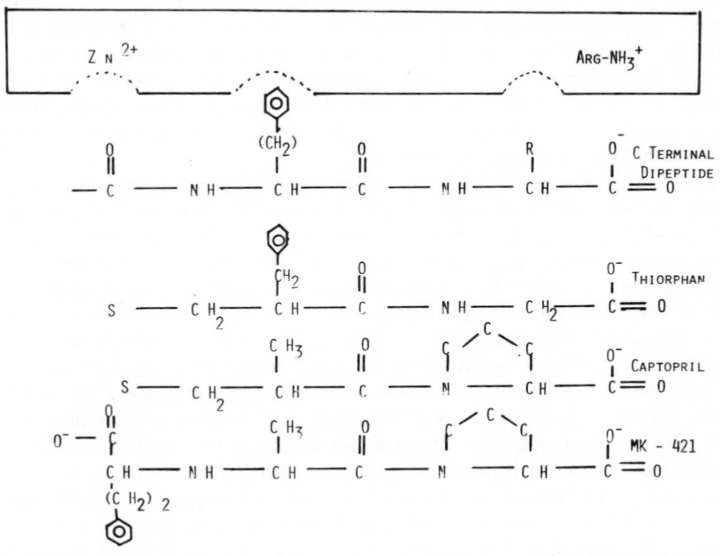

FIGURE 2. Schematic (single dimension) diagram illustrating interaction between inhibitors and the postulated active center of a peptidyl dipeptidase. The first structure represents the C-terminal of a pentapeptide enkephalin interacting at its C-terminus, with a hydrophobic (aromatic) and a metallo subsite of the enzyme. The second compound listed is Thiorphan, or 3-mercapto-2-benzylpropanoyl-glycine; the third compound is Captopril, or D-3-thio-2-methylpropanyl proline; and the fourth is MK–421 or *N*-[(S)-1-carboxy-3-phenyl propyl]-L-Ala-L-Pro. The latter two are specific inhibitors of angiotensin-converting enzyme of peripheral tissues, and inhibit PD-A of brain. Note absence of an aromatic group in the C-terminus. The -SH and -CH$_3$ groups of Captopril promote interaction with their respective subsites. For the nature of the amino acid groups associated with the C-terminal subsite and interacting with the -COO$^-$ group see Quiocho and Lipscomb.[30] For other details, see text or Ondetti *et al.*[28] and Patchett *et al.*[29]

Roques *et al.*[31] and Llorens *et al.*[33] to synthesize a new enzyme inhibitor without the need to characterize the enzyme. That purified systems are required also will become evident on the basis of our experience with Thiorphan, since this was shown to affect ACE as well as the non-ACE enzyme. To simplify this description we propose the nomenclature peptidyl dipeptidase A (PD-A) for ACE (rather than dipeptidyl carboxypeptidase or kininase-II) and the term peptidase B (P-B) for the particulate enzyme that is unaffected by ACE inhibitors and which does not recognize angiotensin substrates (recently P-B was purified from rat brain and kidney and shown to be a Thiorphan-sensitive metalloendopeptidase cleaving enkephalins or its surrogates [16, 19]). Evidence for the existence of these separate PD-A and P-B enzymes has been obtained on the basis of purification studies undertaken in our laboratory [16, 19] and that of others.[15] In the method described briefly herein, the enzymes were shown to be separable by immunoaffinity procedures. One enzyme recognized antibody to purified rabbit lung ACE and was identical in most of its properties (specificity, effect of inhibitors, molecular weight, pH optimum) to ACE purified from peripheral tissues and serum.[19, 36] The other was distinct since it did not bind to antibody, or cleave typical ACE substrates, and was not inhibited by ACE inhibitors.[19] Since P-B acted on kinin-9 with release of its C-terminal dipeptide Phe-Arg, the term P-B appears more appropriate than "enkephalinase" since the enzyme may have a broad specificity and not be limited to one class of neuropeptides.

In addition to these enzymes, we have described some properties of soluble and membrane-bound aminopeptidases. Tyr, the N-terminus of E_5, is one of the earliest products detected upon incubation with homogenates, supernatant fractions, or synaptosomal plasma fractions, emphasizing the need to study aminopeptidases as potential enkephalinases. Soluble aminopeptidases were purified in this laboratory a decade ago [34, 35] and have been shown to cleave the Tyr-Gly bond of enkephalins [13, 36] (see later). Membrane-bound forms in brain were ignored until recently,[14] although such forms actively participate in some digestive and transport processes of cells lining the gut (brush border).[7, 34] The discovery of receptors makes the study of membrane-bound enzymes a logical choice with respect to metabolism of neurotransmitters at their target sites. The use of SPM, however, may be unduly restrictive since these represent only one of the many membranes present in synaptosomes and ignores the role of others in the processing and transport of neuropeptides. One feature of interest to opiate peptides is the role played by aminopeptidase at the SPM or other cellular locations in either inactivation or conversion of opiate peptides to form either fragments acting in a feedback manner on other enkephalinases (for example, desTyr-enkephalin is an inhibitor of the P-B type of enzyme) or fragments with psychoactive properties (desTyr-γ-endorphin is a neuroleptic-like peptide in man, as discussed in this volume).

The recent discovery of other enkephalin forms with actions more potent than that of E_5 *in vitro,* and in some instances *in vivo,* is an important development. We have chosen to call these materials enkephalin surrogates since they were discovered and assayed using the same experimental paradigms. These include those found in the CNS (dynorphins, Met-enkephalin-Arg-Phe and a variety of enkephalins with C-terminal extensions of Arg or a basic amino acid attached to one or more neutral amino acids) [6, 37–39] and those found in adrenal medullary (chromaffin) cells (peptide E of 3200 daltons, BAM 12-22P).[3–6, 40] In bovine adrenals the larger enkephalin forms are derived from a 27,000-dalton precursor of which the C-terminal is Met-enkephalin-Arg-Phe (E_7).[41] It can be concluded that enkephalins are derived largely from nonendorphin precursors since the latter are absent from chromaffin cells, and are low or absent in brain areas richest in E_5 or its surrogates. Endorphins can be cleaved to release Met-enkephalin *in vitro,* but this is unlikely to represent a major pathway in the CNS, and cannot account for production of Leu-enkephalin or dynorphins.[7]

In this report we summarize recent studies on the conversion of E_7 to form pentapeptide enkephalins by PD-type enzymes, along with other data on the stability of enkephalin analogues or surrogates in the presence of different categories of enkephalinases in order to illustrate the approaches available for the enhancement of their *in vivo* actions. For this purpose, we used procedures described elsewhere [16, 19, 21, 35, 36, 42-47] or included in brief form in the text or in legends to tables or figures.

MULTIPLICITY OF ENKEPHALINASES

Evidence for presence of more than one enzyme degrading E_5 was obtained by studies on soluble supernatant fractions and on extracts of particulates. Those present in the cytosol are chiefly aminopeptidases acting on acylated naphthylamides (termed arylamidases) [13, 35] and that can be separated by ion-exchange from others that hydrolyze substrates, such as Leu-Gly-Gly, but which do not inactivate E_5 and are unaffected by puromycin.[45] Detergent extracts of rat brain particulates, in contrast, contain puromycin-sensitive and -insensitive aminopeptidases acting on E_5 which can be separated by ion-exchange and purified by additional procedures (FIG. 3). That present in peak I and eluted by buffer prior to application of the salt gradient was purified further on CM-

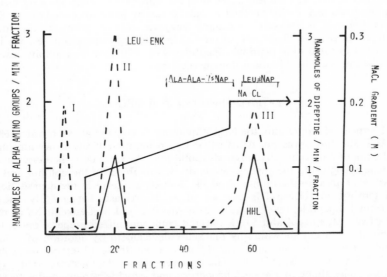

FIGURE 3. Separation of enkephalinases extracted by means of a detergent-containing buffer on a DEAE-cellulose column eluted with a 0–0.2 M NaCl gradient as described elsewhere.[59] The *dashed line* represents enkephalinase action assayed with Leu-enkephalin and a quantitative ninhydrin procedure, and the *solid line* represents hydrolysis of hippuryl-His-Leu (HHL) assayed by a fluorimetric procedure. *Bars* represent areas of activity found with arylamide substrates Ala-Ala or Leu-β-naphthylamide assayed fluorimetrically. Enzyme in peak II was used for further purification, as illustrated in FIGURE 6.

cellulose and shown to cleave Tyr^1-Gly^2 of E_5 by a process unaffected by puromycin but inhibited by bestatin or EDTA. In contrast, that present in peak III (Fig. 3) was purified by immunoaffinity to remove ACE-like enzymes and, when subjected to further DEAE-cellulose chromatography, acted on Leu-β-naphthylamide as well as E_5 and was sensitive to inhibition by bestatin and puromycin and by EDTA. The K_m of aminopeptidase in peaks I and III, however, was 0.7 mM or 10-fold higher than that found for the cytosolic enzyme (0.06 mM). It is of interest that the K_m for membrane-bound aminopeptidases is higher than for peptidyl dipeptidases, supporting the notion that the latter were more relevant.[20] Despite the lower affinities, it is an inescapable fact that the SPM enzyme rapidly cleaves the Tyr-Gly bond so that factors besides affinity apply (see later). The puromycin-insensitive enzyme of peak I has not previously been described, but appeared to be highly specific for E_5 and did not cleave smaller substrates. Previously, Traficante et al.[12] described a highly specific aminopeptidase in human (cytosolic) fractions. The evident heterogeneity of enkephalinases in detergent extracts of brain membranes is demonstrated by the fact that peaks II and III (Fig. 3) contained enzyme active towards the peptidyl dipeptidase substrate hippuryl-His-Leu; also, fractions between peaks II and III hydrolyzed the dipeptidyl aminopeptidase substrate Ala-Ala-β-napththylamide. The latter enzyme may represent one isolated by Gorenstein and Synder[15] cleaving the Gly-Gly bond of E_5. It might be noted that brain and pituitary contain a family of dipeptidyl aminopeptidases which could play a number of roles in neuropeptide turnover.[7] Since Tyr-Gly has not been observed as a major product of catabolism by brain homogenates or SPM preparations, it is unlikely that these enzymes play a primary role in the inactivation process. To study further other relevant enkephalinases, we have succeeded in separating peptidyl dipeptidases of relatively high affinity towards enkephalins as detailed in the following sections.

PEPTIDYL DIPEPTIDASE A (PD-A)

The peak II, containing the largest quantity of enzyme active towards HHL, an ACE substrate, was purified further by an immunoaffinity procedure based on the use of antibody active towards rabbit lung ACE, as described elsewhere.[19] Enzyme recognizing the specific antibody was retained by the column and was active when used in the immobilized (IgG—enzyme) form in the degradation of angiotensin-I to release His-Leu, or of E_5 to release Tyr-Gly-Gly and the C-terminal dipeptide, or of E_7 to release Arg-Phe and Met-enkephalin as products (TABLE 1, FIGS. 4 and 5). It differed from solubilized preparations studied previously[42] in not showing any marked enhancement by addition of chloride anions. The K_m values also are different from those observed for soluble ACE from other tissues.[48, 49] These observations demonstrate that bound enzymes may differ in physical properties and provide a new model to study the properties of membrane-bound forms present in brain, kidney, and lung. Das and Soffer[50] were the first to establish that lung ACE antibody crossreacts with ACE of other tissues: in the case of brain, despite the fact that IgG—enzyme is a noncovalent complex, enzyme could not be eluted from the column in the active form by high salt—urea combinations, indicating high affinity and tight binding. Evidently, the sites involved in linking the enzyme to the antibody do not interfere with catalysis. Inactive protein eluted from the

TABLE 1

SUBSTRATE SPECIFICITIES AND SOME PROPERTIES OF PURIFIED RABBIT BRAIN
PEPTIDYL DIPEPTIDASE A AND PEPTIDASE B

Substrate	Product Detected	K_m (μM)	
		PD-A	P-B
Leu-enkephalin	Tyr-Gly-Gly	100	80
Met-enkephalin-Arg-Phe	Arg-Phe	150	110
Angiotensin-I	His-Leu	180	—
Kinin-9	Phe-Arg	200	130
Hippuryl-His-Leu	His-Leu	2200	—
pH optimum (E_5)		7.9	7.3
Mol. wt. (kilodaltons)		130	n.d.

NOTE: Products were determined by HPLC as described and illustrated in FIGURES
4 and 7, or in the case of HHL by a fluorimetric procedure. The pH optima
shown were for Leu-enkephalin, and the M_r is for protein eluted from Sepharose-IgG
column using 1N NaCl and 1N NH$_4$OH and estimated by electrophoresis on poly-
acrylamide slab gel.[46] n.d. = not determined.

column gave a single band $M_r = 125$ kilodaltons, as compared with that of
standard marker proteins when examined by a slab-gel acrylamide (electrophoretic) procedure. This indicated that brain PD-A is comparable in M_r to

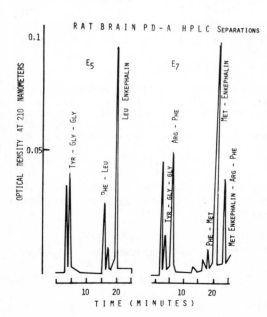

FIGURE 4. High-pressure liquid chromatographic (HPLC)
profile of Leu-enkephalin (E_5)
and of Met-enkephalin-Arg-Phe
breakdown after 60-min incubation at 37° C with purified
rabbit brain PD-A. Separation
was performed on a C_{18}, 10-μ
Bondapak column (Waters Associates, Waltham, MA), eluted
with a gradient formed between
0.1 M KH$_2$PO$_4$ buffer, pH 3.0,
and acetonitrile 0–60% v/v[19],
monitored at 210 nm. The first
peak represents the injection
artifact. Peaks were identified
by their retention times as compared to standards and by subsequent amino acid analysis.
Incubation mixture of 0.1 ml,
40 mM TRIS HCl buffer, pH
7.6, contained 45 nmol E_5 or
14 nmol E_7 and enzyme equivalent to 0.4 nmol HHL hy-
drolyzed/min for E_5 or 0.08
nmol HHL/min for E_7. Profiles
shown represent actual scans of
the low-sensitivity pen of a two-
pen recorder.

that of ACE purified from peripheral tissues or serum.[49] Immobilized preparations were stable for periods of more than 1 year when stored at −20° C and were used to examine kinetics of E_5/E_7 breakdown. Analysis of products by an HPLC procedure for E_5 showed that only Tyr-Gly-Gly and the C-terminal peptide were products indicating absence of other enzyme contaminants (FIGS. 4 and 5). Breakdown of E_7· resulted in its conversion to the E_5 form as an intermediate. In the case of both E_5 and E_7 breakdown, PD-A was inhibited by MK-421 (K_i 0.5 and 1.4 nM, respectively) and also by Thiorphan, but at a 7×10^3 higher concentration (K_i 8.6 µM). In this respect, Thiorphan was more potent than enkephalin fragments desTyr-enkephalin and its C-terminal dipeptide (TABLE 2). In view of the potent effects of MK-421 on enkephalin metabolism *in vitro*, it will be of interest to discover whether this or

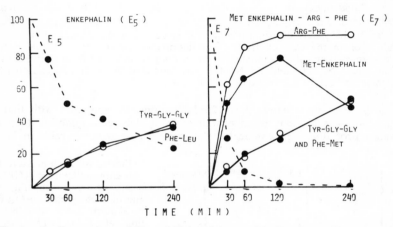

FIGURE 5. Comparison of E_5 and E_7 breakdown with time by purified brain PD-A to illustrate precursor–product relationships. The *dotted lines* represent percent change in substrates, and the *solid lines* the products released as a percent of original substrate. Note that Met-enkephalin is formed as an intermediate of E_7 breakdown. For details of the incubation and HPLC procedures used to measure substrates and products see FIGURE 4.

similar agents act on enkephalinergic systems when used for treatment of essential hypertension [27, 51] since there is evidence linking enkephalins to regulation of blood pressure (see Benuck et al.[16, 43]).

PEPTIDASE B (P-B OR ENDOPEPTIDASE)

Examination of the effluent obtained from peak II (FIG. 3) following the removal of PD-A by immunoaffinity revealed the presence of a second enzyme, which we propose naming P-B (FIG. 6). This enzyme also cleaved the Gly-Phe bond of E_5, but was unaffected by ACE inhibitors and was inactive when incubated with HHL (TABLES 1, 2 and 3). A similar enzyme was present also in rabbit kidney in exceptionally high concentrations relative to PD-A

TABLE 2

COMPARISON OF VARIOUS PEPTIDES OR DERIVATIVES ON THE INHIBITION OF
MET-ENKEPHALIN (E_5) OR MET-ENKEPHALIN-ARG-PHE (E_7) BREAKDOWN BY PURIFIED
PEPTIDYL DIPEPTIDASES

Inhibitor	Substrate	PD-A (μM)		PD-B (μM)	
		I_{50}	K_i	I_{50}	K_i
MK-421	E_5	0.003	0.0005	>1,000	—
MK-421	E_7	0.05	0.0014	>1,000	—
Captopril	E_5	0.27	0.05	>1,000	—
Thiorphan	E_5	20	3.6	0.075	0.03 *
Thiorphan	E_7	25	18	0.2	0.15 *
Gly-Gly-Phe-Met	E_5	>2000	—	50	9
Phe-Met	E_5	1000	180	100	18
Phe-Leu	E_5	100	18	100	18
Phe-Ala	E_5	n.d.	—	50	9
Ala-Phe	E_5	n.d.	—	500	90
Tyr-Ala	E_5	n.d.	—	10	2

NOTE: The K_i values were calculated from the formula $I_{50} = K_i(1 + S/K_m)$ on the assumption of linear kinetics or plotted by the method of Dixon (*). I_{50} is the amount of substance inhibiting release of Tyr-Gly-Gly (E_5) or Arg-Phe (E_7) by 50% as determined by HPLC (see FIGURE 4). n.d. = not determined. For structures of inhibitors see FIGURE 2.

and provided a convenient alternative source.[43] Kidney enzyme incubated with E_5 released Tyr-Gly-Gly and the C-terminal dipeptide by a mechanism insensitive to the action of ACE inhibitors (FIG. 7). In the case of E_7, for both brain and kidney enzyme, the products included Phe-Met-Arg-Phe, indicating cleavage of the Gly[3]-Phe[4] site by an endopeptidase (FIG. 7, TABLE 3). The presence of this membrane-bound endopeptidase raises a number of

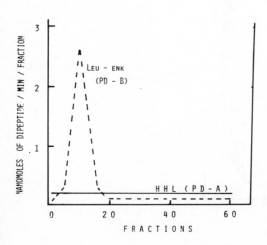

FIGURE 6. Separation of PD-A and P-B enzymes by the use of Sepharose coupled to rabbit lung ACE antibody by the methods described in the text. The *dotted line* represents activity found with Leu-enkephalin as substrate, as analyzed by HPLC, and the *solid line* with HHL as substrate measured fluorimetrically. For other details, see FIGURES 3 and 4.

TABLE 3

BREAKDOWN OF ENKEPHALINS E₅ AND E₇ BY A PURIFIED RABBIT BRAIN PEPTIDASE B

	Products as Percent of Substrate:				
	E₅ (Leu-Enkephalin)		E₇ (Met-Enkephalin-Arg-Phe)		
Products	60 min	120 min	30 min	60 min	120 min
Arg-Phe	—	—	14	24	37
Phe-Leu (Met)	5.3	10	2.8	10	20
Tyr-Gly-Gly	7.1	13	11	17	23
Phe-Met-Arg-Phe	—	—	15	18	23
Tyr-Gly-Gly-Phe Met	—	—	15	21	33

NOTE: Release of products with time of incubation at 37° C for E₅ or E₇ enkephalins incubated with purified brain PD-B. Incubation mixture of 0.4-ml 40-mM Tris–HCl buffer, pH 7.6, contained 57 nmol E₇ or 180 nmol E₅ and 40 μg enzyme protein. At the time intervals indicated, 50-μl aliquots were withdrawn, fixed with 3% w/v perchloric acid, and then analyzed by HPLC (see FIGURES 4 and 7). Under these conditions, actual enzyme rates were 5.3 nmol Tyr-Gly-Gly released/min/mg protein for E₅ (Leu-enkephalin) and 6.3 nmol Arg-Phe/min/mg protein For E₇ (Met-enkephalin-Arg-Phe).

questions on its role in neuropeptide turnover. Further evidence for endopeptidase action was provided by the cleavage of enkephalin analogues (TABLE

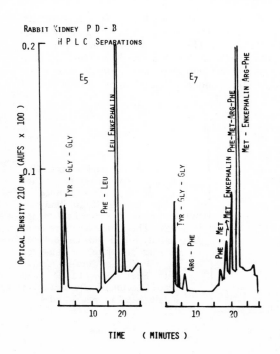

FIGURE 7. HPLC profile of Leu-enkephalin (E₅) and Met-enkephalin-Arg-Phe (E₇) breakdown products after 30-min incubation at 37° C with purified kidney P-B enzyme. Conditions of incubation were identical to those of FIGURE 4, except for the presence of Phe-Met-Arg-Phe as a product of E₇ breakdown. For other details see FIGURE 4.

4). The endopeptidase evidently has a restricted specificity since it did not act on the C-terminus of the decapeptide angiotensin-I.

One method for delineating different enkephalinases is by the use of specific inhibitors. ACE inhibitors, even at concentrations of above 10 μM, were ineffective in contrast to Thiorphan (K_i 9 nM) and enkephalin fragments Gly-Gly-Phe-Met and the C-terminal dipeptides of E_5 (TABLE 2). Our values for K_i of Thiorphan using brain or kidney PD-B are slightly higher than those reported by Llorens *et al.*[33] for mouse striatal membranes incubated in the presence of an aminopeptidase inhibitor.

TABLE 4

BIODEGRADATION OF SELECTED ENKEPHALIN ANALOGUES BY PURIFIED KIDNEY OR
BRAIN ENZYMES AS CORRELATED TO POTENCY

Modification	Cytosolic AP	PD-A	P-B	Relative Potency
None	100	100	100	100
Leu[5]	82	94	n.d.	100
Arg[6]-Phe[7]	95	980	120	700
D-Ala[2]	1	100	100	100
D-Ala[3]	43	0	0	—
D-Phe[4]	60	0	0	—
D-Met[5]	60	0	0	—
D-Ala[2], Met·NH$_2$[5] (Dalamid)	4	0	40	500
D-Met[2], Pro·NH$_2$[5]	1	0	0	1000
D-Ala[2], MePhe[4], Met(0)OH (FK 33–824)	1	0	0	500
D-Ala[2], F$_5$Phe[4], Met·NH$_2$[5]	1	0	0	1000 *
N$^\alpha$, N^e, bis D-Ala[2]-Lys[5], dimer	7	0	120	400 *

NOTE: Incubation was carried out for 1 hr at 37° C with purified rat brain cytosolic aminopeptidase (AP), or rabbit PD-A, or kidney P-B (endopeptidase). Incubation mixture of 25 μl of 40-mM Tris CHl, pH 7.6, contained approximately 4 nmol peptide or analogue, 0.1–5 μg protein. Breakdown was evaluated by disappearance of original substrate or measurement of released products. Potencies are those found *in vivo* or *in vitro* * (see Refs. 3, 8, 55, and 58).

SPM AND ENKEPHALIN DEGRADATION

SPM provides a model to examine those metabolic processes thought to be linked intimately to ligand interactions at the receptor site. We found that purified SPM prepared by procedures described earlier herein degraded E_5 with release of Tyr and the residual tetrapeptide as the initial products, followed later by appearance of the C-terminal dipeptide and Phe (as detected by an HPLC procedure, see FIGURE 8). In presence of bestatin, a known aminopeptidase inhibitor,[52] however, a different picture was observed since the major products with time of incubation were Tyr-Gly-Gly and the C-terminal dipeptide; cleavage at the Gly[3]-Phe[4] site was affected only slightly by MK-421 a PD-A inhibitor, but was inhibited by Thiorphan with a K_i of 0.2 μM (TABLE 5).

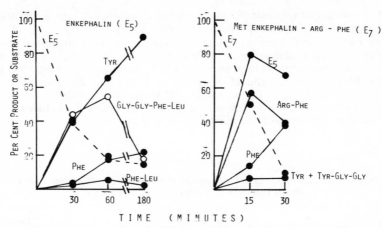

FIGURE 8. Comparison of E_5 and E_7 breakdown with time of incubation at 37° C with purified rat brain synaptosomal plasma membranes (SPM). Incubation conditions were identical to those of FIGURE 5, except for presence of 60 μg membrane protein. For other details see FIGURE 4.

That these preparations, nevertheless, contained a PD-A enzyme was demonstrated by the potent inhibition of E_7 breakdown by MK-421 ($K_i = 8$ nM) (TABLE 5). This result is paradoxical since it was shown earlier that purified PD-A can degrade E_5 with release of Tyr-Gly-Gly (FIGS. 4 and 5). We have no explanation why SPM PD-A behaved towards E_5 in a manner different from that of purified (immobilized) rabbit kidney and brain enzymes. The expression of PD-A activity by SPM towards E_7 (release of Arg-Phe, inhibition by MK-421) excludes presence of an inhibitory substance within the membrane. It is apparent that conversion of E_7 by rat SPM is mediated largely by the PD-A enzyme, but that the pathway for E_5 inactivation is different. This may involve either an aminopeptidase or an enzyme with properties similar to P-B.

TABLE 5

EFFECTS OF INHIBITORS ON BREAKDOWN OF MET-ENKEPHALIN (E_5) OR MET-ENKEPHALIN-ARG-PHE (E_7) BY PURIFIED RAT BRAIN SPM

Addition	Substrate	Product Detected	I_{50} (μM)	K_i (μM)
MK-421	E_5	Tyr-Gly-Gly	>1000	—
MK-421	E_7	Arg-Phe	0.011	0.008
Thiorphan	E_5	Tyr-Gly-Gly	0.2 *	0.17
Thiorphan	E_7	Arg-Phe	11	7.8

NOTE: Incubation conditions were identical to those of FIGURE 4, except for presence of 0.1 mM bestatin in the case of E_7 (to prevent breakdown of Arg-Phe) and 60 μg of SPM membrane protein. K_i values were calculated from the formula $I_{50} = K_i (1 + S/K_m)$.

* Substrate concentration 10 nmol.

Our results indicate further that the pathway mediated by this enzyme (in presence of bestatin) is sensitive to Thiorphan, but not to MK-421.

Comment is required on the disparity of K_i values observed in this study for rat brain SPM in presence of bestatin and Thiorphan as compared with those observed by Llorens *et al.*[33] for mouse striatal membranes incubated in presence of puromycin or other inhibitors. They used trace levels of substrate, 10^{-8} M as compared with 10^{-4}–10^{-5} M in the present study. Regional differences may be a factor since the striatal area may contain a higher concentration of P-B-like enzyme relative to that of other enkephalinases. Kinetics also may be a factor in studies using substrate at levels 10^3-fold lower than the K_m (22 μM as measured by their procedure, or 100 μM by the HPLC procedure used in our study). Of interest in this respect is a low value of 2 nM for Thiorphan when tested on P-B of rabbit kidney using a substrate concentration of 10^{-6} M labeled E_5 (John Norman and Mildred Phillipps, Ciba Geigy, Arsdley, NY, personal communication). Although it is not established whether purified P-B preparation is identical to the membrane enzyme acting at the Gly-Phe bond of E_5, both are inhibited by Thiorphan and are not affected significantly by ACE inhibitors. The isolation of homogeneous P-B enzyme from membranes can facilitate advances in this area and provide a rapid method for testing new inhibitors without the need of adding others (bestatin or puromycin).[16]

DEGRADATION OF ENKEPHALIN ANALOGS

The rapid degradation of enkephalins together with their short half-life *in vivo* stimulated interest in the synthesis of stable and possibly orally active forms. In our previous studies on breakdown of analogues it was established that the presence of a D-amino acid in position 2 retarded breakdown by homogenate aminopeptidases,[7, 8] but the question of their stability towards action of other enkephalinases was not investigated. In an extension of such studies we have reexamined some of the same analogues using cytosolic arylamidase from rat brain, and purified PD-A and P-B enzymes obtained from particulates. The most stable analogues were those with two or more modifications, as, for example, FK 33-824, D-Met^2 Pro$\cdot$NH$_2$^{5} and the D-Ala^2, F$_5$Phe^4, Met$\cdot$NH$_2$^{5} enkephalins (TABLE 4). The presence of modifications on position 4 (MetPhe, F$_5$Phe) may be required to prevent breakdown by membrane-bound endopeptidases in addition to PD-enzymes. In contrast D-Ala^2-enkephalinamide and the decapeptide dimer were degraded by the P-B preparation, and this was attributed to an action by an endopeptidase. In other studies we have observed slow breakdown of D-Ala^2-enkephalinamide by whole brain SPM with release of Tyr-D-Ala-Gly and Phe-Met$\cdot$NH$_2$, indicating cleavage at the Gly-Phe site. Since some enkephalin fragments (Gly-Gly-Phe-Met or Leu, Phe-Met, Phe-Leu) act as inhibitors of enkephalinases the possibility exists that larger enkephalin forms themselves also have inhibitory properties. To examine this possibility we have tested a series of mixed agonist peptides prepared by K. Ramakrishnan and P. S. Portoghese (University of Minnesota) for their effects on two enkephalinases and on rat brain SPM preparations. The suitability as potential probes of des-Tyr enkephalin or its fragments linked covalently to a morphine agonist such as benzomorphan has not previously been examined. Although themselves devoid of opioid properties (P. S. Portoghese, personal communication), these compounds exhibited some inhibitory properties, especially where $R_1 = (\pm)\text{-CH}_2\,\text{NHCOCH}_3$ (TABLE 6). The I_{50} values are comparable to those found for early inhibitors of ACE and further chemical modification to enhance potencies may be justified.

It is beyond the scope of this report to review the clinical or other applications of enkephalins and related opiate peptides. Such aspects have been covered by Krieger and Martin,[53] Verebey *et al.*[54] and by Olsen *et al.*[55] The enkephalin analogue, FK 33-824, (TABLE 6) has been shown to be analgesic in various animal species [55, 56] and to affect behavior in addicted monkeys and circling movements in rats.[55, 57] Recently, Roubicek *et al.*[9] observed clinical improvement in mental patients given 1–2 mg intramuscularly for periods up to 1 week. Enkephalins were found also to affect conditioned avoidance response

TABLE 6

EFFECT OF MIXED BENZOMORPHAN–ENKEPHALINS AS INHIBITORS OF BRAIN ENZYMES
AND OF AN SPM FRACTION OF RAT BRAIN

Substitutions ——R——		Relative Potency as I_{50} (mM)		
		PD-A	P-B	SPM
$(-)\text{-CO-Gly-Gly-Phe-Met}\cdot\text{NH}_2$		0.7	0.8	>2
$(+)\text{-CO-Gly-Gly-Phe-Met}\cdot\text{NH}_3$		0.6	0.9	>2
$(-)\text{-CO-Gly}\cdot\text{NH}_2$		1	2	>2
$(-)\text{-CO-NH}_2$		>2	>1	0.3
$(\pm)\text{-CH}_2\text{-NH-CO-CH}_3$		0.4	0.3	0.7
$(+)\text{-CO-Gly-Gly-Phe-Met}\cdot\text{NH}_2$		1	>2	>2

NOTE: Effects of a mixed agonist–peptide on cleavage of Met-enkephalin expressed as relative I_{50} values when incubated with rabbit brain PD-A or P-B enzymes, or with purified rat brain SPM. The structure of benzomorphan is shown in the insert, and the nature of substituents in position R in the Table. Analogues were prepared by P. S. Portoghese and K. Ramakrishnan (University of Minnesota). Values given are the means of two determinations. For details of incubation see FIGURE 4 and TABLES 3 and 5. Breakdown of E_5 was determined by the HPLC procedure.

when given systematically in low doses.[55] Two analogues, D-Ala²F₅Phe-enkephalin and the decapeptide dimer, also were found to induce profound immobilization and to affect behavior in animals (TABLE 4).[8, 55] Progress in clinical applications has been slow, but may accelerate with the availability of specific μ agonists or enkephalin surrogates of high potency in opioid test systems.[4, 60] In these respects, metabolic studies can be viewed as important in guiding the chemist and clinician to the development and use of new classes of opioid drugs.

CONCLUSIONS

1. There is a multiplicity of enzymes in brain metabolizing Met- or Leu-enkephalin (E_5) or a heptapeptide surrogate, Met-enkephalin-Arg-Phe (E_7).
2. Membrane-bound aminopeptidases acting on the Tyr-Gly bond have a

lower substrate affinity as compared to one purified from the cytosol. One membrane form was unaffected by puromycin and appeared to be highly specific for E_5. Another is comparable to the arylamidase of the cytosol.

3. Two enkephalinases can be separated and purified from detergent extracts of rodent brain which act on the Gly-Phe bond of E_5 or of E_7. One enzyme, termed PD-A, was shown to be identical to angiotensin-converting enzyme of other tissues; the other, termed P-B was a metalloendopeptidase, was unaffected by ACE inhibitors, MK-421 or Captopril, and did not convert angiotensin-I by release of the C-terminal dipeptide. MK-421 was the most effective PD-A inhibitor of the series tested.

4. Purified rat brain SPM degrades E_5 at the Tyr-Gly bond, but in the presence of aminopeptidase inhibitor acts on the Gly-Phe bond with the release of C-terminal dipeptide. This action is inhibited by Thiorphan, des-Tyr-enkephalin, and Phe-Leu or Phe-Met, but only slightly by MK-421. In contrast, SPM degrades E_7 by a PD-A-type enzyme very sensitive to inhibition by MK-421. Conversion of E_7 leads to formation of Met-enkephalin as an intermediate.

5. Some correlation exists between biodegradation of analogues by PD-A/P-B enzymes or cytosolic aminopeptidase and potency. Enkephalin fragments (des-Tyr-enkephalin) or analogues, as illustrated for mixed agonist (benzomorphan)–peptide derivatives, can act as inhibitors of PD-A/P-B enzymes or enzymes present in SPM.

ACKNOWLEDGMENTS

We are indebted to Richard Soffer, Cornell University Medical College, New York, NY, for the supply of antiserum to rabbit lung ACE; to David Cushman, Squibb Institute for Medical Research, Princeton, NJ, for Captopril; to A. A. Patchett, Merck and Co., Rahway, NJ, for MK-42I; to W. Cash and B. Petrack, CIBA-Geigy Corp., Ardsley, NY, for Thiorphan; to P. S. Portoghese, University of Minnesota College of Pharmacy, Minneapolis, MN for benzomorphan analogues; and to Abba Kastin and David H. Coy, Veterans Administration Hospital and Tulane University School of Medicine, New Orleans, LA, for selected enkephalin analogues.

REFERENCES

1. JACQUET, Y. & N. MARKS. 1976. The C-fragment of B-lipotropin, an endogenous neuroleptic or an antipsychotogen. Science **194**: 632–635.
2. BLOOM, F., D. SEGAL, N. LING & R. GUILLEMIN. 1976. Endorphins: Profound effects in rats suggest new etiological factors in mental illness. **194**: 630–632.
3. ROSSIER, J., Y. AUDIGIER, N. LING, J. CROS & S. UDENFRIEND. 1980. Met-enkephalin-Arg⁶-Phe⁷, present in high amounts in brain of rat, cattle, and man is an opioid agonist. Nature **288**: 88–91.
4. KILPATRICK, D. L., T. TANIGUCHI, B. N. JONES, A. S. STERN, J. E. SHIRLEY, J. HULLIHAN, S. KIMURA, S. STEIN & S. UDENFRIEND. 1981. A highly potent 3200-dalton adrenal opioid peptide that contains both a (Met) and (Leu) enkephalin sequence. Proc. Natl. Acad. Sci. USA **78**: 3265–3268.
5. MIZUNO, K., N. MINAMINO, K. KANAGAWA & H. MATSUO. 1980. A new family of endogenous "big" Met-enkephalins from bovine adrenal medulla: Purification and structure of docasa (BAM-22P) and eicosapeptide (BAM-20P) with very potent opiate activity. Biochem. Biophys. Res. Commun. **97**: 1283–1290.

6. STERN, A. S., R. V. LEWIS, S. KIMURA, J. ROSSIER, L. D. GERBER, L. BRINK, S. STEIN & S. UDENFRIEND. 1979. Isolation of the opioid heptapeptide Met-enkephalin (Arg^6, Phe^7) from bovine adrenal medullary granules and striatum. Proc. Natl. Acad. Sci. USA **76**: 6880–6883.

7. MARKS, N. 1977. Conversion and inactivation of neuropeptides. In Peptides in Neurobiology. H. Gainer, Ed.: **5**: 221–258, Plenum Press. New York.

8. GRYNBAUM, A., A. J. KASTIN, D. H. COY & N. MARKS. 1977. Breakdown of enkephalins and endorphin analogs by brain extracts. Brain Res. Bull. **2**: 479–484.

9. ROUBICEK, J., E. KREBS & W. POELDINGER. 1981. Classification of endorphins/enkephalins in brain: Physiology and pathology (based on EEG and clinical study of synthetically modified methione enkephalins. Progr. Neuro-Psychopharmacol. **4**: 507–518.

10. HAMBROOK, J. M., B. A. MORGAN, M. J. RANCE & C. F. C. SMITH. 1976. Mode of deactivation of the enkephalins by rat and human plasma and rat brain homogenates. Nature **262**: 782–783.

11. MARKS, N., A. GRYNBAUM & A. NEIDLE. 1977. On the degradation of enkephalins and endorphins by rat and mouse brain extracts. Biochem. Biophys. Res. Commun. **4**: 1552–1559.

12. TRAFICANTE, L. J., J. ROTROSEN, J. SIEKIERSKI, H. TRACER & S. GERSHON. 1980. Enkephalin inactivation by N-terminal tyrosine cleavage: Purification and partial characterization of a highly specific enzyme from human brain. Life Sci. **26**: 1697–1706.

13. SCHNEBLI, H. P., M. A. PHILLIPPS & R. K. BARCLAY. 1979. Isolation and characterization of an enkephalin degrading aminopeptidase from rat brain. Biochem. Biophys. Acta **569**: 89–98.

14. HERSH, L. B. 1981. Solubilization and characterization of two rat brain membrane-bound aminopeptidases active on Met-enkephalin. Biochemistry **20**: 2345–2350.

15. GORENSTEIN, C. & S. R. SYNDER. 1979. Two distinct enkephalinases: Solubilisation, partial purification and separation from angiotensin converting enzyme. Life Sci. **25**: 2065–2070.

16. BENUCK, M., M. J. BERG & N. MARKS. 1982. Rat brain and kidney metalloendopeptic enkephalin heptapeptide conversion to form a cardioactive neuropeptide, Phe-Met-Ary-Phe-amide. Biochem. Biophys. Res. Commun. **107**: 1123–1129.

17. SCHWARTZ, J. C., S. DE LA BAUME, B. MALFROY, G. PATEY, R. PERDRISOT, J. P. SWERTS, M. C. FOURNIE-ZALUSKI, G. GACEL & B. P. ROQUES. 1980. Properties, variations and possible synaptic functions of "enkephalinase," a newly characterized dipeptidyl carboxypeptidase. Adv. Biochem. Psychopharmacol. **22**: 219–235.

18. SULLIVAN, S. S., H. AKIL, D. BLACKER & J. D. BARCHAS. 1980. Enkephalinase: Selective inhibitors and partial characterization. Peptides **1**: 33–35.

19. BENUCK, M. & N. MARKS. 1980. Characterization of a distinct membrane bound dipeptidyl carboxypeptidase inactivating enkephalin in brain. Biochem. Biophys. Res. Commun. **95**: 822–828.

20. MALFROY, B., J. P. SWERTS, A. GUYON, B. P. ROQUES & J. C. SCHWARTZ. 1978. High-affinity enkephalin-degrading peptidase in brain is increased after morphine. Nature **276**: 523–526.

21. MARKS, N., L. SACHS & F. STERN. 1981. Conversion of Met-enkephalin-Arg^6-Phe^7 by a purified brain carboxypeptidase (cathepsin A). Peptides **2**: 159–164.

22. KOSTERLITZ, H. W. 1980. Possible function of the enkephalins. Adv. Biochem. Pharmacol. **22**: 633–642.

23. WISLER, M., P. RUBINI & R. SCHULTZ. 1981. The preference of punative proenkephalins for different types of opiate receptors. Life Sci. **29**: 1219–1227.

24. HERTZ, A., V. HÖLLT, CH. GRAMSCH, & B. R. SEIZINGER. 1982. Differential distributtion, release and modulation of dynorphin and B-endorphin. Adv. Biochem. Psychopharmacol. **33**: 51–59.
25. COY, D. H. & A. J. KASTIN. 1980. Tyrosine-modified analogs of methionine-enkephalin and their effects on the mouse vas deferens. Peptides **1**: 175–177.
26. GACEL, G., M. C. FOURNIE-ZALUSKI, E. FELLION & B. P. ROQUES. 1981. Evidence of the preferential involvement of μ receptors in analgesia using enkephalins highly selective for peripheral μ or δ receptors. J. Med. Chem. **24**: 1119–1124.
27. GROSS, D. M., C. S. SWEET, E. H. ULM, E. P. BACKLUND, D. MORRIS, A. A. WEITZ, D. L. BOHM, H. C. WENGER, T. C. WASSIL & C. A. STONE. 1981. Effect of N- (s)-carboxy-3-phenylpropyl -L-Ala-Pro and its ethyl ester (MK-421) on ACE in vitro and angiotensin 1 pressor responses in vivo. J. Pharmacol. Exp. Ther. **216**: 552–557.
28. ONDETTI, M. A., B. RUBIN & D. W. CUSHMAN. 1977. Design of specific inhibitors of angiotensin converting enzyme: A new class of active antihypertensive agents. Science **196**: 441–444.
29. PATCHETT, A. A., E. HARRIS, E. W. TRISTRAM, M. J. WYVRATT, M. T. WU, D. TAUB, E. R. PETERSON, T. J. IKELER, J. TEN BROEKE, L. G. PAYNE, D. L. ONDEYKA, E. D. THORSETT, W. J. GREENLEE, N. S. LOHR, R. D. HOFFSOMMER, H. JOSHUA, W. V. RUYLE, J. W. ROTHROCK, S. D. ASTER, A. L. MAYCOCK, F. M. ROBINSON, R. HIRSCHMANN, C. S. SWEET, E. H. ULM, D. M. GROSS, T. C. VASSIL & C. A. STONE. 1980. A new class of angiotensin converting enzyme inhibitors. Nature **288**: 280–283.
30. QUIOCHO, F. A. & W. N. LIPSCOMB. 1971. Carboxypeptidase A: A protein and an enzyme. Adv. Protein Chem. **25**: 1–78.
31. ROQUES, B. P., M. C. FOURNIE-ZALUSKI, E. SOROCA, J. M. LECONTE, B. MALFROY, C. LLORENS & J. C. SCHWARTZ. 1980. The enkephalinase inhibitor thiorphan shows antinociceptive activity in mice. Nature **288**: 286–288.
32. PATEY, G., S. DE LA BAUME, J. C. SCHWARTZ, C. GROS, B. ROQUES, M. C. FOURNIE-ZALUSKI & F. S. LUCAS. 1981. Selective protection of methionine enkephalin released from brain slices by enkephalinase inhibitors. Science **212**: 153–155.
33. LLORENS, C., G. GACEL, J. P. SWERTS, R. PERDRISOT, M.-C. FOURNIE-ZALUSKI, J. C. SCHWARTZ & B. P. ROQUES. 1980. Rational design of enkephalinase inhibitors: Substrate specificity of enkephalinase studied from inhibitory potency of various dipeptides. Biochem. Biophys. Res. Commun. **96**: 1710–1716.
34. MARKS, N. 1968. Peptide hydrolases of the CNS. Int. Rev. Neurobiol. **11**: 57–90.
35. MARKS, N., R. K. DATTA & A. LAJTHA. 1968. Partial resolution of brain arylamidase and aminopeptidases. J. Biol. Chem. **243**: 2882–2889.
36. MARKS, N., M. BENUCK & L. SACHS. 1981. Multiplicity and specificity of tissue enkephalinases: Role in turnover of neuropeptides. *In* Chemisms of the Brain. R. Rodnight, H. S. Bachelard & W. L. Stahl, Eds. 136–146. Churchill Livingston. London.
37. HUANG, W. Y., R. C. CHANG, A. J. KASTIN, D. H. COY & A. V. SCHALLY. 1979. Isolation of structure of pro-methionine-enkephalin: Potential enkephalin precursor from porcine hypothalamus. Proc. Natl. Acad. Sci. USA **76**: 6177–6180.
38. GOLDSTEIN, A., S. TACHIBANA, L. I. LOWNEY, M. HUNKAPILLER & L. HOOD. 1979. Dynorphin-(1–13), an extraordinary potent opioid peptide. Proc. Natl. Acad. Sci. USA **76**: 6666–6670.
39. MINAMINO, N., K. KANAGAWA, A. FUKADA & H. MATSUO. 1980. A new opioid octapeptide related to dynorphin from porcine hypothalamus. Biochem. Biophys. Res. Commun. **95**: 1475–1481.
40. MIZUNO, K., N. MINAMINO, K. KANAGAWA & H. MATSUO. 1980. A new endoge-

nous peptide from bovine adrenal medulla: Isolation and amino acid sequence of a dodecapeptide (BAM-12P). Biochem. Biophys. Res. Commun. **95:** 1482–1488.

41. LEWIS, R. V. 1982. Biosynthesis of the enkephalins in adrenal medulla. Adv. Biochem. Psychopharmacol. **33:** 167–174.

42. BENUCK, M. & N. MARKS. 1978. Subcellular localization and partial purification of a chloride-dependent angiotensin converting enzyme from rat brain. J. Neurochem. **30:** 729–734.

43. BENUCK, M., M. J. BERG & N. MARKS. 1981. A distinct peptidyl dipeptidase that degrades enkephalin: Exceptionally high activity in rabbit kidney. Life Sci. **28:** 2643–2650.

44. SERRA, S., A. GRYNBAUM, A. LAJTHA & N. MARKS. 1972. Peptide hydrolases in spinal cord and brain of the rabbit. Brain Res. **44:** 579–592.

45. SACHS, L. & N. MARKS. 1982. A highly specific aminopeptidase of rat brain cytosol: Substrate specificity and effect of inhibitors. Biochim. Biophys. Acta. In press.

46. BOEHME, D. H. & N. MARKS. 1982. Protracted form of Canavan's disease: Case history and protein kinase activity of membrane fractions. Acta Neuropathol. In press.

47. MARCHBANKS, R. M. 1974. Isolation and study of synaptic vesicles. Res. Methods Neurochem. **2:** 79–98.

48. STEWART, T. A., J. A. WEARE & E. G. ERDOS. 1981. Purification and characterization of human converting enzyme (kininase II). Peptides **2:** 145–152.

49. SOFFER, R. L. 1981. Angiotensin converting enzyme. In Biochemical Regulation of Blood Pressure. R. L. Soffer, Ed.: 123–164. John Wiley. New York.

50. DAS, M. & R. L. SOFFER. 1976. Pulmonary angiotensin-converting enzyme antienzyme antibody. Biochemistry **15:** 5088–5094.

51. ONDETTI, M. A. & D. W. CUSHMAN. 1981. Inhibitors of angiotensin converting enzyme. In Biochemical Regulation of Blood Pressure. R. L. Soffer, Ed.: 115–204. John Wiley. New York.

52. BARCLAY, R. K. & M. A. PHILLIPPS. 1980. Inhibition of enkephalin-degrading aminopeptidase activity by certain peptides. Biochem. Biophys. Res. Commun. **96:** 1732–1738.

53. KRIEGER, D. T. & J. B. MARTIN. 1981. Brain peptides. N. Engl. J. Med. **304:** 944–951.

54. VEREBEY, K., J. VOLAVKA & D. CLOUET. 1978. Endorphins in psychiatry—an overview and a hypothesis. Arch. Gen. Psychiat. **35:** 877–888.

55. OLSEN, G. A., R. D. OLSEN, A. KASTIN & D. H. COY. 1979. Endogenous opiates: through 1978. Neurosci. Behav. Rev. **3:** 285–299.

56. ROEMER, D., H. BNESCHER, R. HILL, J. PLESS, W. BAUER, E. CARDINAUX, A. CLOSSE, D. HAUSER & R. HUGUENIN. 1977. A synthetic enkephalin analogue with prolonged parenteral and oral analgesic activity. Nature **268:** 547–549.

57. KAAKKOLA, S. 1980. Contralateral circling behavior induced by intranigral injection of morphine and enkephalin analogue FK 33–824 in rat. Acta. Pharmacol. Toxicol. **47:** 385–393.

58. RONAI, A. Z., I. P. BERZETEI, S. BAJUSZ & J. I. SZEKELY. 1981. The in vitro pharmacology of D-Met^2, Pro^5-enkephalinamide. J. Pharm. Pharmacol. **33:** 534–535.

59. MARKS, N., A. SUHAR & M. BENUCK. 1981. Peptide processing in the CNS. In Neurosections and brain peptides. J. Martin, S. Reichlin & K. Bicks, Eds. Adv. Biochem. Pharmacol. **28:** 49–62.

60. ROSENFELD, J. P. & P. KERESZTES NAGY. 1980. Differential effects of intracerebrally microinjected enkephalin analogs on centrally versus peripherally induced pain, and evidence for a facial versus lower body analgesic effect. Pain **9:** 171–181.

OPIATE RECEPTORS AND OPIOID PEPTIDES: AN OVERVIEW

Eric J. Simon

Departments of Psychiatry and Pharmacology
New York University Medical Center
New York, New York 10016

It is my assignment to present an overview of the area of opiate receptors and opioid peptides. This is a not inconsiderable challenge, in terms of both the selection of topics to fit into the allotted space and the level of previous knowledge of the field to be expected of my audience.

After reflection I have decided to review as concisely as possible the physiology and distribution of opiate receptors and of opioid peptides. I then plan to concentrate on two areas that have received considerable attention recently. One is the question of the existence of more than one type of opiate receptor; the other is the evidence for possible functions of the endogenous opioid system and, in particular, those aspects of endorphin distribution and actions that have given rise to the hypothesis of their possible involvement in mental disease.

DEMONSTRATION AND PROPERTIES OF OPIATE RECEPTORS

The direct demonstration of specific saturable binding of opiates to nervous tissue was reported simultaneously in 1973 by Simon *et al.*[1] and by Terenius [2] and Pert and Snyder.[3] This discovery was the culmination after many years of pharmacologic and biochemical research, research that had already resulted in the postulation of opiate receptors some decades earlier. The ability to assay specific opiate-binding sites directly with labeled opiates and opiate antagonists of high specific activity has permitted us to learn a great deal about these sites and to provide evidence that they are the pharmacologically relevant opiate receptors. Receptors are defined as specific sites to which a drug must bind in order.to trigger biochemical or biophysical steps that result in the observed pharmacologic response.

Opiate-binding sites are present in the CNS and in some innervations of peripheral organs. They are tightly bound to cell membranes in the vicinity of synapses. They have been found in all vertebrates so far examined and recently in some invertebrates as well.[4]

Binding is saturable and reversible. Binding affinity is high, with a K_d ranging from 10^{-10} to 10^{-8} M for active opiate analgesics. It is stereospecific, that is, only the active enantiomer of an opiate binds with high affinity. All of these properties are consistent with the notion that we are dealing with pharmacologically relevant opiate receptors. The most convincing evidence comes from the excellent correlation between binding affinities and pharmacologic activity of opiates that vary in potency over five to six orders of magnitude. This has been shown for analgesia [5] as well as for the now classical *in vitro* bioassay system, the guinea pig ileum.[6]

327

0077-8923/82/0398-0327 $01.75/0 © 1982 NYAS

Opiate binding is very sensitive to a variety of proteolytic enzymes and reagents that react with functional groups and amino acids of protein. In particular, sulfhydryl reagents have been studied in some detail and all such reagents have been found to inhibit specific opiate binding. Evidence is thus quite convincing for the participation of one or more proteins, containing an SH group, in the binding process. The fact that opiate receptors are highly sensitive to some phospholipases (but not all)[1, 7] as well as to low concentrations of detergents suggests that phospholipids also have a role, possibly by holding the receptor site in its active conformation.

A unique and very specific effect on opiate binding is exerted by sodium ions and, to a lesser extent, by lithium. All other cations, including the closely related alkali metals, potassium, rubidium and cesium, tend to inhibit the binding of all ligands to the opiate receptor in a dose-related manner. Sodium, however, while it inhibits the binding of opiate agonists,[1] actually stimluates the binding of antagonists, as much as twofold in the case of naloxone.[8, 9] This effect is reversible and can be seen with as little as 5 mM Na+. We have accumulated considerable evidence [9, 10] indicating that Na+ acts as an allosteric effector, shifting the equilibrium towards a conformer of the receptor that binds antagonists with greater affinity than agonists. The physiological significance of this conformational plasticity of the opiate receptor is not yet understood.

A word should be said about the state of the art of receptor isolation and purification. This work is of considerable importance for our understanding of the chemical and subunit structure of the opiate receptor and ultimately its function. Initially, these studies were slowed down by the difficulty of solubilizing the receptor, that is, removing it from its tight association with cell membranes into aqueous solution. We accomplished a first important step in our laboratory in 1975 when we were able to solubilize a macromolecular complex of ^{3}H-labeled etorphine from rat brain membranes with the nonionic detergent, BRIJ-36T. This complex had properties consistent with the postulate that it was an etorphine–receptor complex. However, solubilization in the absence of etorphine or dissociation of the etorphine did not yield a receptor able to bind opioid ligands in solution. These experiments were repeated by Zukin and Kream [11] with identical results. These workers also showed that an enkephalin–macromolecular complex was solubilized by the same method and that it was possible to bind a portion of the peptide covalently to the receptor by crosslinking with dimethyl suberimidate.

The solubilization of opiate receptors that retain their binding activity in solution was achieved only within the last year and, as usual, in several laboratories. We reported the solubilization in excellent yield (40–50%) of active opiate-binding sites from brain membranes of the toad, *Bufo marinus,* using digitonin.[12, 13] Simonds et al.,[14] using a new detergent called CHAPS, reported the solubilization of opiate-binding sites from N108-15 neuroblastoma × glioma hybrid cells as well as from rat brain. Bidlack and Abood,[15] using Triton X-100, have reported solubilization and considerable purification of opiate receptors from rat brain. More recently in our laboratory we have had success solubilizing active opiate receptors from mammalian sources.[16] Reasonable yields have been obtained from rat brain, cow striatum, and human frontal cortex.

These solubilization studies have already permitted us to demonstrate a receptor constituent that had previously escaped us. By use of a variety of lectin agglutinins immobilized on Sepharose we found that opiate receptors from four species (man, cow, rat, toad) are retained by columns of wheat germ agglutinin.[17] This provides evidence that the opiate receptor is a glycoprotein containing N-acetylglucosamine and, very likely, other sugars.

DISTRIBUTION OF OPIATE RECEPTORS

I have already stated that opiate receptors are found mainly in the CNS and in the innervation of certain smooth muscle systems such as the gut and the vas deferens. They have also been found in some other tissues such as the pituitary and adrenal glands. Their location in these endocrine tissues, whether on nerve or non-nerve cells, is not clear.

Within the CNS, opiate receptors have a very distinct distribution which is relatively similar in all the species so far studied. Such studies were first done in our laboratory [18] using human brains obtained at autopsy from the Office of the Chief Medical Examiner of New York City. More than 50 regions were dissected, homogenized, and tested for stereospecific ³H-etorphine binding. Similar studies were done in monkey brain with ³H-naloxone by Kuhar et al.[19] More recently, fine mapping studies in rat brain using autoradiography were done by Kuhar's group [20-22] and confirmed in our laboratory by Pearson et al.[23]

Almost all of the regions showing high levels of binding were associated with the limbic system. In fact, the only limbic structure that failed to exhibit high binding was the hippocampus. Moderate to high opiate binding is also displayed by all regions that have been implicated in pain perception or modulation, such as the periventricular and periaqueductal gray, the somatic thalamus, and the dorsal horn of the spinal cord, especially the substantia gelatinosa. High receptor levels are also found in some other areas such as the caudate nucleus and parts of the cortex where their function is not at all clear.

The question of the pre- or postsynaptic location of opiate receptors has been studied in a number of ways. Electrophysiological studies, especially those of Zieglgansberger and his group,[24] have suggested postsynaptic effects, since opiates can inhibit electrical potentials stimulated by glutamate, an amino acid known to act on postsynaptic receptors. On the other hand, La Motte et al.[25] found that dorsal rhizotomy in monkeys resulted in a loss of opiate binding by as much as 50%. These authors admitted that they could not rule out transsynaptic effects, although a presynaptic location of the receptor appeared more likely. In our studies on organotypic tissue cultures in collaboration with Stanley Crain [26] we were able to show the presence of high levels of opiate receptors in the neuritic outgrowth from dorsal ganglia cultured in the absence of spinal cord. These results clearly confirm the notion that opiate receptors can be located presynaptically, in this case on primary afferent fibers.

DISCOVERY OF OPIOID PEPTIDES

The existence of opiate receptors in all vertebrate species examined raised the important question as to why receptors for plant-derived substances should be present and have survived the eons of evolution. A physiological role for opiate receptors that confers a selective advantage on the organism seemed probable and the existence of natural ligands for opiate receptors with opiate-like properties was postulated. An examination of the various known neuro-transmitters, hormones, and other substances present in the CNS did not reveal any that exhibited high affinity for the opiate receptor. This prompted investigators in several laboratories to embark on the tedious search for an as yet unknown substance with opioid properties in extracts of animal brain. This search was successful first in the laboratories of Hughes and Kosterlitz [27] and of Terenius and Wahlström.[28] At about the same time Goldstein and his collaborators [29] reported opioid activity in extracts of pituitary glands.

These studies culminated in the identification of two opioid substances from extracts of pig brain by Hughes et al.[30] Virtually all of the opioid activity was found to reside in two pentapeptides, Tyr-Gly-Gly-Phe-Met and Tyr-Gly-Gly-Phe-Leu, which they named methionine (Met) and leucine (Leu) enkephalin (from the Greek, meaning in the head). This group also reported the interesting observation that the sequence of Met-enkephalin was present in the pituitary hormone, β-lipotropin (βLPH) as residues 61–65. This hormone had been isolated by C. H. Li in 1965 and was found to exhibit weak lipolytic activity, from which it got its name. This report, along with A. Goldstein's finding of opioid activity in the pituitary, led Guillemin to examine carefully extracts from pig hypothalami and pituitary glands, remaining from his Nobel-prize-winning isolation of hypothalamic releasing factors. Two polypeptides with opioid activity were isolated and sequenced.[31] They proved to have structures identical to sequences 61–76 and 61–77 of βLPH. In the meantime researchers in two laboratories [32, 33] had found that the so-called C-terminal fragment of βLPH, originally isolated from camel pituitaries by Li's group, had potent opioid activity. The intact βLPH molecule was devoid of activity. The proliferation in the number of endogenous opioid peptides led me to suggest the term endorphin (a contraction of "endogenous" and "morphine"), which has been widely accepted. The C-terminal fragment was renamed β-endorphin by Li, while LPH 61–76 and 61–77 were named α- and γ-endorphin, respectively, by Guillemin.

Since that time a number of other endorphins have been identified. Kangawa et al.[34] found a peptide in pig hypothalamus extracts which they have called α-neoendorphin. Only the first 8 amino acids of this 15-amino-acid peptide have been sequenced and the sequence found to be: Tyr-Gly-Gly-Phe-Leu-Arg-Lys-Arg-. Goldstein had already pointed out in his early reports that, in addition to β-endorphin, pituitary extracts contain an opioid peptide, the basic nature of which suggested that it contains a number of arginine and lysine residues. This polypeptide was recently isolated and characterized and has been named dynorphin because of its great potency.[35] The original report presented the sequence of the first 13 amino acids of this 17-amino acid peptide. However, the entire sequence is now known and is Tyr-Gly-Gly-Phe-Leu-Arg-Arg-Ile-Arg-Pro-Lys-Leu-Trp-Asp-Asn-Gln.[36] Although both α-neoendorphin and dynorphin have Leu-enkephalin at their N-terminals, neither is thought to be a Leu-enkephalin precursor since both are more potent in various assays than Leu-enkephalin. The possibility that Leu-enkephalin may be a breakdown product of one of the longer peptides has not been totally ruled out but is thought to be unlikely. This is based on the difference in their distributions and on what is known about Leu-enkephalin biosynthesis in the adrenal medulla.

Several other opioid peptides have been reported but will not be discussed here because of space limitations.

PROPERTIES OF OPIOID PEPTIDES

The properties of the opioid peptides can best be summarized by stating that their pharmacologic effects are remarkably similar to those of the plant-derived and synthetic opiate alkaloids. Responses to these peptides include analgesia, respiratory depression, hypothermia, development of tolerance and physical dependence upon chronic administration, and a number of behavioral changes. Like opiates, the endorphins and enkephalins interact with the endocrine system, producing increases in the release of growth hormone, prolactin, and ACTH, and decreases in the release of luteinizing hormone (LH) and follicle-stimulating hormone (FSH). Effects of the enkephalins are short-lived, presumably due to their rapid degradation by peptidases. The duration of activity of enkephalin analogues, resistant to enzymatic degradation, is much longer. The longer-chain endorphins produce analgesia and other effects that can last 3 to 4 hours.

Catatonia in rats upon intraventricular injection of β-endorphin was the major behavioral response noted simultaneously by two groups.[37, 38] It is particularly noteworthy for this Conference that the two groups of investigators derived from this observation essentially opposite hypotheses for involvement of endorphins in schizophrenia. The group at the Salk Institute suggested that catatonic symptoms might result from the presence in the CNS of an excess of endorphins, while the New York group viewed this effect as very similar to the response to certain neuroleptics. Thus, a deficiency of opioid peptides, which might function as endogenous neuroleptics, could account for symptoms of schizophrenia. The former hypothesis justified the administration of opiate antagonists (naloxone and naltrexone) to schizophrenic patients, while the latter hypothesis was the rationale for administering opioid peptides and their analogues. De Wied and coworkers [39] have reported other behavioral effects of endorphins, especially on the extinction of avoidance behavior, that resemble those of haloperidol and other neuroleptics.

Opioid peptides have been found to inhibit the release of various neurotransmitters, a property of opiates known for many years. Thus Met-enkephalin has been shown to inhibit both electrically and high K^+-induced, Ca^{++}-dependent release of norepinephrine from slices of rat cerebral cortex.[40] Inhibition of acetylcholine and dopamine release from rat brain slices by enkephalin has also been demonstrated.[41] D-Ala^2-Met-enkephalinamide and β-endorphin inhibit the K^+-evoked release of substance P from slices of rat spinal trigeminal nerve nuclei.[42] These results are indicative of a neuromodulator role for opioid peptides and favor a presynapic location of opiate receptors. A model for such a role is shown in FIGURE 1. Substance P is shown here as the transmitter, the release of which is regulated by enkephalin, because of the putative role of substance P as the major transmitter in pain pathways.

Additional evidence supporting the candidacy of opioid peptides as neurotransmitters or neuromodulators comes from the findings that they are largely located at nerve terminals [43] and that they can be released from nervous tissue in response to depolarization in a Ca^{++}-dependent manner.[44–46]

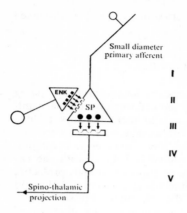

Small diameter
primary afferent

ENK

SP

Spino-thalamic
projection

I

II

III

IV

V

FIGURE 1. Schematic representation of possible physiologic inhibition by enkephalin of substance P release in the dorsal horn of the spinal cord. Roman numerals to the right refer to the laminae of Rexed. A small-diameter primary afferent fiber is shown with its substance-P-containing terminal forming an excitatory synapse with a spinal cord neuron originating in lamina IV or V; the axon of this cell projects rostrally as a secondary afferent fiber. An enkephalin-containing interneuron is shown making an axoaxonic inhibitory synapse with the substance-P-containing primary afferent terminal. (From Jessel and Iversen.[42] Reprinted by permission.)

DISTRIBUTION OF OPIOID PEPTIDES

Phylogenetically, opioid peptides are widely distributed. One or more have been found in all vertebrate species studied and in some invertebrates, such as the earthworm [47] and the leech.[48] Recently, there have even been reports of β-endorphin-like immunoreactivity in single-celled organisms, such as *Tetrahymena* and *E. coli*. However, the material responsible for this immunoreactivity has not been identified.

The distribution of opioid peptides within the CNS has been studied in considerable detail, largely by immunohistochemical techniques. Most of this research has been carried out with the enkephalins and β-endorphin, for α- and γ-endorphin are now thought by most investigators to be breakdown products of β-endorphin. Dynorphin, α-neoendorphin and other peptides are very new, and, while some anatomic studies have been done, they will not be discussed here.

The distribution of the enkephalins and of β-endorphin are summarized schematically in FIGURE 2. It can be seen that the enkephalins are widely distributed throughout the brain and spinal cord. Their distribution is non-uniform and is, in fact, rather well correlated with the distribution of opiate receptors. There are some exceptions, such as the globus pallidus, which has the highest enkephalin content, while it is relatively low in opiate receptors. Certain cortical areas dense in opiate receptors have low levels of enkephalin. All of the areas associated with the limbic system are high in enkephalins. The only exception is the hippocampus, which is low in enkephalins as well as in opiate receptors.

While much of the immunofluorescence due to enkephalins is found at nerve terminals,[43] the use of colchicine to arrest axonal transport permitted Hökfelt and colleagues [50] to visualize enkephalin immunoreactivity in cell bodies. More than 20 cell groups containing enkephalin have been observed in the brain and spinal cord of rats.

The distribution of β-endorphin in the CNS is considerably more limited. Floyd Bloom and coworkers [51] and Stanley Watson *et al.*[52] have provided convincing evidence that β-endorphin is present in a single set of neurons in the arcuate region of the hypothalamus. In other regions with relatively high β-endorphin concentrations, such as the periventricular thalamus, periaqueductal gray, medial amygdala, locus coeruleus and others, the β-endorphin-like immunoreactivity occurs not in cell bodies but in fibers which are considered to be long axonal projections from the arcuate region of the hypothalamus.

The strikingly different distribution of the enkephalins and β-endorphin provided the first suggestion that the biosynthesis of enkephalins is not via βLPH and β-endorphin. There is now considerable evidence for a biosynthetic pathway for enkephalins that is quite different from that of β-endorphin.

Outside of the CNS the opioid peptides have been found in a number of tissues such as the intestinal tract, the pituitary (high in β-endorphin), and the adrenals (high in enkephalins).

MULTIPLE OPIATE RECEPTORS

This is an area of investigation that has recently evoked considerable interest. The question of how many opiate receptors exist, and their functions and endogenous ligands, is of great theoretical as well as practical importance. The latter is especially true if receptors with a degree of functional specificity can be found. The synthesis of highly specific ligands for one receptor class would then become possible and could provide drugs of clinical importance, such as analgesics with low addiction potential. The existence of several endogenous opiate receptor ligands and the finding that multiple receptors exist for classical neurotransmitters such as acetylcholine and catecholamines stimulated an examination of the possible existence of two or more opiate receptors.

Pharmacologic differences between morphine and certain synthetic analogues observed by Martin and collaborators [53] in chronic spinal dog preparations

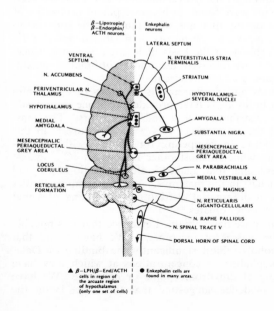

FIGURE 2. Localization of the enkephalins and of β-endorphin in rat brain. (From Barchas et al.[49] Reprinted by permission.)

suggested the existence of three types of opiate receptors, which they named μ for morphine, κ for ketocyclazocine, and σ for SKF 10047.

After the discovery of the enkephalins Kosterlitz's group [54] found an interesting paradox in the potency of opiates and enkephalins in two bioassay systems. Opiates were more potent than enkephalins in inhibiting electrically induced contractions in the guinea pig ileum, while the reverse was true in the isolated mouse vas deferens. They concluded that two different receptor types predominate in the two tissues: A receptor in the guinea pig ileum that prefers morphine and its congeners, which they called μ (in analogy to Martin's μ receptor), and one that prefers enkephalins in the mouse vas deferens, which they called δ (for deferens).

The same group found evidence for a similar or identical receptor heterogeneity from receptor binding studies in guinea pig brain homogenate. When labeled opiates were used, unlabeled opiates competed more effectively for binding than enkephalins, while unlabeled enkephalins were better competitors for the binding of labeled enkephalins. These findings have been confirmed in our laboratory [55] and that of others.[56] However, such competition studies do not rule out other explanations such as binding to a single class of receptors. The difference in competitive efficacy could then be explained by a difference in the functional groups and/or types of chemical bonds by which different classes of ligands bind to the receptors. This possibility is given credence by the biochemical similarity of the μ and δ receptors. Thus, each has a single SH group with a similar half-time of inactivation by N-ethylmaleimide, and both putative receptor types are equally sensitive to proteases and phospholipases and a number of reagents including phenoxybenzamine.

There are now, however, several lines of evidence that support the distinctness of these receptor classes. One approach makes use of the ability of receptor ligands to protect against irreversible receptor inactivation. Robson and Kosterlitz [57] used phenoxybenzamine as the irreversible inhibitor while we used NEM.[58] In both cases enkephalins were found to be more potent protectors of ^{3}H-enkephalin binding, whereas opiate alkaloids were found to be superior in protecting binding when it was measured by means of a labeled opiate (^{3}H-naloxone). This is difficult to explain on the basis of a single receptor, since, once inhibitor and protective agent are removed, the amount of binding remaining should not depend on the ligand used to measure it.

Cross competition experiments and measurements of ratios of enkephalin to naloxone binding in different brain areas have provided evidence most easily explained by differences in the distribution of μ and δ receptors. The most striking result was obtained for the thalamus of rats [55] and humans.[59] In this area naloxone is almost as effective in competing for binding with ^{3}H-Leu-enkephalin as with ^{3}H-naloxone, while in most other regions its IC_{50} against Leu-enkephalin is 10 to 20 times higher than against itself. The ratio of μ ligand to δ ligand binding is also the highest in the thalamus. Autoradiographic studies have also led to the conclusion of differential distribution of binding sites that prefer enkephalins and those that prefer opiates.[60, 61]

Very recently in our laboratory we have obtained evidence that it is possible to inhibit selectively one of the classes of receptors.[62] We have found that ethanol and other aliphatic alcohols inhibit significantly the binding of Dala^2 D-Leu^5 enkephalin (or Leu-enkephalin) at concentrations at which they have little or no effect on the binding of dihydromorphine or naloxone. We have accumulated several pieces of evidence suggesting that the effect is on the receptor and not on the peptide ligand. Perhaps the most compelling evidence comes from experiments with NG108-15 cells in culture. These cells have been reported to contain essentially only receptors of the δ type. In these cells the selective inhibition of enkephalin binding is not seen. There is, in fact, somewhat greater inhibition of naloxone and dihydromorphine binding. These data indicate that it is possible to inhibit one of the putative subclasses of opiate receptors selectively with reagents that are not ligands of the receptors. Other types of evidence for the distinctiveness of μ and δ receptors have been obtained, but space limitations do not permit us to summarize them.

Evidence for the existence of κ receptors, originally postulated by Martin, is now also becoming available. Using highly specific ligands for μ receptors and the relatively specific δ ligand D-Ala²D-Leu⁵-enkephalin, both Chang et al.[63] and Kosterlitz and coworkers [64] have been able to show the presence of binding sites in the brain that have high affinity for benzomorphans, such as ethylketocyclazocine and bremazocine.

The σ binding site, postulated by Martin to be responsible for the psychotomimetic effects of SKF-10047 and related opiates, may also exist, but evidence for this from binding data is still preliminary and controversial. Nevertheless, Zukin and Zukin [65] have very interesting results which suggest that the PCP binding site discovered by them [66] and by Vincent et al.[67] may also be the σ opiate receptor.

CONCLUDING REMARKS

It is clearly impossible to review a field as active as this one in one short paper. I have had to choose aspects of the field I wanted to include and hope that I have chosen aspects that are of interest to the readers of this volume. This paper is meant to form a framework for the papers to follow, which seek to implicate the endogenous opioid system in the etiology of mental diseases.

It should be obvious from this discussion that we know quite a lot about the structures, properties, metabolism, and distribution of the opioid peptides and their receptors. However, we know disappointingly little about the most important question, namely, how this system functions and what role it plays in the CNS and in other tissues in which it is found. There is strong circumstantial evidence, but no proof, that some opioid peptides may function as neurotransmitters or neuromodulators. The evidence for this was summarized earlier.

What provoked investigators to postulate a role for endogenous opioids in mental disease? First of all, there is the inevitable sequence of events that follows the discovery of new substances. Such substances are invariably investigated with respect to a possible role in diseases of unknown etiology. More often than not evidence for such a role in at least one such disease is reported and is sufficiently compelling to stimulate much work in order to prove or lay to rest the initial claim. In the present case there was a series of intriguing reports. The catatonic effects of β-endorphin, discussed earlier, stimulated the administration of opiate antagonists to schizophrenic patients. The observation by Terenius and coworkers that the levels of opioid substances of unknown structure were increased in the spinal fluid of schizophrenic patients also seemed to suggest an overabundance of endorphins.

Experiments in which endorphins were administered to patients with mental disease, both schizophrenia and affective disorders, seemed to show some improvement in the patients' clinical symptoms. These experiments, it must be noted, by the authors' own admission, were not well controlled. Nevertheless, the results clearly called for more carefully controlled studies to be done. The recent studies by De Wied and coworkers are intriguing. They demonstrate ameliorating effects on schizophrenic symptoms by des-Tyr-γ endorphin (DTE). This peptide has properties similar to those of haloperidol and has been suggested to be an endogenous neuroleptic, the shortage of which may produce schizophrenia. What makes this result so puzzling is the fact that DTE is neither a ligand of the opiate receptor nor of the class of dopamine receptors (antagonist receptors) that bind neuroleptics with high affinity. All of these results are surely beyond the scope of this review and will undoubtedly be discussed in detail and far more competently by others.

Let me end by stating that this is an area of research that is very difficult, but potentially very rewarding. It has been extremely difficult to make a connection between known neurotransmitters and disease. In fact, in only a very few cases is such a connection established with virtual certainty (dopamine in Parkinson's disease, acetylcholine receptors in myasthenia gravis, and possibly dopamine in schizophrenia). It is obviously even more difficult to implicate a novel system of peptides and their receptors, whose function is as yet unknown, in human disease. Nevertheless, these studies must be pursued, as must the basic research that will lead to an understanding of the function of the opioid system.

REFERENCES

1. SIMON, E. J., J. M. HILLER & I. EDELMAN. 1973. Proc. Natl. Acad. Sci. USA **70:** 1947–1949.
2. TERENIUS, L. 1973. Acta Pharmacol. Toxicol. **32:** 317–320.
3. PERT, C. B. & S. H. SNYDER. 1973. Science **179:** 1011–1014.
4. STEFANO, G. B., R. M. KREAM & R. S. ZUKIN. 1980. Brain Res. **181:** 440–445.
5. STAHL, K. D., W. VAN BEVER, P. JANSSEN & E. J. SIMON. 1977. Eur. J. Pharmacol. **46:** 199–205.
6. CREESE, I. & S. H. SNYDER. 1975. J. Pharmacol. Exp. Ther. **194:** 205–219.
7. PASTERNAK, G. W. & S. H. SNYDER. 1973. Mol. Pharmacol. **10:** 183–193.
8. PERT, C. B., G. PASTERNAK & S. H. SNYDER. 1973. Science **182:** 1359–1361.
9. SIMON, E. J., J. M. HILLER, J. GROTH & I. EDELMAN. 1975. J. Pharmacol. Exp. Ther. **192:** 531–537.
10. SIMON, E. J. & J. GROTH. 1975. Proc. Natl. Acad. Sci. USA **2:** 2404–2407.
11. ZUKIN, R. S. & R. M. KREAM. 1979. Proc. Natl. Acad. Sci. USA **76:** 1593–1597.
12. RUEGG, U. T., J. M. HILLER & E. J. SIMON. 1980. Eur. J. Pharmacol. **64:** 367–368.
13. RUEGG, U. T., S. CUENOD, J. M. HILLER, T. GIOANNINI, R. D. HOWELLS & E. J. SIMON. 1981. Proc. Natl. Acad. Sci. USA **78:** 4635–4638.
14. SIMONDS, W. F., G. KOSKI, R. A. STREATY, L. M. HJELMELAND & W. A. KLEE. 1980. Proc. Natl. Acad. Sci. USA **77:** 4623–4627.
15. BIDLACK, J. M. & L. G. ABOOD. 1980. Life Sci. **27:** 331–340.
16. HOWELLS, R. D., T. GIOANNINI, J. M. HILLER & E. J. SIMON. 1982. J. Pharmacol. Exp. Ther. In press.

17. GIOANNINI, T., B. FOUCAUD, J. M. HILLER, M. E. HATTEN & E. J. SIMON. 1982. Biochem. Biophys. Res. Commun. **105:** 1128–1134.
18. HILLER, J. M., J. PEARSON & E. J. SIMON. 1973. Commun. Chem. Pathol. Pharmacol. **6:** 1052–1062.
19. KUHAR, M. J., C. B. PERT & S. H. SNYDER. 1973. Nature **245:** 447–450.
20. ATWEH, S. F. & M. J. KUHAR. 1977. Brain Res. **125:** 43–67.
21. ATWEH, S. F. & M. J. KUHAR. 1977. Brain Res. **129:** 1–12.
22. ATWEH, S. F. & M. J. KUHAR. 1977. Brain Res. **134:** 393–405.
23. PEARSON, J., L. BRANDEIS, E. SIMON & J. HILLER. 1980. Life Sci. **26:** 1047–1052.
24. ZIEGLGANSBERGER, W. & J. P. FRY. 1976. *In* Opiates and Endogenous Opioid Peptides. H. W. Kosterlitz, Ed.: 231–238. Elsevier/North-Holland Biomedical Press. Amsterdam.
25. LA MOTTE, C., C. B. PERT & S. H. SNYDER. 1976. Brain Res. **112:** 407–412.
26. HILLER, J. M., E. J. SIMON, S. M. CRAIN & E. R. PETERSON. 1978. Brain Res. **145:** 396–400.
27. HUGHES, J. 1975. Brain Res. **88:** 295–308.
28. TERENIUS, L. & A. WAHLSTRÖM. 1975. Acta Physiol. Scand. **94:** 74–81.
29. TESCHEMACHER, H., K. E. OPHEIM, B. M. COX & A. GOLDSTEIN. 1975. Life Sci. **16:** 1771–1776.
30. HUGHES, J., T. W. SMITH, H. W. KOSTERLITZ, L. A. FOTHERGILL, B. A. MORGAN & H. R. MORRIS. 1975. Nature **258:** 577–579.
31. LING, N., R. BURGIS & R. GUILLEMIN. 1976. Proc. Natl. Acad. Sci. USA **73:** 3942–3946.
32. BRADBURY, A. F., D. G. SMYTH, C. R. SNELL, N. J. M. BIRDSALL & E. C. HULME. 1976. Nature **260:** 793–795.
33. COX, B. M., A. GOLDSTEIN & C. H. LI. 1976. Proc. Natl. Acad. Sci. USA **73:** 1821–1823.
34. KANGAWA, K., H. MATSUO & M. IGANASHI. 1979. Biochem. Biophys. Res. Commun. **86:** 153–160.
35. GOLDSTEIN, A., S. TACHIBANA, L. I. LOWNEY, M. HUNKAPILLER & L. HOOD. 1979. Proc. Natl. Acad. Sci. USA **76:** 6666–6670.
36. GOLDSTEIN, A., W. FISCHLI, L. I. LOWNEY, M. HUNKAPILLER & L. HOOD. 1981. Proc. Natl. Acad. Sci. USA. **78:** 7219–7223.
37. BLOOM, F., D. SEGAL, N. LING & R. GUILLEMIN. 1976. Science **194:** 630–632.
38. JACQUET, Y. F. & N. MARKS. 1976. Science **194:** 632–635.
39. DE WIED, D., B. BOHUS, J. M. VAN REE, G. L. KOVACS & H. M. GREVEN. 1978. Lancet **i:** 1046.
40. TAUBE, H. D., E. BOROWSKI, T. ENDO & K. STARKE. 1976. Eur. J. Pharmacol. **38:** 377–380.
41. SUBRAMANIAN, N., P. MITZNEGG, W. SPRUGEL, W. DOMSCHKE, S. DOMSCHKE, E. WUNSCH & L. DEMLING. 1977. Naunyn-Schmiedeberg's Arch. Pharmacol. **299:** 163–165.
42. JESSEL, T. M. & L. L. IVERSEN. 1977. Nature **268:** 549–551.
43. ELDE, R., T. HÖKFELT, O. JOHANSSON & L. TERENIUS. 1976. Neuroscience **1:** 349–351.
44. OSBORNE, H., V. HOLLT & A. HERZ. 1978. Eur. J. Pharmacol. **48:** 219–221.
45. HENDERSON, G., J. HUGHES & H. W. KOSTERLITZ. 1978. Nature **271:** 677–679.
46. IVERSEN, L. L., S. D. IVERSEN, F. E. BLOOM, T. VARGO & R. GUILLEMIN. 1978. Nature **271:** 679–680.
47. ALUMETS, J., R. HAKANSON, F. SUNDLER & J. THORELL. 1979. Nature **279:** 805–806.
48. ZIPSER, B. 1980. Nature **283:** 857–858.

49. BARCHAS, J. D., H. AKIL, G. R. ELLIOTT, R. B. HOLMAN & S. S. WATSON. 1978. Science **200**: 964–973.
50. HÖKFELT, T., R. ELDE, O. JOHANSSON, L. TERENIUS & L. STEIN. 1977. Neurosci. Lett. **5**: 25–31.
51. BLOOM, F., E. BATTENBERG, J. ROSSIER, N. LING & R. GUILLEMIN. 1978. Proc. Natl. Acad. Sci. USA **75**: 1591–1595.
52. WATSON, S. J., J. D. BARCHAS & C. H. LI. 1977. Proc. Natl. Acad. Sci. USA **74**: 5155–5158.
53. MARTIN, W. R., C. G. EADES, J. A. THOMPSON, R. E. HUPPLER & P. E. GILBERT. 1976. J. Pharmacol. Exp. Ther. **197**: 517–532.
54. LORD, J. A. H., A. A. WATERFIELD, J. HUGHES & H. W. KOSTERLITZ. 1977. Nature **267**: 495–499.
55. SIMON, E. J., K. A. BONNET, S. M. CRAIN, J. GROTH, J. M. HILLER & J. R. SMITH. 1980. *In* Advances in Biochemical Psychopharmacology. E. Costa & M. Trabucchi, Eds. **22**: 335–346. Raven Press. New York.
56. CHANG, K.-J. & P. CUATRECASAS. 1979. J. Biol. Chem. **254**: 2610–2618.
57. ROBSON, L. E. & H. W. KOSTERLITZ. 1979. Proc. Roy. Soc. Lond. Ser. B. **205**: 425–432.
58. SMITH, J. R. & E. J. SIMON. 1980. Proc. Natl. Acad. Sci. USA **77**: 281–284.
59. BONNET, K. A., J. GROTH, T. GIOANNINI, M. CORTES & E. J. SIMON. 1981. Brain Res. **221**: 437–440.
60. GOODMAN, R. R., S. H. SNYDER, M. J. KUHAR & W. S. YOUNG, III. 1980. Proc. Natl. Acad. Sci. USA **77**: 6239–6242.
61. HERKENHAM, M. & C. B. PERT. 1980. Proc. Natl. Acad. Sci. USA **77**: 5532–5536.
62. HILLER, J. M., L. M. ANGEL & E. J. SIMON. 1981. Science **214**: 468–469.
63. CHANG, K.-J., E. HAZUM & P. CUATRECASAS. 1981. Proc. Natl. Acad. Sci. USA. **78**: 4141–4145.
64. KOSTERLITZ, H. W., S. J. PATERSON & L. E. ROBSON. 1981. Br. J. Pharmacol. **73**: 939–949.
65. ZUKIN, R. S. & S. R. ZUKIN. 1981. Mol. Pharmacol. **20**: 246–254.
66. ZUKIN, S. R. & R. S. ZUKIN. 1980. Proc. Natl. Acad. Sci. USA **76**: 5372–5376.
67. VINCENT, J. P., B. KARTALOVSKI, P. GENESTE, J. M. KAMENKO & M. LADZUNSKI. 1980. Proc. Natl. Acad. Sci. USA **76**: 4678–4682.

DISCUSSION OF THE PAPER

J. KAUFMAN (*Johns Hopkins University, Baltimore, MD*): To what do you attribute the effect of alcohol on the receptor? It seems such an innocuous reagent.

E. J. SIMON: It is not only innocuous, but we are also quite sure that it does not react with the opiate binding site. At the moment our hypothesis is the simplest one, and that is that alcohol does what it has been thought to do for some years, which is to increase the fluidity of the cell membrane. For reasons that we do not quite understand, the opiate δ receptors are more sensitive to this change than are the μ receptors. Perhaps for some reason their conformation is not as rigid and gets disturbed by this perturbation of the membrane.

UNIDENTIFIED SPEAKER: Is it possible that the alcohol does not distinguish between receptors, but between peptides and alkaloids? Also, have you any labeled β-endorphin?

SIMON: We carefully looked into that question, but I did not have time to give you the evidence. We feel that the effect is on the receptor and not on the peptides, because FK, the Sandoz peptide, which is a μ-preferring peptide, is much less inhibited than, for instance, enkephalin. Also, in NG 108 cells, the neuroblastoma glioma hybrids which are reputed to have virtually only δ type receptors, the difference in inhibition between the alkaloid and enkephalin disappears. If anything, the alkaloid is a little bit more inhibited. So we do not think that the inhibition is an effect on the peptide. It is an effect on the receptor.

As to your second question, we do not have any labeled β-endorphin and therefore have done no β-endorphin binding. We have done only the binding of FK and enkephalin.

K. VEREBEY (NY State Division of Substance Abuse Services, Brooklyn): Dr. Simon, since you did not have time to discuss the distribution of the receptors and their behavioral correlations, please make a brief statement on that issue.

SIMON: It is clear that for purposes of this discussion there are very high levels of both enkephalin and opiate receptors in the limbic system, which is clearly the area where affect and emotion occur. And, while Mark Gold cautioned about being too eager to interpret the distribution—he is quite right, one has to be careful—it is still encouraging to find such high levels of these receptors and their ligands in these areas.

That is about all you can say about what distribution may mean. Clearly, at this conference we are faced with the very difficult task of discussing the possible involvement of this system in mental disease. It is an area of great importance and great difficulty. One of these days I think that we are going to get some real answers.

MULTIPLE OPIATE RECEPTORS AND THEIR DIFFERENT LIGAND PROFILES *

Martin W. Adler

Department of Pharmacology
Temple University School of Medicine
Philadelphia, Pennsylvania 19140

Despite the fact that the analgesic and euphorigenic properties of opium and its principal alkaloid, morphine, have been known for centuries, it was only in the last few years that we were able to achieve some insight into how that drug exerts its effects. In an attempt to find agents that have greater analgesic potency than morphine, but fewer undesirable features such as addiction liability, respiratory depression, and constipation, a large number of structurally related compounds were synthesized. Other agents bore little, if any, structural relationship to morphine, but shared many properties with the opium alkaloid. With the work of Goldstein [1] and the identification of the opiate receptor in 1973 in the laboratories of Simon,[2] Terenius,[3] and Snyder,[4] we had the first biochemical evidence that a specific receptor molecule was involved in opiate effects.

The discovery of the two pentapeptides (Met- and Leu-enkephalin) and β-endorphin led us to wonder whether all endogenous ligands interact with the same receptor. Indeed, can all opiate drug effects be attributed to actions on a single receptor? Clearly, the answer to these questions has great theoretical and practical importance, for the implication of more than one receptor type would set the stage for the design of drugs with only certain specific opiate effects. Interestingly enough, several investigators [5-8] postulated the existence of multiple receptors even before the biochemical discovery of the receptor in 1973. These suggestions of receptor heterogeneity culminated with the proposal by Martin [9, 10] that there were three opiate receptor types: μ, κ, and σ. Of course, we have ample evidence that receptor subtypes can coexist within a given system (for example, acetylcholinergic, noradrenergic, histaminergic). Although the availability of specific antagonists is a prime prerequisite for the "proof" of subtypes, other lines of evidence, such as differences in pA_2,[11] are strongly indicative of such a subdivision. Perhaps the most useful technique at the present time involves an examination of the profiles of drug action. By profiling a wide variety of opioids, both exogenous and endogenous, we can begin to sort them out according to their common actions on various systems. This is not to say that simply because two drugs produce the same overall effect on a particular measure, these drugs act on the same receptor. For example, they could be acting at two different receptors that normally have opposing functions, with one drug producing an agonist effect at one of the receptors and the other drug producing an antagonist effect at the second receptor. (An illustration of this is seen in the autonomic nervous system, where a parasympathetic drug will frequently produce a response similar to that seen following the administra-

* This work was supported by Grant DA 00376 from the National Institute on Drug Abuse.

0077-8923/82/0398-0340 $01.75/0 © 1982 NYAS

tion of an adrenergic blocking agent). Nevertheless, if a series of compounds can be categorized according to their similarities and differences in effects on several systems, the implication is that such a category may well represent a different receptor type.

Important for the profile and, in fact, for determining whether a response is receptor-mediated is the demonstration of stereospecificity. One would expect that the effect would reside wholly or predominantly in only one member of an enantiomer pair. Another critical step in profiling drug actions at a receptor is the determination of sensitivity to antagonist blockade. In the case of the opioids, our knowledge in this area has been restricted, to a great extent, to the use of the competitive, reversible antagonist, naloxone (or naltrexone, a compound with actions almost identical to those of naloxone). Although the enantiomers of naloxone can be used to verify receptor specificity, naloxone has at least some degree of antagonist properties at all postulated opiate receptor subtypes.[12, 13] Indeed, many investigators believe that sensitivity to naloxone antagonism is an absolute criterion for defining opiate receptors. On the basis of pharmacologic principles and experience with other receptor systems this seems to be an unnecessarily restrictive condition. Nevertheless, naloxone sensitivity is a valuable first approach. It should be noted that naloxone seems to have considerably less activity at the σ receptor than at the others. Recently, more specific and long-acting, irreversible antagonists for the μ receptor have been synthesized (β-CNA,[14] β-FNA,[15] naloxazone [16]). Rounding out the profile is the examination of development of tolerance and cross-tolerance to the opioids. One would certainly expect to see cross-tolerance among members of a group that act on the same receptor type; lack of cross-tolerance would implicate the involvement of different receptors.

TABLE 1 illustrates some of the characteristics of the three opioid prototype drugs as defined by Martin [9, 10] using the chronic spinal dog model. In this scheme, morphine is thought to act primarily at the μ receptors, ethylketazocine at κ receptors, and SKF10,047 (N-allylnormetazocine) at σ receptors. Much of the history of this approach is discussed in a recent paper by Martin.[17]

Our work in categorizing opiates using the flurothyl seizure test in rats began about the time that Martin's classification appeared. We had earlier reported [18] that the morphine-abstinence syndrome could be characterized by a decrease in seizure threshold. Since the symptoms of abstinence are often the opposite of the acute effects of the drug, we reasoned that morphine would be anti-convulsant in the rat. As expected, a dose-related anticonvulsant response to

TABLE 1

SOME CHARACTERISTICS OF OPIOID PROTOTYPES IN CHRONIC SPINAL DOG *

	Morphine	Ketazocine	N-allylnormetazocine
Body temperature	Hypothermia	Slight hypothermia	Slight hyperthermia
Pupils	Miosis	Miosis	Mydriasis
Respiratory rate	Increased	No effect	Increased
Flexor reflex	Marked depression	Marked depression	Slight depression
Skin twitch reflex	Marked depression	Modest depression	No depression

* After Martin et al.[9] and Martin.[17]

acute morphine administration was found.[19] We then decided to use the rat flurothyl seizure as a test to evaluate a wide variety of opioids. The procedure involves administration of hexafluorodiethylether (flurothyl) to a rat placed into a closed jar. Convulsions are produced by inhalation of the flurothyl, the time from onset of the infusion to occurrence of a clonic convulsion with loss of posture constituting the measure of seizure threshold. Details of the procedure may be found in other papers from this laboratory.[20] We found that the opioids could be divided into four groups on the basis of their effect on flurothyl seizure threshold and the ability of naloxone to block the effect.[21] The classification is summarized in TABLE 2. Stereospecificity and tolerance development are also shown. The effects were stereospecific for the two groups that showed anticonvulsant activity. For example, only the *l* form of methadone was effective as an anticonvulsant, and the *l* form of cyclazocine was more effective than was the *d* form. Receptor specificity is further demonstrated by the fact that the antagonism to the anticonvulsant effect of the first group by naloxone occurred only with the *l* form of naloxone, *d*-naloxone having been ineffective. In the case of pentazocine, the *d* form was more effective as a proconvulsant than was the *l* form of the drug, although both enantiomers had activity.

Of obvious interest is the question of whether or not the endogenous opioid peptides alter the seizure threshold, and if so, into which category(ies) they fall. We have shown [22] that intracerebroventricularly (ICV) administered β-endorphin, D-Ala²-D-Leu⁵-enkephalin and D-Ala²-Met-enkephalinamide all produce an anticonvulsant effect on this test that is similar to that seen with a drug such as etorphine (FIG. 1). Naloxone antagonized the anticonvulsant effect of all of these drugs, but it was less effective in blocking the anticonvulsant effect of β-endorphin than in blocking etorphine or the pentapeptides. These results can be seen in TABLE 3.

Another simple, yet effective, means of separating the opioids into groups is based on their effects on body temperature. A report from our laboratory [23] noted that the opioids could be subdivided into several groups according to effects on the body temperature of rats at an ambient temperature of 20° C. Naloxone blockade was an important element in determining this classification. The groupings are somewhat similar to those found with the flurothyl seizure threshold test. Thus, the well-known dual effect of morphine on body temperature in the rat [24] (that is, low-dose hyperthermia; high-dose hypothermia) is shared by drugs such as methadone and levorphanol. On the other hand, ethylketazocine (EK) produced a very marked hypothermia, while SKF 10,047 had virtually no effect on body temperature at 20° C.[23] Although naloxone blocked both phases of the morphine dual effect, it only partially blocked the EK-induced drop in temperature. With respect to the endogenous substances, we found that D-Ala²-Met-enkephalinamide produced naloxone-sensitive hyperthermia at low doses and hypothermia at high doses, responses like those to morphine, methadone, and levorphanol. In the cat, Clark and Ponder,[25, 26] using the tools of naloxone blockade and alteration of ambient temperature, have also found support for the multiple-receptor hypothesis. Ethylketazocine and pentazocine appear to act on the same receptors, which are distinct from those stimulated by morphine. D-Ala²-Met-enkephalinamide, which predominantly produced a dose-related hyperthermia, was hypothermic at high dosages and at low ambient temperature. Both the hypo- and hyperthermia could be antagonized by naloxone, thus implicating yet another receptor type different from

TABLE 2

CLASSIFICATION OF OPIOIDS ON THE BASIS OF THE RAT FLUROTHYL SEIZURE THRESHOLD TEST

Group	Compounds	Dose Range (mg/kg, s.c.)	Characteristics of Group
I	Morphine sulfate Methadone hydrochloride Etorphine hydrochloride Levorphanol tartrate Phenazocine hydrobromide Buprenorphine hydrochloride	12.5 – 64.0 1.25 – 5.0 0.005– 0.02 2.5 – 20.0 0.5 – 5.0 0.004– 12.5	Anticonvulsant; dose-related; sensitive to naloxone blockade; stereospecific (l-enantiomer more effective); tolerance develops; cross-tolerance with other members of the group
II	SKF 10,047 (N-allylnormetazocine) Cyclazocine	10.0 – 40.0 1.0 – 5.0	Anticonvulsant; dose-related; not blocked by naloxone (10 mg/kg); stereospecific (l-enantiomer more effective); no tolerance
III	Ethylketazocine methanesulfonate Ketazocine methanesulfonate Moxazocine tartrate Cyclorphan hydrochloride Normorphine hydrochloride Norcyclazocine Nalbuphine hydrochloride Naloxone hydrochloride Nalorphine hydrochloride	0.5 – 50.0 0.5 – 20.0 12.5 – 50.0 1.0 – 80.0 50.0 –100.0 6.25 – 25.0 5.0 – 20.0 1.0 – 10.0 25.0 –100.0	Small effect, not significant, not dose-related
IV	Meperidine hydrochloride Pentazocine hydrochloride Normeperidine hydrochloride Anileridine hydrochloride	12.5 – 50.0 12.5 – 50.0 1.56 – 50.0 6.25 – 25	Proconvulsant effect; dose-related; potentiated or not blocked by 10 mg/kg naloxone; stereospecific (d-pentazocine more effective than l); no tolerance

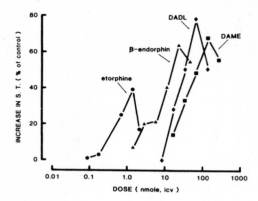

FIGURE 1. Dose-related effect of etorphine, β-endorphin, D-Ala²-D-Leu⁵-enkephalin (DADL) and D-Ala²-Met-enkephalinamide (DAME) on seizure threshold (S.T.) in rats.

that for morphine, which causes only naloxone-sensitive hyperthermia in the cat.

Pupillary effects of opioids are a well-recognized characteristic of this group of drugs. In the chronic spinal dog model, Martin *et al.*[9] showed that pupils were constricted by μ and κ agents, while σ-receptor agonists produced dilation. In the rat, morphine caused a dose-related mydriasis accompanied by fluctuation of pupil size.[27] Utilizing the rat pupil, we determined that representatives from each of our four groups produced different effects in terms of pupillary size, fluctuation, eye movement, and sensitivity to naloxone blockade. These differences are shown in TABLE 4. With respect to the enkephalins, D-Ala-D-Leu-, Met-, and Leu-enkephalin all produced mydriasis in mice,[28] and D-Ala²-Met-enkephalinamide caused miosis in rabbits.[29] It is interesting to note that Met- and Leu-enkephalin produced pupillary mydriasis and fluctuation after intraperitoneal administration in rats.[30] The effects, in all ways including naloxone blockade, are similar to those of morphine.

TABLE 3

NALOXONE BLOCKADE OF ANTICONVULSANT EFFECTS OF INTRACEREBROVENTRICULARLY ADMINISTERED OPIOIDS

Naloxone (mg/kg, s.c.)	Saline Solution (7 μl)	Etorphine (0.8 μg)	DADL (40 μg)	DAME (40 μg)	β-Endorphin (80 μg)
0	385 ± 11	547 ± 38	653 ± 43	624 ± 27	623 ± 33
0.001	—	491 ± 33	631 ± 29	—	—
0.01	—	392 ± 29 *	481 ± 51 *	695 ± 19	552 ± 51
0.1	—	395 ± 24 *	371 ± 19 †	374 ± 12 †	495 ± 37 *
1.0	—	—	—	379 ± 36 †	454 + 36 *
10.0	387 ± 6	—	—	—	348 + 5 †

* Significantly different from animals given no naloxone: * $p < 0.05$, Student's t test (two-tailed).

† Significantly different from animals given no naloxone: $p < 0.02$; Student's t test (two-tailed).

TABLE 4

EFFECTS OF REPRESENTATIVE OPIOIDS ON THE RAT PUPIL

Drug	Dose (mg/kg, s.c.)	Mydriasis	Fluctuation	Nystagmus	Stereospecificity	Naloxone Reversal
Morphine sulfate	32.0	++	+	0		1 mg/kg
Methadone HCl	2.5	++	+	0	+	1 mg/kg
Pentazocine HCl	25.0	++	0	0	+	1 mg/kg (partial)
Cyclazocine	5.0	+	0	+	+	10 mg/kg (partial)
Ethylketazocine methanesulfonate	10.0	+	++	0		10 mg/kg (partial)

Looking at the electroencephalographic effects of these compounds and the susceptibility of the resulting actions to naloxone blockade provides another basis upon which opioids can be differentiated from one another.[31] This categorization can be seen in TABLE 5. Note that the enkephalins and β-endorphin produced responses that are essentially indistinguishable from those of morphine.

TABLE 5

EFFECTS OF OPIOIDS AND ENDOPIOIDS ON EEG OF THE RAT

Drug and Route of Administration	EEG Behavioral Dissociation *	Biphasic Profile †	Naloxone Sensitivity
Morphine (SC)	+	+	++
Ethylketazocine (SC)	+	+	+++
Cyclazocine (SC)	+	−	+
N-Allylnormetazocine (SC)	+	−	+
Morphine (ICV)	+	+	++
D-Ala²-Met-enkephalinamide (ICV)	+	+	++
D-Ala²-D-Leu⁵-enkephalin (ICV)	+	+	++
β-Endorphin (ICV)	++	+	+

* EEG-behavioral dissociation refers to the high-voltage, slow-frequency EEG (EEG slowing) produced by narcotics in the awake, stuporous rat (in contrast to EEG slowing in a sleeping rat).

† Biphasic profile refers to initial phase of EEG synchrony and stupor followed by a period of EEG activation and behavioral arousal.

Analgesic tests have also been used to discriminate among opiate receptors. Tyers [32] showed in rats and mice that μ-receptor agonists were very effective in tests which use heat as the nociceptive stimulus, while κ agonists were inactive, except at doses high enough to produce sedation and motor incapacitation. On tests that employ nonheat noxious stimuli, such as paw pressure and chemical writhing, however, both μ and κ agonists had activity. In the chronic spinal dog model,[9] μ-receptor agonists depressed both the flexor reflex (a pressure test) and skin twitch response (a heat test), whereas κ-receptor agonists depressed the flexor reflex, but did not markedly alter the skin twitch response. Pure sigma-receptor agonists seem to have little analgesic activity regardless of the test used.

Reference should also be made to a number of behavioral tests, some of them quite complex, that can distinguish among the opioids. Such measures range from rather simple locomotor activity [33] and Y-maze performance in rats [34] to discriminative stimulus tests in rats, monkeys, and pigeons.[35, 36] Drug discrimination procedures involve training animals, in any of several types of response–choice paradigms, to discriminate between a drug and saline solution or a second drug. Opioids have been classified into groups according to their ability to generalize or not generalize to other opioids on the basis of these tests. It has been suggested that their discriminative stimulus effects in animals bear a striking similarity to the subjective effects of these drugs in man.[37] Much of the work using discriminative properties of narcotics to determine the characteristics of opioid receptor subtypes is summarized in a recent comprehensive review by Herling and Woods.[37] The results of these studies provide yet further evidence that three or four types of opiate receptors probably exist.

Thus far, information has been presented on qualitative and quantitative acute effects of opioids and endopioids, stereospecificity, and naloxone sensitivity, all of which have helped to categorize and profile these groups of drugs. As previously mentioned, an important additional means of profiling drugs entails the study of the development of tolerance and the testing of cross-tolerance to other drugs. Although our knowledge on this aspect of testing is relatively meager, we can list some findings in this area. In regard to seizure thresholds in rats, tolerance developed to the anticonvulsant effects of levorphanol and cross-tolerance occurred to morphine. No cross-tolerance was seen to cyclazocine or meperidine.[21] Tolerance and cross-tolerance to the analgesic effects of opioids are seen among many members of this class of drugs. The reason for the more ubiquitous cross-tolerance in regard to analgesia compared with other actions is not known, but may well be indicative of the involvement of more than one receptor type in the analgesic effect. Cross-tolerance between morphine and the endorphins and between β-endorphin and the enkephalins has been demonstrated.[38-40]

Thus, on consideration of such factors as the actions produced by these compounds, the sensitivity of these effects to naloxone blockade, stereospecificity of the effect, and tolerance and cross-tolerance, it is readily apparent that the opioids can be divided into groups. The first group consists of drugs such as morphine, methadone, and levorphanol. In the chronic spinal dog model, these drugs produce a series of effects such as sedation, decreased body temperature, constriction of the pupils, and marked depression of the flexor reflex; in the rat, they are analgesic and anticonvulsant, they depress respiration, produce mydriasis accompanied by fluctuation, have a dual effect on body temperature (low-dose hyperthermia, high-dose hypothermia), are similarly perceived as discriminative stimuli, and produce biphasic EEG and behavioral profiles consisting of an initial phase of EEG synchrony and stupor followed by a period of EEG activation and behavioral arousal. Drugs in this group fully suppress the abstinence syndrome in withdrawn morphine-dependent monkeys [41] and dogs.[17] In all cases, the effects are blocked by naloxone, the *l* isomer is the active form of the drug, and tolerance has been observed to the effects of these compounds on all measures tested. In addition, cross-tolerance also seems to exist among members of this group.

The second group includes agents like ketazocine and ethylketazocine, which constrict the pupils of the chronic spinal dog, and which produce sedation, a slight decrease in body temperature, and a marked depression of the flexor reflex; in the rat, agents in this group have little or no effect on seizure threshold, decrease body temperature, are analgesic, and cause mydriasis with marked fluctuation. This group of drugs will not substitute for morphine in the dependent monkey [42-44] and will neither suppress abstinence nor precipitate withdrawal in the morphine-dependent dog.[17]

The third group, containing *N*-allylnormetazocine and cyclazocine, is characterized in the chronic spinal dog by a dilation of pupils, a slight elevation of body temperature, and a modest depression of the flexor reflex; in the rat, these drugs are anticonvulsant, they have little (cyclazocine) or no effect on body temperature, and they dilate the pupils and are somewhat analgesic. Although there is some overlap among this group and the other two in terms of discriminative effects, the dose of naloxone needed to antagonize drugs in this grouping is considerably greater. These drugs will precipitate abstinence in the morphine-dependent dog.[17]

The drugs profiled above seem to group together quite consistently, with only minor differences across tests and across species. It should be obvious that they are analogous to the μ-κ-σ classification of Martin. There are other compounds whose categorization is more difficult in terms of agreement among laboratories and tests. These drugs include pentazocine and meperidine. Whether or not separate receptors are involved with their actions, we do not as yet know.

As to where the endogenous opioid peptides fit, this is strictly a matter of conjecture at the moment. Virtually all of the evidence indicates that the enkephalins produce *in vivo* effects that are virtually inseparable from those seen with morphine and related opioids. Beta-endorphin may have slightly different properties, but the evidence is not clear on this point. Dynorphin is now being evaluated, since the 1–17 structure has only recently been identified by Goldstein.[45] One must also contend with the apparent inconsistency seen between *in vitro* testing compared with the *in vivo* tests. *In vitro* binding, as well as guinea pig ileum and mouse vas deferens assays, generally indicates the presence of several receptors, but these may or may not be identical to those detected with *in vivo* tests. For example, the μ category appears to be the same in the two types of tests, as does the σ. However, the δ classification achieved *in vitro* does not correspond to a known *in vivo* category. Further research will undoubtedly clarify the situation. Of prime importance is the discovery of more specific agonists and, even more importantly, the discovery of more specific antagonists.

ACKNOWLEDGMENT

I gratefully acknowledge the help of Ellen B. Geller in preparing this manuscript.

REFERENCES

1. GOLDSTEIN, A., L. I. LOWNEY & B. K. PAL. 1971. Stereospecific and nonspecific interactions of the morphine congener levorphanol in subcellular fractions of mouse brain. Proc. Natl. Acad. Sci. USA **68:** 1742–1747.
2. SIMON, E. J., J. M. HILLER & I. EDELMAN. 1973. Stereospecific binding of the potent narcotic analgesic [³H] etorphine to rat brain homogenate. Proc. Natl. Acad. Sci. USA **70:** 1947–1949.
3. TERENIUS, L. 1973. Stereospecific interaction between narcotic analgesics and a synaptic plasma membrane fraction of rat cerebral cortex. Acta. Pharmacol. Toxicol. **32:** 317–320.
4. PERT, C. B. & S. H. SNYDER. 1973. Opiate receptor: Demonstration in nervous tissue. Science **179:** 1011–1014.
5. PORTOGHESE, P. S. 1965. A new concept on the mode of interaction of narcotic analgesics with receptors. J. Med. Chem. **8:** 609–616.
6. MARTIN, W. R. 1967. Opioid antagonists. Pharmacol. Rev. **19:** 463–521.
7. SMITS, S. E. & A. E. TAKEMORI. 1970. Quantitative studies on the antagonism by naloxone of some narcotic and narcotic-antagonist analgesics. Br. J. Pharmacol. **39:** 627–638.
8. TAKEMORI, A. E., G. HAYASHI & S. E. SMITS. 1972. Studies on the quantitative antagonism of analgesics by naloxone and diprenorphine. Eur. J. Pharmacol. **20:** 85–92.
9. MARTIN, W. R., C. G. EADES, J. A. THOMPSON, R. E. HUPPLER & P. E. GILBERT. 1976. The effects of morphine- and nalorphine-like drugs in the nondependent and morphine-dependent chronic spinal dog. J. Pharmacol. Exp. Ther. **197:** 517–532.
10. GILBERT, P. E. & W. R. MARTIN. 1976. The effects of morphine- and nalorphine-like drugs in the nondependent, morphine-dependent and cyclazocine-dependent chronic spinal dog. J. Pharmacol. Exp. Ther. **198:** 66–82.
11. TALLARIDA, R. J., A. COWAN & M. W. ADLER. 1979. pA₂ and receptor differentiation: A statistical analysis of competitive antagonism. Life Sci. **25:** 637–654.
12. MARTIN, W. R. 1976. Naloxone. Ann. Int. Med. **85:** 765–768.
13. LORD, J. A. H., A. A. WATERFIELD, J. HUGHES & H. W. KOSTERLITZ. 1977. Endogenous opioid peptides: Multiple agonists and receptors. Nature **267:** 495–499.
14. PORTOGHESE, P. S., D. L. LARSON, J. B. JIANG, A. E. TAKEMORI & T. P. CARUSO. 1978. 6-N,N-bis(2-chlorethyl)amino-17-(cyclopropylmethyl)-4,5-epoxy-3, 14-dihydroxymorphinan (chlornaltrexamine), a potent opioid receptor alkylating agent with ultralong narcotic antagonist activity. J. Med. Chem. **21:** 598–599.
15. PORTOGHESE, P. S., D. L. LARSON, L. M. SAYRE, D. S. FRIES & A. E. TAKEMORI. 1980. A novel opioid receptor site directed alkylating agent with irreversible narcotic antagonistic and reversible agonistic activities. J. Med. Chem. **23:** 233–234.
16. PASTERNAK, G. W., S. R. CHILDERS & S. H. SNYDER. 1979. Multiple opiate receptors: Evidence for mediation of analgesia by a subpopulation of receptors. *In* Endogenous and Exogenous Opiate Agonists and Antagonists. E. L. Way, Ed.: 113–116. Pergamon Press. New York.
17. MARTIN, W. R. 1981. Multiple opioid receptors. Life Sci. **28:** 1547–1554.
18. ADLER, M. W., C. LIN, K. P. SMITH, R. TRESKY & P. L. GILDENBERG. 1974. Lowered seizure threshold as a part of the narcotic abstinence syndrome in rats. Psychopharmacologia **35:** 243–247.
19. ADLER, M. W., C. H. LIN, S. H. KEINATH, S. BRAVERMAN & E. B. GELLER. 1976. Anticonvulsant action of acute morphine administration in rats. J. Pharmacol. Exp. Ther. **198:** 655–660.

20. ADLER, M. W. 1975. Pharmacology of flurothyl: Laboratory and clinical applications. *In* Current Developments in Psychopharmacology. W. B. Essman and L. Valzelli, Eds. Vol. **2**: 30–61. Spectrum Publications. New York.
21. COWAN, A., E. B. GELLER & M. W. ADLER. 1979. Classification of opioids on the basis of change in seizure threshold in rats. Science **206**: 465–467.
22. TORTELLA, F. C., A. COWAN & M. W. ADLER. 1981. Comparison of the anticonvulsant effects of opioid peptides and etorphine in rats after icv administration. Life Sci. **10**: 1039–1045.
23. GELLER, E. B., C. HAWK, R. J. TALLARIDA & M. W. ADLER. 1982. Postulated thermoregulatory roles for different opiate receptors in rats. Life Sci. In press.
24. LOTTI, V. J., P. LOMAX & R. GEORGE. 1966. Heat production and heat loss in the rat following intracerebral and systemic administration of morphine. Int. J. Neuropharmacol. **5**: 75–83.
25. CLARK, W. G. & S. W. PONDER. 1980. Effects of centrally administered pentazocine and ethylketocyclazocine on thermoregulation in the cat. Brain Res. Bull. **5**: 615–618.
26. CLARK, W. G. & S. W. PONDER. 1980. Thermoregulatory effects of (D-ala²)-methionine-enkephalinamide in the cat. Evidence for multiple naloxone-sensitive opioid receptors. Brain Res. Bull. **5**: 415–420.
27. KLEMFUSS, H., R. J. TALLARIDA, C. H. ADLER & M. W. ADLER. 1979. Morphine-induced mydriasis and fluctuation in the rat: time and dose relationships. J. Pharmacol. Exp. Ther. **208**: 91–95.
28. KORCZYN, A. D., Y. ESHEL & O. KEREN. 1980. Enkephalin mydriasis in mice. Eur. J. Pharmacol. **65**: 285–287.
29. DRAGO, F., G. GORGONE, F. SPINA, G. PANISSIDI, A. DAL BELLO, F. MORO & U. SCAPAGNINI. 1980. Opiate receptors in the rabbit iris. Naunyn-Schmiedeberges Arch. Pharmakol. **315**: 1–4.
30. TORTELLA, F. C., A. COWAN & M. W. ADLER. 1980. Pupillary effects of leucine and methionine enkephalin in rats after intraperitoneal administration. Peptides **1**: 237–241.
31. TORTELLA, F. C., A. COWAN & M. W. ADLER. 1980. EEG and behavioral effects of ethylketocyclazocine, morphine and cyclazocine in rats: Differential sensitivities towards naloxone. Neuropharmacology **19**: 845–850.
32. TYERS, M. B. 1980. A classification of opiate receptors that mediate antinociception in animals. Br. J. Pharmacol. **69**: 503–512.
33. IWAMOTO, E. T. 1981. Locomotor activity and antinociception after putative mu, kappa and sigma opioid receptor agonists in the rat: Influence of dopaminergic agonists and antagonists. J. Pharmacol. Exp. Ther. **217**: 451–460.
34. COWAN, A. 1981. Simple in vivo tests that differentiate prototype agonists at opiate receptors. Life Sci. **28**: 1559–1570.
35. WOODS, J. H., S. HERLING, R. S. VALENTINO, D. W. HEIN & E. H. COALE, JR. 1980. Narcotic drug discrimination by rhesus monkeys and pigeons. Problems of Drug Dependence 1979. NIDA Res. Mono. **27**: 128–134.
36. TEAL, J. J. & S. G. HOLTZMAN. 1980. Discriminative stimulus effects of prototype opiate receptor agonists in monkeys. Eur. J. Pharmacol. **68**: 1–10.
37. HERLING, S. & J. H. WOODS. 1981. Discriminative stimulus effects of narcotics: Evidence for multiple receptor-mediated actions. Life Sci. **28**: 1571–1584.
38. HUIDOBRO-TORO, J. P. & E. L. WAY. 1980. Rapid development of tolerance to the hyperthermic effect of β-endorphin, and cross-tolerance between the enkephalins and β-endorphin. Eur. J. Pharmacol. **65**: 221–231.
39. SZEKELY, J., A. RONAI, Z. DUNAI-KOVACS, E. MIGLECZ, S. BAJUSZ & L. GRAF. 1977. Cross-tolerance between morphine and β-endorphin in vivo. Life Sci. **20**: 1259–1264.

40. TSENG, L. F., H. H. LOH & C. H. LI.   1976.   β-endorphin: Cross-tolerance to and cross-physical dependence on morphine. Proc. Natl. Acad. Sci. USA **73:** 4187–4189.
41. DENEAU, G. A. & M. H. SEEVERS.   1964.   Drug dependence. *In* Evaluation of Drug Activities: Pharmacometrics. D. R. Laurence and A. L. Bacharach, Eds. Vol. **I:** 167–179. Academic Press. London.
42. VILLARREAL, J. E. & M. H. SEEVERS.   1972.   Evaluation of new compounds for morphine-like physical dependence in the rhesus monkey. Bull. Probl. Drug Dependence **34** (addendum 7): 1040–1053.
43. SWAIN, H. H. & M. H. SEEVERS.   1974.   Evaluation of new compounds for morphine-like physical dependence in the rhesus monkey. Bull. Probl. Drug Dependence **36** (addendum 1): 1168–1195.
44. SWAIN, H. H. & M. H. SEEVERS.   1976.   Evaluation of new compounds for morphine-like physical dependence in the rhesus monkey. Bull. Probl. Drug Dependence **38** (addendum 2): 768–787.
45. GOLDSTEIN, A., W. FISCHLI, L. I. LOWNEY, M. HUNKAPILLER & L. HOOD.   1981.   Porcine pituitary dynorphin: Complete aminoacid sequence of the biologically active heptadecapeptide. Proc. Natl. Acad. Sci. USA **78:** 7219–7223.

DISCUSSION OF THE PAPER

E. J. SIMON (*New York University Medical Center, New York*): Thank you, Dr. Adler, for a very lucid overview of the *in vivo* methods of distinguishing the receptor subtypes.

UNIDENTIFIED SPEAKER: How does a miosis-producing drug produce mydriasis?

M. W. ADLER: I wish I knew, but we have some ideas about it. In the cat it was recently shown by Dr. Sharpe from the Addiction Research Center in Lexington that by injecting morphine into the Edinger-Westphal nucleus of the cat's brain, he can produce mydriasis. He thinks that morphine performs a blocking function on the neurons innervating the constrictor muscles.

We have some preliminary evidence that if morphine is injected into the Edinger-Westphal nucleus of the rat, both mydriasis and fluctuation are produced, just as they are when the compound is given subcutaneously, but we don't know the exact mechanism. That is something we are working on now.

G. KING (*Pointe Claire, Quebec, Canada*): It has been known that in many systems the body temperature can have a profound effect on seizure susceptibility. You have shown that morphine causes hypothermia and decreases susceptibility to flurothyl seizures. Meperidine, which would appear to be also a μ receptor agonist, on the other hand, causes slight hyperthermia and increases susceptibility to seizures. To what extent can you separate the body temperature effects and the anticonvulsant effects?

ADLER: Although there must be some relationship, there is no question that they are separable. For example, even stronger than the morphine group as anticonvulsants are the σ compounds, cyclazocine and SKF 10,047. They produce essentially no effects on body temperature and yet they are more potent anticonvulsant compounds.

M. S. GOLD (*Fair Oaks Hospital, Summit, N.J.*): Do you see any differences between local and systemic injections?

ADLER: We have not done localized intracerebral injections. However, we have done the intracerebroventricular (ICV) administration and have found that there are marked differences between the two types of injection with respect to some, but not most, effects. For example, if the anticonvulsant compounds are given into the lateral ventricle, an anticonvulsant effect is seen. However, as we will report very shortly, the proconvulsant compounds, given into the ventricles, are not always proconvulsant. Some may produce no effect or even be anticonvulsant. This may be due to a distributional factor after the drug goes out of the ventricles, reaching those areas that are more involved in the anticonvulsant as opposed to proconvulsant activity. We also believe that all of the opioids have a balance between excitatory and inhibitory properties and, because of this, the balance may be shifted when they are given intracerebroventricularly as compared to systemically. So there are some differences, but we are not sure what causes those differences.

SIMON: I would like to add that there is now some *in vitro* evidence for κ receptors. Dr. Costa's group, using a very specific μ ligand peptide from Reckitt-Colman and using D-Ala-D-Leu-enkephalin for blocking δ receptors, showed leftover receptors that have properties that are consistent with κ, that is, that bind benzomorphans very well.

ADLER: Yes; there is now evidence, as Dr. Simon pointed out, in the rat brain that there are κ binding sites. We have some evidence for that in our laboratory, but the evidence that Dr. Simon cites is very strong. The more we can correlate the findings of *in vitro* pharmacologic studies with those of *in vivo* studies, the more likely it is that the binding sites are receptors.

SIMON: The difficulty in finding κ binding sites is simply that they react just as well with μ ligands as they do with κ. Specific blocking must be done to find κ sites.

UNIDENTIFIED SPEAKER: Does it make any difference whether naloxone is given before, with, or after the opioid?

ADLER: Yes and no. There is some quantitative difference, but no qualitative difference. However, one of the reasons why you still may see the statement in the literature that naloxone blocks only the hypothermic effects of morphine and not the hyperthermic effects is that in those studies naloxone was given just before or with it. At the time morphine was still exerting its effect, naloxone had worn off because it has a half-life of about 18 minutes in the rat. So, we give the naloxone twice—at the beginning of the test period and 1 hour later. Both the hyperthermia and the hypothermia can be blocked this way.

There are some differences resulting from time of naloxone administration in terms of the development of tolerance and dependence. Some of the work, for example, that has been done on this at Boston University shows some differences. It seems to depend on the length of time of exposure of the receptors to morphine.

UNIDENTIFIED SPEAKER: A group in Chicago has attempted to potentiate analgesia with a peptidase blocker. Since you are doing *in vivo* experiments with several effects, have you attempted to replicate the whole-body effect of the peptidase inhibitors?

ADLER: No, we have not. The problem is that these compounds are broken down by a variety of enzymes and enzymes systems and to inhibit just one does not seem to have very much effect *in vivo*.

ROLE OF OPIOID PEPTIDES IN DISORDERS OF ATTENTION IN PSYCHPATHOLOGY

M. S. Buchsbaum, V. I. Reus, G. C. Davis,
H. H. Holcomb, J. Cappelletti, and E. Silberman

Biological Psychiatry Branch
National Institute of Mental Health
Bethesda, Maryland 20205

Disorders of attention are among the most prominent and consistent psycho-pathologic findings in schizophrenia.[1,2] Four lines of evidence suggest that opioid peptides may mediate disorders of attention in man:[3] (1) pain perception is dependent upon endorphinergic neuronal mechanisms[4] and is intimately associated with attention; (2) schizophrenics are relatively pain-insensitive;[5] (3) opiates and opiate antagonists affect attentional performance;[3,6] and (4) schizophrenic thought disorders may be modified by opiates and their antagonists.[5]

In examining the effects of opiate peptides on attention, we have also considered adrenocorticotropin (ACTH). Since ACTH and β-lipotropin (a precursor of β-endorphin) are synthesized in the large prohormone pro-opio-melanocortin and are released and jointly influenced by similar feedback signals, the effects of opioids and ACTH require careful differentiation. ACTH, melanocyte-stimulating hormone (MSH), vasopressin, and oxytocin also modulate adaptive processes by affecting motivational, learning, and memory processes.[7]

In an effort to extend previous studies of opioid peptides and related neuro-transmitters, we have studied the influence of ACTH, morphine, and opioid antagonists on both attention and pain. In this report we have attempted to link clinical and physiological studies by employing somatosensory, visual, and auditory evoked potentials. In particular, we have used the N120 peak of the evoked potential (EP) as an index of attention. The amplitude of the N120 peak increases with pain sensitivity and selective attention, responds to pharma-cological manipulation by opiates, opiate antagonists and peptides, and is diminished in schizophrenia.

THE EVOKED POTENTIAL AND ATTENTIONAL DYSFUNCTION IN SCHIZOPHRENIA

The EP technique provides several advantages in pain and schizophrenia research. In psychophysical tasks, whether of reaction time or pain ratings, there is a whole series of neurophysiological events and anatomic locations between the stimulus reception by sense organ and stimulus response by motor system. Slow reaction time or low pain ratings could be the result of phenomena ranging from primary cortical atrophy to deficient social motivation or inter-fering delusions.

Careful use of EP technology may help to isolate dysfunctional neural events. If two drugs or experimental manipulations affect the same EP component,

0077–8923/82/0398–0352 $01.75/0 © 1982 NYAS

then some commonality of mechanism is more strongly suggested than would be by similar effects on a psychophysical task. With the EP technique, psychomotor performance is unnecessary, permitting the testing of catatonic, disturbed, paralyzed or unconscious patients. Further, not only have unmedicated schizophrenics been found to have impaired fine motor coordination,[8] but also abnormalities of the motor system itself, including pathologic muscle fibers, have been reported [9, 10] and EMG studies of schizophrenics' reaction time [11] suggest that peripheral factors may be partly contributory to differences previously held to be due solely to central dysfunction.

Cortical localization of attention and pain processing may also be possible with new techniques for evoked potential topographic mapping.[12-14] Since attentional deficits appear in schizophrenics when either visual or auditory stimuli are used,[15] one might expect any overlap in function between pain, light and sound processing to occur in various association or polysensory cortex areas. Such an overlap could be plotted using topographic techniques.

The N120 Component

In the average EP to light, sound and shock, the N120 component (negative at 120 milliseconds post stimulus) is probably the earliest to appear at the same latency and configuration for all three modalities. While its cortical distribution maximum peaks over occipital cortex for visual EPs and somatosensory cortex for somatosensory EP, the configuration over somatosensory, parietal and temperoparietal cortex is quite similar, more so than the preceding positive peak, P100.

Effects of Attention

The amplitude of the N120 component appears to index the process by which "stimuli are selected or rejected on the basis of their simple physical attributes." [16] The N120 and its sensitivity to attentional task demands have been extensively studied and are well reviewed elsewhere.[17] In a naturalistic situation, such as an insect bite or thorn in the toe, a pain stimulus has to be selected from a background of other sensory stimuli (such as leaves moving, bird calls, or the feel of warm stones underfoot). Thus, the modality-selective sensitivity of N120 would appear to be a reasonable choice for examining the overlap of cortical distribution between EPs for visual and auditory attention tasks and pain stimuli.

In a typical selective attention experiment we have carried out, subjects are seated in a quiet, darkened room. A series of brief lights and tones of four different intensities in a random sequence are presented at 1-second intervals, each stimulus 64 times.[18] The subjects first receive training in the correct identification of the intensity of the visual and auditory stimuli; [19] then subjects are instructed to count the number of visual stimuli that were of the same intensity in a row, ignoring intervening tones. Then, the same stimulus sequence is repeated, and subjects are instructed to count the tone stimuli, ignoring intervening lights. The visual EP measured while the subject is counting light pairs is normally of larger amplitude than the visual EP recorded while the subject is counting tone pairs in the second series. This difference is a physiological measure of the effect of the attentional task. In some cases, a third condition is used where subjects are requested to do continuous mental arithmetic (subtracting 7 serially from 2000) while the stimulus sequence is presented.

The EEG is recorded, amplified (3 dB points 0.3 and 110 Hz), and digitized at 250 samples/second. In the ACTH and pain experiments the EEG was analogue-filtered with a high-frequency cutoff at 40 Hz. For the cortical mapping experiments described below, EPs were not analogue-filtered, but were first "detrended" using linear regression and then digitially filtered to remove frequencies below 4 Hz and above 30 Hz, as described elsewhere (with a different bandpass).[20] Eye movements and artifacts were monitored using lead Fpl; trials exceeding a threshold were automatically excluded from the average for all leads.

For the pain stimulation experiments, 1-msec single shocks of four intensities were similarly presented at 1-second intervals in a random order for a total of 64 presentations to the right forearm.[21]

The N120 component was measured for all EPs by integrating the area between 116 and 152 msec and expressed as the mean absolute deviation in microvolts, as described elsewhere.[22]

Cortical Mapping

For the cortical maps, in addition to the 12 electrodes normally on the left side (10–20 system) or midline (C_z-P_z-O_z), four additional electrode locations were included to provide greater resolution of the posterior cortex.[14] These were placed at the centers of squares formed by connecting P_3-P_z-O_z-O_1 (PO), C_3-C_z-P_z-P_3 (CP) and T_3-C_3-P_3-T_3 (FTC). The 16 values were then used to interpolate values over the entire scalp areas as described elsewhere.[14]

Psychophysical Pain Assessment

To provide validating evidence for the evoked potential measures of pain sensitivity, we studied psychophysical pain response in healthy and well-trained normal volunteers. We used the same stimuli as in the somatosensory EP recordings. Brief electrical stimuli were administered to the skin of the left forearm with a computer-controlled constant-current stimulator. A total of 93 stimuli (ranging from 1 to 31 mA) were applied and categorized by the subject as "noticeable," "distinct," "unpleasant," or "very unpleasant." An index, termed "insensitivity," is a measure of the overlap or variation in judgments of noticeable–distinct with unpleasant–very unpleasant. It is reported as percent error and indicates confusion of the distinct/unpleasant distinction.[23] We have developed this measure as a nonparametric analogue of signal detection analysis. Using this method, we have observed significant reductions in a subject's sensitivity after morphine or aspirin administration.[21]

The N120 Component in Schizophrenia and Pain Sensitivity

Patients with schizophrenia tend to have smaller-amplitude EPs than do normal controls under a variety of experimental conditions (see the reviews by Shagass et al.[24] and by Buchsbaum [25, 26]). In our studies of individuals

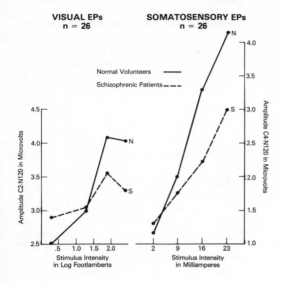

FIGURE 1. Mean visual and somatosensory EPs at four intensities of stimulation in 26 unmedicated schizophrenics and 26 age- and sex-matched normal controls. Note diminished amplitude at high-intensity in patient group.[3]

resting without any task, the N120 amplitude was reduced in unmedicated schizophrenics (FIG. 1) for both visual and somatosensory stimulation.[3] This reduction in the N120 component was most marked at the highest stimulus intensities; only the N120 component showed this intensity-related difference. The pattern of lower-amplitude intensity slopes has previously been reported in visual EPs in schizophrenics.[27] Among normal individuals, persons who are relatively pain-insensitive on the psychophysical task show this pattern (FIG. 2),

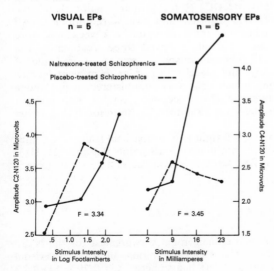

FIGURE 2. Mean visual and somatosensory EP amplitudes, as in FIGURE 1, in five schizophrenic patients on and off chronic naltrexone administration. Note increased amplitude at high intensity with this opiate antagonist and similar shift of the amplitude/intensity function across both sensory modalities.[5]

suggesting that the schizophrenic group is relatively pain-tolerant. Indeed, on our psychophysical task, schizophrenics were pain-insensitive.[5] This pain-insensitivity in schizophrenics has been reported for both clinical and experimental pain (reviewed by Davis et al.[28]). The pain-insensitivity suggests to us some abnormality in the endorphin system and is consistent with reports of CSF endorphin elevation in schizophrenia.[29]

The N120 Component and the Opioid System

Both the N120 component and the P200 component are reduced in amplitude after the administration of morphine,[22] but only the N120 is more reduced for painful stimuli (16- and 23-mA shocks) than for nonpainful stimuli (2 and 9 mA). The opioid antagonist naloxone increases N120 amplitude, again more at higher than lower intensities,[30] but only in individuals categorized as pain-insensitive. This suggested that schizophrenics, who are pain-insensitive and have low N120 amplitudes, might show a marked response to opiate antagonists. In a subsequent study, we found that oral naltrexone administered to five schizophrenics induced a threefold increase in the N120 amplitude associated with most intense stimulation. Furthermore, naltrexone also enhanced the N120 component for visual EPs. This suggests that the nervous system may possess an opioid-sensitive mechanism for modulating multiple modes of intense stimulation (FIG. 2).

ACTH and ACTH 4-9

N120 attention effects were studied in nine patients with affective disorders (five men and four women, mean age 48.5 years, SD = 16.8). Eight patients satisfied research diagnostic criteria (RDC)[31] for primary major depressive disorder. Seven had bipolar affective disorder and two were unipolar. All patients were off psychoactive medications for a minimum of 2 weeks and were living on an NIMH inpatient unit. Patients received three treatments in a random order: 60 units of ACTH subcutaneously, 40 mg of an analogue of ACTH 4-9 (Organon 2766) orally, and placebo. In order to prevent investigators and patients from knowing which drug was administered, a pill and a subcutaneous injection was given on all three occasions, one or both being a placebo. Patients were tested on the visual/auditory EP attention task 2 hours after drug administration.

The EEG was recorded from left and right temporoparietal leads (the center of a triangle P_3-T_3-T_5, termed W_3),[32] amplified (3 dB points 0.3 and 110 Hz), analogue-filtered, and digitized at 250 samples/sec in the first series of experiments.

Attention Effects on Placebo

As previously reported, attentional enhancement was greatest for the N120 component at the lowest intensity. The mean attentional increase for visual EPs at 2 footlamberts for the right and left hemispheres was 0.79 ± SD 1.23 and 0.85 ± 0.06 μV, respectively. Both were significant task effects (paired t's p < 0.05). Statistically significant attentional enhancement was also found for P100, left hemisphere, 30 footlamberts (1.14 μV).

The attention effect was relatively uniform in its appearance across subjects; seven of nine showed a positive change score at the lowest intensity and eight of nine showed a positive score for the average of the two lowest intensities for N120—on either the right or left hemisphere.

Effect of ACTH

ACTH tended to shift the appearance of the attention enhancement for modality selection to higher intensities, as shown in TABLE 1. This appeared for both visual and auditory EPs, and ACTH–placebo differences were confirmed by paired t tests on difference scores for visual EPs. Auditory EPs showed their only significant attentional enhancement on ACTH, although the placebo–ACTH difference only reached the p < 0.10 level.

TABLE 1

ATTENTION INCREASE WTIH TASK, RIGHT TEMPEROPARIETAL LEAD—
LIGHT-ATTENTION VERSUS TONE-ATTENTION

	Placebo	ACTH	2766	Placebo	ACTH	2766
P100						
Low	.77	—.18*	—.05	—.67	.51	+.37
High	.16	.12	.31	.81	.08	+.81
N120						
Low	.79†	.56	—.23*	—.30	.59	+.37
High	—.31	1.02*, †	—.57	.54	1.33†	+1.59
P200						
Low	—.78	—.18	.46*	.00	+.24	—.09
High	—.98	—1.12	—.25	—.10	—.48	—.66

* Significantly different from placebo by paired t test (drug effect).
† Significantly different from zero by paired t test (indicates task effect).

Similar results were observed for the comparison of the light-attention condition with the mental-arithmetic condition. While attention enhancement decreased in intensity on placebo, it increased from 1.28 μV at the low intensity to 2.42 at the high intensity with ACTH (linear trend effect F = 4.42, 2, 10 d.f., p < 0.05).

Effect of Organon 2766

Unlike ACTH, Organon 2766 had little effect on P100 or N120, but did enhance visual EP P200 attention effects for low intensities (TABLE 1) for the selective attention task. This was confirmed by a drug effect (mean placebo effect, 0.22 μV; ACTH, 0.37 μV; and Organon 2766, 0.30 μV, F = 8.15, p < 0.05) and a drug by intensity interaction (F = 11.66, p < 0.05). For the comparison of EPs during light-attention with those during mental arithmetic,

TABLE 2

ATTENTION INCREASE WITH TASK—LIGHT-ATTENTION MINUS MENTAL ARITHMETIC

	Visual EP			Auditory EP		
	Placebo	ACTH	2766	Placebo	ACTH	2766
P100						
Low	1.89	−.24	.28	+.10	−.15	−.30
High	−.95	2.41*	−.42	−.34	−.47	−.47
N120						
Low	1.44	1.28	0.38	−.01	−.81	−.29
High	.43	2.42*	0.28	−.31	−.31	−.20
P200						
Low	−.17	.64	−.09	+.27	+.16	+.78
High	−.20	.34	.21	+.13	+.12	+.45

NOTE: On left side visual P100 was only component to reach $p < 0.05$ significance.
* Significant drug by intensity interaction, 2, 10 d.f.

(ANOVA with placebo, ACTH and 2766, drug by intensity interactions) P100 and N120 reached significance (TABLE 2), but results with 2766 tended to resemble those with placebo.

Comparison of Cerebral Topography of the N120 Component of the Somatosensory EP and Visual EP in Selective Attention

The topography of the somatosensory EP was studied in seven normal volunteers. With wrist stimulation, the peak at the top of the somatosensory cortex (FIG. 3) for the low intensity is expected. As stimulus intensity increases

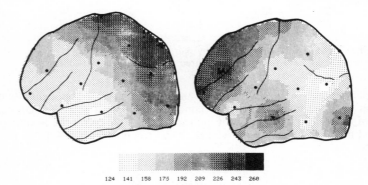

124   141   158   175   192   209   226   243   260

FIGURE 3. Somatosensory evoked potentials in normal volunteers and patient with schizophrenia. (*Left*) topographic distribution of N120 somatosensory EP in seven normal volunteers. Stimulation level of 16 mA used here is generally judged unpleasant in psychophysical tests. (*Right*) topographic distribution in a 19-year-old catatonic schizophrenic patient off all medication for 2 weeks. The parietal area, which shows attentional effect (FIG. 6), also shows absence of N120 component for pain stimulation. (Scale is in microvolts × 100.)

from the 2-mA level, normally reported as light touch, to the 16- and 23-mA level, reported as unpleasant, pricking and painful, the distribution spreads into posterior and superior parietal areas.

Six patients with schizophrenia (mean age 22, five males, one female) all off medication for 2 weeks or more and 12 age- and sex-matched normal volunteers served as subjects in the visual/auditory selective attention task. All patients satisfied RDC criteria [31] for schizophrenia. For normal volunteers, the map shows two areas of attentional enhancement, one at the frontal pole and a second in the parietal area (FIGS. 4 and 5). This is dissimilar to the low-intensity distribution seen for the somatosensory EP, but an area of overlap appears at the intensity level where subjective reports of pain occur.

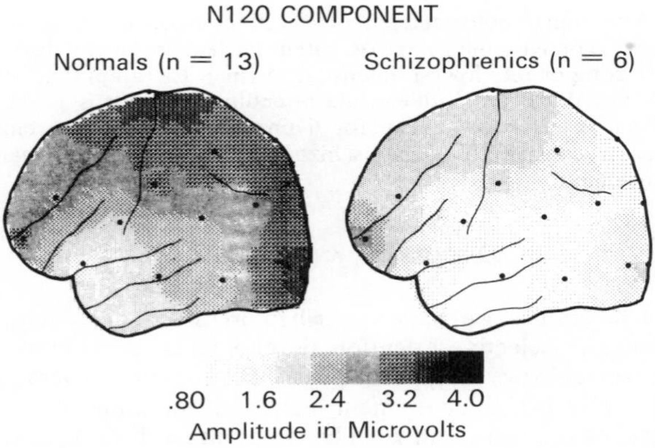

N120 COMPONENT

Normals (n = 13)   Schizophrenics (n = 6)

.80 1.6 2.4 3.2 4.0
Amplitude in Microvolts

FIGURE 4. Visual EP distribution. Topographic distribution of mean EP amplitude for N120 component. Note distribution not only over vertex of cortex, but also extending in a posterior direction into the parietal and occipital lobe. Patients with schizophrenia show markedly smaller amplitudes. Compare distribution to that in FIGURE 5. Parietal area is not enhanced, suggesting some similarity to schizophrenia. (Scale is in microvolts × 100.)

We have recently begun a program designed to study how specific drugs alter pain perception and attention tasks. Naltrexone, 150 mg orally, was administered to a patient suffering from episodic psychoses of undetermined origin. The patient was tested twice on the EP procedures, 7 days apart, while maintained on cimethidine. On the first occasion, testing began 2½ hours after taking 150 mg naltrexone; then the patient was retested after she had been off naltrexone for 5 days.

EPs to somatosensory stimuli and to the visual/auditory attention task were recorded. Results indicate that naltrexone strikingly enhanced somatosensory evoked potentials (FIG. 6), and similarly enhanced the attentional effect visual EPs (FIG. 7). This enhancement was, however, in the frontal rather than the parietal area, thus resembling a pattern of attentional effects in schizophrenics (FIG. 5).

An unusual somatosensory EP distribution was also observed in a young, unmedicated, catatonic schizophrenic (FIG. 3).

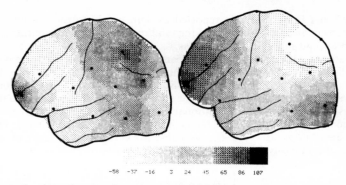

-58 -37 -16   3   24   45   65   86 107

FIGURE 5. Attentional enhancement of N120 component in schizophrenics and normal subjects. Topographic map of attention enhancement for visual evoked response, N120 component, lowest intensity. Visual EP amplitude while attending to lights minus visual EP amplitude while attending to tones is given. (*Left*) mean for 12 normal subjects; (*right*) mean for 6 unmedicated schizophrenics. Note that the frontal area is constant, but that schizophrenics lack temperoparietal areas of attention enhancement.

DISCUSSION AND SUMMARY

The series of studies we have described in this report indicate some EP features common to selective attention psychological paradigms, pain perception, and pharmacologic manipulation of the opioid system, especially in schizophrenia. The N120 component increased in amplitude with selective attention, opiate antagonists, and ACTH. In contrast, it decreased in amplitude with inattention, opiate agonists, and schizophrenia. These data and our earlier auditory data [3] are consistent with those of Arnstein et al.,[33] who have recently reported that naloxone enhances electrophysiologic measurements of attention on a negative auditory EP component.

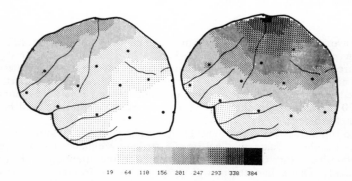

19   64 110 156 201 247 293 338 384

FIGURE 6. Effect of naltrexone on somatosensory EP. Topographic map of somatosensory EP, N120 component in patient with intermittent psychosis (see text). (*Left*) baseline EP map and (*right*) EP map 2 hours after naltrexone. Note marked increase in N120 amplitude with administration of naltrexone (150 mg) orally.

ACTH appears to act similarly to naloxone on the attention-related N120 component of the evoked potential. In animal studies, ACTH has some characteristics of an endogenous naloxone-like compound. Jacquet and Wolf[34] reported that ACTH 1–24 injections into the periaqueductal gray matter resulted in a behavioral syndrome characterized by fearful hyperactivity and explosive motor behavior similar to that noted during opiate withdrawal. Injection of ACTH 1–24 into the cerebral ventricles of rats is also associated with hyperalgesia on the hot-plate test; this effect is potentiated by naloxone and antagonized by morphine.[35] Antagonism between morphine and ACTH 1–24 has been reported by Zimmerman and Krivoy.[36] In man, administration of naloxone to volunteers seems to elevate ACTH and cortisol and to promote a slight hyperalgesia.[37]

ACTH fragments and peptides sharing extensive homology with that hormone affect several aspects of analgesia[38] and "selective attention" (see the review by Pigache and Rigter[39]). Differences between ACTH 1–24, ACTH

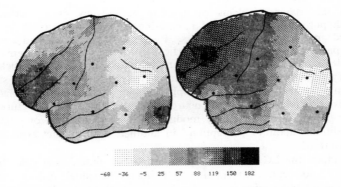

-68   -36   -5   25   57   88   119   150   182

FIGURE 7. Effect of naltrexone on visual EP N120 component, low intensity, in same patient as in FIGURE 6. (*Left*) baseline and (*right*) after 150 mg naltrexone orally. Marked increase in N120 attention effect (as described in text and FIG. 5) appears with naltrexone.

4–9 and morphine and opiate antagonists may be related to each compound's preferential affinity for a particular class of opiate receptors and their different adrenocorticoid effects.

Drugs that promote nonadrenergic activity are best known for their attention-enhancing characteristics. Amphetamine, which is used in the treatment of the attention deficit disorder in children, increases the amplitude of the N120 component of the EP in selective attention tasks.[40, 41] One of the main sites of action of this noradrenergic agonist is the locus coeruleus (LC), where it increases the release of norepinephrine.[42] Electrophysiologic studies indicate that morphine inhibits LC activity.[43, 44] Binding studies also provide for a high concentration of opioid receptors in this catecholamine nucleus.[45]

Finally, naloxone, a potent opiate antagonist which binds to these receptors, reverses opioid suppression of LC activity.[43, 44, 46] Thus, the attention-enhancing effects of naloxone may be mediated by reversing endorphin suppression of noradrenergic activity in the LC or other physiologically similar pathways. The relationship of CNS peptides, especially endorphins and ACTH, to noradrenergic neurons is reviewed by Versteeg.[47]

The studies in cerebral topography are preliminary, but there is an overlap between areas where EP amplitude is enhanced with selective attention and pain. The frontal cortex and the superior and middle parietal lobe are two such areas. The parietal area seems especially relevant insofar as EPs are enhanced there in normal attending subjects, but not in patients with schizophrenia. This anatomic region may be relevant to attention dysfunction in schizophrenia,[48] and could be responsible for the diminished pain perception observed in this population. Lewis et al.[49] supported our suggestion of a role for opioid peptides in attention [3] by examining the topographic distribution of naloxone-binding sites in the primate cortex. They found a parallel between successively later stages of sequential processing pathways compatible with the "affective filtering of sensory stimuli." It is premature to speculate on the relationship between EP topography observed during selective attention or pain studies and the topographic distribution of opiate receptors in the cortex.

One of the major problems confronting our review of the attention/endorphin hypothesis is the task of integrating studies of anatomic systems, clinical syndromes and behavioral tasks. Psychologists have studied complex attentional paradigms associated with cortical processing in schizophrenics and college students; pharmacologists, however, have studied pain-related behavior in laboratory animals. Even in our laboratory, we previously segregated studies of attention and pain. Recent neurophysiologic studies indicate that this separation is artificial since the same neurotransmitters, anatomic structures and information-processing systems may modulate pain perception in one environmental condition,[5] auditory perception [3] in another, and abstract symbol perception [6] in a third.

For example, the LC apparently plays important modulating roles in the transmission of nociceptive information by acting on the spinal cord and nucleus raphe magnus in some circumstances. It also regulates levels of attention, arousal, and anxiety by acting on the cortex and limbic system. Clinical studies which alter pain and attention will promote complex changes in norepinephrine activity that would not be interpretable from urine and cerebrospinal fluid metabolite measurements. We anticipate that the use of specific pharmacological probes coupled with positron emission tomography and EP topographic mapping will promote clearer physiological modeling in this area of investigation.

REFERENCES

1. VENABLES, P. H. 1973. Input regulation and psychopathology. In Psychopathology. M. Hammer, K. Salzinger and S. Sutton, Eds.: 261–284. John Wiley. New York.
2. GARMEZY, N. 1977. The psychology and psychopathology of attention. Schizophr. Bull. 3: 360–369.
3. DAVIS, G. C., M. S. BUCHSBAUM & W. E. BUNNEY, JR. 1980. Alterations of evoked potentials link research in attention dysfunction to peptide response symptoms of schizophrenia. In Neural Peptides and Neuronal Communications. E. Costa and M. Trabucchi, Eds.: 473–487. Raven Press. New York.

4. PERT, A., C. B. PERT, G. C. DAVIS & W. E. BUNNEY, JR. 1981. Opiate peptides and brain function. *In* Handbook of Biological Psychology, Vol. IV. H. M. van Praag, M. H. Lader, O. J. Rafaelsen and E. J. Sachar, Eds.: 547–582. Marcel Dekker. New York.

5. DAVIS, G. C., M. S. BUCHSBAUM, D. P. VAN KAMMEN & W. E. BUNNEY, JR. 1979. Analgesia to pain stimuli in schizophrenics reversed by naltrexone. Psychiatr. Res. **1:** 61–69.

6. LIPINSKI, J., R. MEYER, C. KORNETSKY & B. M. COHEN. 1979. Naloxone in schizophrenics: Negative results. Lancet **i:** 1292–1293.

8. GOODE, D. J., A. A. MANNING, J. F. MIDDLETON & B. WILLIAMS. 1981. Fine motor performance before and after treatment in schizophrenic and schizoaffective patients. Psychiatr. Res. **5:** 247–255.

9. MELTZER, H. Y. 1976. Neuromuscular dysfunction in schizophrenia. Schizophr. Bull. **2:** 106–135.

10. MELTZER, H. Y. 1979. Biology of schizophrenia subtypes: A review and proposal for method of study. Schizophr. Bull. **5**(3): 460–479.

11. SCHNEIDER, R. D. & V. GROSSI. 1979. Differences in muscle activity before, during, and after responding in a simple reaction time task: Schizophrenics vs. normals. Psychiatr. Res. **1:** 141–145.

12. DUFFY, F. H., J. L. BURCHFIEL & C. T. LOMBROSO. 1979. Brain electrical activity mapping (BEAM): A method for extending the clinical utility of EEG and evoked potential data. Ann. Neurol. **5:** 309–321.

13. LEHMANN, D. & W. SKRANDIES. 1980. Reference-free identification of components of checkerboard-evoked multichannel potential fields. Electroencephalogr. Clin. Neurophysiol. **48:** 609–621.

14. BUCHSBAUM, M. S., F. RIGAL, R. COPPOLA, J. CAPPELLETTI, C. KING & J. JOHNSON. 1982. A new system for gray-level surface distribution maps of electrical activity. Electroencephalogr. Clin. Neurophysiol. **53:** 237–242.

15. NEUCHTERLEIN, K. H. 1977. Reaction time and attention in schizophrenia: A critical evaluation of the data and theories. Schizophr. Bull. **3:** 373–428.

16. SCHWENT, V. L., E. SNYDER & S. A. HILLYARD. 1976. Auditory evoked potentials during multichannel selective listening cues. J. Exp. Psychol. **2:** 313–325.

17. HILLYARD, S. A. 1978. Sensation, perception and attention: Analysis using ERPs. *In* Event-Related Brain Potentials in Man. E. Callaway, P. Tueting and S. H. Koslow, Eds.: 223–321. Academic Press. New York.

18. BUCHSBAUM, M. S., R. COPPOLA, E. S. GERSHON, D. P. VAN KAMMEN & NURNBERGER, J. I. 1981. Evoked potential measures of attention and psychopathology. Adv. Biol. Psychiat. **6:** 1–5.

19. SCHECHTER, G. A. & M. S. BUCHSBAUM. 1978. The effects of attention, stimulus intensity and individual differences on the average evoked response. Psychophysiology **10:** 392–400.

20. LAVINE, R. A., M. S. BUCHSBAUM & G. SCHECHTER. 1980. Human somatosensory evoked responses: Effects of attention and distraction on early components. Physiol. Psychol. **8:** 405–408.

21. BUCHSBAUM, M. S., G. DAVIS, R. COPPOLA & D. NABER. 1981a. Opiate pharmacology and individual differences. I. Psychophysical pain measurements. Pain **10:** 357–366.

22. BUCHSBAUM, M. S., G. DAVIS, R. COPPOLA & D. NABER. 1981b. Opiate pharmacology and individual differences. II. Somatosensory evoked potentials. Pain **10:** 367–377.

23. CLARK, W. C. & L. MEHL. 1973. Signal ˌ ˀction theory procedures are not equivalent when thermal stimuli are judged. J. Exp. Psychol. **97:** 148–153.

24. SHAGASS, C., E. M. ORNITZ, S. SUTTON & P. TUETING. 1978. Event related potentials and psychopathology. *In* Event-Related Brain Potentials in Man.

E. Callaway, P. Tueting and S. H. Koslow, Eds.: 443–496. Academic Press. New York.

25. Buchsbuam, M. S. 1977. The middle evoked response components and schizophrenia. Schizophr. Bull. **3:** 93–104.

26. Buchsbaum, M. S. 1979. Neurophysiological aspects of the schizophrenic syndrome. *In* Disorders of the Schizophrenic Syndrome. L. Bellak, Ed.: 152–180. Basic Books. New York.

27. Landau, S. G., M. S. Buchsbaum, W. Carpenter, J. Strauss & M. Sacks. 1975. Schizophrenia and stimulus intensity control. Arch. Gen. Psychiat. **32:** 1239–1245.

28. Davis, G. C., M. S. Buchsbaum & W. E. Bunney, Jr. 1979. Research in endorphins and schizophrenia. Schizophr. Bull. **5:** 244–250.

29. Buchsbaum, M. S., G. C. Davis & D. P. Van Kammen. 1980. Diagnostic classification and the endorphin hypothesis of schizophrenia: Individual differences and psychopharmacological strategies. *In* Perspectives in Schizophrenia Research. C. F. Baxter and T. Melnechuk, Eds.: 177–191. Raven Press. New York.

30. Buchsbaum, M. S., G. C. Davis & W. E. Bunney, Jr. 1977. Naloxone alters pain perception and somatosensory evoked potentials in normal subjects. Nature **270:** 620–622.

31. Spitzer, R. L., J. E. Endicott & E. Robins. 1975. Research Diagnostic Criteria (RDC) for a Selected Group of Functional Disorders. New York: Biometrics Research, New York State Psychiatric Institute.

32. Matsumiya, Y., V. Tagliasco, C. T. Lombroso & H. Goodglass. 1972. Auditory evoked response: Meaningfulness of stimuli and interhemispheric asymmetry. Science **175:** 790–792.

33. Arnstein, A., D. S. Segal, H. Neville & S. Hillyard. 1981. Naloxone augments electrophysiological measures of selective attention. Soc. Neurosci. **7:** 659.

34. Jacquet, Y. & G. Wolf. 1981. Morphine and ACTH 1–24: Correlative behavioral excitations following microinjections in rat periacqueductal gray. Brain Res. **219:** 214–218.

35. Bertolini, A., R. Poggiolo & W. Ferrari. 1979. ACTH induced hyperalgesia in rats. Experientia **35:** 1216–1217.

36. Zimmerman, E. & W. Krivoy. 1974. Antagonism between morphine ACTH 1–24 in the isolated spinal cord of the frog and in the acute rat. Proc. Soc. Exp. Biol. **146:** 575–579. New York.

37. Volavka, J., J. Bauman & J. Pevnick *et al.* 1980. Short-term hormonal effects of naloxone in man. Psychoneuroendocrinology **5:** 225–234.

38. Walker, J. M., G. G. Bernston, C. A. Sandman, A. J. Kastin & H. Akil. 1981. Induction of analgesia by central administration of ORG 2766, an analog of ACTH 4–9. Eur. J. Pharmacol. **69:** 71–79.

39. Pigache, R. & H. Rigter. 1981. Effects of peptides related to ACTH on mood and vigilance in man. *In* Frontiers of Hormone Research, Vol. **8:** 193–207. S. Karger. Basel.

40. Buchsbaum, M. S., R. Coppola, E. S. Gershon, D. P. Van Kammen & J. I. Nurnberger. 1981. Evoked potential measures of attention and psychopathology. Adv. Biol. Psychiat. **6:** 186–194.

41. Nurnberger, J. I., E. S. Gershon, D. C. Jimerson, M. S. Buchsbaum, P. Gold, G. Brown & M. Ebert. 1981. Pharmacogenetics of d-amphetamine response in man. *In* Genetic Research Strategies for Psychobiology and Psychiatry. E. S. Gershon, S. Matthysse, X. O. Breakefield and R. D. Ciaranello, Eds.: 257–268. Boxwood Press. Pacific Grove, CA.

42. Axelrod, J. 1970. Amphetamine, physiological disposition and its effect on catecholamine storage. *In* Amphetamines and Related Compounds. E. Costa and S. Garattini, Eds. Raven Press. New York.

43. BIRD, S. J. & M. J. KUHAR. 1977. Iontophoretic application of opiates to the locus coeruleus. Brain Res. **122:** 523–533.
44. KORF, J., B. S. BUNNEY & G. K. AGHAJANIAN. 1974. Noradrenergic neurons: Morphine inhibition of spontaneous activity. Eur. J. Pharmacol. **25:** 165–169.
45. PERT, C. B., M. J. KUHAR & S. H. SNYDER. 1976. Opiate receptor: Autoradiographic localization in rat brain. Physiology **73:** 3729–3733.
46. PEPPER, C. M. & G. HENDERSON. 1980. Opiates and opioid peptides hyperpolarize locus coeruleus neurons in vitro. Science **209:** 394–396.
47. VERSTEEG, D. H. G. 1980. Interaction of peptides related to ACTH, MSH and Beta-LPH with neurotransmitters in the brain. Pharmacol. Ther. **11:** 535–557.
48. MESULAM, M. M. & N. GESCHWIND. 1978. On the possible role of neocortex and its limbic connections in the process of attention and schizophrenia. *In* The Nature of Schizophrenia. L. C. Wynne, R. L. Cromwell and S. Matthysse, Eds.: 161–166. John Wiley & Sons. New York.
49. M. E. LEWIS, M. MISHKIN, E. BRAGIN, R. M. BROWN, C. PERT & A. PERT. 1981. Opiate receptor gradients in monkey cerebral cortex: Correspondence with sensory processing hierarchies. Science **211:** 1166–1170.

[NOTE: This paper will be discussed with the next one, which is by Glenn C. Davis *et al.*]

ALTERED PAIN PERCEPTION AND CEREBROSPINAL ENDORPHINS IN PSYCHIATRIC ILLNESS

Glenn C. Davis,*† Monte S. Buchsbaum,‡ Dieter Naber,‡
David Pickar,‡ Robert Post,‡ Daniel van Kammen,‡
and William E. Bunney, Jr.‡

* Department of Psychiatry
Case Western Reserve School of Medicine,
Psychiatry Research Program
Cleveland Veterans Administration Medical Center
Cleveland Ohio 44106
‡ Biological Psychiatry Branch
National Institute of Mental Health
Bethesda, Maryland 20205

INTRODUCTION

Clinical descriptions of insensitivity to pain among patients with schizophrenia have been reported for centuries. Similarly, patients with affective illness have been reported to experience pain differently in affective episodes than they do in well periods. While previous explanations for these phenomena have depended heavily upon metapsychological theory, the recent discovery of opiatelike substances (endorphins) has prompted the suggestion that these phenomena might be mediated by the neural networks integrating pain perception.

In this paper, we suggest that abnormalities in pain appreciation may be useful as psychophysiological markers in schizophrenia and affective illness. Alterations in pain perception may direct us toward the underlying neurochemistry which mediates the symptoms, or possibly even toward the etiology, of these illnesses. Alternatively, characteristic abnormalities in pain appreciation may be a consequence of the psychotic state and may provide independent confirmation of specific diagnoses.

We will also describe in this paper a psychophysical pain-rating task. This task has test–retest reliability,[1] and is sensitive enough to demonstrate individual differences in sensitivity to pain,[1] diurnal variation in pain sensitivity,[2] differences with respect to age and gender,[1] the analgesic effects of morphine [1] and aspirin,[3] and the hyperalgesic effects of naloxone.[4] We also describe the use of the somatosensory evoked potential as a correlate of subjectively reported pain perception. The amplitude of the waveform of the evoked potential at a latency of 120 milliseconds, like the pain-rating task, is sensitive to individual differences in pain appreciation, differences in age and sex, diurnal variation, the analgesic effects of morphine and aspirin, and the hyperalgesic effects of naloxone.[1-5]

Having described the measurement techniques, we will summarize our studies of pain sensitivity in affectively ill and schizophrenic individuals. Evidence supporting the hypothesis that endorphins mediate the insensitivity to

† Address for correspondence: Glenn C. Davis, M.D., Psychiatry Service, Cleveland Veterans Administration Medical Center, 10701 East Boulevard, Cleveland, Ohio 44106.

0077-8923/82/0398-0366 $01.75/0 © 1982 NYAS

pain found in these illnesses will be discussed. We also report cerebrospinal fluid opiate-binding levels (a measure of total opioid activity) in normal, schizophrenic, and affectively ill patients.

PAIN MEASUREMENT TECHNIQUE

The somatosensory stimuli utilized in these studies are mild electric shocks administered to the dorsal surface of the left forearm. Prior to entering an experiment, the subject is given a series of shocks in ascending order, both to familiarize the subject with the range of intensities as well as to make consent more informed.

The experimental procedure includes three shocks at each milliamperage increment from 1 to 31 mA in a random sequence (for a total of 93 shocks lasting approximately 4 minutes). Subjective judgments of shock intensity vary from person to person; the lowest intensities are generally barely noticed, while the highest intensities are found noxious. The somatosensory rating task requires that subjects rate shocks in one of four categories: noticeable, distinct, unpleasant, or very unpleasant.

Three measures derived from subjects' responses have been found to be useful: the "distinct/unpleasant response criterion," the "distinct/unpleasant error rate" (called also "insensitivity"), and "pain counts."

The first measure, termed "response criterion," is the milliamperage level required for the subject to judge the stimulus as noxious (thus, this measure is roughly comparable to the more familiar "pain threshold"). This response criterion is the milliamperage level at which the subject is most accurate in distinguishing between "distinct" and "unpleasant" stimuli.

The "error rate" or "insensitivity" is expressed as a percentage, that is, the total errors at the response criterion, divided by the total number of subject responses. The error rate provides a measure of overlap between intensity categories.

"Pain counts" is the total number of "unpleasant" and "very unpleasant" responses the subject makes during the task. Thus pain counts is the frequency of noxious judgments.

The first two measures are nonparametric analogues of variables derived from signal detection analysis as applied to pain assessment (see Buchsbaum *et al.*[1] for an extensive description of this paradigm). This nonparametric approach takes advantage of the useful distinction suggested by signal detection theorists between observer sensitivity (related to perceptual integrity) and response bias (influenced by affective and cognitive factors). Furthermore this approach avoids the controversial parametric assumptions of signal detection theory as applied to pain judgment.[6, 7] The theoretical advantages of nonparametric signal detection analysis are discussed in McNichol.[8]

SOMATOSENSORY EVOKED POTENTIAL TECHNIQUE

The use of evoked potential correlates of pain sensitivity provides additional measures that supplement reliance on analysis of the subjective reports of subjects (for example, the pain-rating task). Because psychomotor performance is unnecessary to the collection of evoked potentials, it is possible to test unconscious, disturbed, or paralyzed patients. Cortical localization of somatosensory processing may also be possible. The recordings of somatosensory EPs in this paper are at Cz and C4, both parietal locations; Cz is at the vertex polysensory associational area and C4 is roughly located in the arm region of the sensory homunculus. Furthermore, specific EP components at known poststimulus latencies can be related to psychophysical parameters such as our pain measures of "response criterion" and "insensitivity." Finally, evoked potential parameters are very sensitive to drug effects and thus allow stronger assessment of pharmacologic change.

To measure the somatosensory evoked potential, four stimulus levels (2, 9, 16, and 23 mA) judged as ranging from barely perceptible to unpleasant by most individuals are presented 64 times, each at 1-second intervals in a random order. From multiple presentations of these four stimulus levels, a computer produces four cortical average evoked potential waveforms. It is the analyses of the amplitudes and amplitude/intensity functions of components of these waveforms that has been found to relate to pain sensitivity.

The largest and most commonly occurring components in these evoked responses are a sequence of positive, negative and positive deflections at about 100, 120 and 200 milliseconds after the shock stimulus (called P100, N120 and P200). The pattern of increasing amplitude (particularly for the N120) with increasing stimulus intensity is associated with pain sensitivity and hyperalgesia,[1, 5] while a pattern of diminished rate of increase is associated with analgesia and insensitivity.[1] In this paper, unless otherwise stated, the C4 or Cz N120 is the component of interest since it is so strongly related to individual differences in pain sensitivity and narcotic effects. For further details of the importance of somatosensory EP measures of pain sensitivity in other studies relating stimulus/intensity see Buchsbaum,[9] von Knorring and Johansson,[10] and Coger et al.[11]

CEREBROSPINAL FLUID OPIATE-BINDING

There are several strategies for measuring endorphins in man: there are specific radioimmunoassays for endorphins such as methionine enkephalin or β-endorphin or the "radioreceptor" assay for total opiate-like binding. The advantage of the first approach is that a relevant peptide is identified and may be specifically related to a particular physiology. The advantage of the second approach is that when a particular physiological function may be mediated by one or more unknown endorphins, we can examine whether there are increases in total opioid substances.

In our studies of pain appreciation we have chosen the latter approach since we are not sure which endorphins may be relevant to critical perceptual processing. Measurement of total opiate-like binding in cerebrospinal fluid obtained in patients who were medication-free at least 2 weeks was accomplished according to the method of Naber et al.[12]

PAIN APPRECIATION IN AFFECTIVE ILLNESS

Hemphill and associates[13] and Hall and Stride,[14] using heat pain, Merskey,[15] using a pressure algometer, and von Knorring,[16] using electrical stimulation, all found that depressed patients have increased pain thresholds and pain tolerance compared with those variables in normal subjects. There are many similarities between the phenomenology of pain and affective illness: patients with chronic pain and patients with depression typically report loss of appetite, sleep disturbances, decreased libido, inability to concentrate or to take an interest in things, and loss of ability to function at work. Of interest, patients with chronic pain may have a higher frequency of clinical depression and depressive spectrum disorders in first-degree relatives than control subjects.[17]

We have studied 76 affectively ill patients hospitalized on the research wards of the National Institute of Mental Health. These patients were diagnosed using the Research Diagnostic Criteria of Spitzer *et al.*[18] and had been medication-free for at least 2 weeks at the time they participated in somatosensory testing. A small portion of the population with affective disorders was studied during a manic episode: criteria for inclusion in the manic sample required only a global rating of 2 or more on the Bunney–Hamburg rating scale.[19] Age- and sex-matched normal control subjects were recruited from the local community and served as paid volunteers.

Our findings are similar to those cited earlier: depressed patients are more insensitive to experimental pain than are age- and sex-matched controls (for a complete exposition of this study see Davis *et al.*[20]) Depressed patients as a group rated significantly fewer stimuli as unpleasant and very unpleasant than did control subjects (the measure called pain counts). In the overall group the response criterion and insensitivity measures also reflected insensitivity when compared with control subjects' responses. Male depressed patients exhibited pain insensitivity for both unipolar and bipolar depressions. It is of interest that both diagnostic groups were analgesic on the pain counts measure, while only the bipolar patients had elevated error rates and only unipolar patients had elevated response criterions. These data suggest that the insensitivity observed in men with unipolar and bipolar depression may be mediated by different mechanisms. Depressed female patients did not demonstrate pain insensitivity nor were there differences in perception between those with unipolar and bipolar depressions.

Depressed patients as a whole and when divided into unipolar and bipolar subgroups showed pain insensitivity assessed by the evoked potential technique. Depressed patients had lower amplitude/intensity slopes for the N120 than did control subjects.

Although only a small number of actively manic patients was tested (n = 10), these patients were very different from control subjects in pain appreciation. Both male and female manic depressive patients showed pain insensitivity. This was particularly true for males with bipolar depression, who were analgesic on all pain measures. Furthermore manic patients showed markedly lower slopes than did normal subjects and these slopes were lower than those of depressed male counterparts.

The analgesia (relative to normal subjects) found in depressed male patients is in sharp contrast to the high incidence of the complaint of pain in this group. It may be that we are measuring the body's attempt to compensate for increased pain in depression mediated by other mechanisms. We have hypothesized that affective illness is associated with increased pain by virtue of impaired affective inputs to pain appreciation.[20] Our experimental pain measurement technique does not measure affective components of pain appreciation as well as it measures perceptual integrity. If our hypothesis were true, then we would expect that the patients experiencing *increased* clinical pain would be *insensitive* to experimental pain. In fact, in a subgroup of 13 depressed patients, those reporting greater somatic distress (such as headaches or stomach aches) during the 3 days before sensory testing were found to be *more* pain insensitive than those with a low somatic distress score. This suggests that depressed patients experiencing somatic distress may be recruiting endorphins in an attempt to reduce the distress.

Could this insensitivity among depressed patients be due to heightened endorphin activity in relevant somatosensory neuron networks? Certainly opiate receptors and opioid peptides have been located at critical somatosensory sites in the dorsal horn of the spinal cord, in the midbrain and thalamus. A strong case has been made for a pain-inhibitory role for endorphin neurotransmitters at several levels of the nervous system.[21] Furthermore, painful stimulation causes release of endorphins into the ventricles.[22] Patients with chronic pain treated with Zimelidine, a serotonin reuptake inhibitor, experienced relief of pain and a decrease in their CSF endorphin levels.[23] Terenius et al.[24] have reported increased opiate-binding in the cerebrospinal fluid of depressed and manic patients. Furthermore, Almay et al.[25] reported that patients with pain syndromes and depression have elevated opiate-binding material in their cerebrospinal fluid.

We studied opiate binding activity in the cerebrospinal fluid of 35 normal subjects. These subjects participated in our somatosensory tasks on a day different from that on which lumbar puncture was carried out. The subjects were divided in half on the basis of their CSF opiate-binding activity, which created high and low binding groups. We divided the subjects because our earlier work suggested that pain-insensitive subjects show consistent effects to naloxone and morphine administration while relatively sensitive subjects do not.[1, 4] Thus, on the basis of prior studies, we predicted that those subjects with higher CSF endorphin levels would show insensitivity on pain rating and evoked potential measures. In fact, we found that subjects with higher CSF endorphin levels had greater "insensitivity" than did those with lower levels (11.9 versus 11.1) and significantly lower amplitude/intensity slopes for N120 (0.99 versus 1.65 μV/mA, $p < 0.05$, t test). Individual differences in pain sensitivity appear to be partially dependent upon the activity of endorphin neurons in normal volunteers. This finding was also reported by von Knorring et al.[26] in patients with chronic pain; patients with high levels of opiate binding in CSF had higher pain threshold and tolerance levels than did patients with lower CSF levels.

We studied the CSF opiate-binding activity in 24 depressed patients. The group was divided in half, as just described for the normal subjects. Again, the group with high CSF endorphins had significantly greater insensitivity than did the low endorphin group (13.8 versus 7.3, $p < 0.05$), but there was no difference in their amplitude intensity slopes. Furthermore, there were no differences between the normal subjects and the depressed patients with respect to the means of CSF endorphin levels overall.

To summarize: depressed patients, especially depressed males, showed insensitivity to pain in an experimental pain paradigm. Normal and depressed subjects with higher CSF endorphins appear to be more insensitive than those with low endorphin levels in the CSF. While some studies suggest that endorphins may be elevated in depressive illness, we were unable to replicate this finding. Thus, the insensitivity found among our patients may not relate to endorphins or may reflect normal recruitment of endorphin neurons rather than excess activity.

PAIN APPRECIATION IN SCHIZOPHRENIA

Perceptual dysfunction has been a theme of investigations of the psychology of schizophrenia.[27, 28] Abnormal visual, auditory, and olfactory sensation in schizophrenia involves not only sensory thresholds, but also the integration of sensory information as well. It is therefore not surprising that the normal perception of pain appears disturbed in schizophrenia. Even severe and acute clinical conditions usually experienced as exquisitely painful may be less strongly appreciated in psychotic patients. Marchand *et al.*[29] reported that pain did not accompany acute perforated peptic ulcer, acute appendicitis, or fracture of the femur in 21%, 37%, and 42%, respectively, of 79 psychotic patients presenting with these surgical disorders. In an earlier study Marchand [30] found that 82% of psychotic patients with myocardial infarction presented without pain.

Pain insensitivity has been reported not only in clinical conditions, but also in experimental studies of pain in schizophrenic patients. Many investigators have demonstrated that schizophrenics have higher thresholds and diminished reactivity to painful stimuli.[31–34]

We have reported on the insensitivity to pain of 17 medication-free hospitalized schizophrenics compared with 17 age- and sex-matched normal control subjects.[35] Schizophrenics were less pain-sensitive than were control subjects on the pain counts and error rate measures. In fact, 4 of the 17 schizophrenics tested had pain count scores lower and insensitivity scores higher than any of the age- and sex-matched controls.

Schizophrenics had lower mean amplitudes and lower amplitude/intensity slopes than did control subjects: these differences were significant for the N120 as well as for most other evoked potential components.

In a separate experiment,[35] naltrexone, an oral narcotic antagonist, was administered in a placebo-controlled study for a period of not less than 2 weeks. Naltrexone administration was associated with a diminished response criterion and error rate, both findings compatible with a hyperalgesic effect. Naltrexone produced larger amplitudes at the higher stimulus intensities (more painful stimuli), which was significant for the N120 component.

In summary, schizophrenics as a group are more insensitive or analgesic than are normal control subjects, both on the pain-rating task and in their evoked potentials. Presumptive evidence that endorphins may mediate this effect is contained in a pilot study of naltrexone. Naltrexone, which blocks opioid activity, increased the sensitivity to pain of schizophrenic patients on both the pain-rating task and the evoked potential pain paradigm.

We have studied CSF opiate binding in 26 schizophrenic individuals. When pain measures were compared between high and low opiate-binding groups (divided as described in the preceding section), no differences in percent error and N120 amplitude or amplitude intensity measures could be detected. Interestingly, the high binding group had a significantly more sensitive response criterion. In general, opiate binding was lower than in normal and affectively ill patients, although not significantly. The most simple interpretation of these data implies that schizophrenics do not demonstrate a normal association between CSF endorphins and pain sensitivity. A more speculative expression of this conclusion can be phrased as follows: the normal relationships of endorphins to sensitivity to pain seem disturbed in schizophrenia.

A role for endorphins in the symptoms of schizophrenia has been suggested by a number of investigators and tested experimentally by the administration of narcotics, narcotic antagonists, and endorphins to schizophrenic patients. Furthermore, a number of investigators have measured endorphins in the plasma and CSF of schizophrenic patients, with variable results.[36–40] The variability of findings may be due to the fact that schizophrenia is likely heterogeneous in etiology. We have suggested that pain insensitivity might be used as a means of selecting a subgroup of schizophrenics. The subgroup of schizophrenics could then be studied clinically and biologically using narcotic antagonists and tissue endorphin levels.

CONCLUSION

In this paper, we have reviewed a number of studies using an experimental pain paradigm to test somatosensory function in patients with affective illness and schizophrenia. It appears that a portion of affectively ill patients have activated endorphin mechanisms which contribute to insensitivity to experimental pain. This insensitivity appears to be neither qualitatively nor quantitatively different from insensitivity among nondepressed normal volunteers. It may represent the recruitment of normal mechanisms for reducing pain in patients experiencing increased somatic distress via other neural mechanisms.

On the other hand, schizophrenics are not only pain-insensitive, but also do not demonstrate normal relationships between CSF endorphins and pain measures. The disturbance in appreciation of pain may be endorphin-mediated since naltrexone reversed the insensitivity. The disturbance in pain appreciation found in schizophrenic individuals may be a reflection of a far more broad-based disturbance in perceptual functioning related to defective selective attention (see Davis et al.[41] and Buchsbaum et al.[42]).

REFERENCES

1. BUCHSBAUM, M. S., G. C. DAVIS, R. COPPOLA & D. NABER. 1981. Pain **10:** 357–366.
2. DAVIS, G. C., M. S. BUCHSBAUM & W. E. BUNNEY, JR. 1978. Life Sci. **23:** 1449–1460.
3. BUCHSBAUM, M. S. & G. C. DAVIS. 1979. *In* Human Evoked Potentials. D. Lehmann and E. Calloway, Eds.: 43–54. Plenum Press. New York.
4. BUCHSBAUM, M. S., G. C. DAVIS & W. E. BUNNEY, JR. 1977. Nature **270:** 620–622.
5. BUCHSBAUM, M. S., G. C. DAVIS, R. COPPOLA & D. NABER. 1981. Pain **10:** 367–377.
6. MCNICHOL, D. 1972. A Primer of Signal Detection Theory. George Allen & Unwin. London.
7. ROLLMAN, G. 1977. Pain **3:** 187–211.
8. MCNICHOL, D. 1972. A Primer of Signal Detection Theory. George Allen & Unwin. London.
9. BUCHSBAUM, M. S., G. C. DAVIS & F. K. GOODWIN et al. 1980. *In* Clinical Neurophysiological Aspects of Psychopathological Conditions. C. Perris, L. von Knorring & D. Kemali, Eds.: 63–70. S. Karger. Basel.
10. VON KNORRING, L. & F. JOHANSSON. 1979. Psychiat. Res. **1:** 225–230.
11. COGER, R. W., B. KENTON, J. PINSKY, et al. 1980. Psychiat. Res. **2:** 279–294.

12. NABER, D., D. PICKAR, R. A. DIONNE, D. L. *et al.* 1980. Subst. Alcoh. Act. Misuse 1: 83–92.
13. HEMPHILL, R. E., K. R. L. HALL & T. G. CROOKES. 1952. J. Mental Sci. 98: 433–440.
14. HALL, K. R. L. & E. STRIDE. 1954. Br. J. Med. Psychol. 27: 48–60.
15. MERSKEY, H. 1965. J. Psychosomat. Res. 8: 405–519.
16. VON KNORRING, L. 1975. The experience of pain in patients with depressive disorders. A clinical and experimental study. Umeå University Medical Dissertations, Umeå, Sweden.
17. SCHAFFER, C. B., P. T. DONLON & R. M. BITTLE. 1980. Am. J. Psychiat. 137: 118–120.
18. SPITZER, R. L., J. ENDICOTT & E. ROBBINS. 1975. Psychopharmacol. Bull. 3: 22–25.
19. BUNNEY, W. E. JR. & D. A. HAMBURG. 1963. Arch. Gen. Psychiat. 9: 280–294.
20. DAVIS, G. C., M. S. BUCHSBAUM & W. E. BUNNEY, JR. 1979. Am. J. Psychiat. 136: 1148–1151.
21. PERT, A., C. B. PERT, G. C. DAVIS & W. E. BUNNEY, JR. 1981. *In* Handbook of Biological Psychiatry, Vol. IV. H. M. van Praag, M. H. Lader, O. J. Rafaelsen & E. J. Sacher, Eds.: 547–582. Marcel Dekker. New York.
22. AKIL, H., D. E. RICHARDSON, J. HUGHES & J. D. BARCHAS. 1978. Science 201: 463–465.
23. JOHANSSON, F., L. VON KNORRING, G. SEDVALL & L. TERENIUS. 1980. Psychiat. Res. 2: 167–172.
24. TERENIUS, L., A. WAHLSTRÖM, L. LINDSTRÖM & E. WIDERLÖV. 1976. Neurosci. Lett. 3: 157–162.
25. ALMAY, B. G. L., R. JOHANSSON & L. VON KNORRING *et al.* 1978. Pain 5: 153–162.
26. VON KNORRING, L., B. G. L. ALMAY, F. JOHANSSON & L. TERENIUS. 1978. Pain 5: 359–365.
27. VENABLES, P. H. 1973. *In* Psychopathology. M. Hammer, K. Salzinger & S. Sutton, Eds.: 261–284. John Wiley & Sons. New York.
28. GARMEZY, N. 1978. J. Psychiat. Res. 14: 3–34.
29. MARCHAND, W. E., B. SAROTA & H. C. MARBLE *et al.* 1969. N. Engl. J. Med. 260: 580–585.
30. MARCHAND, W. E. 1955. N. Engl. J. Med. 253: 51–55.
31. MALMO, R. B. & C. SHAGASS. 1949. Psychosomat. Med. 11: 9–24.
32. MALMO, R. B., C. SHAGASS & A. A. SMITH. 1951. J. Personal. 19: 359–375.
33. HALL, K. R. L. & E. STRIDE. 1954. Br. J. Med. Psychol. 27: 48–60.
34. SAPPINGTON, J. 1973. Percept. Mot. Skills 37: 498–490.
35. DAVIS, G. C., M. S. BUCHSBAUM, D. L. VAN KAMMEN & W. E. BUNNEY, JR. 1979. Psychiat. Res. 1: 61–66.
36. LINDSTRÖM, L. H., E. WIDERLÖV, L.-M. GUNNE *et al.* 1978. Acta Psychiat. Scand. 57: 153–164.
37. RIMON, R., L. TERENIUS & R. KAMPMAN. 1980. Acta Psychiat. Scand. 61: 395–403.
38. ROSS, M., P. A. BERGER & A. GOLDSTEIN. 1979. Science 205: 1163–1164.
39. EMRICH, H. M., V. HOLLT & W. KISSLING *et al.* 1979. Pharmakopsychiatr. 12: 269–276.
40. TERENIUS, L. 1968. *In* Characteristics and Function of Opioids. J. M. van Ree & L. Terenius, Eds.: 143–158. Elsevier/North Holland Biomedical Press. Amsterdam.
41. DAVIS, G. C., M. S. BUCHSBAUM & W. E. BUNNEY, JR. 1980. *In* Neural Peptides and Neuronal Communications. E. Costa & M. Trabucchi, Eds.: 473–487. Raven Press. New York.
42. BUCHSBAUM, M. S., V. I. REUS, G. C. DAVIS, H. H. HOLCOMB, J. CAPPELLETTI & E. SILBERMAN. Ann. N.Y. Acad. Sci. 398: 352–365. This volume.

ROLE OF OPIOID PEPTIDES IN DISORDERS OF ATTENTION IN PSYCHOPATHOLOGY

M. S. Buchsbaum, V. I. Reus, G. C. Davis, H. H. Holcomb,
J. Cappelletti, and E. Silberman

ALTERED PAIN PERCEPTION AND CEREBROSPINAL ENDORPHINS IN PSYCHIATRIC ILLNESS

Glenn C. Davis, Monte S. Buchsbaum, Dieter Naber, David Pickar,
Robert Post, Daniel Van Kammen, and William E. Bunney, Jr.

DISCUSSION OF THE PAPERS

UNIDENTIFIED SPEAKER: Dr. Davis, have you looked at CSF opiate binding in placebo responders?

G. C. DAVIS: No, we have not done specific placebo experiments. Our own approach is that of studying individual differences in pain sensitivity. Since the degree of placebo responsiveness is one type of individual difference, these two phenomena may be related.

We certainly need to do experiments to determine whether placebo responsiveness is one component of the individual differences we are measuring.

QUESTION: Would you expect persons who are placebo reactors to have higher CSF opiate bindings?

DAVIS: I do not know.

UNIDENTIFIED SPEAKER: I am curious to know about the drug history of your patients during these tests. It seems to me that it might be difficult to distinguish what is just an attentional deficit due to chlorpromazine or some other antipsychotic drug.

DAVIS: That's a fair observation. All of our patients had been drug-free for at least 2 weeks, and many for more than a month.

UNIDENTIFIED SPEAKER: Was the dose of naltrexone used in your study administered orally?

DAVIS: Yes.

UNIDENTIFIED SPEAKER: The dose seems rather high. You used between 150 and 300 mg/day for 3 weeks.

DAVIS: No; we used between 200 and 800 mg/day.

UNIDENTIFIED SPEAKER: That seems very high. How were the dosages chosen? Did you see any side effects or did you see symptomatic improvement in the schizophrenic patients?

DAVIS: In our small sample of patients we did not see dramatic clinical effects. While several patients improved, we have no independent validation that these patients comprised a subgroup. I was not in charge of the management of these patients, so I cannot tell you the incidence of adverse effects.

Certainly, no *major* side effects were seen. One patient required dental work and was taken off of the naltrexone so that analgesics could be given.

UNIDENTIFIED SPEAKER: Dr. Buchsbaum, what is the reliability of your method of obtaining positron emission tomography (PET) images? How does this relate to the resolution power of your particular positron tomograph?

M. S. BUCHSBAUM: We have not yet done test–retest reliability studies on the PET procedure since it is such an expensive and complicated procedure. We have not had the resources to repeat the test on the same normal volunteer in two separate sessions.

However, in terms of reliability, in our first series we have studied eight schizophrenics and approximately eight normal volunteers, age- and sex-matched, with the PET procedure. The first set of tests was done with the schizophrenics and the normal subjects resting quietly in a dark room with as much silence as possible.

In a paper submitted for publication we report a marked increase in glucose use in the frontal cortex of normal volunteers in comparison with that of the schizophrenic group, and this was statistically reliable.

Now, since the time of this report we have examined a series of patients with our pain stimulation technique, collecting evoked potentials from the 16 cortical locations and simultaneously administering the fluordeoxyglucose for PET scanning.

In these studies we have now completed observations on eight normal subjects and only two schizophrenics. While we cannot really use a statistical comparison, the data show a tremendous increase in frontal lobe glucose use with the electric shock in the normal group compared with the two schizophrenics. The schizophrenic who was quite symptomatic had no increase in frontal lobe glucose utilization at all with the electric shock, while the schizophrenic in remsision looked quite normal.

The resolution limit of the PET scan is a technical issue; it is 1.7 centimeters full width half-max, which means that you can make out the caudate nucleus and the thalamus if you have a lot of imagination. If you have experience in administering electric shocks, then you can see the thalamus a lot more clearly. In one illustration I showed you the thalamus could be seen as one cross-sectional image. Thus, the resolution is adequate to see some of these pain structures, certainly the primary somatosensory area in the cortex, the frontal lobe, and the thalamus; I am not sure whether the medulla can be seen or not. The exact glucose quantification of those small structures may not be as accurate as we would hope. Perhaps we will have large enough effects to be able to show a statistically significant comparison.

DAVIS: Another limiting factor in PET work is the amount of radiation to which patients may be exposed. Thus, true test–retest reliability may not be determined at this state of the art.

C. KORNETSKY (*Boston University School of Medicine, Boston, MA*): I found the work on attention to be quite interesting for it reminded me of some work I did a few years ago with Joe Lapinsky in which we treated schizophrenic patients with naloxone. Basically, we found that the patients did not improve at all with the naloxone treatment. However, we did test them also with the continuous performance test, which was the only test that we ran that showed significant improvement in these schizophrenic patients. At the time we did not think too much of it, and just mentioned it in a note.

DAVIS: While you did not pay much attention to the finding, we did, and we cite your paper with regard to its findings on attention. In preliminary studies with the continuous performance task we were unable to demonstrate a naloxone effect.

Nevertheless, we believe that the issue of the narcotic antagonist's effect on selective attention in schizophrenics is very important. It is an outcome measure in my current studies of the effects of narcotic antagonists on schizophrenia.

UNIDENTIFIED SPEAKER: I would like to congratulate the NIH researchers both for their good work and for their restraint (some groups who are working with PET have implied that they can diagnose certain illnesses on the basis of the patterns).

Now, my question has to do with the specificity of the effects that are seen in the diagrams that were drawn yesterday by Dr. Clouet and others. It's quite obvious that interconnections in the brain are multiple, and although a lot of attention has been paid to endorphins in the last decade, if antagonists of other brain neurotransmitters were used, would there be any changes in the N120, for instance?

H. H. HOLCOMB: The drugs that we found most effective so far in effecting the N120 attentional enhancement, aside from the one or two little pilot studies we have done with naloxone or naltrexone, have been amphetamines and caffeine. Those are the two that have the largest effect on the attentional enhancement.

So, some of the effect that we might be seeing with naloxone could be related to indirect effects on the noradrenergic system, and the two things are then working together to enhance the N120.

DAVIS: We are certainly not single-substance investigators. The existing clinical evidence that narcotic antagonists might have therapeutic effect may suggest a neuroleptic interaction. Dr. Pickar may also address this possibility in his paper. Naloxone has a small, statistically significant effect on thought disorder symptoms, but it appears only in neuroleptic-stabilized individuals. Medication-free patients do not seem to show this effect.

We are very interested in the dopamine–endorphin–enkephalin interaction. It may be that narcotic antagonists facilitate neuroleptic effects.

UNIDENTIFIED SPEAKER: Were your patients a particular subtype of schizophrenic?

DAVIS: We do not have an adequate sample size to do subgrouping. Nevertheless, you might say it was a typical NIMH patient sample, and it contained a large percentage of paranoid patients. At the NIMH, schizophrenic patients are generally younger and are late-onset schizophrenics.

ENDORPHIN LEVELS IN OPIOID-DEPENDENT HUMAN SUBJECTS: A LONGITUDINAL STUDY *

C. P. O'Brien,[†] L. Terenius,[‡] A. Wahlström,[‡]
A. T. McLellan,[†] and W. Krivoy [§]

† Department of Psychiatry
University of Pennsylvania, and
Philadelphia Veterans Administration Medical Center
Philadelphia, Pennsylvania 19104

‡ Department of Pharmacology
University of Uppsala
Uppsala Sweden

§ National Institute on Drug Abuse
Addiction Research Center
Lexington, Kentucky 40597

The discovery of specific opiate receptors [1-3] and endogenous opiates [4-6] raised hopes that the biochemical changes produced by opioid dependence would soon be better understood. Thus far, however, studies of endorphins in opioid-dependent subjects have produced inconclusive results. Several investigators reported no alteration in total brain enkephalin content in rats after acute morphine treatment or after chronic treatment for up to 10 days or after naloxone-precipitated withdrawal.[7-9] However, enkephalin content of a specific brain region, the striatum, was significantly decreased in rats after 24 hours of abstinence produced by abrupt cessation of morphine treatment.[10] Striatal enkephalin reduction was also seen in rats treated with high doses of morphine for a month or longer.[11] These chronically treated animals also showed reduction in β-endorphin-like immunoreactivity in the septum, midbrain, and pituitary, but not in the hypothalamus. Follow-up studies by the same investigations, using high-affinity agonists (etorphine, levorphanol) instead of morphine, failed to reproduce the endorphin changes despite high degrees of tolerance/dependence. This raises the possibility that the morphine effects were due to nonspecific factors.

Reduction in regional enkephalin levels is consistent with the report [13] that chronic morphine treatment activates a high-affinity enkephalin-hydrolyzing enzyme. Although confirmation so far is lacking, this finding highlights the need for techniques for studying endorphin turnover rates during dependence and withdrawal.

Studies of endorphin activity have been conducted in three groups of human addicts. Clement-Jones and colleagues [14] found cerebrospinal fluid (CSF) β-endorphin activity to be elevated in five of the six addicts studied during mild withdrawal. Twelve patients in withdrawal gave 22 plasma samples, and 19 of these samples showed elevated β-endorphin-like immunoreactivity. Methionine-enkephalin levels were not elevated in either plasma or CSF of these patients,

* This work was supported by Grant DA 01505 from the National Institute on Drug Abuse and by the Veterans Administration Medical Research Service.

0077–8923/82/0398–0377 $01.75/0 © 1982 NYAS

but electroaccupuncture was followed by a significant rise in CSF methionine-enkephalin. In another study, Ho and colleagues [15] studied plasma from 19 men with unspecified levels of addiction to heroin. Plasma samples were tested using an immunoassay reactive to a spectrum of compounds including β-endorphin, β-lipotropin, the 31-K prohormone, and an unidentified plasma factor. The addict plasma had about one-third the immunoreactivity of control samples. In a third study, Holmstrand and colleagues [16] found great variability in radioreceptor endorphin assays of CSF from 17 opiate addicts. These subjects were studied after 3 drug-free weeks and again after 3 weeks of methadone maintenance treatment. Those with abnormal endorphin levels tended to show the best clinical response to methadone treatment.

The present study is based on the assumption that if there are changes in the endorphin system caused by opioid dependence, the changes are likely to be dynamic rather than static. Accordingly, repeated measures of endorphin activity have been made in a population of opioid addicts as they progress through measurable clinical states. These states are agonist maintenance (methadone), withdrawal, the drug-free state, and antagonist maintenance (naltrexone). Thus, subjects can be compared with themselves at different times or in different states as well as with others. Endorphin activity has been measured by receptor-binding assay [5] and by appropriate immunoassay as indicated. The study is ongoing and herein we report preliminary results.

METHOD

Opiate-dependent subjects were recruited from the Drug Dependence Treatment and Research Center of the Philadelphia Veterans Administration Hospital. All were males, 21 to 55 years of age, who met the criterion of being physically dependent on opiates for 1 year or more. Excluded were volunteers with history of regular nonopiate use, organic mental disorder, neurologic disorder, major affective disorder, or schizophrenic disorder. All subjects were given a full explanation of the procedure and only permitted to sign the consent form after they had passed a quiz indicating comprehension of the information.[17] A detailed lifetime drug history and a rating on the Addiction Severity Index [18] were obtained prior to entering the study. Before each sampling procedure, self-ratings of opiate withdrawal and affect were obtained. Observer ratings of anxiety, depression, and opiate-withdrawal signs were also obtained. Drug history was verified by regular urine testing during outpatient treatment and during hospitalization.

Samples were obtained from patients in one or more of the following clinical states:

Agonist maintenance (methadone): level dose for at least 2 weeks.

Withdrawal: abrupt cessation of methadone; samples were obtained 24 to 96 hours after the last dose of methadone.

Antagonist Maintenance: subjects were stabilized on naltrexone, 50 mg per day, for at least 2 weeks.

Drug-free: subjects were detoxified and verified to be drug-free by urine testing for at least 1 month.

Cerebrospinal fluid was obtained between the hours of 0830 and 0930 by lumbar puncture with the patient in the lateral decubitus position. A 22-gauge spinal needle was inserted into L3–L4 after local anesthesia with 2% lidocaine. Sixteen ml of CSF was collected in four tubes and centrifuged in a refrigerated centrifuge, and the supernatant was frozen to −60° C. Plasma samples were collected immediately after completion of spinal tap.

All CSF samples were extracted with methylene chloride [16] and separated into two fractions (FI and FII) on Sephadex G-10 columns prior to radio-receptor assay, using the method described by Terenius and Wahlström.[5] Samples from patients receiving naltrexone were also assayed by radioimmuno-assay (RIA) for dynorphin (1–13) and methionine-enkephalin. Antisera raised by bovine thyroglobulin conjugates of tritium-labeled methionine-enkephalin and iodine-125-labeled dynorphin (1–13) were used in a standard RIA proce-dure.[10] Plasma samples also were analyzed for methadone by RIA.[19] The remainder of the CSF and plasma have been kept frozen for future endorphin analysis.

RESULTS

Thus far, 51 samples have been obtained from 27 opioid-dependent (or postdependent) subjects. All were males with a mean age of 30 years who had been addicted to opiates for an average of 10 years. Results of the radio-receptor assays are shown in FIGURES 1 and 2. Values for endorphin fractions are expressed in methionine-enkephalin equivalents (pmol/ml). The previously reported [20] levels of FI and FII in 38 samples from 19 normal subjects of both sexes are also shown.

The levels of FI are not significantly different among the groups, although there is more variance among the addicts. FII levels are generally much higher

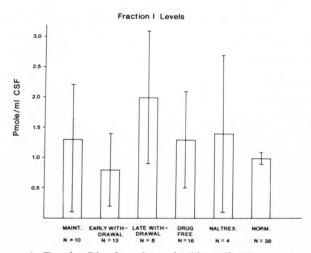

FIGURE 1. Fraction I levels as determined by radioreceptor assay.

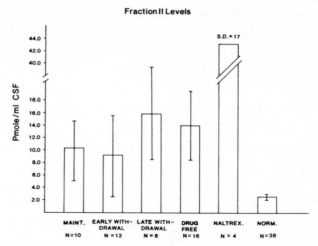

FIGURE 2. Fraction II levels as determined by radioreceptor assay.

in the addicts than in normal subjects, with naltrexone-treated subjects showing values 20–100 times greater than those found in normal subjects. When the samples from naltrexone-treated subjects were analyzed by RIA, values for methionine-enkephalin and dynorphin (1–13) were not significantly different from control values.

Pearson product–moment correlations with FI and FII were calculated for the following variables: age, years addicted, methadone dose, methadone plasma level, hours since last dose, affect scores, subjective withdrawal scores, and objective withdrawal scores. Number of years addicted was consistently and positively related to FI ($r = 0.44$; $p = 0.002$). Patients maintained on higher doses of methadone tended to manifest significantly greater withdrawal signs and symptoms, higher affect scores, and lower endorphin levels (FI versus methadone plasma level: $r = 0.5$; $p = .04$; FII versus methadone level: $r = 0.5$; $p = 0.03$). FIGURES 1 and 2 show the endorphin values for early (24–48 hr) and later (48–96 hr) withdrawal. Higher withdrawal symptoms were related to lower FII ($r = 0.6$; $p < 0.04$), and there was a trend for both fractions to become higher in the withdrawal group as hours passed since the last dose of methadone. However, about half of the subjects received low doses of diazepam or doxepin during withdrawal. The increase in endorphin as withdrawal progressed was only present in subjects who received no diazepam. When subjects receiving diazepam were analyzed separately, the only relationship that remained significant for those subjects was the consistent positive correlation between number of years addicted and levels of FI.

COMMENTS

Studies of any biological variable in addicted persons must take into account the radical changes that occur in these patients relative to the time and size of their last dose. We have elected to study subjects in four different states of the addiction cycle which are definable and possess clinical relevance. As shown in FIGURES 1 and 2, results of radioreceptor assays of both CSF endorphin fractions show generally higher values and much greater variance in the clinical states as compared with findings in the normal group. Levels of both endorphin fractions show a trend toward being lower in early withdrawal than in either maintenance or late withdrawal. Because of the large variance, more subjects are needed before the significance of the changes can be adequately assessed.

Better definition of patients and clinical states may also help to clarify these relationships. For example, the role of small doses of nonopioids (diazepam or doxepin) was not appreciated when the first samples were obtained. Since addicts in withdrawal have a very low pain threshhold and usually exhibit fear of spinal taps, obtaining volunteers in withdrawal was difficult. In some patients, a low dose of diazepam was used to allay anxiety. Subsequently, it was discovered that relationships between last dose of methadone and endorphin levels were different in subjects who received the diazepam. This observation is consistent with reports of diazepam-induced release of opioid activity in rodents.[21]

Since the variables are confounded, it is not clear whether the diazepam or the anxiety (which led to the administration of diazepam) might have affected endorphin levels. Of course, in all recent work, ancillary medications have been prohibited, even though this caused some volunteers to leave the study.

By far the most striking finding was the greatly elevated FII levels in the patients receiving naltrexone. The levels of this endorphin fraction were found to be increased 20–100 times over those found in normal subjects. This large increase led us to wonder whether naltrexone or naltrexone metabolites active at opiate receptors were interfering with the radioreceptor assay. When samples of naltrexone and all available naltrexone metabolities * were added to CSF samples and run through our extraction procedure, almost all of the added naltrexone and metabolites were recovered. This suggests that the extraction procedure was successful for the available metabolites of naltrexone. However, we have recently analyzed FII samples by electrophoresis and high-performance liquid chromatography (HPLC), which showed that the large FII elevations as measured by radioreceptor assay were not due to a peptide. Thus, the possibility remains that an unextracted naltrexone metabolite is responsible for the elevation of FII. In this preliminary report, therefore, we are uncertain as to the source or the significance of the FII elevations in the naltrexone-treated patients.

An elevation in endorphin activity produced by the opioid antagonist naltrexone is entirely in keeping with the feedback hypothesis. Such a finding is also consistent with the report of naloxone-induced endorphin elevation [22] and antagonist-induced increases in opiate receptor activity.[23-25] The possibility of consistently high endorphin levels in naltrexone-maintained patients suggests the need for further study of these persons. Does the presence of naltrexone block *all* of the effects of elevated endorphins? Might a short-acting antagonist such as naloxone produce endorphin effects that outlast the antagonist? Thus, some supposed naloxone effects might be cause by reflex elevations of endorphins.

* Naltrexone-3-glucuronide, 6-β-naltrexol, 2-hydroxy-3-methoxynaltrexol; courtesy of National Institute on Drug Abuse.

In methadone-maintained subjects, CSF endorphin levels, as determined by radioreceptor assay, were also higher than normal. The feedback hypothesis would have predicted the opposite: suppressed endorphins during agonist maintenance. Perhaps the "suppression" of endogenous opiate activity occurs via down regulation of receptor sensitivity or reduction in number of receptors. In consequence, the data suggest a "rebound" effect on endorphin levels during late withdrawal. However, our sample is not yet adequate to be clear about this.

SUMMARY

Endorphin levels were measured in 51 cerebrospinal fluid samples from 27 opioid-dependent or postdependent subjects. Radioreceptor assay showed the endorphin levels to be higher than those found in normal subjects. These high levels were found even while subjects were on methadone maintenance. The duration of opioid dependence was positively correlated with fraction I values. Both fractions tended to be lower during early withdrawal than late withdrawal. In naltrexone-maintained patients, radioreceptor assay showed FII to be greatly elevated, but electrophoresis and HPLC indicated that the elevations were not due to a peptide. Thus, the possibility of unextracted naltrexone metabolites remains at least a partial explanation for this apparent FII elevation.

ACKNOWLEDGMENTS

The plasma methadone levels were determined by Dr. Charles Inturrisi, Cornell Medical College. Drs. George Woody, Robert Greenstein, Martin Marcovici, and Bradley Evans assisted in the clinical aspects of this project.

REFERENCES

1. PERT, C. B. & S. H. SNYDER. 1973. Opiate receptor: Demonstration in nervous tissue. Science 179: 1011–1014.
2. SIMON, E. J., J. M. HILLER & I. EDELMAN. 1973. Stereospecific binding of the potent narcotic analgesic ³H-etorphine to rat brain homogenate. Proc. Natl Acad. Sci. USA 70: 1947–1949.
3. TERENIUS, L. 1973. Characteristics of the "receptor" for narcotic analgesics in synaptic plasma membrane fractions from rat brain. Acta Pharmacol. Toxicol. 33: 377–384.
4. TERENIUS, L. & A. WAHLSTRÖM. 1974. Inhibitor(s) of narcotic receptor binding in brain extracts and in cerebrospinal fluid. Acta Pharmacol. (Kbh.) (Suppl. 1) 33: 55.
5. PASTERNAK, G. W., R. GOODMAN & S. H. SNYDER. 1975. An endogenous morphine-like factor in mammalian brain. Life Sci. 16: 1765–1769.
6. HUGHES, J., T. W. SMITH, H. W. KOSTERLITZ, L. FOTHERGILL, B. A. MOYAN & H. R. MORRIS. 1975. Identification of two related pentapeptides from the brain with potent opiate agonist activity. Nature 258: 577–579.
7. FRATTA, W., H. Y. T. YANY, J. HONG & E. COSTA. 1977. Stability of met-enkephalin content in brain structures of morphine dependent or foot-shock stressed rats. Nature 268: 452.

8. CHILDERS, S., R. SIMINTOV & S. H. SNYDER. 1977. Enkephalin: Radio-immuno-assay and radioreceptor assay in morphine dependent rats. Eur. J. Pharmacol. **46:** 289.
9. WESCHE, D., V. HOLLT & A. HERZ. 1977. Radio-immunoassay of enkephalins. Regional distribution in rat brain after morphine treatment and hypophysectomy. Naunyn-Schmiedebergs' Arch. Pharmakol. **301:** 79.
10. BERGSTRÖM, L. & L. TERENIUS. 1979. Enkephalin levels decrease in rat striatum during morphine abstinence. Eur. J. Pharmacol. **60:** 349.
11. PRZEWLOCKI, R., V. HOLLT, T. DUKA, G. LKEBER, C. GRAMSCH, I. HAARMANN & A. HERZ. 1979. Long term morphine treatment decreases endorphin levels in rat brain and pituitary. Brain Res. **174:** 357.
12. WUSTER, M., R. SCHULZ & A. HERZ. 1980. Inquiry into endorphinergic feedback mechanisms during the development of opiate tolerance/dependence. Brain Res. **189:** 403–411.
13. MALFROY, B., J. P. SWERTZ, A. GUYON, B. P. ROQUES & J. C. SWARTZ. 1978. High affinity enkephalin degrading peptidase in brain is increased after morphine. Nature **276:** 523.
14. CLEMENT-JONES, V., L. MCLAUGHLIN, P. J. LOWRY, G. M. BESSER & L. H. REES. 1979. Acupuncture in heroin addicts: Changes in met-enkephalin and endorphin in blood and cerebrospinal fluid. Lancet **ii:** 380.
15. HO, W. K. K., H. L. WEN & N. LING. 1980. Beta endorphin-like immuno-activity in the plasma of heroin addicts and normal subjects. Neuropharmacology **19:** 117.
16. HOLMSTRAND, J., L. M. GUNNE, A. WAHLSTRÖM & L. TERENIUS. 1981. CSF-endorphins in heroin addicts during methadone maintenance and during withdrawal. Pharmacopsychiatria **14**(4): 126–128.
17. GRABOWSKI, J. G., C. P. O'BRIEN & J. MINTZ. 1979. Increasing the likelihood that consent is informed. J. Exp. Anal. Behav. **24:** 283–284.
18. MCLELLAN, A. T., L. LUBORSKY, C. P. O'BRIEN & G. E. WOODY. 1980. An improved diagnostic evaluation instrument for substance abuse patients: The Addiction Severity Index. J. Nerv. Ment. Disord. **168:** 26–33.
19. LING, G. F. F., J. G. UMANS & C. E. INTURRISI. 1981. Methadone: Radioimmunoassay and pharmacokinetics in the rat. J. Pharmacol. Exp. Ther. **217:** 147–151.
20. LINDSTRÖM, L. H., E. WIDERLÖV, L. M. GUNNE, A. WAHLSTRÖM & L. TERENIUS. 1978. Endorphins in human cerebrospinal fluid: Clinical correlations to some psychotic states. Acta Psychiat. Scand. **57:** 153–164.
21. WUSTER, M., T. DUKA & A. HERZ. 1980. Diazepam-induced release of opioid activity in the rat brain. Neurosci. Lett. **16:** 335–337.
22. NABER, D., D. PICKAR, G. C. DAVIS, R. M. COHEN, D. C. JIMERSON, M. A. ELCHISAK, E. G. DEFRAITES, N. H. KALIN, S. C. RISCH & M. S. BUCHSBAUM. 1981. Naloxone effects on β-endorphin, cortisol, prolactin, growth hormone, HVA and MHPG in plasma of normal volunteers. Psychopharmacologie **74:** 125–128.
23. TANG, A. H. & R. J. COLLINS. 1978. Enhanced analgesic effects of morphine after chronic administration of naloxone in the rat. Eur. J. Pharmacol. **47:** 473–476.
24. SCHULZ, R., M. WUSTER & A. HERZ. 1979. Supersensitivity to opioids following the chronic blockade of endorphin by naloxone. Arch. Pharmacol. **306:** 93–96.
25. ZUKIN, R. S., E. GARDNER & A. R. GINTZLER. 1981. Mechanisms of supersensitivity in the enkephalinergic system. International Narcotics Research Conference, Kyoto, Japan. Abstracts. 8.

DISCUSSION OF THE PAPER

E. SIMON (*New York University School of Medicine, New York*): What evidence do you have that the great amount of receptor inhibition that you found with the naltrexone-treated patients is in fact attributable to opioids and does not present a poison of the opioid receptor?

We had many problems with plasma and plasma extracts. We have found inhibition of opiate binding, some of which is even irreversible.

C. O'BRIEN: There is no indication of any irreversible effect, but perhaps Dr. Wahlström will answer your question.

A. WAHLSTRÖM: I don't really know what you mean by poisoning of the receptor, but we have a purification procedure before we measure the receptor binding, and I can't imagine that there are any other substances that could poison the receptor. Could you suggest some?

SIMON: Yes. We have used supernatant from homogenates, for instance, and we get clear-cut irreversible inhibition, and we have not identified it. Also, phospholipase and heavy metals and other substances will poison the receptor.

M. J. KREEK (*Rockfeller University, New York*) As you know, Dr. O'Brien, we are carrying out similar studies here in New York. Not able to obtain CSF, we have to content ourselves with plasma; we also are looking specifically at β-endorphin. We have found one thing that I think dovetails very nicely with what you have seen, that is, that there are very few differences between the chronic methadone-maintained patients and the otherwise healthy patients with respect to β-endorphin levels in peripheral plasma.

However, unlike what you found with fraction II (containing a mixture of opioid fragments), which seemed to be lowered maximally at 4 hours after dose, we found that β-endorphin levels were essentially normal at 4 hours after a methadone dose.

Secondly, in our work in the rat, in which we have studied the effects of chronic methadone or chronic naltrexone treatment on β-endorphin content, we have seen no effects due to methadone. However, the effects of chronic naltrexone administration have correlated very well with your clinical findings on total opioid activity, that is, you are seeing an increase in opioid-related compounds in CSF and we have seen a depletion of β-endorphin in the hypothalamus. Those two findings are highly complementary.

Finally, in your diazepam-medicated patients, did you study prolactin, ACTH, or cortisol levels, or any other markers of acute stress, to see whether those are also diminished by benzodiazepines?

O'BRIEN: Dr. Kreek, I may have misled you about the timing. We have the subject stop taking methadone and do spinal taps at 24, 48, 72 or 96 hours later. Of course, for 36 to 48 hours later methadone can still be detected in plasma. Early withdrawal is usually around 36 to 48 hours, and that is when we find that there is a tendency for lower endorphin levels with a trend toward subsequent increases.

I should also mention that a group of Swedish addicts were studied by Lindström, Terenius and Wahlström, in which plasma methadone and CSF endorphin levels on maintenance were examined. In this study, the plasma methadone levels didn't correlate well with CSF endorphin level as measured by the radioreceptor assay. In our study it was the *time* since the last dose of methadone that correlated best, but the time period is much longer than 4 hours—the time course is more like 36 to 100 hours.

UNIDENTIFIED SPEAKER: Would you define detoxification? How is it accomplished? How long does it take? How is it done?

O'BRIEN: Normally we do not even put the person in the hospital, until the methadone dosage is down to 20 milligrams. Then, the amount of methadone is withdrawn gradually, at the rate of 5 milligrams or less per day from there. Occasionally, we use clonidine or other agents to help with the detoxification.

Now, our endorphin study did not use a gradual withdrawal. Here we are trying to set up an experimental situation in which there may be some detectable changes. So, in some cases individuals who have been taking fairly high doses of methadone stop the dose abruptly. As the plasma levels decline, symptoms may take 48 hours or more to develop. We looked for objective signs, not just subjective complaints. The subjects were volunteers who were willing to remain off methadone until clear physical signs developed. Thus, this was an abrupt detoxification for experimental purposes. We would not, of course, use this method for purely clinical reasons.

J. VOLAVKA (*New York University School of Medicine, New York*): Why were you puzzled by the increase of these opioids on naltrexone? Wouldn't you expect accumulation of the opioids after displacing them from the receptor with the antagonist? What did you expect?

O'BRIEN: This is exactly what we expected on the basis of your work reported in *The New England Journal of Medicine* several years ago. We thought that if ACTH increases, then endorphin should increase. Herz and coworkers, in a study in animals, showed that administration of naloxone increases enkephalin in the striatum. On the receptor side, Dr. Zukin and her colleagues recently reported that treating rats with naltrexone causes an increase in opiate receptor sensitivity beginning about 2 days after naltrexone administration and peaking at about 8 days. So we did expect to find some increases in endorphin levels in patients chronically treated with opiate antagonists. There are problems, as I discussed in the paper, in being certain that naltrexone metabolites which are active at opiate receptors are not being mistaken for endorphins. Thus, the significance and magnitude of this finding remains uncertain and we must continue to investigate in the area.

SIMON: Dr. O'Brien, have you ever tried to see whether this activity is inhibited by peptidases?

O'BRIEN: No, we have not studied peptidase inhibition on the increased activity seen in naltrexone-treated patients. It is another strategy that should be considered.

H. D. KLEBER (*Yale Medical School, New Haven, CT*): It is interesting to try to put your findings together with what we know clinically. I wonder whether the large increase in CSF endorphin that occurs after naltrexone administration in any way explains why we have so much trouble getting patients to continue to take naltrexone, especially during the first 2 to 4 weeks. If these patients are followed and retention rates on naltrexone are studied, we find a leveling off after about a month. But at that point, you've lost about 60% of the persons who started the therapy. I wonder whether perhaps endorphins are being stripped from the hypothalamus, producing a very dysphoric experience at that point.

O'BRIEN: One of the things I like about discussion periods is that you can be a little more speculative.

Although we do not really know, we suspect that while we are causing an increase in fraction II, some of it may actually be having some effect. Naltrexone has few subjective effects in normal subjects if the dose is increased slowly. Postaddicts, however, have spontaneously testified to having greater interest in sexual activity while on naltrexone therapy. Some of them have lost weight and others have had traumatic injuries, like breaking a hand or a foot, and did not have any problems with pain. Thus, one may speculate that some of the possible increase in endorphins is having an effect. This might have been thought to be an agonist effect, but, in fact, it may really be due to a feedback endorphin increase due to blocking of some opiate receptors.

K. A. BONNET (*New York University Medical Center, New York*): I would like to compliment you on a nice piece of work, Dr. O'Brien. We've done a number of studies, and our study group is now up to about 86 addicts in whom we have determined plasma β-endorphins and ACTH, taking serial samples in many cases. Our findings agree with yours, for we were also unable to see any systematic changes with respect to the stage of withdrawal or of abstinence in terms of β-endorphin or ACTH levels.

One of our strategies differs from yours, however, when we examine addicts presenting for withdrawal we consider the secondary drug of abuse and in fact can find considerable differences in β-endorphin relative to ACTH levels in plasma depending on the secondary rather than one the primary drug of abuse.

O'BRIEN: What secondary drugs?

BONNET: We had selected heroin addicts to study, but, of course, while all were on heroin, many were taking other drugs as well. We assumed that most addicts supplemented with whatever else he or she could find. If we took addicts who were on secondary drugs, along with the heroin, and rank-ordered their β-endorphin and ACTH levels, we found that the differences were considerably greater in some groups taking secondary drugs. Persons who were taking a combination of drugs showed a considerable change in β-endorphin and ACTH levels compared to control values or values in the simple heroin addict. The simple heroin addict presenting for detoxification did not show a considerable change compared with the control subjects.

O'BRIEN: We did not collect data on that because we felt that opiate dependence by itself is complicated enough. We confined ourselves to persons who have gotten on methadone and we have a reliable history on them. Once they are stabilized in one of the states of the addiction career that I described, we do the spinal tap. If they start using "speed" or cocaine or sedatives, then they are excluded from the study.

H. M. EMRICH (*Max Planck Institute for Psychiatry, Munich, FRG*): In Munich, in cooperation with Dr. Herz's laboratory, we measured β-endorphin in the plasma of patients during heroin maintenance and withdrawal. We found no difference during maintenance compared with normal control values, whereas there was about a 25% increase during the first week of withdrawal in β-endorphin activity. So possibly there is a difference between the early phases concerning blood levels and CSF.

J. J. KAUFMAN (*Johns Hopkins University, Baltimore, MD*): I have two points. One is a suggestion for medication that you might use to get the samples from patients who are very difficult to handle. You could explore the use of general anesthetics. You could obtain the control values easily in the patients who can be handled, taking a CSF sample first, putting the patient under a general anesthetic, and then taking another sample to see whether it affects the endorphins violently. You might use a gentle anesthetic like nitrous oxide. You might have to switch to dissosciative ones like Ketamine, but you might find one that does not affect the endorphin system, but that works in a different way and thus let you obtain samples. That is a matter of experiment.

The second point is that in the late 1960s Al Kurland, who was Director of the Maryland Center for Psychiatric Research, had a prisoner parolee population of former narcotic addicts. They were to remain drug-free as part of their parole conditions. If they didn't, they were not returned to jail, but were given naloxone prophylactically. Dr. Kurland himself took a large dose of naloxone before he gave it to a patient. He was one of the first I knew who did that, and he said the most striking effect was that he lost his appetite for 3 days. I am curious as to whether that was really an endorphin-related effect or whether this increased libido and loss of appetite might not be due also to an aberration of some of the more common neural transmitters.

So I would like to know, Dr. O'Brien, if you have studied neurochemically whether giving naltrexone under the same conditions that cause an increase in interest in sex or a decrease in appetite has an effect on the neural transmitters and their metabolites as well as increasing or decreasing the endorphin levels.

O'BRIEN: Some studies have been done on this, but I do not have the results at my fingertips right now. Certainly transmitters such as dopamine, acetylcholine, and serotonin have been reported to be influenced by opiate agonists. The effects of the "pure" antagonists are largely unsettled at present. There are reported effects of naltrexone and naloxone on feeding behavior and libido.

KAUFMAN: I'm not asking for the behavioral effects—I would like to know the neurochemical profile, where the measure is not subjective, but objective.

O'BRIEN: I do not think that such profiles are available at present.

UNIDENTIFIED SPEAKER: Did you look for any correlations between CSF opiate levels and HVA levels in drug-free periods or in normal people?

O'BRIEN: We have only analyzed about half of our samples so far for HVA and 5HIAA. Regarding HVA, there is a weak correlation in that HVA is highest during early withdrawal and it subsides over 36–72 hours. The endorphins tend to rise over this period; but we need more samples to be clear about this.

UNIDENTIFIED SPEAKER: Is it a positive or a negative correlation?

O'BRIEN: It has been a negative correlation. First there is a high amount of the catecholamine metabolite and a low amount of endorphin, but this reverses as time goes on.

PART X. POTENTIAL ROLE OF ENDOGENOUS OPIOIDS IN SCHIZOPHRENIA
AND AFFECTIVE DISORDERS

DEPRESSIVE PHENOMENOLOGY AND
LEVELS OF CEREBROSPINAL FLUID ENDORPHINS *

Hans Ågren,† Lars Terenius,‡ and Agneta Wahlström ‡

† Department of Psychiatry
‡ Department of Pharmacology
University of Uppsala
Uppsala, Sweden

INTRODUCTION

Brain endorphins may serve as transmitters in neuronal systems mediating reward and satisfaction. It is possible that disease states characterized by dysphoria or euphoria are accompanied by endorphin dysfunction.

To investigate this possibility, we studied the effect of the opiate antagonist naloxone in five clinically depressed patients.[1] Two patients responded with a worsening of symptoms. Endorphin content was measured in a receptor assay, and found to be elevated in comparison with levels seen in healthy volunteers.

We now report a larger series of 55 depressive patients fulfilling RDC (Research Diagnostic Criteria) for Major Depressive Disorder, diagnosed and rated following the SADS (Schedule for Affective Disorders and Schizophrenia [2]). The same receptor assay [3] has been maintained in the present series. Several practical considerations have lead to continued use of this assay rather than a specific radioimmunoassay. First, a radioimmunoassay may also detect biologically inert material. Secondly, potent endorphins with longer chain-lengths than the enkephalins have been and are being isolated and characterized from biological tissues.[4, 5] These peptides usually have higher metabolic stability and they may be functionally significant. It therefore seemed prudent at the time to use the receptor assay, in expectation of the chemical identity of the measured activity. Thus, there is evidence that Fraction I activity is confined within intermediate-sized (1000–2000 MW) hydrophilic peptides whereas Fraction II contains peptides of the same or lower molecular weight, which are more hydrophobic.

ANALYTICAL METHODS

The patients were prepared for spinal taps in a standardized manner. A total of 13 ml lumbar CSF were withdrawn at 8–9 AM with the patient in a supine position. The fluid was kept frozen at —20° C or lower until analysis. A 4–5 ml aliquot was filtered through an Amicon PM-10 ultrafilter (nominal cut-off 10,000 daltons) and the eluate was passed over a Sephadex G-10 column 50 × 2 cm) with 0.2 M acetic acid at a flow rate of 1 ml/min. Forty

* This work was supported by the Swedish Medical Research Council (21X–05095), the Bror Gadelius Memorial Fund for Psychiatric Research, and the National Institute on Drug Abuse, Washington, D.C. (5 RO1 DAO 1503).

388

5 ml samples were collected and the elution position of the salt peak was determined by flame photometry. Fraction I (defined as three samples of 5 ml prior to the salt peak) and Fraction II (four samples of 5 ml after the peak)[3] were collected and lyophilized. Combined samples were reconstituted in one ml of water and 100 μl aliquots were assayed for displacing activity against tritium-labelled dihydromorphine being allowed to interact with rat brain synaptic plasma membranes. Each sample was tested in triplicates. Details of the assay are given elsewhere.[7] Displacement activity was read against a standard curve and expressed as equivalents of methionine-enkephalin.

The assay of cortisol in 24-hour urine and the dexamethasone suppression test performed on the patients investigated have been described earlier (Ågren and Wide.[19])

METHODS OF INTERVIEWING PATIENTS

All patients were interviewed using the SADS,[2] for which some reliability data have been published.[9] The interviews lasted between 1 and 2 hours and were all conducted by the same rater in Swedish with the SADS manual in English as a guide. All patients were admitted to a research ward for a minimum of 5 days, during which a number of psychobiological investigations were performed. No diagnostic medication was given prior to the lumbar puncture. All patients were off neuroleptic or antidepressant medication for at least 10 days before investigation.

Consent had been obtained from the Ethics Committee at the Medical Faculty of Uppsala University to perform lumbar puncture as part of a routine investigatory program.

STATISTICAL METHODS

Rating scores from the SADS interview, diagnostical dummy codes, patient bodily characteristics, sex, illness duration variables as well as biological measures were stored in a computer file at the Uppsala University Computing Center, operating an IBM 4341.

Statistical programs from the SAS (Statistical Analysis System, Inc.) package like the Correlation, Stepwise, and Plot procedures were employed.

In performing a multiple regression analysis between the two endorphin fractions in turns as the independent variables and the scored depressive symptoms and other patient variables as a large number of independent variables, or predictors, certain precautionary measures have to be taken in order to reduce the so-called capitalization of chance that is always a problem in these kinds of multivariate approaches (discussed in Ågren[8]).

Using a split-half technique, we correlated endorphin values univariately (Pearson r) with all patient variables at hand in the undivided sample and in two randomly split halves (odds and evens in terms of serial number) of the patient population. Those variables displaying a trend correlation ($p < 0.10$) when correlating the endorphin measures with the undivided group, and retaining their r values reasonably well in both split sample halves, were selected for further analysis. For instance, if a variable showed a good cor-

TABLE 1

ENDORPHINS FRACTION II AND SELECTED DEPRESSIVE SYMPTOMS—UNI- AND MULTIVARIATE CORRELATIONS *

| | | | Univariate Correlations | | | Multivariate Correlations | | | | | | | | |
| | | | A Undivided Sample n=54 | | B Split Sample | | C Split Sample, Odds n=27 | | | D Split Sample, Evens n=27 | | | E Undivided Sample n=54 | | |
SADS No.	SADS Item	Score	r	p	Odds r	Evens r	b	F	p	b	F	p	b	F	p
248	Number of Suicide Attempts during Present Depression	0-2	0.28	0.043	0.24	0.32	X			2.73	4.53	0.044	X		
249 + 250	Seriousness of Intent (0-6)+Medical Lethality (0-6) at Worst Suicide Attempt during This Episode	0-12	0.31	0.023	0.37	0.24	0.64	5.06	0.034	X			0.52	9.92	0.0028
263	Somatic Anxiety Worst Week	1-6	0.27	0.045	0.34	0.22	1.45	4.46	0.045	X			1.03	7.14	0.010
269	Phobias (yes/no)	0-1	0.31	0.025	0.33	0.27	X			3.49	5.45	0.029	X		
332	Overt Anger Worst Week	1-6	-0.26	0.054	-0.20	-0.35	X			-1.94	6.52	0.018	-1.26	5.36	0.025
	Intercept						+3.86			+11.2			+8.07		
	R^2						0.269			0.369			0.281		
	F						4.41			4.48			6.52		
	df						2,24			3,23			3,50		
	p						0.023			0.013			0.0008		

* Eight symptom variables had been included in the initial regression equations of both split groups before the backward stepwise procedure started (criteria for inclusion was a univariate correlation in the undivided group with $p < 0.10$ and a retained level of r in both split samples; the weakest r was not less than 24% of that of the undivided sample).

relation (even p < 0.01) in the undivided group, but was highly unstable after splitting (for instance, p < 0.01 in one group but p = 0.50 in the other), it was not considered trustworthy as representing anything other than a chance fluctuation.

The independent variables selected in this way are thought to play some role in explaining the total variance in the CSF endorphin measures, and not to represent wholly fluctuations due to chance and the so-called Type I statistical errors. These variables were used as the independent terms (*x*'s) in backward stepwise multiple regression analyses with Fraction I and II, in turns, as the dependent variables (*y*). The final selection would retain those independent variables that showed a probability of less than 0.10 that their b coefficient did not significantly differ from null.

RESULTS

The concentrations (mean ± 1 SD) of CSF Fraction I and II were 2.1 ± 1.3 and 10.1 ± 5.0 pmoles/ml CSF (median values 1.7 and 9.1 pmoles/ml), respectively. The distributions were skewed with outliers in the upper tails. The Kolmogorov-Smirnov test for deviation from a Gaussian distribution revealed non-normal distributions for both fractions (D = 0.14 and 0.15; p < 0.01 for both).

These values should be compared with results obtained from healthy volunteers (means ± 1 SD): Fraction I 1.0 ± 0.4 and Fraction II 2.5 ± 1.5 pmoles/ml (n = 19).[10] These values are not significantly different from those in the present study.

Fractions I and II displayed a highly significant intercorrelation (Pearson r = 0.525, n = 54, p = 0.0001; Spearman r_s = 0.488, p = 0.0002), as depicted in FIGURE 1.

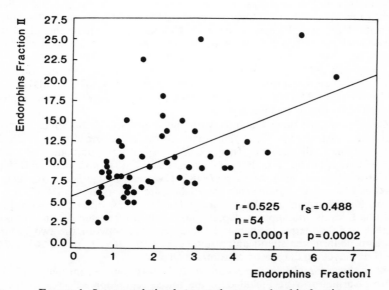

FIGURE 1. Intercorrelation between the two endorphin fractions.

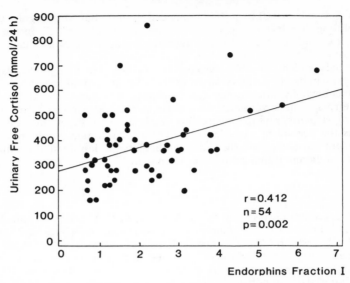

FIGURE 2. Linear correlation between endorphins Fraction I (pmoles/ml CSF) and urinary free cortisol (mmoles/24h urine).

Endorphins Fraction I, but not Fraction II, correlated positively and highly significantly with various measures of corticosteroid output, most clearly with urinary free cortisol (UFC). Correlation with plasma cortisol measured at 8 AM after 1 mg dexamethasone given orally at 11:30 PM the night before reached the 5% level of significance (r = 0.355, n = 33, p = 0.043). Correlation with UFC was higher, as seen in FIGURE 2, and here the number of cortisol analyses matched those of the endorphin analyses (Pearson r = 0.412, n = 54, p = 0.0020; Spearman r_s = 0.344, n = 54, p = 0.011).

There was no correlation between any endorphin fraction and other biological variables measured on the patients investigated (HVA, MHPG, and 5HIAA in CSF, MHPG in 24-hour urine, MAO activity in blood platelets, plasma TSH response to TRH injection).

Correlating Fractions I and II with the diagnostic dichotomies unipolar/bipolar depression (n = 37/18), primary/secondary depression (n = 38/17), pure unipolars/all others (n = 12/43), spectrum unipolars/all others (n = 6/49), sporadic unipolars/all others (n = 7/48), and with-schizotypal/without-schizotypal features (n = 7/48) revealed a significant tie between Fraction I and the unipolar/bipolar dichotomy (Pearson r = 0.285, n = 55, p = 0.036; Spearman r_s = 0.347, p = 0.0095). This difference with higher Fraction I levels in unipolar depressions is shown graphically in FIGURE 3, where a nonparametric median test for differences between the two groups is shown to confirm the significant result (χ^2 = 4.01, df = 1, p = 0.045). Fraction II displayed no diagnostic relations at all.

A backward multiple regression analysis was then performed, with independent variables to be included in the initial regression selected in the way described above.

As for Fraction I, five variables withstood the univariate selection procedure (for undivided group: p < 0.10; r in the "worst" group less than 27% smaller than that in the undivided group). In the final backward regression no variables remained below the 10% level of significance.

For Fraction II, however, interesting results emerged. The selection procedure admitted nine variables to further analysis (r in the "worst" split less than 24% smaller than that in the undivided group).

Columns A and B in TABLE 1 show the univariate correlations (Pearson r) between five of those nine variables inserted in the initial equation, for the undivided sample (A) as well as both split groups (B). Columns C and D show the final result in both splits after the backward stepwise procedure had eliminated most of the variables. It can be seen that the end result in each split retained one suicide measure correlating positively with Fraction II (Seriousness + Medical Lethality of Worst Suicidal Attempt in one group and Number of Suicidal Attempts in the other) and one anxiety measure correlating negatively (Somatic Anxiety Worst Week in one group and Phobias, yes/no, in the other). The overall multiple correlation was quite high in both splits (*odds*: $R^2 = 0.269$, $F = 4.41$, df $= 2,24$, p $= 0.023$; *evens*: $R^2 = 0.369$, $F = 4.48$, df $= 3,23$, p $= 0.013$).

When those five independent variables that remained in the two splits were inserted in a stepwise regression for the whole sample, the finally selected variables were those listed in Column E. Exactly the same selection was the result if the original nine variables were used in a backward stepwise regression with the whole sample. Thus, the independent variables Seriousness of Intent + Medical Lethality at Worst Suicide Attempt during Present

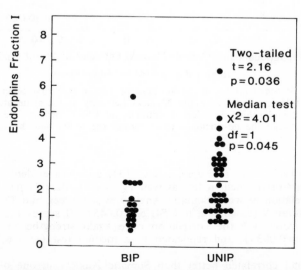

FIGURE 3. Difference between unipolar and bipolar depression (all patients in present or recent depressive phase) in regard to endorphins Fraction I (pmoles/ml CSF).

or Recent Depressive Episode as well as Somatic Anxiety Worst Week cor-
related positively and Overt Anger Worst Week negatively with endorphins
Fraction II. These three variables explained 28% of the total variance in
Fraction II ($R^2 = 0.281$, $F = 6.52$, $df = 3,50$, $p = 0.0008$).

The Suicide score is plotted against Fraction II in FIGURE 4. Individuals
scoring 0 were those 37 patients who had never attempted suicide. The
univariate regression line shows a significant correlation ($r = 0.309$, $n = 54$,
$p = 0.023$). If the 17 patients who had tried to commit suicide were viewed
together and compared with the no-suicide group, the correlation actually

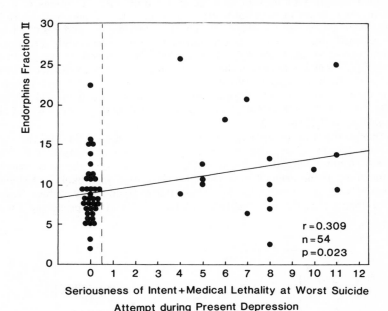

FIGURE 4. Summed scores on Seriousness of Intent at Worst Suicidal Attempt
during Present Depression (0–6) and Medical Lethality at the same attempt (0–6)
correlated with endorphins Fraction II (pmoles/ml CSF). Broken line denotes the
comparison between the no-suicidal-attempt group (score 0) and the suicide group
(scores > 2).

strengthened (ANOVA: $F = 6.69$, $p = 0.013$), and was evident in the very
robust nonparametric median test as well ($\chi^2 = 4.91$, $df = 1$, $p = 0.027$).

The correlation between Somatic Anxiety Worst Week and Fraction II is
shown in FIGURE 5 ($r = 0.274$, $n = 54$, $p = 0.045$). If scores 1–3 were compared with scores 4–6 the correlation once again strengthened (ANOVA:
$F = 9.42$, $p = 0.0034$), and replicated in a median test ($\chi^2 = 6.12$, $df = 1$,
$p = 0.013$).

Phobia had correlated better than Somatic Anxiety in one of the splits.
If this variable was correlated with Fraction II in the undivided sample, the
result was significant ($r = 0.305$, $n = 54$, $p = 0.025$). In FIGURE 6, this
difference in Fraction II is clearly shown, as evidenced by a two-tailed t-test

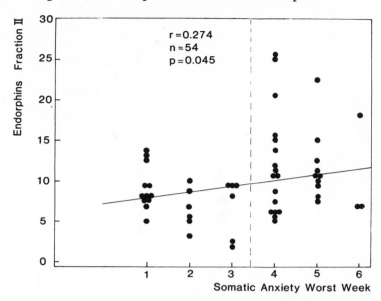

FIGURE 5. Correlation between rated Somatic Anxiety Worst Week of Present Depression (scores 1–6) and endorphins Fraction II (pmoles/ml CSF). Broken lines denotes a comparison described in the text between patients with anxiety scores $\leqq 3$ and scores $\geqq 4$.

($t = 2.31$, $n = 54$, $p = 0.025$) as well as a median test ($\chi^2 = 4.59$, $df = 1$, $p = 0.032$). Of the 22 patients with phobic symptoms during their depression nearly all were agoraphobics.

The item Overt Anger Worst Week correlated univariately and negatively close to the 5% level of significance with Fraction II, as shown in FIGURE 7 ($r = -0.264$, $n = 54$, $p = 0.054$).

DISCUSSION

The broad actions of morphine on mood and behavior suggest that endogenous opioids may be associated with psychiatric disturbances. The field has been reviewed.[11] Inaccurate sensitivity to pain has also been reported to occur in depression.[12, 13] Fink and co-workers reported [14] that the narcotic antagonist cyclazocine had antidepressant activity in an open clinical trial. Terenius *et al.* observed [1] that whereas naloxone given intramuscularly at 0.4–0.8 mg t.i.d. for 1 to 2 weeks had no therapeutic effects, abrupt discontinuation of treatment led to worsening of symptoms in two of the six trials. In another study, chronic naltrexone treatment induced a depression-like syndrome.[15] Our early pilot study [1] indicated that CSF endorphins as assayed with the present procedure were sometimes elevated in depression but there were also cases with low levels. This suggested to us that this biological variable might relate to some form of behavior rather than a traditional diagnostic category.

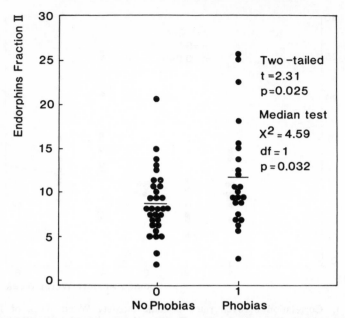

FIGURE 6. Difference in CSF levels of endorphin Fraction II (pmoles/ml) between patients without and with phobic symptoms (almost all were agoraphobics). N = 31 and 23.

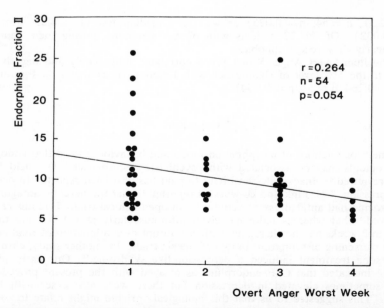

FIGURE 7. Correlation between Overt Anger Worst Week of Present Depression (scores 1–6) and endorphins Fraction II (pmoles/ml CSF).

One general problem of interpretation of CSF analyses of chemical markers is the relevance of the measured activities for central events. In our particular case another problem is the lack of knowledge about the chemical identity of the measured activities. Until the chemical structures of the active agents are known, we cannot for instance attribute the observed activities to any particular endorphin system. Also, the interrelation between Fractions I and II and their relative significance are unknown. We are fully aware of these limitations, and special emphasis is presently given to the identification of Fraction II endorphins, some progress already being made for Fraction I.[6]

Hypercortisolism has been found to be a concomitant of depressions with melancholic features in several recent investigations, and the dexamethasone suppression test has been hailed as a laboratory test for melancholia.[16] One of us has found a significant correlation between poor cortisol suppression after dexamethasone and scored "endogeneity" of RDC Major Depressions.[8, 19] Increased urinary free cortisol (UFC) occurred in depressives with little overt anger.[8, 19] The ties between endorphins Fraction I and cortisol measures found in the present study, the most evident being a positive correlation with UFC, was surprising but very compatible with the known stimulatory influence of endorphins on the secretion of hypothalamic-releasing hormones and the concomitant increase in ACTH and corticosteroid output.

Endorphins as analyzed in the CSF do seem to play roles in some brain mechanisms involved in affective disorders. The difference in Fraction I between uni- and bipolar patients is particularly interesting in view of the paucity of other findings of biochemical differences between these affective subpopulations. The results could tentatively be interpreted to the effect that unipolar depression is a disorder involving endorphin dysfunction.

The ties between Fraction II and suicide, anxiety, and anger (irrespective of affective subdiagnosis) are also of great theoretical interest, and can be compared with other findings of ties between CSF monoamine metabolites and suicidal behavior and anxiety. For example, lower levels of the serotonin metabolite 5HIAA have been correlated with suicidal attempts [8, 17] and anxiety,[8, 18] and lower excretion of the noradrenaline metabolite MHPG in 24-hour urine has been connected with suicidal behavior.[8, 20] However, no connections between endorphin and monoamine metabolite levels in CSF have as yet been discovered.

ACKNOWLEDGMENT

The technical assistance of Ms. Inga Hansson is gratefully acknowledged.

REFERENCES

1. TERENIUS, L., A. WAHLSTRÖM & H. ÅGREN. 1977. Naloxone (Narcan®) treatment of depression. Clinical observations and effects on CSF endorphins and monoamine metabolites. Psychopharmacology **54:** 31–33.
2. ENDICOTT, J. & R. L. SPITZER. 1979. Use of the Research Diagnostic Criteria and the Schedule for Affective Disorders and Schizophrenia to study affective disorders. Am. J. Psychiatry **136:** 52–56.
3. TERENIUS, L. & A. WAHLSTRÖM. 1975. Morphine-like ligand for opiate receptors in human CSF. Life Sci. **16:** 1759–1764.
4. STERN, A. S., B. N. JONES, J. E. SHIVELY, S. STEIN & S. UDENFRIEND. 1981. Two adrenal opioid polypeptides: Proposed intermediates in the processing of proenkephalin. Proc. Natl. Acad. Sci. USA **78:** 1962–1966.

5. GOLDSTEIN, A., S. TACHIBANA, L. L. LOWNEY, M. HUNKAPILLER & L. HOOD. 1979. Dynorphin-(1-13), an extraordinary potent opioid peptide. Proc. Natl. Acad. Sci. USA **76:** 6666–6670.
6. WAHLSTRÖM, A. & L. TERENIUS. 1980. Chemical characteristics of endorphins in human cerebrospinal fluid. FEBS Letters **118:** 241–244.
7. TERENIUS, L. 1974. A rapid assay of affinity for the narcotic receptor in rat brain: Application to methadone analogues. Acta Pharmacol. Toxicol. **34:** 88–91.
8. ÅGREN, H. 1981. Biological Markers in Major Depressive Disorders: A Clinical and Multivariate Study. Acta Univ. Ups., Abstracts of Uppsala Dissertations from the Faculty of Medicine 405.
9. ENDICOTT, J. & R. L. SPITZER. 1978. A diagnostic interview. Arch. Gen. Psychiatry **35:** 837–844.
10. LINDSTRÖM, L. H., E. WIDERLÖV, L.-M. GUNNE, A. WAHLSTRÖM & L. TERENIUS. 1978. Endorphins in human cerebrospinal fluid. Clinical correlations to some psychotic states. Acta Psychiatr. Scand. **57:** 153–164.
11. VEREBEY, K., J. VOLAVKA & D. CLOUET. 1978. Endorphins in psychiatry. An overview and a hypothesis. Arch. Gen. Psychiatry **35:** 877–888.
12. VON KNORRING, L. & M. ESPVALL. 1974. Experimentally induced pain in patients with depressive disorders. Acta Psychiatr. Scand., Suppl. 255.
13. DAVIS, G. C., M. D. BUCHSBAUM & W. E. BUNNEY. 1979. Analgesia to painful stimuli in affective illness. Am. J. Psychiatry **136:** 1148–1151.
14. FINK, M., J. SIMEON, T. M. ITIL & A. M. FREEDMAN. 1970. Clinical antidepressant activity of cyclazocine—a narcotic antagonist. Clin. Pharmacol. Ther. **11:** 41–48.
15. HOLLISTER, L. E., K. JOHNSON, D. BOUKHABZA & H. K. GILLESPIE. 1981. Aversive effects of naltrexone in subjects not dependent on opiates. Drug and Alcohol Dependence **7:** 1–5.
16. CARROLL, B. J., M. FEINBERG, J. F. GREDEN, J. TARIKA, A. A. ALBALA, R. F. HASKETT, N. MCI. JAMES, Z. KRONFOL, N. LOHR, M. STEINER, J. P. DE VIGNE & E. YOUNG. 1981. A specific laboratory test for the diagnosis of melancholia. Arch. Gen. Psychiatry **38:** 15–22.
17. ÅSBERG, M., L. TRÄSKMAN & P. THORÉN. 1976. 5HIAA in the cerebrospinal fluid: A biochemical suicide predictor? Arch. Gen. Psychiatry **33:** 1193–1197.
18. BANKI, C. M. 1977. Correlation of anxiety and related symptoms with cerebrospinal fluid 5-hydroxyindoleacetic acid in depressed women. J. Neural Transm. **41:** 135–143.
19. ÅGREN, H. & L. WIDE. Patterns of depression reflected in pituitary-thyroid and pituitary-adrenal endocrine changes. Psychoneuroendocrinology. In press.
20. ÅGREN, H. 1982. Depressive symptom patterns and urinary MHPG excretion. Psychiatr. Res. **6:** 185–196.

DISCUSSION OF THE PAPER

J. C. VOLAVKA (*New York University School of Medicine, New York*): I have a question. Did either you or Dr. Ågren look at the 5-hydroxy-indole-acetic acid in the same patients or is it in different patients?

A. WAHLSTRÖM (*Uppsala University, Sweden*): It is in the same patients.

VOLAVKA: What is the relationship between the 5HIAA and the fractions? Do we have any direct correlation?

WAHLSTRÖM: There was no correlation between any endorphin fractions (I or II) and 5HIAA.

ENDORPHINS IN THE CEREBROSPINAL FLUID OF PSYCHIATRIC PATIENTS

David Pickar,* Dieter Naber,† Robert M. Post,*
Daniel P. van Kammen,* Walter Kaye,‡ David R. Rubinow,*
James C. Ballenger,§ and William E. Bunney, Jr.*

Biological Psychiatry Branch
‡ *Laboratory of Clinical Science*
National Institute of Mental Health
National Institutes of Health
Bethesda, Maryland 20205

† *Psychiatric Clinic of the University of Munich*
Munich, Federal Republic of Germany

§ *Department of Psychiatry*
University of Virginia
Charlottesville, Virginia 22903

INTRODUCTION

Biological psychiatry has pursued hypothesized relationships between the endogenous opioid system and behavior to a large degree by focusing on possible endogenous opioid (endorphin) diatheses in psychiatric illness.[1] Partly on the basis of the behavioral effects of exogenous opiates in man and those of endogenous opioids in animals, alterations in the endogenous opioid system have been hypothesized to be related to schizophrenia [2, 3] as well as to the affective disorders.[4, 5] Three principal strategies have been used clinically to test endorphin hypotheses: the administration of the pure narcotic antagonist, naloxone,[3, 6, 7] the administration of opioid peptide agonists,[8–11] and the measurement of endogenous opioids in body fluids such as plasma [12–14] and cerebrospinal fluid (CSF).[15–19] Each of these strategies has inherent strengths and liabilities; the measurement of endorphins themselves is the only nonpharmacologic approach and the one that is based on laboratory methodologies.

Two major assay techniques have been employed to measure endorphins in clinical studies: the radioimmunoassay (RIA) [12, 14, 16, 18, 19] and the radio-receptor assay (RRA).[13, 15–17, 20] RIA determinations have the advantage that they detect levels of specific opioids (e.g., β-endorphin, or Met-enkephalin, etc). The major limitation with the RIA method lies in the fact that the antibodies commonly used show cross-reactivity to other peptide molecules while they themselves may not possess opiate-like activity (e.g., β-lipotropin); results of RIA, therefore, usually represent a composite of substances, with levels expressed as immunoreactivity.[21, 22] A further limitation with the RIA is that there are a number of endogenous opioid peptides already discovered,

0077-8923/82/0398-0399 $01.75/0 © 1982 NYAS

and despite differing anatomic locations of these compounds, there are little data indicating that any single one (e.g., β-endorphin, Met-enkephalin, Leu-enkephalin, dynorphin, etc.) is more closely related to behavior or psychiatric illness than another. The principal theoretical advantage to the RRA is that determinations are based on biological activity, i.e., stereospecific binding to the opiate receptor.[20] This RRA approach, while limited in providing information regarding an individual opioid peptide, does permit an assessment of "functional" opioid activity, which may then reflect overall tone or activity of the endogenous opioid system. Biochemical separation techniques have been used with both RIA [19] and RRA [15, 17] to enhance specificity for specific opioids or groups of opioids.

While the measurement of endorphins has been applied to both CSF and plasma, CSF analysis may more directly reflect activity of CNS endorphin systems. Evidence that opioid activity in CSF reflects brain opioid system activity may be gained from the results of several experiments. It has been shown, for example, that electrical stimulation of the periaqueductal gray matter produces both naloxone-reversible analgesia in patients with chronic pain and increases levels of β-endorphin-like [23] and enkephalin-like [24] material in ventricular CSF. Electroacupuncture, a treatment hypothesized to be mediated through the endogenous opioid system, has been shown to produce elevations in lumbar CSF enkephalin-immunoreactivity [25] and in RRA-determined opioid activity.[26] Recently, levels of certain fractions of CSF taken prior to general surgery have been found to be predictive of the amount of post-operative morphine required by patients to relieve pain.[27] A diurnal rhythm of CSF opioid activity has been demonstrated in non-human primates with a pattern of increased morning and decreased afternoon levels,[28] a rhythm similar to that of cortisol and ACTH [29] as well as to the reported diurnality in human pain sensitivity.[30]

In this paper we describe our research testing endorphin hypotheses in schizophrenia and affective disorders [16, 31] and in anorexia nervosa [32] using the strategy of measuring opioid activity and β-endorphin–immunoreactivity (ir) in the CSF.

METHODS

Patient Populations

All psychiatric patients in this study were inpatients on clinical research wards of the NIH and granted informed consent to participate in this study of levels of CSF endorphins. Patients met Research Diagnostic Criteria (DRC) [33] for either schizophrenia, major depressive disorder, mania or DSM III criteria [34] for anorexia nervosa. In addition to psychiatric patients, a group of normal volunteers granted informed consent for participation and served as a control group. These normal subjects were free from medical or psychiatric illness. All patients and normals were maintained medication-free for at least 14 days prior to study. Demographic data of these subject populations are presented in TABLE 1.

CSF Sampling

For all patients and control subjects CSF was obtained by lumbar punctures performed between 8:00 and 9:00 A.M. All subjects were at bedrest since awakening and fasting since the previous evening's meal. Immediately following collection, CSF samples were frozen at −70° C. Analysis was performed on samples obtained from a pool of the first through twelfth milliliters of withdrawn CSF.

Radioreceptor Assay (RRA)

Levels of CSF opioid activity were determined by the RRA methodology of Naber *et al.*[20] This technique is based on the competition between [³H]-[D-Ala²]enkephalin-(L-Leu-amide)[5] and biologically active opioid ligands using

TABLE 1

DEMOGRAPHY OF PATIENTS STUDIED

Group	N	Age in Years (mean ± SD)	Male	Female
Normal	41	31 ± 13	27	14
Schizophrenic	27	34 ± 13	13	14
Schizoaffective	14	30 ± 13	8	6
Depressed	35	41 ± 14	14	21
Manic	13	34 ± 13	3	10
Anorexia nervosa	5	24 ± 5	—	5
Recovered anorectics	8	23 ± 4	—	8
Controls for anorectics	7	25 ± 5	—	7

crude rat brain membranes. This assay methodology has been presented previously in detail including results from gel chromatography and opioid specificity analysis.[20] Non-opioid peptides such as ACTH, β-lipotropin and MSH have been shown to produce negligible radioligand displacement at physiologic concentrations. All samples analyzed by the RRA were assayed in triplicate blind to clinical information; samples from the different diagnostic groups and control subjects were assigned in a balanced fashion to individual assays by nonlaboratory personnel. CSF from all subjects were analyzed by the RRA for opioid activity.

β-Endorphin Radioimmunoassay (RIA)

After completing RRA analysis, additional CSF was available from some subjects to perform RIA for β-endorphin. This assay was performed with reagents and antibody supplied by New England Nuclear; rabbit antiserum was prepared against synthetic human β-endorphin. The antibody demonstrates $<50\%$ cross-reactivity with β-lipotropin, $<.004\%$ with Met- or Leu-enkephalin, $<.01\%$ with α-endorphin or α-MSH. Samples were assayed blind to clinical information, in duplicate and assigned in a balanced fashion throughout one assay.

RESULT AND COMMENT

Schizophrenia

Patients who met RDC for schizoaffective type schizophrenia were considered separately from other schizophrenic types (i.e., undifferentiated, catatonic, etc.) since they had shown significant mood-related symptomatology as part of their illness. Overall, schizophrenics showed significantly less CSF opioid activity than did the normal control group: mean $\pm$ SEM were 2.92 ± 1.9 pmol/ml, and 4.01 ± 2.3 pmol/ml, respectively; $p < .05$, independent t-test, two-tailed-Welch's method for comparing groups of unequal variances, while schizoaffective patient (3.96 ± 2.5 pmol/ml) showed no significant deviation from normals or other schizophrenics. Further analysis revealed that the schizophrenic-normal difference was accounted for primarily by sex: a nearly twofold decrease in CSF opioid activity was found in male schizophrenics in comparison to normal male subjects ($p < .005$), whereas levels in female schizophrenics and normal female subjects were similar. Analysis of CSF by RIA for β-endorphin in representative subsamples of these groups, however, revealed no significant or near significant differences between any of the schizophrenic groups and normal subjects in β-endorphin (ir) (FIG. 1), suggesting that the observed difference between male schizophrenics and normal male subjects may be related to opioids other than β-endorphin.

There were no significant correlations between CSF opioid activity or β-endorphin (ir) and age, number of previous hospitalizations, or nurses' ratings of psychosis. Levels of CSF opioid activity and β-endorphin (ir) were not significantly related.

Comment

In its most simple form the endorphin-schizophrenia hypothesis states that an excess in endogenous opioid system activity is related to symptomatology of schizophrenia. The basis for this hypothesis is indirect: cyclazocine, a mixed agonist/antagonist is known to produce naloxone-reversible dysphoria and auditory hallucinations in normal subjects, intraventricularly administered β-endorphin in rats produces an unusal behavioral syndrome reminiscent of catatonia, and preliminary studies reported that the administration of the "pure" narcotic antagonist, naloxone, was associated with reductions in auditory hallucinations in schizophrenic patients.[3] Over the last half-decade there have been numerous studies addressing endorphins in schizophrenia; results from this work, however, have not consistently supported the "excess endorphin" hypothesis.[3, 7] Many studies have now used the naloxone strategy: while some groups have found results suggestive of therapeutic effects of naloxone, others have not.[3] Recently, a World Health Organization collaborative study [7] reported that schizophrenic patients who were concurrently treated with neuroleptics showed significant naloxone-associated reductions in physician-rated symptomatology whereas medication-free schizophrenics showed significant naloxone-associated worsening in the BPRS subscale, "withdrawal-retardation." The results from double-blind studies of the intravenous administration of the opioid peptide, β-endorphin, have been inconclusive. Berger *et al.*[9] reported significant but clinically nonapparent improvement in ratings of schizophrenic

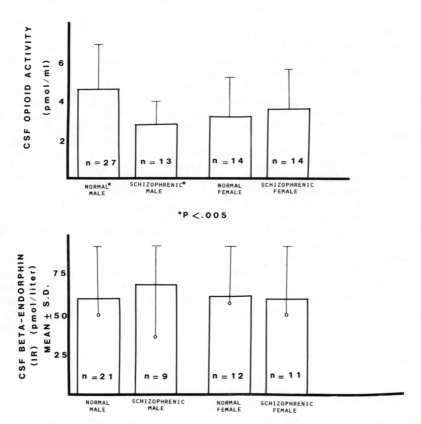

FIGURE 1. CSF opioid activity and β-endorphin (ir) in CSF of schizophrenic patients and normal control subjects.

patients following β-endorphin administration; Pickar *et al.*[11] and Gerner *et al.*[10] reported no significant behavioral effects.

The RRA method of Terenius *et al.*[15] has been used most extensively in studying levels of opioids in the CSF of medication-free schizophrenics. This method differs from the RRA employed in our study primarily in that, prior to RRA analysis, CSF is separated into two fractions (I and II) by gel chromatography. Although further biochemical specification of these fractions is needed, reported elution profiles suggest that Fraction I is composed of opioid(s) intermediate in size between β-endorphin and the enkephalins which, in turn, co-elute with Fraction II. Using this method, individual medication-free chronic [35] and "symptom rich" [15, 17] schizophrenics have been reported to have elevated Fraction I levels beyond the "normal range." More recently, Rimon et al.[36] have reported that acute medication-free schizophrenic patients showed a statistically significant group elevation in Fraction I levels compared to normal subjects, while chronic schizophrenics were found to have significantly lower levels than acute schizophrenics. All previous studies using β-endorphin RIA analysis of CSF from schizophrenics have studied patients who were concurrently receiving neuroleptics. In one study, acute patients were found to have elevated levels of β-endorphin (ir) while chronic patients had decreased levels, each in comparison with controls.[18] In another study, no differences between schizophrenics and normal subjects were found.[12]

The results of our study do not support the notion of excess endogenous opioid system activity in schizophrenia. On the contrary, our data indicate the possibility of decreased endogenous opioid system activity, at least in male schizophrenics. The fact that we found no differences between schizophrenics and normal subjects with regard to β-endorphin (ir) may suggest that the observed decrease in CSF opioid activity in the male schizophrenics may be related to opioid(s) other than β-endorphin. In this regard our data are consistent with other studies that have used the RRA of Terenius et al.[15, 17, 35, 37] since deviations in opioid activity in non-β-endorphin CSF fractions have been found in both acute and chronic schizophrenic patient groups. The lack of correlation between β-endorphin (ir) and RRA determined opioid activity suggest that intact β-endorphin may not be a major contributing factor to total opioid activity.

Our data may be consistent with the results of the WHO collaborative project in which naloxone administration produced worsening in medication-free schizophrenics, rather than improvement. While further analysis of our data with regard to clinical variables is in progress, a current working hypothesis includes the notion that decreased endogenous opioid activity in some patients may be related to anhedonic features of the schizophrenic illness such as emotional withdrawal and poor interpersonal relatedness.

Depression and Mania

Results of RRA and β-endorphin RIA analyses of CSF revealed no significant differences between depressed or manic patients and normal volunteers, or significant differences between depressed and manic groups for each variable (TABLE 2). In four manic-depressive patients in whom paired samples were available from closely associated depressed and manic periods, however, CSF opioid activity has higher in mania than during depression in each subject: mean $\pm$ SD were 3.81 ± 0.68 pmol/ml and 1.91 ± 0.51 pmol/ml for mania and depression, respectively ($p < .05$, paired t-test, two tailed).

In examining possible relationships between CSF opioid activity and symptomatology in depressed patients, a significant correlation was found between research ward nurses' ratings [37] of anxiety on the day prior to LP and CSF opioid activity ($r = .46$, $p < .05$). These ratings reflect assessment

TABLE 2

CSF OPIOID ACTIVITY AND β-ENDORPHIN (IR) IN AFFECTIVELY ILL PATIENTS
AND CONTROLS

Group	Opioid Activity (pmol/ml)		β-Endorphin (ir) (pmol/l)	
	N	mean ± SD	N	mean ± SD
Depressed	35	3.95 ± 2.4	28	65 ± 31
Manic	13	3.97 ± 1.9	12	58 ± 27
Normal	41	4.01 ± 2.3	33	59 ± 39

of anxiety from the perspective of observed behavior in a research ward setting.

As part of studies investigating abnormalities of the hypothalamic-pituitary-adrenal (HPA) axis in affective illness, determinations of urinary free cortisol were made by RIA in subgroups of depressed patients and normal volunteers (means of two 24 hr urines). These determinations were made from urine samples during the same medication-free period as were the lumbar punctures. We observed that CSF opioid activity was significantly related to mean urinary free cortisol excretion (MUFC) in the depressed patients ($r = .47$, $p < .05$) but not in the normal volunteers ($r = -.01$, NS) (FIG. 2). In the subgroup of depressed patients in whom both β-endorphin (ir) and MUFC was available for analysis, a direct relationship was also found ($r = .32$), which, although not reaching statistical significance, was in contrast to the slight negative relationship between normals and CSF β-endorphin (ir) and MUFC ($r = -.10$). MUFC was significantly higher in depressed patients (80.0 ± 8.5 mg/24-hr) than in normal volunteers (56.4 ± 4.3 mg/24-hr) ($p < .05$) (FIG. 2).

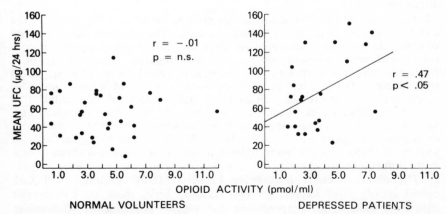

FIGURE 2. The relationship between mean urinary free cortisol (MUFC) and CSF opioid activity in depressed subjects and normal control subjects.

Comment

The notion that the endogenous opioid system may be involved in affective disorders stems largely from the considerable mood-altering properties of exogenous opiates coupled with animal experimentation relating the endogenous opioid system to reinforced behavior.[4, 5, 38] Specifically, the ability or inability to experience pleasure has been suggested to be related to relative increases and decreases in endogenous opioid system activity. In this regard, enhanced opioid activity might be expected to be related to mania while decreased activity related to depression. Reflecting this view, most clinical studies of mania have involved naloxone administration, while those in depression have used the strategy of administering opiate agonists (exogenous as well as endogenous).[39]

Following initial clinical studies in which naloxone was found to have therapeutic effect in manic patients,[6] there have been several studies that have found no significant behavioral effects of naloxone in manic patients.[7, 40] There have been two reports suggesting that opioid activity differs with state change in manic-depressive illness. Lindström *et al.*[17] reported CSF Fraction I opioid activity to be elevated during mania in comparison to depression in several manic-depressive patients. Pickar *et al.*[13] found significant elevations in plasma opioid activity during mania compared with depression in a cycling medication-free manic-depressive patient. Although there has been little study of depressed patients with either naloxone or endorphin measurement strategies, several studies have reported the effects of opiate agonist administration in depression. Antidepressant effects of intravenously administered β-endorphin in open or single blind studies have been reported.[8, 41] Of the two studies using double-blind methodologies, one reported significant β-endorphin–associated improvement in depressed patients,[10] while the other [11] reported no significant behavioral effects. The acute administration of exogenous opiates has been tried in individual depressed patients; [42] data to date do not support antidepressant effects. Chronic oral opiate (methadone) administration has been reported in a refractorily ill depressed patient with some antidepressant effects observed.[38]

The results of our CSF study do not point to an abnormality *per se* in the endorphin system in either depression or mania. The increased opioid activity observed during mania compared to depression in individual patients is consistent with some previous reports, and also suggests the possibility of a relative increase and decrease in the endogenous opioid system activities across state change. The relationship between nurses' ratings of anxiety and CSF opioid activity in depressed patients is of interest, although it is difficult to know the significance of this finding. It is possible that this relationship may be part of a common stress response. It is also possible that relative alterations in endogenous opioid activity are related directly to the biological basis of anxiety, perhaps through interrelationship with other neurotransmitters such as the noraadrenergic system.

The observed direct relationship between MUFC excretion and CSF opioid activity is of interest for two reasons. First, there are considerable data from basic science experiments that suggest physiological relationships between the HPA axis and the endogenous opioid system.[43, 44] Second, activation of the HPA axis has been a major focus of research in depression for a number of years.[45, 46] Our data suggest that while the endogenous opioid system itself may not be abnormal in depression, it may be related to abnormality of the HPA axis found in this illness.

Anorexia Nervosa

We used three patient groups in our study of CSF opioid activity in anorexia nervosa: anorectic patients currently hospitalized for treatment of weight loss (N = 5), recovered anorectics (at least 80% of ideal body weight) brought into the hospital for study (N = 8), and normal female control subjects studied during the first week of their menstrual cycle (N = 8). Ill anorectics were studied initially at minimum weight and again following refeeding prior to hospital discharge (80% of ideal body weight). Each anorectic showed greater CSF opioid activity when at minimal weight in comparison with levels

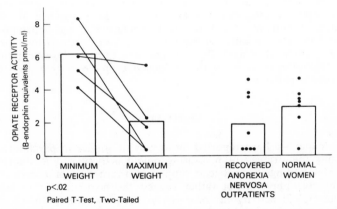

FIGURE 3. CSF opioid activity from patients with anorexia nervosa at minimum weight, at maximum weight after refeeding, in recovered anorexia nervosa patients, and female control subjects.

following refeeding (p < .02, paired t-test, two-tailed). The mean CSF opioid activity at minimal weight was also significantly greater than the mean levels of recovered anorectics and normal control subjects (p < .01, independent t-test, two tailed), while recovered anorectic patients had levels comparable to those of controls.

Comment

There is considerable evidence from animal experimentation suggesting that the endogenous opioid system may play a role in eating behavior. β-Endorphin has been found to stimulate food intake in satiated rats when injected into the ventro-medial hypothalamus.[47] Naloxone given intraperitoneally reduced food intake in starved rats,[48] and abolished overreating in genetically obese mice and rats.[49] To date there have been few clinical studies of anorexia with regard to a possible endorphin diathesis, although there is a large body of work relating anorexia to abnormalities in neuroendocrine systems.

We observed pronounced elevations in CSF opioid activity in the anorectic patients when at minimal weight in comparison to levels found after refeeding, as well as those of recovered anorectics and controls. These data do not support a simple relationship between opioid activity and eating, since levels were highest when subjects were at minimum weight. It is well known clinically, however, that even in the starved condition anorectic patients demonstrate major preoccupation with food and eating behavior, although the caloric intake is decreased. Furthermore, periods of increased food intake as well as gorging of food (bulemia) are known to occur in these patients. It is a possibility that the high levels of CSF opioid activity observed in the anorectics at minimal weight may reflect some alterations in endogenous opioid system-eating behavior relationship. It is also a possibility that the elevations in CSF opioid activity during starvation represent a stress response, since the opioid system has been hypothesized to play a role in aiding survival in famine by conservation of nutrients and water and decreasing energy-expending activities.[50] Recently, abnormalities of the HPA axis were reported to occur during periods of minimum weight in anorectics.[51] Further investigations might focus on relationships between the endogenous opioid system and the HPA axis in anorectic patients.

SUMMARY

In this paper we have reported the results of studies in psychiatric patient groups using the strategy of measuring opioid activity and β-endorphin (ir) in CSF. Our findings do not lend support to the notion of excess endorphin activity in schizophrenia, but rather suggest the possibility of a decrease in endogenous opioid activity in some schizophrenic patients. In affectively ill patients our data suggest that there may be a relative change in endogenous opioid system activity across state change in manic-depressive illness. We also found a relationship between nurses' ratings of anxiety and CSF opioid activity in depressed patients, although it is unknown whether this directly relates to the pathophysiology of this symptom, or is related to stress response. The relationship between CSF opioid activity and HPA axis activity, as reflected by urinary free cortisol excretion, supports the notion of important physiologic relationships between these systems and raises the issue of a role for the endogenous opioid system in the abnormal activation of this system in depression. Finally, the finding of increased CSF opioid activity in anorexia nervosa patients when a minimum weight coupled with data relating endogenous opioids to eating behavior raises interesting questions regarding a possible involvement of the endogenous opioid system involvement in this illness.

REFERENCES

1. USDIN, E., W. E. BUNNEY, JR. & N. S. KLINE, Eds. 1979. Endorphins in Mental Health Research. Macmillan. New York.

2. BLOOM, F., D. SEGAL, N. LING & R. GUILLEMIN. 1976. Endorphins: Profound behavioral effects in rats suggest new etiologic factors in mental illness. Science **194:** 630–632.
3. DAVIS, G. C., M. S. BUCHSBAUM & W. E. BUNNEY, JR. 1979. Research in endorphins and schizophrenia. Schizophr. Bull. **5:** 244–250.
4. BYCK, R. 1976. Peptide transmitters: A unifying hypotheses for euphoria, respiration, sleep and the action of lithium. Lancet **2:** 72–73.
5. BELLUZZI, J. D. & L. STEIN. 1977. Enkephalin may mediate euphoria and drive reduction reward. Nature **266:** 566–568.
6. JANOWSKY, D. S., L. L. JUDD & D. SEGAL. 1979. Effects of naloxone in normal, manic and schizophrenic patients: Evidence for alleviation of manic symptoms. *In* Endorphins in Mental Health Research. E. Usdin, W. E. Bunney, Jr., & N. S. Kline, Eds.: 435–447. Macmillan. New York.
7. PICKAR, D., F. VARTANIAN, W. E. BUNNEY, JR., H. D. MAIER, M. T. GASTPAR, R. PRAKASH, B. B. SETTHI, B. BELGAER, M. TSULTULKOUSA, G. JUNGHUNZ, T. N. NEDOPIL, W. VERHOEVEN & H. VAN PRAAG. 1982. Short-term naloxone administration in schizophrenic and manic patients: A World Health Organization Collaborative Study. Arch Gen. Psychiatry. **39:** 313–319.
8. KLINE, N. S. & H. E. LEHMANN. 1979. β-Endorphin therapy in psychiatric patients. *In* Endorphins in Mental Health Research. E. Usdin, W. E. Bunney, Jr. & N. S. Kline, Eds.: 500–517. Macmillan. New York.
9. BERGER, P. A., S. J. WATSON, H. AKIL, G. R. ELLIOT, P. T. RUBIN, A. PFEFFER-GAUM, K. L. DAVIS, J. D. BARCHAS & C. H. LI. 1980. β-Endorphin and schizophrenia. Arch. Gen. Psychiatry **37:** 635–640.
10. GERNER, R. H., D. H. CATLIN, D. A. GORELICK, K. H. KUI & C. H. LI. 1980. β-endorphin: Intravenous infusion causes behavioral change in psychiatric patients. Arch. Gen. Psychiatry **37:** 642–647.
11. PICKAR, D., G. C. DAVIS, S. C. SCHULZ, I. EXTEIN, R. WAGNER, D. NABER, P. W. GOLD, D. P. VAN KAMMEN, F. K. GOODWIN, R. J. WYATT, C. H. Li & W. E. BUNNEY, JR. 1981. Behavioral and biological effects of acute β-endorphin injection in schizophrenic and depressed patients. Am. J. Psychiatry **138:** 160–166.
12. EMRICH, H. M., V. HOLLT, W. KISSLING, M. FISHLER, H. LASPE, H. HEINEMANN, D. VAN ZERSSEN & A. HERZ. 1979. β-Endorphin-like immunoreactivity in cerebrospinal fluid and plasma of patients with schizophrenia and other neuropsychiatric disorders. Pharmakopsychiatr. Neuropsychopharmakol. **12:** 267–276.
13. PICKAR, D., N. R. CUTLER, D. NABER, R. M. POST & W. E. BUNNEY, JR. 1980. Plasma opioid activity and manic-depressive illness. Lancet **1:** 937.
14. ROSS, M., P. A. BERGER & A. GOLDSTEIN. Plasma β-endorphin immunoreactivity in schizophrenia. Science **200:** 974–981.
15. TERENIUS, L., A. WAHLSTRÖM & C. JOHANSSON. 1979. Endorphins in human cerebrospinal fluid and their measurement. *In* Endorphins and Mental Health Research. E. Usdin, W. E. Bunney, Jr. & N. S. Kline, Eds.: 553–650. Macmillan. New York.
16. NABER, D., D. PICKAR, R. M. POST, D. P. VAN KAMMEN, R. N. WATERS, J. C. BALLINGER, F. K. GOODWIN & W. E. BUNNEY, JR. 1981. Endogenous opioid activity and β-endorphin-immunoreactivity in CSF of psychiatric patients and normal volunteers. Am. J. Psychiatry. **138:** 1457–1462.
17. LINDSTRÖM, L. H., W. WIDERLÖV, L. M. GUNNE, A. WAHLSTRÖM & L. TERENIUS. 1978. Endorphins in human cerebrospinal fluid: Clinical correlations to some psychotic states. Acta Psychiatr. Scand. **57:** 153–164.
18. DOMSCHKE, W., A. DICKSCHAS & P. MITZNEGG. 1979. CSF β-endorphin in schizophrenia. Lancet **2:** 1024.

19. JEFFCOATE, W. J., L. McLOUGHLIN, J. HOPE, C. H. REES, S. J. BATTER, P. J. LOWRY & G. M. BESSER. 1978. β-Endorphin in human cerebrospinal fluid. Lancet 2: 119–121.

20. NABER, D., D. PICKAR, R. A. DIONNE, D. L. BOWIE, B. A. EWELS, T. W. MOODY, M. G. SOBLE & C. B. PERT. 1980. Assay of endogenous opiate receptor ligands in human CSF and plasma. Substance and Alcohol Actions/Misuse 1: 83–91.

21. SIMANTOV, R., S. R. CHILDERS & S. SNYDER. 1977. Opioid peptides: Differentiation by radioimmunoassay and radioreceptor assay. Brain Res. 135: 358–369.

22. PICKAR, D., D. NABER, R. M. POST, D. P. VAN KAMMEN, J. C. BALLENGER & W. E. BUNNEY, JR. 1981. Measurement of Endorphins in CSF. In Modern Problems in Pharmacotherapy: The Role of Endorphins in Neuropsychiatry. H. M. Emrich, Ed.: 246–262. A. G. Karger. Basel.

23. HOSOBUCHI, Y., J. ROSSIER, F. E. BLOOM & R. GUILLEMIN. 1979. Stimulation of human periaqueductal gray for pain relief increases immunoreactive β-endorphin in ventricular fluid. Science 203: 279–289.

24. AKIL, H., D. E. RICHARDSON, J. HUGHES & J. D. BARCHAS. 1978. Enkephalin-like material elevated in ventricular cerebrospinal fluid of pain patients after focal stimulation. Science 201: 463–465.

25. SJÖLUND, B., L. TERENIUS & M. ERIKSSON. 1977. Increased cerebrospinal fluid levels of endorphin after electro-acupuncture. Acta Physiol. Scand. 100: 382–384.

26. CLEMENT-JONES, V., P. J. LOWRY, L. McLOUGHLIN, G. M. BESSER, L. H. REES & H. L. WEN. 1979. Acupuncture in heroin addicts: Changes in met-enkephalin and β-endorphin in blood and cerebrospinal fluid. Lancet 2: 380–382.

27. TANSON, A., P. HARTVIG, G. DAHLSTRÖM, A. WAHLSTRÖM AND L. TERENIUS. 1980. Endorphins and on-demand pain relief. Lancet 2: 769.

28. NABER, D., R. M. COHEN, D. PICKAR, N. S. KALIN & W. E. BUNNEY, JR. 1981. Episodic secretion of opioid activity: Evidence for a diurnal rhythm. Life Sci. 28: 931–935.

29. GALLAGHER, T. F., K. YOSHIDA, H. D. ROFFWARG, D. K. FUKUSHIMA, E. D. WEITZMAN & L. HELLMAN. 1973. ACTH and cortisol secretory patterns in man. J. Clin. Endocrinol. Metab. 36: 1058–1073.

30. DAVIS, G. C., M. S. BUCHSBAUM & W. E. BUNNEY, JR. 1978. Naloxone decreases diurnal variation in pain sensitivity and somatosensory evoked potentials. Life Sci. 23: 1449–1460.

31. RUBINOW, D. R., R. M. POST, D. PICKAR, D. NABER, J. C. BALLENGER, P. W. GOLD & W. E. BUNNEY, JR. 1981. Relationship between urinary free cortisol and CSF opioid binding activity in depressed patients and normal volunteers. Psychiatry Res. 5: 87–93.

32. KAYE, W., D. PICKAR, D. NABER & M. EBERT. CSF opioid activity in anorexia nervosa.

33. SPITZER, R. L., J. E. ENDICOTT & E. ROBINS. 1975. Research Diagnostic Criteria (RDC) for a Selected Group of Functional Disorders, 2nd edit. Biometrics Research. NY State Psychiatric Institute. New York.

34. DIAGNOSTIC AND STATISTICAL MANUAL OF MENTAL DISORDERS (Third Edition). 1980. The American Psychiatric Association, Washington, D.C.

35. TERENIUS, L., A. WAHLSTRÖM, C. LINDSTRÖM & E. WIDERLÖV. 1976. Increased CSF levels of endorphins in chronic psychosis. Neurosci. Lett. 3: 157–162.

36. RIMON, R., L. TERENIUS & R. KAMPMAN. 1980. Cerebrospinal fluid endorphins in schizophrenia. Acta Psychiatr. Scand. 61: 395–403.

37. BUNNEY, W. E., JR. & D. A. HAMBURG. 1963. Methods for reliable longitudinal observations of behavior. Arch. Gen. Psychiatry 9: 267–276.

38. PICKAR, D., I. EXTEIN, P. W. GOLD, D. NABER, R. S. SUMMERS & F. K. GOODWIN.

1982. Endorphins in Affective Disorders. *In* Endorphins and Opiate Antagonists in Psychiatric Illness. N. S. Shah & A. G. Donald, Eds.: 375–397. Plenum Press. New York.
39. COHEN, M. R. & D. PICKAR. 1981. Pharmacologic challenges to the endogenous opioid system in affective illness. J. Clin. Psychopharmacology **1:** 223–231.
40. DAVIS, G. C., I. EXTEIN, V. REUSS, W. HAMILTON, R. M. POST & F. K. GOODWIN. 1980. Failure of naloxone to reduce manic symptoms. Am. J. Psychiatry **137:** 1583–1585.
41. ANGST, J. V. AUTENRIETH, F. BREM, M. KOUKKOU, H. MEYER, H. H. STASSEN & U, STORCK. 1979. Preliminary results of treatment with β-endorphin in depression. *In* Endorphins in Mental Health Research. E. Usdin, W. E. Bunney, Jr. & N. S. Kline, Eds.: 518–528. Macmillan. New York.
42. EXTEIN, I., D. PICKAR, M. S. GOLD, P. W. GOLD, A. L. C. POTTASH, D. R. SWEENEY, R. REBAR, D. MARTIN & F. K. GOODWIN. 1981. Methadone and morphine in depression. 1981. Psychopharm. Bull.: 1729–1733.
43. MAINS, R. E., B. A. EIPPER & N. LING. 1977. Common precursor to corticotropins and endorphins. Proc. Natl. Acad. Sci. USA **74:** 3014–3016.
44. GUILLEMIN, R., T. VARGO, J. ROSSIER, S. MINICK, N. LING, C. RIVIER, W. VALE & F. BLOOM. 1977. β-Endorphin and adrenocorticotropin are secreted concomitantly by the pituitary gland. Science **197:** 1337–1369.
45. CARROL, B. J., G. C. CURTIS & J. MENDELS. 1976. Neuroendocrine regulation in depression: II. Discrimination of depressed from non-depressed patients. Arch. Gen. Psychiatry **33:** 1051–1058.
46. SCHLESSER, M. A., G. WINOKUR & B. M. SHERMAN. 1980. Hypothalamic-pituitary-adrenal axis activity in depressive illness. Arch. Gen. Psychiatry **37:** 737–743.
47. GRANDISON, L. & L. GUIDOTTI. 1977. Stimulation of food intake by muscimol and β-endorphin. Neuropharmacology **16:** 533–536.
48. HOLTZMAN. S. G. 1974. Behavioral effects of separate and combined administration of naloxone and d-amphetamine. J. Pharmacol. Exp. Ther. **189:** 51–60.
49. MARGULES, D. L., B. MOISSET, M. J. LEWIS, H. SHIBUYA & C. B. PERT. 1978. β-Endorphin is associated with overeating in genetically obese mice (ob/ob) and rats (fa/fa). Science **202:** 988–991.
50. MARGULES, E. L. 1979. β-Endorphin and endoloxone: Hormones of the autonomic nervous system for the conservation or expenditure of bodily resources and energy in anticipation of famine or feast. Neurosci. Biobehav. Rev. **3:** 155–162.
51. GERNER, R. H. & H. E. GWIRTSMAN. 1981. Abnormalities of dexamethasone suppression test and urinary MHPG in anorexia nervosa. Am. J. Psychiatry **138:** 650–653.

DISCUSSION OF THE PAPER

R. A. MASLANSKY (*New York, NY*): I wonder whether anybody has reported ectopic endorphin production like the ACTH syndrome?

D. PICKAR (*NIMH, Bethesda, MD*): Are you looking for an endorphin illness?

MASLANSKEY: Yes.

PICKAR: To my knowledge, no one has definitively found it. There are unusual cases in children involving autonomic/hypothalamic dysfunction and psychosis which are reported to be improved by naloxone. These are probably the closest which you will get. There is no known malignancy or tumor associated with hypersecretion of endorphins as with ACTH in the lung, etc. but it is not impossible.

G. KING (*Pointe Claire, Quebec, Canada*): I would like to know whether you have looked at correlation between CSF opioid activity and response to tricyclic antidepressants in your depressed patients because carbamazepine has a great number of structural resemblances to the tricyclics and may be acting like a tricyclic.

PICKAR: Although carbamazepine is related to tricyclics, we have tended to focus on its antiseizure properties as relating to its clinical effects in patients, although it is possible that more classical tricyclic effects are also involved.

To date, we have only limited data regarding tricyclics and CSF opioid activity.

KING: Well, is there any information which says that carbamazepine is any more effective than tricyclics?

PICKAR: No. There are two areas which carbamazepine appears to be particularly useful. One is its general antimanic properties, particularly in non-lithium-responsive manics and/or rapid cyclers and the other is in the treatment of refractory depressed patients. No cross-over study with tricyclics and carbamazepine has, to my knowledge, been performed.

H. M. EMRICH (*Max Planck Institute for Psychiatry, Munich, FRG*): Anorectic patients have a high level of cortisol and also animals under hunger metabolism show very high levels of ACTH and cortisol. So, probably, your data reflect this fact.

The question would be, have you measured β-endorphin immunoreactivity in the anorectic patients?

PICKAR: We did not because we did not have enough CSF in these patients; we are currently studying another group of these patients, and perhaps at a later date will have more information in this area.

It is interesting to speculate that stress-induced increases in opioid activity may be behaviorally meaningful. It is possible that some aspects of anorexia nervosa behavior are mediated by enhanced endogenous opioid functioning resulting from the stress of starvation.

β-ENDORPHIN IMMUNOREACTIVITY IN THE PLASMA OF PSYCHIATRIC PATIENTS RECEIVING ELECTROCONVULSIVE TREATMENT *

Charles E. Inturrisi, George Alexopoulos, Robert Lipman,
Kathleen Foley, and Jean Rossier †

*Departments of Pharmacology and Psychiatry and Neurology
Cornell University Medical College
New York, New York 10021*

† *Laboratoire de Physiologie Nerveuse
Centre National de la Recherche Scientifique
Gif-sur-Yvette, France*

The endorphins have been implicated in the pathogenesis of various psychiatric disorders. In man several studies have focused on the behavioral effects seen following the administration of endorphins or an opiate antagonist such as naloxone. The development of sensitive analytical procedures has made it possible to measure circulating levels of endorphins.

Using a radioreceptor assay Pickar et al.[1] presented a case report of a manic-depressive person whose manic phase was associated with significantly higher plasma levels of opioid activity than was found during her depressed state. Emrich et al.[2] reported that plasma immunoreactive β-endorphin (ir-β-ep) was elevated in three depressed patients after electroconvulsive therapy (ECT). ECT has powerful but as yet not understood antidepressant effects.

The objectives of our study were:

(1) to determine the basal ir-β-ep levels in the plasma of drug-free depressed patients;

(2) to determine the effect of single and repetitive ECT treatment on ir-β-ep; and

(3) to determine whether a relationship exists between ECT-induced alterations of ir-β-ep and therapeutic outcome.

MATERIALS AND METHODS

Subjects

The subjects of the ECT study were 13 patients hospitalized in the psychiatric facilities of the Westchester Division of the New York Hospital-Cornell Medical Center. Data are reported on 11 patients in whom at least one ECT study was completed. Seven were men, and four were women. Their ages ranged from 40 to 87 years, with a mean age of 68. Each patient had been diagnosed by two psychiatrists as having a recurrent primary unipolar affective disorder according to the Research Diagnostic Criteria.[3] None of the patients had received psychotropic drugs for at least 10 days prior

* This work was supported in part by Grant DA–01457 from the National Institute on Drug Abuse.

0077–8923/82/0398–0413 $01.75/0 © 1982 NYAS

to study. ECT was prescribed by each patient's physician. Sixteen psychiatrically normal subjects also participated in the study. Eleven were men and five women. They ranged in age from 21 to 47 years, with a mean age of 29.

Study Design

Each patient underwent ECT between 1:00 and 2:00 PM, after the intravenous administration of atropine sulfate (1.1 mg), pentobarbital sodium (200 mg), and succinylcholine chloride (45 mg). A 15-ml venous blood sample was collected into a heparinized plastic syringe just prior to ECT and a second blood sample was collected at 15 minutes after the completion of ECT treatment.

Normal subjects provided a 15-ml blood sample collected in the same manner as that for patients between 1:00 and 2:00 P.M. Patient and normal blood samples were centrifuged in a refrigerated unit within 5 minutes of collection and the plasma frozen at -20 C until the time of assay for ir-β-ep.

Peptides

α-Endorphin, γ-endorphin, and synthetic human β-endorphin (β-ep) were purchased from Peninsula Laboratories (San Carlos, CA) methionine and leucine enkephalin from Boehringer Mannheim (Indianapolis, IN). Human β-lipotropin (β-LPH) was a gift from Dr. C. H. Li.

Antiserum

Human β-endorphin was coupled to bovine serum albumin and injected into rabbits as described by Guillemin et al.[4]

Preparation of Trace

The β-ep was labeled with ^{125}I using a chloramine-T procedure.[5] The labeled peptide was purified by chromatography on Sephadex G-50 (0.7 × 50 cm) using an acetate buffer (1M acetic acid, 20 mM HCl). An equal volume of 95% ethanol was added to the purified trace prior to storage at 4°C.

Buffers

Buffers used were: 20mM phosphate buffer, pH 7.5, containing 150 mM NaCl + 0.01% thimerosal (buffer A); buffer A + 0.1% gelatin (buffer B); buffer A + 0.1% gelatin + 0.01% crystalline bovine serum albumin (BSA) (buffer C); buffer A + 0.1% gelatin, 0.01% BSA + 0.1% (v/v) Triton X-100 (buffer D); and buffer A + 0.1% gelatin + 0.01% BSA + 0.05% (v/v) Triton X-100 (buffer G).

Extraction of β-ep Immunoreactivity from Plasma

The extraction procedure was adapted from that described by Wardlaw and Frantz.[6] A 50-mg talc tablet (Ormont Drug and Chemical Co., Englewood, NJ) was added to 4 ml of thawed plasma in a polypropylene tube and mixed by rotation for 30 min. After centrifugation ($1500 \times g$, 10 min), the supernatant was removed and the pellet washed with 4 ml of ice-cold deionized water. The immunoreactivity was eluted from the talc pellet by mixing for 15 min with 2 ml of freshly prepared, ice-cold acetone:1N HCl (50:50). After centrifugation ($1500 \times g$, 10 min) the acetone–HCl phase was transferred with a polyethylene pipette to a polypropylene tube. The acetone-HCl extraction was repeated and the supernatants were combined and evaporated to dryness in two steps. The samples were placed in a Savant Speedvac Concentrator/Evaporator centrifuge (Savant Instruments, Inc., Hicksville, NY) and the acetone removed using a water aspirator. The remaining aqueous phase was reduced to dryness by use of the Speedvac refrigerated trap system (Savant Instruments, Inc.). The dried residue was reconstituted in 800 μl of buffer G, and after 30 min at room temperature, during which the sample was repeatedly agitated, the sample was centrifuged as just described to separate any undissolved residue. Endorphin-free plasma (EFP) was prepared in 200-ml batches from thawed, pooled blood bank plasma or pooled plasma collected by us from normal volunteers. One talc tablet was added for each 4-ml plasma aliquot. After mixing for 30 min the supernatant was removed by centrifugation (as just described) and used immediately or stored at −20°C. This procedure removed greater than 95% of the radioactivity of ^{125}I-labeled β-ep added together with unlabeled β-ep at a concentration of 34 pg/ml. EFP was used to prepare blank extracts, to bring samples to a final volume of 4 ml, and to prepare extracted standard curves. Extracted standard curves were prepared using dilutions of β-ep in buffer C. These diluted standards were added to EFP to yield standards that ranged from 8.5 to 1088 pg/ml. The standards were subjected to the talc extraction procedure described earlier for samples.

Radioimmunoassay (RIA) Procedure

One hundred μl of buffer C and 200 μl of the reconstituted extract of a sample or standard was pipetted in triplicate into borosilicate tubes followed by the addition of 200 μl of antiserum in buffer B to achieve a final antiserum dilution of 1:24,000. This antiserum dilution resulted in a mean B_0 equal to 31.4 ± 3.7 (SD) percent of the total added cpm (see *Calculations*). Control tubes received 200 μl of reconstituted extract equivalent to 1 ml of EFP. After incubation for 24 hr at 4°C, 100 μl containing approximately 5600 counts per minute (cpm) of trace in buffer D was added, followed by incubation at 4°C for an additional 24 hr. When the incubation period was completed the tubes were transferred to an ice-water bath for 10 min. Separation of bound and free trace was achieved by the addition of an 0.5-ml aliquot of an iced, stirring suspension of 0.2% dextran and 2.0% charcoal in buffer B. After an additional 12 min in the ice-water bath, the assay tubes were centrifuged for 15 min at $1500 \times g$. A 0.5-ml aliquot of the clear supernatant, containing the antibody-bound trace, was transferred to polypropylene tubes and counted with a Packard Model 5260 gamma counter (Packard Instrument, Downers Grove, IL).

Calculations

The standard curve and sample calculations were made using the radio-immunoassay (RIA) program (Clinical Lab and Nuclear Medicine Pac) supplied with the HP-97 electronic calculator (Hewlett-Packard Co., Cupertino, CA). The program performs calculations for a logit/log plot of RIA data using the equation:

$$\text{logit } B/B_0 = m \log X + b$$

where B is the average of triplicate cpm in standards containing unlabeled β-ep. B_0 is the average of triplicate cpm in the absence of unlabeled β-ep (both numerator and denominator are corrected for nonspecific binding); m is the slope, X the amount or concentration of unlabeled β-ep standard; and b is the point where the regression line intercepts the logit axis.

Stability of β-LPH and β-ep

One hundred and fifty nanograms of β-LPH or 50 ng of β-ep were added to 4 ml of EFP and subjected to the extraction procedure described earlier. The residue was resuspended in 0.5 ml of the previously described acetate buffer modified by the addition of 0.1% (v/v) Triton X-100 and 5% methanol and chromatographed on a Bio-Gel P-60 column (1.5 × 50 cm) as described by Ghazarossian et al.[7] Fractions (1.2 ml) were collected at a flow rate of 5 ml/hr. The fractions were dried and the residue was resuspended in buffer C and analyzed by RIA. The columns were calibrated with β-LPH and β-ep standards. The void volume was determined with BSA.

Other RIA Procedures

We also report on estimates of plasma ir-β-ep obtained by use of the radioimmunoassay kit (NEK-003) supplied by New England Nuclear Corp. (Boston, MA).

Cortisol Assay

Plasma cortisol was determined by use of the Coat-a-count® solid phase radioimmunoassay kit supplied by Diagnostic Products Corporation (Los Angeles, CA).

RESULTS AND DISCUSSION

RIA Standard Curve, Precision, Sensitivity, and Specificity

FIGURE 1 shows a representative standard curve for the β-ep RIA using the logit transformation plot. The linear portion of the curve extends from 8.5 to 1088.0 pg/ml. For nine assays the slope averaged 2.46 ± .27 (SD). The precision of the assay was independent of concentration in the range shown in FIGURE 1. The interassay and intraassay coefficients of variation were 13% and 3%, respectively.

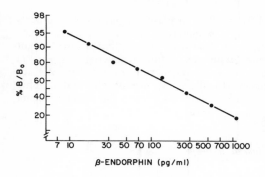

FIGURE 1. RIA standard curve for β-ep extracted from endorphin-free plasma (logit-log plot). *Ordinate:* percentage of B/B₀ (logit scale). *Abscissa:* amount of unlabeled β-ep added per ml of plasma prior to extraction. Each assay tube contained the extract from 1 ml of plasma.

Each assay was calculated using a concurrently extracted standard curve. If we assume that extracted ir-β-ep behaves like the β-ep standards, no correction is necessary for the efficiency of the extraction. Nevertheless, in three separate assays we found recovery of β-ep standards to be 93.6% ± 12.8 (SD) and independent of concentration in the working range (FIG. 1). The antiserum did not recognize α-endorphin, γ-endorphin, methionine enkephalin, or leucine enkephalin (crossreactivity <0.1%). β-LPH crossreacts approximately 25% (wt/wt). The specificity of this antiserum is similar to that of antiserum RB-100-10/76, as reported by Guillemin *et al.*[4] Both antisera were prepared from the same immunogen. Guillemin *et al.*[4] on the basis of a more complete specificity study, concluded that antiserum RB-10010/76 recognizes a specific conformation between the Asn[20] and His[27] (Asn, asparagine:His, histidine) sequence of the C-terminal region of β-ep (1–31).

β-LPH (1–91), which contains β-ep in its primary sequence 61 to 91, is also present in human blood and plasma [6,7] in amounts sufficient to be detected by our antiserum. FIGURE 2 shows the elution pattern of the immunoreactivity obtained following talc extraction of standard β-LPH added to EFP. An immunoreactive component is observed at the elution position of β-LPH, but not at that of β-ep. In a separate study the immunoreactivity of extracts prepared by addition of β-ep to EFP eluted as a single peak identical in elution position to that of authentic β-ep. These results provide no evidence for interconversion and indicate that β-LPH and β-ep are stable in our talc extraction procedure. On the basis of studies to date [6,7] it is reasonable to assume that the immunoreactivity we observed in plasma consists of both

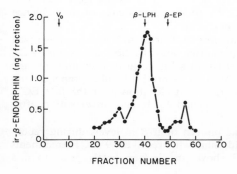

FIGURE 2. Stability of β-LPH during talc extraction. Elution profile is shown of β-LPH added to endorphin-free plasma, extracted, and chromatographed as described in MATERIALS AND METHODS on a Bio-Gel P-60 column. The fractions were assayed using the β-ep RIA. The elution positions of calibration standards of BSA, void volume (V₀), β-lipotropin (β-LPH), and β-endorphin (β-EP) are indicated by arrows.

β-LPH and β-ep. The ratio of β-LPH to β-ep in plasma from normal subjects is approximately 2 (molar basis) or approximately 6 on a wt/wt basis. Since β-LPH has a 25% crossreactivity (wt/wt) with our antiserum we might expect our plasma values (assuming equal extraction recoveries for β-LPH and β-ep) to represent β-LPH and β-ep in a weight ratio of 1.5/1.0. We are attempting to obtain sufficient plasma to allow the use of chromatographic methods to define the immunoreactive components present in patient plasma before and after ECT.

Plasma ir-β-ep

FIGURE 3 presents the mean plasma ir-β-ep values in pg/ml for the normal subjects and the depressed patients. There is no significant difference between the mean ir-β-ep levels of normal subjects and depressed patients prior to the

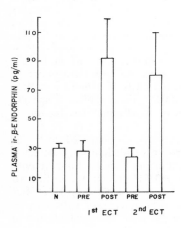

FIGURE 3. The effect of electroconvulsive treatment (ECT) on plasma ir-β-ep concentration. The values are the mean ir-β-ep (+SE) for 16 normal subjects (N) and 11 depressed patients before (pre) and at 15 min after (post) their first and second ECT.

first ECT treatment. Following the first ECT treatment the mean ir-β-ep level was significantly (p < 0.05) increased to an average value three times greater than that prior to treatment. Forty-eight hours later, just prior to the second ECT, ir-β-ep levels had returned to pre-ECT levels. The second ECT treatment also resulted in a significant increase. We found no evidence of an influence of age (range, 21–87 years) or gender on ir-β-ep.

FIGURE 4 shows individual pre- and post-ECT ir-β-ep levels for the seven depressed patients who provided samples after both the first and second ECT treatments. The ir-β-ep values are plotted on a log scale to accommodate the range of values. The interindividual variation in pre-ECT values ranged from 8 to 62 pg/ml. Each patient shows a significant elevation after the first ECT, a return to pre-ECT levels prior to the second ECT, and an elevation after the second ECT.

FIGURE 5 shows an example of the pattern of ir-β-ep levels during repetitive ECT treatment in an 80-year-old man who received 9 ECT treatments during a 1-month period. FIGURE 5 shows the ir-β-ep levels prior to and

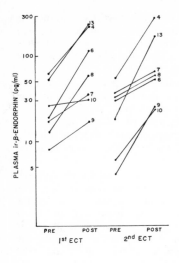

FIGURE 4. Plasma ir-β-ep concentration and electroconvulsive treatment (ECT) in seven depressed patients. The values are the ir-β-ep before (pre) and at 15 min after (post) the first and second ECT. Patients are identified by number.

15 minutes after the first, second, fifth, eighth, and ninth ECT in this patient. As can be seen, the pattern remains fairly constant, with an average increase of 6 times in the value of ir-β-ep following each ECT.

Nine of the eleven patients were asymptomatic following the series of 10 to 12 ECT treatments. Two patients had an incomplete remission. To date we have found no relationship between the outcome of ECT treatment and the transient changes in ir-β-ep following ECT. This conclusion must be tempered by the knowledge that patients with depression of the type seen in this study have a high likelihood of a successful response to ECT. In future studies we plan to extend our observations to include plasma from patients who do not respond to ECT.

β-LPH, β-ep, and ACTH are derived from a common precursor, proopiocortin.[8] Concomitant release of β-ep and ACTH has been reported with various stimuli, including insulin-induced hypoglycemia,[9] acute stress,[10] metyrapone administration,[11] and in such disease states as Addison's disease, Cushing's disease, and Nelson's syndrome.[12]

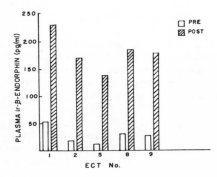

FIGURE 5. Pattern of plasma ir-β-ep concentration during repetitive electroconvulsive (ECT) treatment in a depressed 80-year-old man. The values are ir-β-ep before (pre) and at 15 min after (post) the first, second, fifth, eighth, and ninth ECT.

In rats the secretion of both ir-β-ep and ACTH is inhibited by dexamethasone.[10] Dexamethasone pretreatment also blocks the increase in plasma ir-β-ep, ACTH, and prolactin induced by inescapable electric footshock stress.[13] Levels of ir-β-ep in rat anterior pituitary, but not intermediate lobe, are decreased by long-term dexamethasone administration or acute stress.[14]

Allen et al.[15] have shown a transient elevation of plasma ACTH in depressed patients following ECT that is similar to the ECT-induced increase in plasma ir-β-ep that we find. These studies support the concept that the anterior pituitary contains a readily dischargeable pool of ACTH and ir-β-ep that can be secreted into plasma promptly in response to stressful stimuli. They also suggest that similar hypothalamic regulatory mechanisms govern the release of ACTH and ir-β-ep.

ACTH release is reflected at the adrenal cortex by the release of cortisol. Dent et al.[16] reported a diurnal variation in human plasma ir-β-ep that correlates closely with changes in plasma cortisol, again suggesting a similar secretory pattern for β-ep and ACTH. The most extensively studied and most consistently reported biochemical abnormality in major depressive illness is hypersecretion of cortisol.[17] In a subpopulation of depressed patients, the failure of dexamethasone administration to suppress cortisol secretion (the dexamethasone suppression test or DST) may identify half of the patients suspected clinically of having a unipolar depression and therefore is useful as a confirmatory diagnostic test.[17, 18] Carroll et al.[18] have demonstrated the ability of the DST to identify abnormal responses in depressed patients. They have proposed an "overnight DST procedure" wherein patients receive a 1-mg oral dose of dexamethasone at 11:30 P.M. followed by the collection of a blood sample at 8 A.M., 4 P.M., and 11 P.M. the following day. A criterion value for plasma cortisol is 5 micrograms per deciliter ($\mu g/100$ ml), with plasma cortisol levels exceeding this value at any of the three sample times considered abnormal (that is, dexamethasone failed to suppress plasma cortisol). It has been suggested that these nonsuppressors may belong to a subtype of depressed patients.[19]

It was of interest then to learn whether—as expected from animal studies—dexamethasone will suppress both plasma cortisol and ir-β-ep levels in depressed patients. In the preliminary study reported in TABLES 1 and 2 we used the DST procedure and plasma cortisol response criterion of Carroll et al.[18] We do not yet know what is an appropriate response criterion for a change in plasma ir-β-ep. However, since we anticipated a reduction of ir-β-ep levels below normal in some plasma samples, we used the β-ep RIA kit (New England Nuclear Corp.) as described in MATERIALS AND METHODS. The use of this RIA extended the lower limit of sensitivity of the assay to 5 pg/ml of ir-β-ep (TABLES 1 and 2).

TABLE 1 shows data on plasma cortisol and ir-β-ep before and after dexamethasone administration in two depressed patients (patients A and C). For patient A the administration of dexamethasone at 11 P.M. resulted in suppression of both plasma cortisol and ir-β-ep during the next 24 hours. In patient C dexamethasone failed to suppress plasma cortisol and ir-β-ep in the 8 A.M. sample.

TABLE 2 shows the plasma levels of cortisol and ir-β-ep in a depressed patient in response to dexamethasone before and after successful ECT treatment. Note that before ECT cortisol levels were not suppressed by dexamethasone at 4 and 11 P.M. while after a successful series of ECT treatments,

TABLE 1

PLASMA CORTISOL AND IR-β-ENDORPHIN IN DEPRESSED PATIENTS A AND C:
EFFECT OF DEXAMETHASONE

	Cortisol (μg/100 ml)		IR-β-Endorphin (pg/ml)	
	A	C	A	C
Pre-dexamethasone				
8 am	26	18	22	10
4 pm	6	21	12	11
11 pm	5	7	24	7
Post-dexamethasone				
8 am	3	16	8	7
4 pm	2	8	9	3
11 pm	4	—	7	—

dexamethasone suppressed plasma cortisol at each sample time. It also appears that ir-β-ep was not suppressed by dexamethasone prior to ECT treatment, but was suppressed by dexamethasone at 4 and 11 P.M. after successful ECT. These preliminary results suggest that in some depressed patients both plasma cortisol and ir-β-ep levels respond abnormally to a dexamethasone challenge. The generality of this finding and the utility of plasma ir-β-ep measurements in the diagnosis of unipolar depression and the response to treatment are currently under investigation by our group.

TABLE 2

PLASMA CORTISOL AND IR-β-ENDORPHIN IN A DEPRESSED PATIENT AFTER
DEXAMETHASONE: EFFECT OF SUCCESSFUL ECT TREATMENT

	Cortisol (μg/100 ml)		IR-β-Endorphin (pg/ml)	
	Before	After	Before	After
Post-dexamethasone				
8 am	0	2	0	5
4 pm	16	2	6	2
11 pm	11	2	7	0

REFERENCES

1. PICKAR, D., N. R. CUTLER, D. NABER, R. M. POST, C. B. PERT, W. E. BUNNEY, JR. 1980. Plasma opioid activity in manic-depressive illness. Lancet: 937.
2. EMRICH, H. M., V. HÖLLT, W. KISSLING, M. FISCHLER, H. LASPE, H. HEINEMANN, D. V. ZERSSEN & A. HERZ. 1979. β-Endorphin-like immunoreactivity in cerebrospinal fluid and plasma of patients with schizophrenia and other neuropsychiatric disorders. Pharmakopsychiat. **12:** 269–276.
3. SPITZER, R. L., J. ENDICOTT & E. ROBINS. 1977. Research Diagnostic Criteria (RDC) for a Selected Group of Functional Disorders, 3rd ed. New York State Psychiatric Institute. New York.

4. GUILLEMIN, R., N. LING & T. VARGO. 1977. Radioimmunoassays for α-endorphin and β-endorphin. Biochem. Biophys. Res. Commun. **77:** 361–366.
5. LING, N., J. LEPPÄLUOTO & W. VALE. 1976. Chemical, biological and immunological characterization of mono and diiodothyrotropin releasing factor. Anal. Biochem. **76:** 125–133.
6. WARDLAW, S. L. & A. G. FRANTZ. 1979. Measurement of β-endorphin in human plasma. J. Clin. Endocrinol. Metab. **48:** 176–180.
7. GHAZAROSSIAN, V. E., R. R. DENT, K. OTSU, M. ROSS, B. COX & A. GOLDSTEIN. 1980. Development and validation of a sensitive radioimmunoassay for naturally occurring β-endorphin-like peptides in human plasma. Anal. Biochem. **102:** 80–89.
8. MAINS, R. E., B. A. EIPPER & N. LING. 1977. Common precursor to corticotropins and endorphins. Proc. Natl. Acad. Sci. USA **74:** 3014–3018.
9. NAKAO, K., N. YOSHIKATSU, H. JINGAMI, S. OKI, J. FUKATA & H. IMURA. 1979. Substantial rise of plasma β-endorphin levels after insulin-induced hypoglycemia in human subjects. J. Clin. Endocrin. Metab. **49:** 838–839.
10. GUILLEMIN, R., T. VARGO, J. ROSSIER, S. MINICK, N. LING, C. RIVIER, W. VALE & F. BLOOM. 1977. β-Endorphin and adrenocorticotropin are secreted concomitantly by the pituitary gland. Science **197:** 1367–1369.
11. NAKAO, K., Y. NAKAI, S. OKI, K. HORII & H. IMURA. 1978. Presence of immunoreactive β-endorphin in normal human plasma. J. Clin. Invest. **62:** 1395–1398.
12. SUDA, T., A. S. LIOTTA & D. T. KRIEGER. 1978. β-Endorphin is not detectable in plasma from normal human subjects. Science. **202:** 221–222.
13. ROSSIER, J., E. FRENCH, C. RIVIER, T. SHIBASAKI, R. GUILLEMIN & F. E. BLOOM. 1980. Stress-induced release of prolactin: Blockade by dexamethasone and naloxone may indicate β-endorphin mediation. Proc. Natl. Acad. Sci. USA **77:** 666–669.
14. ROSSIER, J., E. FRENCH, C. GROS, S. MINICK, R. GUILLEMIN & F. E. BLOOM. 1979. Adrenalectomy, dexamethasone or stress alters opioid peptide levels in rat anterior pituitary but not intermediate lobe or brain. Life Sci. **25:** 2105–2112.
15. ALLEN, J. P., D. DENNEY, J. W. KENDALL & P. H. BLACHLY. 1974. Corticotropin release during ECT in man. Am. J. Psychiat. **131:** 1225–1228.
16. DENT, R. R. M., C. GUILLEMINAULT, L. H. ALBERT, B. I. POSNER, B. M. COX & A. GOLDSTEIN. 1981. Diurnal rhythm of plasma immunoreactive β-endorphin and its relationship to sleep stages and plasma rhythms of cortisol and prolactin. J. Clin. Endocrinol. Metab. **52:** 942–947.
17. GOLD, M. S., A. L. C. POTTASH, I. EXTEIN & D. R. SWEENEY. 1981. Diagnosis of depression in the 1980s. J. Am. Med. Assoc. **245:** 1562–1564.
18. CARROLL, E. J., M. FEINBERG, J. F. GREDEN, J. FARIKA, A. A. ALBALA, R. F. HASKETT, N. M. JAMES, Z. KRONFOL, N. LOHR, M. STEINER, J. P. DE'VIGNE & E. YOUNG. 1981. A specific laboratory test for the diagnosis of melancholia. Standardization, validation and clinical utility. Arch. Gen. Psychiat. **38:** 15–22.
19. BROWN, W. A. & I. SHUEY. 1980. Response to dexamethasone and subtype of depression. Arch. Gen. Psychiat. **37:** 747–751.

DISCUSSION OF THE PAPER

H.M. EMRICH (*Max Planck Institute for Psychiatry, Munich, FRG*): I would first like to congratulate you for this excellent data and, of course, we are very happy to see that it is a confirmation of our findings. Furthermore, I would like to mention that Dr. J. W. Holaday (HOLADAY *et al.,* 1981, *In* Modern Problems of Pharmacopsychiatry. T.A. Bam, Ed. Vol 17: 142, Karger, Basel) has shown in animals that ECT induces an activation of the endorphinergic system.

The interesting point in this work, I think, is now the question of the possible role of this activation to the therapeutic effects of ECT. Is the therapeutic effect of ECT really mediated by the activation of endorphins?

There are two approaches to answer this question, one as proposed by you, seeks a correlation between the therapeutic outcome of ECT and the elevation of endorphins. The other approach would be to attempt to prevent the therapeutic effect of ECT by administration of naltrexone. In patients this use of naltrexone would not be ethical.

R. CHIPKIN (*Schering Corp. Bloomfield, NJ*): The first question is did the patients receive any drug between the pre measure and when you do the post measure?

C.E. INTURRISI (*Cornell University Medical College, New York*): They received the drugs that are ordinarily given as pretreatment for ECT, including atropine, pentobarbital, and succinylcholine.

CHIPKIN: Do you have any indication if this treatment might have any effect on the levels of plasma β-endorphin?

INTURRISI: No, we have not examined that question. But Allen *et al.* (reference 15) found that pretreatment for ECT as described above did not alter basal ACTH levels. We presume the same is true for β-endorphin levels.

CHIPKIN: The other question is, do you have any indication as to the specificity of the ECT induced release of β-endorphin?

INTURRISI: At this point I would say that until a correlation can be shown between the changes we observe and a therapeutic effect we must assume that ECT is, *per se*, a stressful stimulus resulting in the release of ACTH and β-endorphin from the pituitary. However, our data would suggest that measures of peripheral endorphins may be of some value. Whether plasma endorphin levels are, like plasma cortisol levels, useful in the diagnosis and treatment of some depressed patients remains to be determined.

UNIDENTIFIED SPEAKER: Why did you measure the endorphin levels at 15 minutes after ECT?

INTURRISI: We know that in man exogenously administered β-endorphin has a relatively short half-life, averaging approximately 37 minutes (Foley *et al.*, 1979, Proc. Natl. Acad. Sci. USA, **76:** 5377). Therefore, assuming that endogenous β-endorphin has a similar half-life, the measurement of the response to ECT should be made soon after the stimulus.

UNIDENTIFIED SPEAKER: I was wondering if after ECT you still have a release of endorphins at 30 minutes, one hour and so on?

INTURRISI: We would like to define the time course of the response, but, for this initial study, we chose 15 minutes after ECT as being a reasonable time. We could sample earlier and a little bit later, but, again, as Allen *et al.* have shown for ECT induced release of ACTH, the peak of plasma ACTH occurs at two and a half minutes and declines over the next hour or so.

UNIDENTIFIED SPEAKER: In a very simplistic way I would assume that when you depolarize the cell you say it releases endorphins and, then, the cell does not recover after ECT right away as in the period following a convulsion.

INTURRISI: If you give multiple ECT stimuli and Allen *et al.* did this in the ACTH study, you can produce a sustained elevation of plasma ACTH. Whether this is true for plasma β-endorphin remains to be determined.

CLINICAL AND EXPERIMENTAL STUDIES OF STRESS AND THE ENDOGENOUS OPIOID SYSTEM

Martin R. Cohen,* † David Pickar,* Michel Dubois,‡ John Nurnberger,*
Yolanda Roth,§ Robert M. Cohen,‖ Elliot Gershon,* and
William E. Bunney, Jr.*

* Biological Psychiatry Branch
‖ Clinical Neuropharmacology Branch
National Institute of Mental Health
Bethesda, Maryland 20205

† Department of Psychiatry
University of Iowa College of Medicine
Iowa City, Iowa 55240

‡ Anesthesia Section
National Institutes of Health Clinical Center
Bethesda, Maryland 20205

§ Surgery Branch
National Cancer Institute
National Institutes of Health
Bethesda, Maryland 20205

Stress is manifested by complex behavioral [1] and physiological alterations.[2] Some hormone alterations, such as increases in plasma levels of growth hormone, cortisol, and prolactin, are such a frequent part of these physiological effects that they are often used as markers of stress-induced states or arousal.[2, 3] However, their relationship to physiological adaptation to stress is more certain than their relationship to behavioral adaptation. Recent animal studies have suggested that an increase in plasma β-endorphin may also be a frequent accompaniment of stress and have suggested a linkage between the stress-induced responses of the endogenous opioid system and the hypothalamus–pituitary–adrenal (HPA) axis.[4] Thus, increases in circulating β-endorphin may also prove to be a marker of human stress or arousal. This is particularly intriguing since behavioral and physiological effects of exogenous opiates have long been recognized,[5] and animal experiments have suggested an important role for the endogenous opioid system in self-regulation of behavior[6] and physiology.[7]

To assess the role of the endogenous opioid system in the human response to stress, we have evaluated the effects of the administration of amphetamines and of surgical stress on plasma β-endorphin immunoreactivity (ir). In animals, amphetamine administration has been shown to simulate or potentiate behavioral effects of stress and amphetamines are utilized clinically in the treatment of disorders of arousal.[1] Surgery has long been recognized as a stress model. Because plasma cortisol is an index of arousal, and to assess the possible stress-induced linkage of the endogenous opioid system and the

424

HPA axis in man, we have also measured plasma cortisol. Finally, we have attempted to evaluate the relationship of plasma β-endorphin levels to stress-induced human behavior.

MATERIALS AND METHODS

Amphetamine Study

Eight normal (free of psychiatric and physical illness) monozygotic twins (including 3 pairs), aged 18 to 39 years, were tested from a larger pool of twins utilized in pharmacogenetic studies. Individuals were permitted to eat breakfast, but began fasting prior to placement of an intravenous catheter in a forearm vein between 0800 and 0930 hr. By means of a random, crossover, double-blind design, placebo or 0.3 mg/kg dextroamphetamine was infused on separate days over a 2-minute period starting 1 hour after catheter placement. Since previous clinical studies had demonstrated cortisol and ACTH responses to intravenous stimulants to be maximum at 30 minutes,[8, 9] blood was obtained for hormone evaluations 5 minutes prior to and 30 minutes post infusion. Blind-observer ratings of mood and behavioral changes were made from video-tapes of the baseline period and the first hour after infusion; these are described elsewhere.[10]

Surgery Study

Nine patients (seven men, two women) underwent laparotomy as part of a National Cancer Institute protocol for the treatment of testicular or ovarian malignancy. Patients were medication-free for at least 72 hours prior to the surgical procedures. Pentobarbital, 100 mg, was administered intramuscularly for premedication. Induction of anesthesia was accomplished with thiopental and succinylcholine and anesthesia was maintained with enflurane, nitrous oxide, and a, muscle relaxant. All patients were intubated and had controlled ventilation. Surgery lasted between 2 and 4 hours. No exogenous opioids were administered prior to or during surgery. However, once patients were conscious (between the first and third hour post awakening), they were given intravenous morphine at 1.5 to 3.5 mg/hr as needed for relief of postoperative pain. This was the standard clinical order used for the first 24 hr of postoperative care in the NIH Clinical Center Surgical Intensive Care Unit (SICU). A patient's morphine requirement was calculated as the total morphine administered during the first 24 postoperative hours. This was obtained from the clinical record maintained by nursing staff. Neither patients or nursing staff were aware that an assessment of morphine administration was to be accomplished. Although medication usage under such conditions might conceivably be determined by multiple factors, its relationship to hormone variables would be relevant to the natural or clinical setting rather than to special laboratory or experimental conditions. Blood samples were collected following premedication and prior to anesthetic induction (presurgery hormone levels were assayed from these samples), 10 minutes after skin incision, and at subsequent 30-minute intervals until skin closure. A patient's mean surgery hormone level was calculated as the mean of values derived from samples obtained during surgery at the times just noted. Details of sample care are reported elsewhere.[11]

Hormone Assays

Plasma cortisol and β-endorphin were determined by radioimmunoassay on unextracted samples with reagents supplied by New England Nuclear Corp. Intraassay variations were 6% and 3.5% and interassay variations were 8% and 5%, respectively. Hormone evaluations for the amphetamine study and for any individual surgery were accomplished in the same assay. There is in the β-endorphin assay 50% crossreactivity to β-lipotropin, <5% to ACTH, < 0.01% to α-endorphin and α-MSH, and < 0.004% to methionine and leucine enkephalin. Thus β-endorphin (all subsequent references in this paper are to immunoreactivity, ir) as determined in these studies is essentially the sum of circulating β-endorphin and β-lipotropin; their ratio was not determined. The lower limit of sensitivity for the β-endorphin assay is 14.4 picomolar. Plasma samples with no detectable β-endorphin were therefore arbitrarily assigned the value of 14.4 picomolar to minimize any reported increase of levels found with surgery. Personnel involved in laboratory determinations were not involved as clinical staff. Their determinations were made blind to behavioral ratings and morphine assessments.

Statistics

The significances of hormonal alterations following amphetamine infusion and surgery were determined by means of paired Student's t tests, df = 7 and 8, respectively. Correlations, unless otherwise noted, were determined by the Pearson product moment (r), variance = r^2, df = 6 and 7, respectively.

RESULTS

Amphetamine Study

Individual hormonal responses to amphetamine infusion are illustrated in FIGURE 1. After administration of amphetamine, plasma β-endorphin rose in six of eight volunteers, a mean ± SEM increase of +6.8 ± 5.3 picomolar (+10.2%) (p < 0.05, two-tail). In contrast, after placebo, levels decreased in

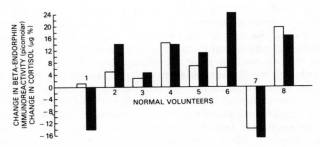

FIGURE 1. Individual changes from baseline values in plasma β-endorphin (picomolar) and cortisol (μg %) 30 minutes after a 0.3 mg/kg dextroamphetamine infusion in eight normal volunteers. *Black bars* = β-endorphin; *white bars* = cortisol.

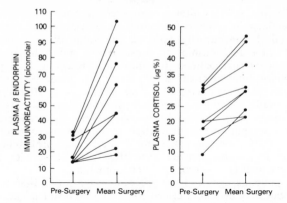

FIGURE 2. Individual patient plasma β-endorphin (ir) and cortisol responses to surgery. Each line connects an individual's presurgery hormone level to his mean surgery hormone level. Presurgery β-endorphin levels below the sensitivity of our radioimmunoassay (< 14.4 picomolar) were arbitrarily assigned the value of 14.4 picomolar to minimize any found increases with surgery. The group means ± SEM were as follows: presurgery β-endorphin ≤ 19.9 ± 2.4 picomolar; mean surgery = 54.9 ± 10.2 picomol; presurgery cortisol = 22.1 ± 2.6 μg %; mean surgery cortisol = 32.4 ± 3.2 μg %.

seven of eight volunteers (mean, −10.7 picomolar). The mean amphetamine–placebo difference was +17.5 picomolar (+26%).

After administration of amphetamine, plasma cortisol levels increased in seven of eight volunteers, a mean ± SEM of +5.3 ± 3.5 μg% (+25.6%) (p < 0.025, one-tail). After placebo administration, cortisol levels decreased in seven of eight volunteers (mean, −3.5 μg%). The mean amphetamine–placebo difference was 8.8 μg% (+42%).

Volunteers' β-endorphin and cortisol responses to amphetamine were significantly correlated (r = +0.76, p < 0.025, one-tail). However, no correlation was found between the hormonal and behavioral responses to amphetamine.

Surgery Study

Individual hormonal responses to surgery are illustrated in FIGURE 2. In all nine patients, plasma β-endorphin and cortisol levels increased after the onset of surgery. The mean increase in β-endorphin was >34.9 picomolar (175%, p < 0.01, two-tail); the mean cortisol increase was 10.2 μg% (46%, p < 0.001, two-tail). These increases were not significantly correlated.

The postsurgical morphine requirements of our patients ranged from 12 to 56 mg (mean ± SEM, 35.2 ± 16.1). There was a significant negative correlation between patients' morphine requirements and their mean surgery β-endorphin levels (r = 0.-0.68, p < 0.05, two-tail) (FIG. 3). Mean surgery cortisol levels were negatively (−0.52), but not significantly related to post-operative morphine requirements. Patients' presurgery β-endorphin levels were also significantly negatively correlated with morphine requirements (r = −0.84, p < 0.01, two-tail) and positively related to their mean surgery β-endorphin levels ($r = 0.71$, $p < 0.05$, two-tail). However, because many of our patients' presurgery β-endorphin levels were below the sensitivity of our assay (14.4 picomolar), and thus arbitrarily assigned the value of 14.4 picomolar, the significance of these relationships to presurgery β-endorphin is questionable. Yet it was apparent that patients fell into two groups with respect to their presurgery β-endorphin levels: those with levels ≤ 16 picomolar (six) and those with levels >28 picomolar (three). Five of the six patients with low β-endorphin required ≥ 44 mg postoperative morphine in contrast to the three patients with high preoperative β-endorphin, who required only ≤ 22 mg morphine. This nonparametric distinction in morphine requirement was significant at $p < 0.05$, one-tail using the Fisher exact probability test. Presurgery cortisol levels also showed a negative correlation with postoperative morphine requirement ($r = -0.65$, $p < 0.05$, one-tail).

Individual patient's ages (21–60 yr) and weights (47.5–85.5 kg) are not detailed here, but may be found elsewhere.[28] A significant negative correlation

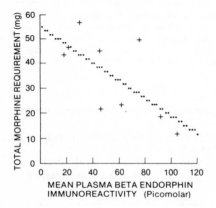

FIGURE 3. Variables of morphine requirement and mean (surgery) plasma β-endorphin plotted two dimensionally in nine patients ($+$). Patient morphine requirement can be predicted by the illustrated linear equation: morphine requirement $= 54.9$–$0.36 \times$ mean (surgery) plasma β-endorphin. Patient morphine requirement is the total amount of morphine used during the first 24 postoperative hours. Mean (surgery) plasma β-endorphin is the mean of plasma β-endorphin levels found in samples taken at 30-minute intervals during surgery.

between the patient's age and postoperative morphine requirement was found ($r = -0.69$, $p < 0.05$, two-tail). Age was not significantly related to mean surgery β-endorphin levels. Patients' weights were correlated, but not significantly, with morphine requirement ($r = 0.55$).

Mean surgery β-endorphin level and age could explain, respectively, 46% and 48% of the variance in individual morphine requirement after surgery. Using both variables in a multiple regression analysis, it was possible to predict 70% of the variance, although this increase of 22% over the variance predicted by either variable alone did not reach statistical significance.

DISCUSSION

The results of these studies confirm previous reports that amphetamine administration [12, 13] and surgery [14] increase plasma cortisol levels in humans. These studies are the first to demonstrate, in human subjects, increases in plasma β-endorphin during these procedures. We have previously demonstrated that enflurane anesthesia alone has no effect on plasma cortisol or β-endorphin levels.[11]

The correlated change in plasma β-endorphin and cortisol following amphetamine administration suggests a stress-induced linkage of the endogenous opioid system and the HPA axis in man. This is consistent with the results of animal stress studies,[4] and the probable common origin of plasma β-endorphin and ACTH.[15] Although we were unable to find a significant relationship between changes in plasma β-endorphin and cortisol after surgery using a mean surgery–presurgery difference, we have previously shown correlated levels of plasma β-endorphin and cortisol using time points inclusive of presurgery, mean surgery, and postsurgery.[11]

In our subject group, we were not able to find any relationship between amphetamine-induced behavioral and plasma hormone changes. However, using a larger group of volunteers, which included the subsample of the presently reported subjects, a significant correlation between an excitation factor subscale and cortisol was able to be demonstrated.[16]

Clinicians have previously noted the great variance in patients' postoperative morphine requirements that we observed in this study.[17] One major explanation of this variance may well be based upon expected individual differences in morphine pharmocokinetics. This is supported by our findings of a significant negative correlation between morphine requirement and age, consistent with the suggested slowing of morphine metabolism in the aged,[18] and a positive (0.55), although not significant correlation, between body weight and morphine requirement. These correlations also support the validity of our morphine measurement as an indicator of patients' physiological need for pain relief. However, we also found a significant negative relationship between mean surgery plasma β-endorphin levels and postoperative morphine requirements. This power of plasma β-endorphin to predict morphine usage suggests that a second, nonpharmacokinetic factor may be involved in differences among patients in postoperative morphine usage.

Using our small study sample, we were not able to demonstrate that the use of both mean surgery β-endorphin level and age could explain more of the variance than either variable alone. However, the almost equally strong predictive power of each of these variables, the increased predictability of morphine requirement with the use of both variables (22%), and the lack of significant correlation between mean surgery levels and age all suggest that the two variables are at least partly independent predictors of a patient's morphine requirements.

The similar, although not quite as strong or significant, negative correlations between plasma cortisol levels and postoperative morphine usage support the possibility that the latter's correlation with plasma β-endorphin may represent a relationship to individual stress or arousal. Stress-induced analgesia is a well-established laboratory phenomenon in animals [19] and in humans.[20] Our negative correlations between stress-induced hormone levels and postoperative morphine requirements support the importance of this mechanism in a clinical setting.

The significant negative relationships between *preoperative* hormone levels and postoperative morphine usage suggest that variability in physical trauma during surgery may not be a major determinant of patient variance in morphine usage. Rather, the patient's physiological arousal prior to surgery, which may be dependent upon innate responsiveness of an arousal system and/or responses to psychological stress, may be the major determinant of postoperative pain and may also predict the degree of physiological response to surgical stress. The latter is supported by the positive correlation between pre- and mean surgery cortisol levels. These studies lend a physiological basis to reports of prediction of postsurgical outcome on the basis of presurgery psychological assessment [21] and to the consistent findings that presurgery psychological intervention may have beneficial effects on the postsurgery course.[22] Classic psychosomatic studies have suggested that psychological adaptation to stress may be reflected in the functioning of the HPA axis, which in turn may be predictive of future behavior.[23, 24] This may well also hold for the endogenous opioid system.

Although endogenous opioids have been implicated in the phenomenon of stress-induced analgesia [20] as well as in other behavioral responses to stress,[25] circulating plasma β-endorphin may not be directly involved in such responses, at least in humans.[26] It is likely, however, that circulating β-endorphin is a marker of central nervous system arousal, which involves endogenous opioid systems, although this marker role may well not be unique to plasma β-endorphin. Thus, patients with low levels of β-endorphin might need larger doses of morphine to activate relatively poorly stress-activated CNS endogenous opioid systems. This last hypothesis is supported by the work of Tamsen et al.,[27] who found in their patients a significant negative relationship between presurgery CSF endogenous opioid levels and calculated postsurgery CSF levels of the self-administered exogenous opiate pethidine.

REFERENCES

1. ANTELMAN, S. & A. CAGGIULA. 1980. *In* Psychobiology of Consciousness. J. Davidson and R. M. Davidson, Eds.: 65–104. Plenum Press. New York.
2. MASON, J. 1975. *In* Emotions: Their Parameters and Measurements. L. Levi, Ed.: 143–167. Raven Press. New York.
3. VERNIKOS-DANELLIS, J. & J. HEYBACH. 1980. *In* Selye's Guide to Stress Research, Vol. 1. H. Selye, Ed.: 206–251. Van Nostrand Reinhold. New York.
4. ROSSIER, J., E. FRENCH, C. RIVIER, N. LING, R. GUILLEMIN & F. BLOOM. 1977. Nature **270:** 618–620.
5. JAFFE, J. H. & W. E. MARTIN. 1975. *In* The Pharmacological Basis of Therapeutics. L. Goodman and A. Gilman, Eds.: 245. Macmillan. New York.
6. BLOOM, F., D. SEGAL, N. LING & R. GUILLEMIN. 1976. Science 194: 630–632.
7. HOLADAY, J. W. & H. H. LOH. 1979. *In* Neurochemical Mechanisms of Opiate Ligands. H. Loh and D. H. Ross, Eds.: 227–257. Raven Press. New York.
8. BESSER, B. M., P. W. BUTLER, J. LANDON & L. REES. 1969. Br. Med. J. **29:** 528–530.
9. CHECKLEY, S. A. 1979. Psychol Med. **9:** 107–116.
10. NURNBERGER, J., E. GERSHON, D. JIMERSON, M. BUCHSBAUM, P. GOLD, G. BROWN & M. EBERT. 1981. *In* Genetic Research Strategies in Psychobiology and Psychiatry. E. Gershon, S. Matthyse, X. Breakefield and R. D. Ciaranello, Eds.: 257–268. Boxwood Press. Pacific Grove, CA.
11. DUBOIS, M., D. PICKAR, M. R. COHEN, Y. ROTH, T. MACNAMARA & W. E. BUNNEY. 1981. Life Sci. **29:** 1249–53.

12. BESSER, G. M., P. W. BUTLER, J. G. RATCLIFFE, L. REES & P. YOUNG. 1970. Br. J. Pharmacol. **39**(1): 196–197.
13. BROWN, W. A., D. P. CORRIVEAU & M. H. EBERT. 1978. Psychopharmacology **58**(2): 189–195.
14. OYAMA, T., K. TANIGUCHI, H. ISHIHARA, A. MATSUKI, A. MAEDA, T. MURAKAWA & T. KUDO. 1979. Br. J. Anaesth. **51**: 141–147.
15. GUILLEMIN, R., T. VARGO, J. ROSSIER, S. MINICK, N. LING, C. RIVIER, W. VALE & F. BLOOM. 1977. Science **197**: 1368–1369.
16. NURNBERGER, J., E. GERSHON, N. SITARAM, J. GILLIN, G. BROWN, M. EBERT, P. GOLD, D. JIMERSON & L. KESSLER. 1981. Psychopharmacol. Bull. **17**: 80–82.
17. DODSON, M., A. HUSSAIN & H. MATHSON. 1977. *In* Pain: New Perspectives in Measurement and Management. A. Harcus, R. Smith and B. Whittle, Eds. Churchill Livingston. New York.
18. STANSKI, D., D. GREENBLATT & E. LOWENSTEIN. 1978. Clin. Pharmacol. Ther. **24**: 52.
19. AKIL, H., D. J. MAYER & J. LIEBESKIND. 1976. Science **191**: 961.
20. WILLER, J., H. DEHEN & J. CAMBIER. 1981. Science **212**: 689.
21. COHEN, F. & R. S. LAZARUS. 1973. Psychosom. Med. **35**: 375–389.
22. SCHLESINGER, H., E. MUMFORD & G. GLASS. 1980. *In* Emotional and Psychological Responses to Anesthesia and Surgery. F. Guerra and J. Aldrete, Eds. Grune and Stratton. New York.
23. WOLFF, C., S. FRIEDMAN, M. HOFER & J. MASON. 1964. Psychosom. Med. **26**: 576.
24. HOFER, M., C. WOLF, S. FRIEDMAN & J. MASON. 1972. Psychosom. Med. **34**: 481.
25. MORLEY, J. & A. LEVINE. 1980. Science **209**: 1259–61.
26. FOLEY, K. M., I. A. KOURIDES, C. E. INTURRISI, R. F. KAIKO, C. G. ZAROULIS, J. B. POSNER, R. W. HOUDE & C. H. LI. 1979. Proc. Natl. Acad. Sci. USA **76**: 5377.
27. TAMSEN, A., P. HARTVIG, B. DAHLSTRÖM, A. WAHLSTRÖM & L. TERENIUS. 1980. Lancet **i**: 769–770.
28. COHEN, M. R., D. PICKAR, M. DUBOIS & W. E. BUNNEY. 1982. Psychiat. Res. **6**: 7–12.

DISCUSSION OF THE PAPER

UNIDENTIFIED SPEAKER: When we compared a variety of methods to measure endorphin in plasma we found that using unextracted plasma (the plasma was stripped of β-endorphin by prior adsorption) that we could not get parallelism with the buffer curve, implying that there was a nonspecific component in plasma which interfered with antigen antibody binding. Could you explain your justification for using unextracted plasma?

M.R. COHEN (NIMH, Bethesda, MD): First, we agree that plasma may well contain components that interfere with antigen-antibody binding in our β-endorphin assay. However for the purposes of these studies, we were content to use an assay procedure that would be capable of showing accurately increases in β-endorphin immunoreactivity (ir). We were not as concerned with measuring absolute plasma β-endorphin (ir) which with the present state of the art of plasma extraction and radioimmunoassay procedures would be a difficult task at best. Thus, comparisons of β-endorphin (ir) prior to and post drug or surgery were always completed using the same 100 μl volume of plasma.

Nonspecific binding in plasma was low enough that samples prior to surgical stress often demonstrated no β-endorphin (ir). Our colleagues have also been able to demonstrate quantitative recovery on the assay of β-endorphin–spiked plasma at the levels assessed in our studies.

UNIDENTIFIED SPEAKER: The dose that you were using, .3 mg/kg is quite a high dose and, actually, higher than that given in most studies in the literature. There may be dose response curve of the behavioral response and endorphin response to the amphetamine. So, maybe, if you were using the usual dosages of amphetamines, something between .1 to .15 mg/kg i.v., the β-endorphin responses might be different, especially when the cortisol responses to amphetamines that are correlated with your β-endorphin responses are dose dependent.

Secondly, I see that you only list some of the studies that were included in the studies previously reported by Elliot Gershon and John Nurnberger concerning the correlation between the prolactin response to amphetamines and behavioral response and mood response to this drug in normal subjects and twin studies; they found some correlation between the baseline levels of prolactin and the prolactin response and the behavioral response. So, I wonder if you were looking at the possible correlation between prolactin and β-endorphins not only with cortisol in these patients.

COHEN: We were only able to study plasma β-endorphin(ir) in a subgroup of the normals whose behavioral and hormonal responses were more extensively studied by John Nurnberger and Elliot Gershon, et al. In this subgroup we were unable to find a correlation between hormonal responses and behavior or between plasma β-endorphin (ir) and stress induced plasma levels of growth hormone or prolactin. The latter finding when considered in the context of the close correlation between stress-induced plasma levels of cortisol and β-endorphin (ir) supports the close-linkage of the hypothalamic-pituitary-axis (HPA) and the endogenous opioid system as well as the specificity of our radioimmunoassay for plasma β-endorphin.

INTRODUCTORY REMARKS

Nathan S. Kline

Rockland Research Institute
Orangeburg, New York 10962

A lot of the interesting observations and sometimes the input to some of the studies arises from clinical treatment of patients. Two years ago I had a patient come into my office, a rather dramatic looking gentleman with long hair and deep set eyes and a rich basso profundo voice, who announced that he was giving me three months to cure him or he was going to commit suicide. In going through his history I noted that my associate, who had just seen him, had failed to put in his occupation. I said, "They must have forgotten to get it." He answered, "No, they asked me twice and I evaded the issue each time." I then said, "Well, what is it that you do?" He replied, "I am a bank robber."

According to his story, he had depression followed by anhedonia, but, so severe that he felt life was not worth living. The only time he could feel anything was when he was at great risk and robbing banks made that possible especially since he could get shot. His motivation for the hold-ups was the fact that they did give him feelings. It is entirely possible that this led to production of β-endorphin. After antidepressant drug treatment he is going to school, has a job and a steady girlfriend so that things are moving along in a good fashion.

Last week I had the duplicate of this patient, a girl in her middle twenties from Pennsylvania, who in the course of a week robbed five department stores. On those nights she was quite excited and was out of her depression. When she was caught, she went back into the depression again.

This raises the question as to whether or not there are a special group of people, some of whom are labeled psychopaths, who suffer from a biological deficit that is manifest by anhedonia. I do not know that any such individuals have been examined for β-endorphin levels. It is a provocative group to look at since one characteristic of many of the psychopaths is that the main deficit seems to be a failure to learn, i.e. a failure of reward and punishment, which could well be related to a neuroendocrine disorder.

Another difficulty arises because in bi-polar depressives we are measuring a condition that tends to be self-limited. It almost looks as if both the depressive and manic phase create endogenous biological antidotes for themselves. Measurement is also complicated because in the use of antidepressant medications, very often the difference between success or failure (in a 2- or 3-week trial) depends on whether the patient is on his or her way *into* a depression or on the *way out*. Some of the difficulties that arise from measuring serum levels, whether of β-endorphin or other biochemical or endocrine levels, is that the depression is not static and seems to be a self-correcting kind of a disorder that varies very much from one time to another.

CLINICAL PHARMACOLOGY OF β-ENDORPHIN IN DEPRESSION AND SCHIZOPHRENIA *

Don H. Catlin,†, ‡ David A. Gorelick,§, ¶ and Robert H. Gerner §

† *Department of Medicine*
‡ *Department of Pharmacology*
§ *Department of Psychiatry*
UCLA Center for the Health Sciences
Los Angeles, California 90024
¶ *Brentwood Veterans Administration Medical Center*
Los Angeles, California 90073

The history of clinical studies with β-endorphin (β-EP) differs in sequence from that of most drugs. Clinical trials of drugs usually begin with studies on the metabolism, biological activity and toxicity in normal volunteers (FDA phase I), then proceed to efficacy studies in diseased subjects (phase II). This has not been the sequence with β-ep in part because of uncertainty in identifying the appropriate diseased population.

This paper reviews the results of our work on the clinical pharmacology of β-EP in depression and schizophrenia. We have focused not only on the efficacy of β-EP in these disease states, but also on other aspects of its clinical pharmacology, for example dosage form, pharmacokinetics, pharmacodynamics, and physiological effects. Because of the unusual history of clinical trials with β-EP, these variables have never been studied in normal subjects. We believe they should not be neglected, because knowledge of the clinical pharmacology of a drug is important in designing valid efficacy studies.

EXPERIMENTAL METHODS

Subjects

We administered β-EP to 18 psychiatric in-patients with diagnoses of schizophrenia (n = 8) or depression (7 unipolar, 2 bipolar, 1 schizoaffective) according to DSM-III.[1] Subject characteristics have been described in detail elsewhere.[2] In addition, 9 normal subjects and 37 psychiatric in-patients (19 unipolar depressed, 8 bipolar depressed, 10 schizophrenic) had lumbar puncture performed for measurement of cerebrospinal fluid (CSF) endorphin levels. All subjects were free of neuroleptic or antidepressant medication for at least 4 days prior to study.

Experimental Design

A double-blind, placebo-controlled, cross-over design was used, with the cross-over interval between experimental sessions ranging from 1 to 8 days. Each session was divided into three consecutive 30-minute periods: A (t = —30

* Research for this paper was supported in part by United States Public Health Service Grants D–01006 (D.H.C.) and RR–05756 (R.H.G.).

434

to 0 min), B (t = 0 to 30 min), and C (t = 30 to 60 min). Saline was always infused during the first (A) and third (B) periods. For the β-EP experimental session, synthetic human β-EP [3] was infused (zero order) during period B. For the placebo experimental session saline was infused during period B. The scheduled dose of β-EP was 10 mg but 6 subjects received less (minimum 3.4 mg) because of technical problems or side-effects. Details of the experimental procedure have been presented.[2]

Dependent Variables

Behavioral data were measured along three time scales: acute-patient self-ratings during the 90-minute infusion session, subacute-psychiatrist's psychopathology rating made 1–2 hours before and 2–4 hours after each infusion session, and chronic–daily nurses' ratings on the Brief Psychiatric Rating Scale (BPRS).[2] The psychiatrist's rating was the sum of 8 items on a modified Bunney-Hamburg scale.[4] The BPRS was analyzed in terms of total score, as well as the separate sums of three depression items (anxiety, depressive mood, helplessness-hopelessness) and three psychosis items (conceptual disorganization, hallucinations, unusual thought content).

Physiological variables were measured as previously described.[5] Plasma prolactin, growth hormone, cortisol and β-EP like immunoreactivity (β-EP-LI) were measured by RIA as previously described.[6, 7] CSF β-EP-LI was measured by RIA [8] on samples collected by lumbar puncture at 0800 after overnight fast and bed rest. The collection tubes were at 0°C., and contained bacitracin. The tubes were stored at −80°C. Three depressed subjects had lumbar puncture performed within 24 hours of receiving β-EP.

Data Analysis

Data from β-EP administration were analyzed in terms of difference scores from pre-β-EP (or placebo) infusion baseline, calculated as the mean of measurements made during and/or before the first saline infusion period. (There were no significant differences between β-EP and placebo infusion baselines for any dependent variable, by paired t-tests). Each variable was analyzed separately using a repeated measures statistical test to compare β-EP and placebo effects: Wilcoxon test for behavioral variables, analysis of variance for physiological variables, and t-tests on area under the time vs. hormone level curve for hormone variables. Comparisons of CSF β-EP-LI levels among subject groups were made by independent t-tests. All probability levels are two-tailed. Unless otherwise specified, sample size is 18.

RESULTS AND DISCUSSION

Pharmacokinetics

The 30-minute zero-order infusion produced rapidly increasing plasma concentrations of β-EP-LI (FIG. 1). At the end of the infusion the mean (n = 5) plasma concentration was 562 ng/ml (range 320–830 ng/ml). Since the endogenous plasma concentration of β-EP-LI (in normal subjects) is less

than 50 pg/ml [9-11] it is readily apparent that the infusion resulted in pharmacological amounts of β-EP entering the central circulation.

There was a biphasic decline in plasma β-EP-LI at the end of infusion
(FIG. 1). The plasma disappearance curves of β-EP-LI following IV bolus
administration of β-EP to rats,[12] rabbits,[12, 13] and man [14, 15] are also curvi-
linear when plotted on logarithmic (concentration) vs. arithmetic (time) coordinates. These data suggest that the pharmacokinetics of intravenously

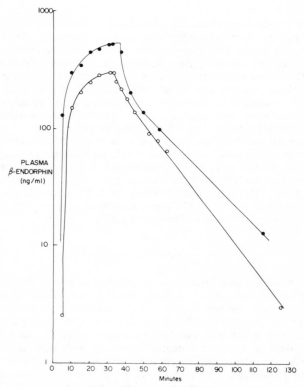

FIGURE 1. Concentration of β-EP-LI in plasma of 2 depressed subjects during
and after a zero-order infusion of 10 mg of β-EP. (Adapted from Catlin et al.[57]
Reproduced by permission of Raven Press.)

administered β-EP conforms to a two (or more) compartment model (cf.
refs. 16 and 17). We fitted the post-infusion plasma concentration data from
five subjects to a two compartment model using a non-linear least squares
regression procedure programmed on a desk top calculator. The mean values
of the elimination rate constants were: α (rate constant of the α
phase) $= 0.35^{-1}$; and β (rate constant of the β phase) $= 0.051^{-1}$. These correspond to an apparent half-life of 2 minutes for the distribution phase ($T\frac{1}{2}_\alpha$)

and of 14 minutes for the elimination phase (T½ β). These values are quite short but similar to the half-lives of other hormonal peptides.[18]

The validity of the estimate of pharmacokinetic parameters depends on the accuracy of the analytical technique. The magnitude of the plasma concentrations of β-EP-LI established by the infusion essentially precludes interference by endogenous substances such as β-LPH or endorphins. However, the metabolism of β-EP in man is not known and it is possible that the plasma β-EP-LI reflects metabolites, particularly in the later phases of the post-infusion disappearance curve. Errors of this type would result in over-estimations of T½ and T½ β.

A zero-order infusion of β-EP has several pharmacokinetic and experimental advantages compared to the rapid IV infusion (bolus) technique. It is desirable to study the effects of a drug when plasma and tissue levels are constant (steady state) because drug effects are likely to be constant at this time, or, if they are not constant, the changes cannot be attributed to time or to changing tissue levels of drug. Bolus administration of a drug cannot produce a steady state. If a drug conforms to first order kinetics [16] and there is no evidence to the contrary for β-EP) the concentration of drug in plasma (C_p) resulting from a zero order infusion is:

$$C_p = \frac{\text{rate of administration}}{\text{clearance}}(1 - e^{-kt})$$

where k is the elimination rate constant and t is the duration of infusion. Since $k = \dfrac{0.693}{T½}$ the shorter the T½ (or T½ β) of a drug, the more rapidly the steady state will be approached. As shown in FIGURE 1 and discussed elsewhere [17] the 30-minute infusion of β-EP nearly achieved the steady state levels of β-EP-LI in plasma. Support for these pharmacokinetic concepts includes the finding that an infusion of ACTH in man can produce greater and more prolonged responses than the bolus technique,[19] and the data of Rapoport *et al.*[20] indicating that brain concentrations of some endorphins will rapidly reach a new steady state after an increase in plasma levels.

Experimental advantages of the infusion technique include the ability to interrupt before the complete dose has been administered in case of toxicity, and the avoidance of side-effects that might be associated with the higher peak levels produced by bolus administration. Such side-effects can lead to breaking of the double-blind design. Only 8 of our 18 subjects reported somatic side-effects (abdominal discomfort, hunger, paraesthesias, dry mouth) during β-EP infusion (4 during placebo infusion). None showed any awareness of the order of drug administration, so that the raters remained blinded to drug condition. In contrast, Pickar, *et al.*[21] found that all 10 of their subjects given β-EP by rayid IV infusion over 5 minutes experienced somatic side-effects, and raters were consistently able to break the drug blind.

Cardiovascular Effects

β-EP produced a biphasic effect on heart rate (HR) and decreased systolic blood pressure (BP) (FIG. 2) but had no effect on diastolic BP (n's = 14). During the first 10 minutes of the infusion HR increased, and then declined

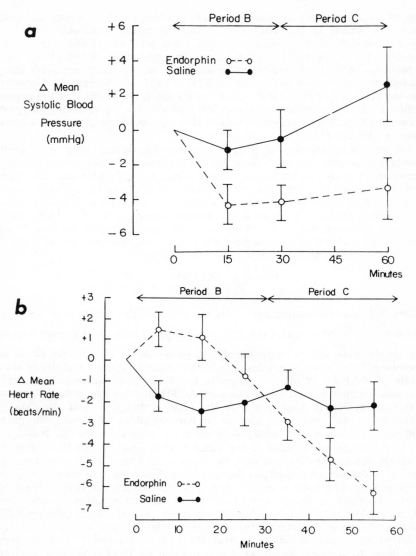

FIGURE 2. Effects of β-EP (○– –○) and placebo (●——●) infusion from t = 0 − 30 min on (a) mean systolic BP difference scores at t = 15,30 and 60 min (p < 0.05), and (b) mean HR difference scores plotted at the mid-point of successive 10-min epochs (p < 0.01). Points are the mean ± SEM for the 14 subjects.

during (t = 10–30 min) and after (t = 30–60 min) the infusion. The mean systolic BP decreased during the infusion and remained lower than the placebo at t = 30 and 60 minutes. By t = 90 minutes there was no difference between the β-EP and placebo infusion.

These effects are similar to the cardiovascular effects of morphine reported in some human studies.[22, 23] Other investigators have not reported any significant cardiovascular effects of β-EP in man,[14, 15, 24] possibly because the studies were not specifically designed to detect physiological changes. Our results are consistent with animal studies showing that IV or intracisternal β-EP decreases blood pressure and heart rate in the rat [25, 26] and cat [27, 28] and produces biphasic heart rate changes (initial increase) in the dog.[29] These effects are presumably mediated by opiate receptors, since they are blocked or reversed by the opiate antagonist naloxone.[25, 26, 29] Other types of experiments also suggest that endorphins may play a role in regulating blood pressure. For example, naloxone increases BP in animal models of shock [30] and the antihypertensive effect of clonidine in spontaneously hypertensive rats is reversed by naloxone.[31]

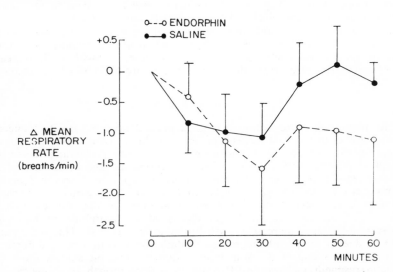

FIGURE 3. Effects of β-EP (O---O) and placebo (●—●) infusion from t = 0 — 30 min on mean respiratory rate difference scores plotted at the mid-point of successive 10-min epochs. Points are the mean ± SEM.

Other Physiological Effects

A prominent characteristic of morphine is the production of respiratory depression. Clinically this is principally manifested by a decrease in tidal volume; respiratory rate also decreases but is a less sensitive measure of respiratory depression. In a subset of nine subjects we assessed the effect of β-EP on respiratory rate by recording each respiratory excursion with a thermistor positioned in the nasal air stream. The mean respiratory rate decreased during and after the β-EP infusion (FIG. 3), but the change was not significantly different from the placebo (p = 0.10).

There is one report that IV β-EP produced a 15 percent decrease in the respiratory rate of withdrawing heroin addicts.[32] Other clinical investigators have not presented data on respiratory effects of β-EP, although some mentioned that vital signs were unchanged.[14, 15, 24] The carbon dioxide rebreathing technique is the most definitive and commonly used method of investigating the respiratory depressant effect of opioids in man. This technique has not been used to assess the effect of β-EP in man, but it was used to show that intracisternally administered β-EP produces marked respiratory depression in dogs.[33]

Another prominent effect on morphine in man in pupillary constriction. We assessed the effect of β-EP on the pupil by visually estimating the diameter of the pupil using a chart of standards. In a subset of 6 psychiatric patients, we found no effect of β-EP or placebo on pupil diameter. In other studies, we have administered up to 30 mg of β-EP IV to patients withdrawing from methadone,[5] and have not observed pupillary constriction. In contrast, one patient reported by Foley et al.[15] demonstrated pupil constriction lasting several hours after receiving 7.5 mg of β-EP intraventricularly.

We found that β-EP also produced a small decrease in oral temperature (n = 7) (p = 0.04). Morphine also decreases temperature slightly in man, but in other species the effects of morphine are complex, with both increases and decreases reported. β-EP decreased temperature in some animal studies.[34]

Hormone Effects

Hormone levels were measured in six depressed subjects.[7] β-EP produced a significant two- to fourfold increase in serum prolactin (p < 0.01), but did not increase cortisol or growth hormone (p's > 0.1). The prolactin increase was present 15 minutes after the start of β-EP infusion, peaked at the end of the infusion (35–40 ng/ml vs. 10 ng/ml during placebo), and was still present 90 minutes after the end of the infusion (FIG. 4). This pattern of hormone responses is consistent with that reported in other human studies with IV β-EP [14, 15, 21] and is also similar to effects of IV morphine in humans.[35] However, β-EP does increase growth hormone in rats.[36, 37] This discrepancy could be due to the peripheral route of administration, to species differences, or to use of insufficient doses in human studies. The rat studies show that prolactin responds to lower β-EP doses than does growth hormone.[36, 37]

Behavioral Effects

β-EP had no significant effect on patient self-ratings during the infusion period (acute time scale), or on the daily nurses' rating on the BPRS (chronic time scale), but did significantly change physicians overall ratings made before and after the infusion sessions (subacute time scale).[2] The depressed subjects improved significantly after β-EP (mean change of +5 scale points) compared with placebo (mean change of +2 scale points (p = 0.05). All 10 depressed subjects improved after β-EP, while only 4 improved after placebo (FIG. 5). No subject had a hypomanic response or rebound increase in depression. Schizophrenic subjects showed a tendency to worsen after β-EP (mean change of −3 scale points) compared with placebo (mean change of +½ scale point) (p = 0.07). Six schizophrenics worsened after β-EP whereas only one did after placebo (p = 0.025 by Fisher's Exact Test). No subject showed catalepsy or other motor abnormalities.

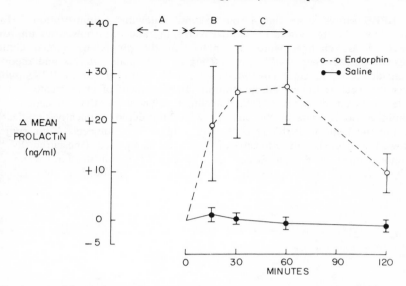

FIGURE 4. Mean change in serum prolactin in 6 depressed subjects receiving 4.3–10 mg/70 kg of β-EP. Each data point is the mean (± SEM) change in serum prolactin compared to the baseline. β-EP was infused at a constant rate between 0 and 30 minutes (O–––O). Corresponding control infusion of saline is indicated by (●—●). (Adapted from Catlin *et al.*[57] Reproduced by permission of Raven Press.)

Our results are not completely consistent with others reported in the literature. Two studies gave β-EP intravenously over 5 minutes to medication-free depressed women. Angst *et al.*[38] gave 10 mg in a non-placebo-controlled design and reported improvement on subjects' self-ratings and physicians' global rating over the period ½–4 hours after administration (no statistical analysis done). Three subjects (two of them bipolar) became hypomanic or manic. Pickar *et al.*[21] gave 4-10 mg in a double-blind, placebo-controlled design and found no significant changes in BPRS scores or physicians' global clinical observations over the 4-hour period following administration.

Our results in depressed subjects, together with those of Angst *et al.*[38] are consistent with the hypothesis that mania is related to excess endorphin activity,[39, 40] and depression to deficient endorphin activity.[40] There is at present, little other direct experimental evidence for this hypothesis. In a woman with rapidly cycling bipolar affective disorder, higher levels of plasm β-EP like radioreceptor activity (BELRA) were found during manic than during depressed episodes, as well as a high inverse correlation ($r = -0.98$) between nurses' rating of depression and BELRA.[41] In 12 patients with manic bipolar affective disorder given naloxone 20 mg by 20-minute IV infusion using a double-blind, placebo-controlled cross-over design, naloxone caused a significant decrease in manic symptoms in 4 of the 12 subjects.[40]

Three studies gave β-EP by IV bolus or rapid infusion (5 min) to 20 medication-free schizophrenic subjects using a double-blind design. Pickar *et al.*[21] gave 10–15 mg to six subjects and found no significant group changes

in BPRS scores over the 4-hour period following administration. However, two subjects showed substantial worsening and one showed an improvement. These changes were also noted on the physicians' global clinical
observations. Berger et al.[14] gave 20 mg to eight male subjects and reported
"statistically significant" (by one-tailed t-test) improvement in BPRS scores
over the week following administration. Improvement of even greater magnitude occurred during the saline acclimatization week that preceded drug
administration. None of the changes were considered "clinically significant."
In the third study, Pethö et al.[42] gave 4 mg to six subjects. Four subjects
showed a decrease in intensity of psychotic symptoms (measured by the
Factor Construct Rating Scale) on the day of administration, while one
subject showed an increase and one no change. In addition, four subjects

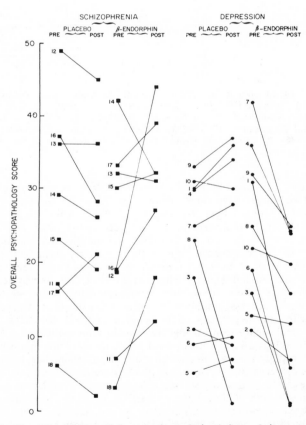

FIGURE 5. Overall psychopathology ratings derived from 8 items on a modified
Bunney-Hamburg scale. Ratings were made 1 hour before and 2 to 4 hours after
β-EP or saline (placebo) infusion in 8 schizophrenic and 10 depressed subjects.
Numbers refer to subject identification numbers given in reference 2. (From
Gerner et al.[2] Reproduced by permission of Archives of General Psychiatry.)

showed a decrease in anxiety or dysphoria. By the fourth day, five subjects had an increase in psychotic symptoms or anxiety.

These results, coupled with our own findings, do not suggest a therapeutic role for β-EP in the treatment of schizophrenia. In fact, there is evidence from our study and several subjects in other studies that β-EP might worsen schizophrenic symptoms. This would be consistent with the general hypothesis that endorphins are implicated in the pathogenesis of schizophrenia.[43]

Such a hypothesis was suggested by early reports that opiate receptor blockade reduced schizophrenic symptoms [43, 44] and that hemodialysis improved schizophrenia by reducing levels of an abnormal endorphin.[45] However, this hypothesis is still extremely speculative, since later studies have failed to confirm improvement in schizophrenia with opiate antagonist treatment [46, 47] or hemodialysis [48] or to detect abnormal β-EP in the blood or dialysate of schizophrenics.[49]

CSF *Endorphin Levels*

CSF β-EP-LI was increased two- to fivefold over baseline levels in the three depressed subjects who were studied after β-EP infusion. The highest level (550 pg/ml) was found in the subject sampled 2 hours after receiving β-EP (187 μg/kg). A level of 470 pg/ml was found in a subject 4 hours after receiving 105 μg/kg and 280 pg/ml in the third subject 17 hours after 125 μg/kg. β-EP-LI was inversely correlated with the β-EP infusion-lumbar puncture interval. There are several possible mechanisms which could explain the increased levels of CSF β-EP-LI. Among these are transport of β-EP or metabolites of β-EP from the blood into the CSF and secretion or release of an immunoreactive endorphin from the CNS into the CSF. Increased CSF β-EP-LI was measured in one subject 17 hours after β-EP administration. This is consistent with a report that in a cancer patient given 7.5 mg of β-EP intracerebroventricularly, the half life of β-EP-LI in CSF was 93 minutes and β-EP-LI could be detected by RIA 21 hours later.[15]

The 9 normal subjects had a mean ($\pm$ SEM) CSF β-EP-LI level of 100 ± 8 pg/ml. This is within the range of CSF β-EP-LI levels in normal subjects reported in two previous studies,[50, 51] but at least fivefold higher than levels reported in two other studies.[52, 53] Some of these discrepancies may be related to differences in sample preparation and storage, and to different specificities and sensitivities of the RIAs used. We found no group mean differences in β-EP-LI levels among the normal, depressed (97 ± 6 pg/ml), and schizophrenic subjects (108 ± 6 pg/ml), nor were there any significant correlations between levels and psychiatric ratings. These findings are consistent with a previous report of no differences in β-EP immunoreactivity among normal, depressed, manic, and schizophrenic subjects.[54]

However, there is one report of a 10-fold higher mean ($\pm$ SEM) β-EP-LI in five acute schizophrenic subjects (2467 ± 1248 pg/ml) compared with seven control subjects (245 ± 24 pg/ml).[55] Terenius *et al.*[56] have reported increased CSF levels of opioid-receptor-active material (Fraction I) in schizophrenics, with levels decreasing to normal when the patients improve clinically.

Summary and Conclusions

We administered synthetic human β-EP by constant rate IV infusion to 10 depressed and 8 schizophrenic psychiatric inpatients according to a double-blind placebo-controlled, cross-over design. Plasma sampling in five subjects showed that significant amounts of β-EP-LI entered the body (mean peak plasma level 562 pg/ml at the end of infusion), with the following apparent plasma half-lives according to a two-compartment pharmacokinetic model: distribution half-life $\approx$ 2 minutes, elimination half-life $\approx$ 14 minutes. Furthermore, in three subjects undergoing lumbar puncture, CSF β-EP-LI levels were elevated two- to fivefold up to 17 hours after β-EP administration. The mean baseline CSF β-EP-LI level was 100 pg/ml in 9 normal subjects, and did not differ significantly in the depressed or schizophrenic subjects.

β-EP produced significant physiological and hormonal effects, including decreased systolic and mean arterial blood pressures and oral temperature, biphasic changes in heart rate and increased serum prolactin levels. There were no significant changes in diastolic blood pressure, respiratory rate, pupil diameter, or serum cortisol and growth hormone levels. β-EP produced significant behavioral effects on the day of infusion. Depressed subjects got significantly better on the infusion day, but not on subsequent days. Schizophrenic subjects did not improve. There were no significant behavioral effects during the infusions themselves, or on subsequent days.

The effects summarized above may be mediated either at CNS sites, or at peripheral sites. The pattern of effects produced by β-EP was similar to, but not identical with, effects expected from an opium alkaloid such as morphine. For example, the cardiovascular and hormonal effects of morphine and β-EP are similar but two prominent effects of morphine, respiratory depression and pupillary constriction, were not observed.

Our work demonstrates that peripherally administered β-EP is pharmacologically active. It supports the general hypothesis that endorphin systems play a role in the regulation of physiological and behavioral processes. In viewing β-EPs potential as a therapeutic agent, three points must be considered: (1) there is a need to conduct Phase I trials in normal subjects; (2) β-EP is still in a very early stage of pharmaceutical development; and (3) analogues that are active by the oral route of administration need to be developed.

Acknowledgments

We thank Dr. C. H. Li for synthetic human β-EP; Drs. R. T. Rubin and R. E. Poland for the prolactin, growth hormone and cortisol assays; Dr. B. Sharp for the CSF β-EP assay; C. Kane and P. Stern for technical assistance; and the staff of ward 2-South.

References

1. Diagnostic and Statistical Manual of Mental Disorders. 1980. Third Edition. American Psychiatric Association. Washington, D.C.
2. Gerner, R. H., D. H. Catlin, D. A. Gorelick, K. K. Hui & C. H. Li. 1980. Arch. Gen. Psychiatry 37: 642–647.

3. LI, C. H., O. YAMASHIRO, L. F. TSENG, *et al.* 1977. J. Med. Chem. **20:** 325–328.
4. BUNNEY, W. E. & D. A. HAMBURG. 1963. Arch. Gen. Psychiatry **9:** 280–294.
5. CATLIN, D. H., K. K. HUI, H. H. LOH & C. H. LI. 1977. Commun. Psychopharmacol. **5:** 493–500.
6. GORELICK, D. A., D. H. CATLIN & R. H. GERNER. 1981. β-Endorphin studies in psychiatric patients. *In* Modern Problems in Pharmacopsychiatry. The Role of Endorphins and Neuropsychiatry. H. Emrich, Ed. Karger. Basel, Switzerland. In press.
7. CATLIN, D. H., R. E. POLAND, D. A. GORELICK, R. H. GERNER, K. K. HUI, R. T. RUBIN & C. H. LI. 1980. J. Clin. Endocrinol. Metab. **50:** 1021–1025.
8. SHARP, B. & A. E. PEKARY. 1981. J. Clin. Endocrinol. Metab. **52:** 586–588.
9. NAKAO, K., Y. NAKAI, S. OKI, K. HORII & H. IMURA. 1978. J. Clin. Invest. **62:** 1395–1398.
10. WARDLAW, S. L. & A. G. FRANTZ. 1979. J. Clin. Endocrinol. Metab. **48:** 176–180.
11. ROSS, M., P. A. BERGER & A. GOLDSTEIN. 1979. Science **205:** 1163–1164.
12. HOUGHTEN, R. A., R. W. SWANN & C. H. LI. 1980. Proc. Natl. Acad. Sci. USA **77:** 4588–4591.
13. MERIN, M., V. HOLLT, R. PRZEWLOCKI & A. HERZ. 1980. Life Sci. **27:** 281–289.
14. BERGER, P. A., S. J. WATSON, H. AKIL, G. E. ELLIOTT, R. T. RUBIN, A. PFEFFERBAUM, K. L. DAVIS, J. D. BARACHAS & C. H. LI. 1980. Arch. Gen. Psychiatry **37:** 635–640.
15. FOLEY, K. M., I. A. KOURIDES, C. E. INTURRISI, R. F. KAIKO, C. G. ZAROULIS, J. B. POSNER, R. W. HOUDE & C. H. LI. 1979. Proc. Natl. Acad. Sci. USA **76:** 5377–5381.
16. GIBALDI, M. & D. PERRIER. 1975. *In* Pharmacokinetics. J. Swarbrick, Ed. Vol. 1. Marcel Dekker, Inc. New York.
17. CATLIN, D. H., D. A. GORELICK & R. H. GERNER. 1981. Studies of β-Endorphin in patients with pain and drug addiction. *In* Hormonal Proteins and Peptides. C. H. Li, Ed. Vol. 10: 311–338. Academic Press. New York.
18. MAKHLOUF, G. 1973. Gastroenterology **65:** 170–173.
19. RENOLD, A. E., P. H. FORSHAM, J. MAISTERRENA & G. W. THORN. 1951. N. Engl. J. Med. **244:** 796–798.
20. RAPOPORT, S. I., W. A. KLEE, K. D. PETTIGREW & K. OHNO. 1980. Science **207:** 84–86.
21. PICKAR, D., G. C. DAVIS, S. C. SCHULTZ, I. EXTEIN, R. WAGNER, D. NABER, *et al.* 1981. Am. J. Psychiatry **138:** 160–166.
22. THOMAS, M., R. MALMCRONA, S. FILLMORE & J. SHILLINGFORD. 1965. Br. Heart J. **27:** 863–875.
23. SAMUEL, I. O., R. S. J. CLARKE & J. W. DUNDEE. 1977. Br. J. Anaesth. **49:** 927–933.
24. HOSOBUCHI, Y. & C. H. LI. 1978. Commun. Psychopharmacol. **2:** 33–37.
25. LEMAIRE, I., R. TSENG & S. LEMAIRE. 1978. Proc. Natl. Acad. Sci. USA **75:** 6240–6242.
26. WEI, E. T., A. LEE & J. K. CHANG. 1980. Life Sci. **26:** 1517–1522.
27. FELDBERG, W. & E. T. WEI. 1978. J. Physiol. **280:** 18.
28. BOLME, P., K. FUXE, L. AGNATI, R. BRADLEY & J. SMYTHIES. 1978. Eur. J. Pharmacol. **48:** 319–324.
29. LAUBIE, M., H. SCHMITT, M. VINCENT & G. REMOND. 1977. Eur. J. Pharmacol. **46:** 67–71.
30. FADEN, A. I. & J. W. HOLADAY. 1979. Science **205:** 317–318.
31. FARSANG, C. & G. KUNOS. 1979. Br. J. Pharmacol. **67:** 161–164.
32. SU, C.-Y., S.-H. LIN, Y.-T. WANG, C. H. LI, L. H. HUNG, C. S. LIN & B. C. LIN. 1978. J. Formosan Med. Assoc. **77:** 133–142.

33. Moss, I. R. & E. Friedman. 1978. Life Sci. **23:** 1271–1276.
34. Nemeroff, C. B., A. J. Osbahr, P. F. Manberg, G. N. Ervin & A. J. Prange. 1979. Proc. Natl. Acad. Sci. USA **76:** 5368–5371.
35. Tolis, G., J. Hickey & H. Guyda. 1975. J. Clin. Endocrinol. Metab. **41:** 797.
36. Dupont, A., L. Cusan, F. Labrie, D. H. Coy & C. H. Li. 1977. Biochem. Biophys. Res. Commun. **75:** 76.
37. Chihara, K., A. Arimura, D. H. Coy & V. Schally. 1978. Endocrinology **102:** 281.
38. Angst, J., V. Autenrieth, F. Brem, et al. 1979. Preliminary results of treatment with β-endorphin in depression. In Endorphins in Mental Health Research. E. Usdin, W. E. Bunney & N. S. Kline, Eds.: 518–528. Oxford University Press. New York.
39. Byck, R. 1976. Lancet **2:** 72–73.
40. Judd, L. L., D. S. Janowsky, D. S. Segal & L. Y. Huey. 1980. Arch. Gen. Psychiatry **37:** 583–586.
41. Pickar, D., N. R. Cutler, D. Naber, R. M. Post, C. B. Pert & W. E. Bunney, Jr. 1980. Lancet **1:** 937.
42. Pethö, B., L. Gráf, I. Karczag, I. Bitter, J. Tolna, K. Baraczka & C. H. Li. 1981. Lancet **1:** 212–213.
43. Gunne, L.-M., L. Lindstrom & L. Terenius. 1977. J. Neural Transm. **40:** 13–19.
44. Watson, S. J., P. A. Berger, H. Akil, M. J. Mills & J. D. Barchas. 1978. Science **201:** 73–76.
45. Palmour, R. M., F. R. Ervin, H. Wagemaker, et al. 1979. Characterization of a peptide from the serum of psychiatric patients. In Endorphins in Mental Health Research. E. Usdin, W. E. Bunney & N. S. Kline, Eds.: 581–593. Oxford University Press. New York.
46. Volavka, J., A. Mallya, S. Baig & J. Perez-Cruet. 1977. Science **196:** 1227–1228.
47. Gitlin, M. J., R. H. Gerner & M. Rosenblatt. 1981. Psychopharmacology **74:** 51–53.
48. Kroll, P. D., F. K. Port & K. R. Silk. 1978. J. Nerv. Ment. Dis. **166:** 291–293.
49. Ross, M., P. A. Berger & A. Goldstein. 1979. Science **205:** 1163–1164.
50. Jeffcoate, W. J., L. McLoughlin, H. Hope, L. H. Rees, S. J. Ratter, P. J. Lowry & G. M. Besser. 1978. Lancet **2:** 119–121.
51. Clement-Jones, V., L. McLoughlin, S. Tomlin, G. M. Besser, L. H. Rees & H. L. Wen. 1980. Lancet **2:** 946–949.
52. Nakao, K., S. Oki, I. Tanaka, K. Horri, Y. Nakai, et al. 1980. J. Clin. Invest. **66:** 1383–1390.
53. Wilkes, M. M., R. D. Stewart, J. F. Bruni, M. E. Quigley, C. S. S. Yen, N. Ling & M. Chretien. 1980. J. Clin. Endocrinol. Metab. **50:** 309–315.
54. Naber, D., D. Pickar, R. M. Post, D. P. van Kammen, R. N. Walters, et al. 1981. Am. J. Psychiatry **138:** 1457–1461.
55. Domschke, W., A. Dickschas & P. Mitznegg. 1979. Lancet **1:** 1024.
56. Terenius, L., A. Wahlström, L. Lindström & E. Widerlöv. 1976. Neurosci. Lett. **3:** 157–162.
57. Catlin, D. H., D. A. Gorelick, R. H. Gerner, K. K. Hui & C. H. Li. 1980. Clinical Studies with Human β-Endorphin. In Polypeptide Hormones. Twelfth Miles International Symposium. R. F. Beers & E. G. Bassett, Eds. No. 12: 337–347. Raven Press. New York.

DISCUSSION OF THE PAPER

COMMENT: I would like to compliment you on your very careful work Dr. Catlin on the measurement of cardiovascular parameters. It would be interesting to find out what happens to catecholamines and, of course, serotonin. I am sure the displacement of biogenic amines is likely to happen and looking at the blood pressure curves and increase in heart rate one is bound to think of possible histamine release by endorphins when the infusion is at a slow rate.

STUDIES OF β-ENDORPHIN IN
PSYCHIATRIC PATIENTS *

Philip A. Berger and Jack D. Barchas

Department of Psychiatry and Behavioral Sciences
Stanford University School of Medicine
Stanford, California 94305

INTRODUCTION TO STUDIES ON ENDORPHINS AND PSYCHOPATHOLOGY

A massive research effort is being made to investigate the role of endorphins in normal and abnormal physiology. Part of this research is focused on the possible role of endorphins in psychopathology. There is controversial evidence for both an excess and a deficiency of endorphin activity in mental illness.

Several types of evidence support the hypothesis that schizophrenia reflects a deficiency of endorphins. Positive reports of the effects of exogenous opiates on schizophrenic symptoms have appeared in the psychiatric literature of the last 130 years; however, none of these reports is based on double-blind study designs.[1] A synthetic analog of enkephalin (ENK), FK 33–824, has been reported to decrease psychotic symptoms in schizophrenic patients. In one uncontrolled pilot study, nine patients received 0.5 mg and 1 mg FK 33–824 for two days.[2] The investigators reported a significant lessening in symptoms in this group, lasting from 1 to 7 days. In a single-blind study, researchers reported that FK 33–824 had a strikingly positive effect on the hallucinations of nine chronic psychotic patients.[3]

Des-tyrosine ¹-γ-endorphin (DTγE) (β-LPH 62–77) is structurally related to endorphins, but is devoid of opiate activity. Burbach and de Wied have reported finding evidence of DTγE in rat pituitary, rat brain, and human spinal fluid.[4] Incubation of β-endorphin (β-END) with homogenates of rat forebrain yielded DTγE, suggesting that it is an endogenously formed compound.[4] A decrease in schizophrenic symptoms was reported in a single-blind study with six patients and in a double-blind study of eight patients following the administration of DTγE.[5] However, a study by Emrich and colleagues reported only slight differences between placebo and DTγE.[6]

Recently, the group from the Netherlands reported that a new compound, des-ENK-γ-endorphin (DEγE; β-LPH 66–77), has behavioral effects in animals similar to those of DTγE, suggesting that this compound might also have antipsychotic activity. DEγE may be formed from DTγE in mammalian brain. Preliminary clinical results suggest that DEγE may also reduce schizophrenic symptoms in a subgroup of schizophrenic patients. In this preliminary report, the antipsychotic effects of DEγE were similar to those of DTγE.[7]

The stiffness that occurs after intraventricular β-END injections in rats has been compared to the catalepsy produced by neuroleptics in these animals.

* This research was supported by the Medical Research Service of the Veterans Administration, by Grant MH 30854 for the NIMH Specialized Research Center, by Grants MH 23861, MH 29491, and MH 30245 from the National Institute of Mental Health, and by Grant DA 02265 from the National Institute on Drug Abuse.

Although not all investigators agree,[8] this suggests that β-END is an endogenous neuroleptic and that schizophrenic symptoms might reflect an endorphin deficiency.[9] Furthermore, in the single-blind study of Kline and Lehmann,[10] three of four schizophrenic patients were reported to benefit from 15 intravenous doses of 1.5 to 9 mg of β-END.

In contrast to those studies suggesting an endorphin deficiency in schizophrenia, several current studies indicate an *increase* in endorphin activity in schizophrenia. In the double-blind crossover study by Gerner *et al.*, the condition of six of eight schizophrenic subjects worsened after β-END treatment, when compared with results of placebo trials.[11] In a second double-blind study, six schizophrenic subjects received β-END 4 to 15 mg intravenously. While there were no statistically significant changes in these six patients, there was a tendency for the schizophrenic patients to worsen after β-END administration.[12]

According to Wahlström *et al.*,[13, 14] endorphin fractions other than β-END and ENK are elevated in the cerebrospinal fluid (CSF) of unmedicated schizophrenic patients. When these patients were medicated, the increased levels returned toward normal. There are also reports of elevated CSF concentrations of β-END in some schizophrenic patients. One group reported that normal subjects had values of 72 fmol/ml, neurologic control subjects had 92 fmol/ml, and chronic schizophrenic patients had 35 fmol/ml, while acute schizophrenics had 760 fmol/ml β-END.[15]

The reported decrease in schizophrenic symptoms after hemodialysis is further evidence that suggests an endorphin excess in schizophrenia. Wagemaker and Cade [16] and Palmour *et al.*[17] have proposed that the patients' improvement results from the removal of leucine⁵-β-END (leu⁵-β-END). Unfortunately, the hemodialysis trial was not double-blind, and there has been no confirmation of elevated leu⁵-β-END concentrations in either the dialysate or the plasma of schizophrenic patients.[18, 19] The observations reported in the study by Bloom *et al.* that rats exhibited catatonic-like behavior when given β-END is further evidence suggesting a possible increase in endorphin activity in schizophrenia.[20]

Finally, a lessening of schizophrenic symptoms has been reported in five controlled double-blind studies after intravenous administration of the opiate antagonist, naloxone hydrochloride. One study [21] reported a decrease in unusual thought content of schizophrenic patients; two of the studies [22, 23] reported a decrease in schizophrenic hallucinations following naloxone administration; and a further study [24] reported an overall amelioration of psychotic symptoms. While some investigators have not been able to duplicate these findings, a recent World Health Organization (WHO) (Geneva, Switzerland) collaborative study involving 32 schizophrenic patients found that naloxone produced a significant reduction in hallucinations.[25]

To date, several studies indicate an endorphin deficiency in patients with depression. In a study by Angst and colleagues, three of six depressed patients became hypomanic after a 10-mg intravenous injection of β-END.[26] This mood swing could be due to low endorphin levels in depressed patients, although other factors such as the stress of the experimental situation or patient expectation may be involved. Kline *et al.* reported positive changes in a variety of psychotic symptoms in depressed patients following intravenous administration of 1 to 9 mg of β-END.[27] However, these trials were not double-blind, and a relatively low dose of β-END was given. β-END also seemed to transiently lessen depression in two investigations.[12, 28]

In a double-blind, placebo-controlled crossover study by Gerner *et al.*, nine depressed patients showed significant improvement 2 to 4 hours after β-END administration when compared with results after placebo trials.[11] These findings support the hypothesis that depressed patients may have a deficit in endorphin activity.

Terenius and colleagues describe two endorphin fractions (labeled fractions I and II) that are neither β-END nor ENKs.[14] Fraction I was reported to be elevated in three of four manic subjects. Interestingly, these patients also had increased levels of fraction II during normal mood states. Judd and coworkers report a reduction in manic symptoms in four of eight manic patients after the administration of 20 mg of naloxone.[29] In another study using generally lower doses of naloxone, investigators found no change in the symptoms of patients with affective disorders.[30] Finally, in a recent collaborative investigation of the WHO, a larger number of manic patients had no change in symptoms following high doses of naloxone.[25]

Janowsky and coworkers [31] observed a recurrence of depressive symptoms in patients with a history of depression after the infusion of the cholinesterase inhibitor, physostigmine. Antimanic properties of physostigmine have also been reported.[32, 33] In an investigation with normal volunteers performed by Risch *et al.*,[34] the physostigmine-induced mood changes, particularly the depressive components, were significantly correlated with elevations in plasma β-END levels. These changes included an increase in depression, hostility, and confusion, and a decrease in arousal and mania. However, the mood and behavioral changes were not correlated with peak increases in cortisol. This study suggests a cholinergically mediated β-END pathway and supports the hypothesis of an increase in endorphin activity as the possible cause of depressive symptoms.

CLINICAL STUDIES

In our search for the possible role of endorphins in mental illness, we employ three strategies. First, we measure endorphin concentrations in various biological fluids. We also administer the opiate and endorphin antagonist, naloxone, in an attempt to lessen schizophrenic symptoms. Third, β-END is given as an experimental treatment for schizophrenia.

β-Endorphin in Biological Fluids

To determine the possible significance of leu⁵-β-END in the hemodialysis treatment of schizophrenia, we reasoned that if schizophrenic patients had extremely high levels of endorphins in their dialysate, then these high levels should be evident in their plasma. In 98 schizophrenic patients and 42 normal subjects, we found strikingly similar plasma concentrations of endorphin-like immunoreactivity using an antibody sensitive to both leu⁵-β-END and met⁵-β-END (2.8 fmol/ml average for the schizophrenic patients, and 2.4 fmol/ml for the normal subjects).[19] We were unable to find increased concentrations of β-END or leu⁵-β-END in the dialysate of ten schizophrenic patients.[19]

Although hemodialysis may eventually be shown to decrease schizophrenic symptoms, our results suggest that this is not likely to be due to the removal of leu⁵-β-END.

In our investigation, we studied more than 60 CSF samples from chronic schizophrenic patients and normal control subjects, and found β-END concentrations measured by radioimmunoassay to be between 3 and 12 fmol/ml. No differences were found between normal and schizophrenic CSF endorphin concentrations.[35] In a study by Emrich et al.,[23] normal subjects and groups of patients with schizophrenia, meningitis, disk herniation, and lumbago all showed approximately the same level of CSF endorphins (10 to 15 fmol/ml). These studies reporting lower concentrations used more sophisticated calibration methods for antisera, more accurate extraction procedures, and more elaborate controls that did studies that report normal β-END CSF concentrations of 72 fmol/ml.[15] These results show great disparity in the CSF endorphin levels of schizophrenic patients, in addition to the levels in normal control subjects. Thus, the question of CSF β-END levels remains unanswered. We are now studying concentrations of dynorphin, ENKs, and other endorphins in schizophrenic patients and normal control subjects.

Naloxone in Schizophrenia

To study the possible role of endorphins in schizophrenia, we administer naloxone in an attempt to decrease schizophrenic symptoms.[22] Our naloxone study involved 14 male veterans who reported frequent hallucinations and had relatively stable psychotic symptoms, either on or off medications. The subjects who gave informed consent to participate in this double-blind, randomized, crossover study received naloxone and placebo infusions given 48 hours apart. Seven of the subjects had not received neuroleptics for at least 2 weeks prior to the study, and the rest were maintained on routine doses of neuroleptics. The patients were interviewed and rated (NIMH Rating Scale) by trained raters at baseline, 15 minutes, and 1, 2, and 4 hours post-infusion.

In 15 trials with the 14 chronic schizophrenic patients, naloxone produced a statistically significant decrease in auditory and visual hallucinations ($p < 0.05$).[36] In 10 of the 15 trials, a reduction in hallucinations was reported, and, in the shortest responses, hallucinations returned in 3 hours. Comparative reading of earlier studies with naloxone reveals conflicting results. Some studies claim naloxone is ineffective in reducing hallucinations. However, these studies use lower doses of naloxone, are not double-blind, and/or examined only a relatively short time period after the infusion.[37–39] Finally, the recent WHO collaborative study found a significant reduction in schizophrenic hallucinations in 32 schizophrenic patients given naloxone, 0.3 mg/kg subcutaneously.[25]

β-Endorphin and Schizophrenia

Our β-END study was designed to test the reported antipsychotic actions of intravenously administered β-END in a placebo controlled, double-blind, crossover design. Because β-END is thought to have opiate agonist activity and since opiate agonists stimulate prolactin (PRL) secretion, we also measured serum PRL concentrations. In addition, we sought preliminary data on the pharmacokinetics of β-END and its effects on the EEG.

Ten male veterans from the Palo Alto Veterans Administration Medical Center gave informed consent to participate in the study. Their ages ranged from 27 to 47 years, with a mean age of 37. Each patient was interviewed and diagnosed by a psychiatrist using the Research Diagnostic Criteria (RDC) [40, 41] as having either chronic schizophrenia or chronic schizoaffective disorder, depressed type. All subjects were free of psychotropic medications for at least 2 weeks prior to the study. Subjects received a single weekly injection on the same day for 3 weeks. The initial injection was always saline solution and the first week was considered an acclimatization period. The next two randomized injections were either saline control or 20 mg of β-END. Both the patients and staff were blind to the content of the injections.

β-END was supplied as a liquid solution (4 mg/ml) in sterile saline solution for the first five patients. For the next five patients, β-END was supplied as a white powder. Immediately prior to administration, the β-END was dissolved in 10 ml of normal saline solution, forced through a filter to remove particulates, and taken up in a human-albumin-coated glass syringe. To minimize possible biases, the 5- to 10-ml saline control was also administered in an albumin-coated glass syringe. Nine of the subjects had the substances administered intravenously as a bolus; one subject was given three slow intravenous injections from non-albumin-coated syringes.

Two investigators rated the patient's symptoms according to the Brief Psychiatric Rating Scale (BPRS) [42] and the Clinical Global Inventory (CGI).[43] Baseline BPRS and CGI ratings were obtained just prior to each injection. The ratings were repeated 3 and 5 hours later, as well as on the third and fifth days after the infusion. CGI ratings alone were performed on the second and fourth days. Our interrater reliability for the BPRS was 0.94 (Pearson product-moment correlation coefficient).

Venous blood was drawn each week for serum PRL determinations at 60, 40, 20 minutes and immediately prior to the infusion, and at 10, 30, 60, 120, and 180 minutes after the infusion. Serum PRL was measured using an established and reliable double antibody and radioimmunoassay technique,[44] with an intraassay variability of 8.9%, interassay variability of 13.8%, and sensitivity of 0.1 ng/tube. Human PRL (hPRL AFP 1562-C) for iodination and standard was provided by Albert F. Parlow (Harbor UCLA Medical Center, Torrance, California). Iodination was performed according to the glucose oxidaselactoperoxidase technique,[45] and the suitability of the ^{125}I-labeled PRL was verified by the talc–resin–trichloroacetic acid (TCA) method.[46] Anti-hPRL (AFP-1) was supplied by the National Pituitary Agency. For these assays, the values are reported in nanograms of hPRL AFP 1562-C per milliliter of serum.

Venous blood was also drawn each week for β-END measurement immediately prior to infusion, and at 2, 5, 10, 30, 60, 120, and 180 minutes postinfusion. The β-END concentrations were measured using a specific and sensitive radioimmunoassay.[47] The detection range of this assay is from 15 fmol/ml to 600 pmol/ml of plasma.

For one patient, an electroencephalogram (EEG) was recorded from central (Cz) and parietal (Pz) electrode sites with disc electrodes referenced to linked ear electrodes for all infusions. The EEG results underwent fast Fourier analysis, which resulted in a power spectrum with 0.5-Hz resolution for the 0- to 32-Hz components. This patient also received a single 10-mg infusion of morphine sulfate under double-blind conditions.

The slow intravenous injection from the non-albumin-coated syringe produced a plasma β-END concentration of 1.3 pmol/ml at 5 minutes and 0.45 pmol/ml at 30 minutes after infusion. Bolus injection in six patients from albumin-coated syringes produced the following mean plasma β-END concentrations: 197.6 $\pm$ 37 (SE) pmol/ml at 2 minutes, 80 $\pm$ 37 (SE) pmol/ml at 30 minutes, and 1.8 $\pm$ 0.4 (SE) pmol/ml at 3 hours. The β-END two-component half-life in human plasma was 15 and 39 minutes. Thus, the patient who received the slow infusion had a plasma β-END concentration only one one-hundredth the mean of that of six other patients. For this reason, his PRL and clinical responses were not included in the data analysis.

For each patient, serum PRL concentrations from the saline control day were subtracted from PRL concentrations from the same time points on the β-END day. A comparison of the PRL concentrations on the saline versus β-END days revealed a statistically significant difference ($p < 0.001$).[48] β-END produced a maximal plasma prolactin concentration of 27 $\pm$ 7 (SE) ng/ml at 30 minutes; prolactin levels returned to normal 5 $\pm$ 1 (SE) ng/ml by 180 minutes.

For one patient, the EEG responses were monitored during each infusion and during one 10-mg infusion of morphine. After the injection of either morphine or β-END, spectral analysis of each treatment revealed changes in the alpha frequency range (8 to 12 Hz). The alpha activity increased rapidly and remained high for at least 50 minutes after the morphine injection. After β-END, there was a rise in alpha activity that was similar to but faster than that produced by morphine, and the increase lasted less than 30 minutes. No changes in alpha activity were observed after the injections of saline solutions.[49]

The patients were rated on the BPRS five times per week and on the CGI seven times per week. A saline infusion was given in the first week to act as an acclimatization period and was not used as a control for the drug condition. In the following two weeks, saline and β-END injections were administered in double-blind conditions and in random order. The degree of change in each patient was quantitated by selecting the lowest postinjection BPRS score and subtracting it from the baseline score. A positive score reflected lessening of symptoms, as the postinjection BPRS was lower than the baseline score; a negative score reflected a relative worsening of symptoms. One of the ten patients withdrew from the study after two injections, and nine of the medication-free schizophrenic patients were able to complete the study. As previously mentioned, one additional patient was not included in the analysis because of his extremely low plasma β-END concentration. Since eight patients exhibited an average improvement of 10 points on the BPRS after the first saline injection, the acclimatization period proved to be particularly important. This compares with an average improvement of four points on the BPRS after the saline control injection and six points after the β-END injection. No improvement was recorded on the CGI during the 3-week period for any patient. These scores are consistent with the impressions of both patients and staff, that is, neither patients nor staff could distinguish the response to β-END from the response to saline solution.

Of the eight patients with adequate plasma concentrations, six patients were found to have a statistically significant improvement in total BPRS scores after β-END injection than they did after the saline injection ($p < 0.05$).[48] One patient showed equal improvement under the two conditions, and one patient had the reverse response.

In an earlier study, a single intravenous injection of 9 mg of β-END produced a plasma concentration of 80 to 90 ng/ml (27.3 pmol/ml).[24, 27] These values readily fit a single-component elimination time with a half-life of about 20 minutes.[27] In our β-END study, we were approximately three times more efficient in achieving an initial plasma concentration per milligram of the compound. The average of our 15- and 39-minute half-lives is similar to the 20-minute half-life reported by Kline et al.,[10] even though our two-component elimination curve differs from the single-component curve that they reported.

The significant increase in serum PRL levels observed in our patients after β-END administration is consistent with opiate agonist activity in man. Elevated PRL levels have been measured in rats after morphine, met-enkephamid, and β-END infusions.[50-53] Morphine and methadone have also been reported to increase human serum PRL concentrations.[54, 55] The mechanism of opiate agonist PRL stimulation has not yet been determined, but it is possible that it is mediated by dopaminergic neurons; dopamine exerts tonic inhibitory control of PRL secretion.[56] The acute response of plasma PRL to a maximal dose of morphine in the rat was not further increased by haloperidol. Ferland et al. claim that this evidence suggests that the effect of morphine on PRL is secondary to inhibition of dopaminergic activity, perhaps through presynaptic inhibitory opiate receptors on dopaminergic neurons.[57]

The effect of morphine on EEG activity is consistent with previous reports.[58, 59] The acute increase in alpha EEG activity produced by both morphine and β-END might be secondary to the peripheral actions of morphine and β-END. However, a direct effect of both compounds on central opiate receptors is a more logical explanation.[49] The fact that the met-ENK analogue FK 33–824 also increases alpha power is further evidence that this effect is mediated by central opiate receptors.[60] Furthermore, there is evidence that in the rabbit, CSF levels of β-END are significantly elevated after intravenous injection, and that four modified opioid peptides enter the CNS after peripheral administration in the rat.[61, 62] This provides additional evidence that β-END administered peripherally enters the mammalian brain.[61]

Kline and Lehmann, in their single-blind study, observed dramatic improvement in three of four patients after β-END administration.[10, 27] They reported that a patient with schizoaffective schizophrenia showed improvement after 1.5-, 3-, 6-, and 9-mg doses of β-END, with the greatest improvement after 9 mg. In this study, one patient with chronic undifferentiated schizophrenia showed no improvement at the 1.5-mg dose level, had diminished hallucinations and more "appropriate behavior" after 3 mg, and showed "marked improvement" after 6 mg. Interestingly, this patient failed to respond to a later dose of 6 mg of β-END. The third patient with a diagnosis of paranoid schizophrenia was "more active" and "less withdrawn" after 6 mg, but did not respond to lower levels of the compound. In these same investigations, the administration of two intravenous injections of 9 mg of β-END had no apparent effect on a patient with catatonic schizophrenia.[10, 27]

In our study, neither patients nor staff were able to distinguish between the effects of β-END and saline solution on the basis of clinical changes. This observation is in accordance with the constant level of pathology recorded on the CGI scale. A statistically significant improvement was observed in BPRS scores after β-END compared with the improvement after saline solution. However, the improvement after β-END just reached statistical significance with a one-tailed test, was not obvious clinically, and was less than the improvement on the BPRS noted during the acclimatization period. Use of a one-tailed statistical test might seem questionable since there is controversial evidence for both a deficiency and an excess of endorphin activity in schizophrenia. However, the reports of Kline *et al.* led us to predict that patients would show improvement after β-END administration; thus, we used a one-tailed test.

Our study design was not optimal for testing the antipsychotic activity of a new compound. We felt the need for a double-blind comparison of a single injection of β-END with saline solution because of the limited availability of β-END and the report of Kline *et al.* of a decrease in schizophrenic symptoms after a single injection of β-END.[10, 27] However, even the comparison of saline solution with a clearly effective neuroleptic such as fluphenazine given to eight patients could yield only slightly positive results or may fail to demonstrate any antipsychotic activity of the neuroleptic. Thus, a single 20-mg injection of β-END produced a statistically significant, yet not clinically obvious improvement in psychotic symptoms. It is now necessary to accomplish further studies with repeated doses of β-END in the same patient to determine whether these apparent improvements will become clinically obvious.

CONCLUSION

Our β-END findings can be summarized as follows: 20 mg of intravenously injected β-END in humans has pharmacologic activity both on PRL and the EEG. β-END shares this PRL-stimulating ability with other opiate agonists in rats and in man. The acute increase in alpha EEG power after intravenous β-END administration was similar to that seen after intravenous morphine sulfate administration. It was also shown that the method of intravenous injection has a profound effect on the plasma concentration of β-END. Slow intravenous infusion from non-albumin-coated syringes yielded markedly lower plasma levels than did the bolus injection from an albumin-coated syringe. Finally, a statistically significant, but not clinically obvious lessening in schizophrenic symptoms was found after a 20-mg intravenous injection of β-END when compared with a saline injection in our double-blind, crossover design.

Endorphin research has led to new and exciting, although conflicting findings in the field of mental illness. Evidence exists for both an excess and a deficiency of endorphin activity in both depression and schizophrenia. The report of a decrease in schizophrenic hallucinations by Gunne *et al.*[63] led to our successful double-blind trial of naloxone in schizophrenic hallucinations.[64] Positive reports of β-END administration in psychiatric patients by Kline and Lehmann, Angst, and others prompted us to perform our double-blind, placebo-controlled, crossover study with intravenously administered β-END. The lack of a clinically obvious patient response in our study was perhaps due to the method of injection. More recent studies with intrathecally administered β-END are promising, and studies using this method would enable researchers to study the effectiveness of β-END at lower doses. Other study designs, such as the use of multiple doses, are necessary to further investigate the activity of β-END in psychiatric patients. Such investigations may yield a new treatment for depression or schizophrenia and should improve our understanding of the role of endorphins in normal and abnormal physiology.

ACKNOWLEDGMENTS

The investigations reported in this paper were accomplished with the help of Huda Akil, Kenneth L. Davis, Glen R. Elliott, Avram Goldstein, James Kilkowski, Helena Kraemer, Choh Hao Li, Adolf Pfefferbaum, Maureen Ross, and Robert T. Rubin.

REFERENCES

1. BERGER, P. A. 1978. Neurosci. Res. Program Bull. **16:** 585–599.
2. NEDOPIL, W. & E. RUTHER. 1979. Pharmakopsychiatr. Neuro-Psychopharmakol. **12:** 277–280.
3. JORGENSON, A., R. FOG & B. VEILIS. 1979. Lancet **1:** 935.
4. BURBACH, P. & D. DE WIED. 1980. *In* Enzymes and Neurotransmitters in Mental Disease. E. Usdin, T. S. Sourkes & M. B. H. Youdim, Eds.: 103–114. Wiley. New York.
5. VERHOEVEN, W. M., H. M. VAN PRAAG, J. M. VAN REE & D. DE WIED. 1979. Arch. Gen. Psychiat. **36:** 294–298.
6. EMRICH, H. M., M. ZAUDIG, W. KISSLING, G. DIRLICH, D. V. ZERSSEN & A. HERZ. 1980. Pharmakopsychiatr. Neuro-Psychopharmakol. **13:** 290–298.
7. VAN PRAAG, H. M., W. M. A. VERHOEVEN, J. M. VAN REE & D. DE WIED. 1981. *In* Proceedings of IIIrd World Conference on Biological Psychiatry, Stockholm. G. Struwe, Ed. Abstract S311. Elsevier/North-Holland. Amsterdam.
8. SEGAL, D. S., R. G. BROWN, A. ARNSTEN & D. C. DERRINGTON. 1978. *In* Characteristics and Function of Opioids. J. M. van Ree & L. Terenius, Eds.: 413–414. Elsevier/North-Holland. Amsterdam.
9. JACQUET, Y. R. & N. MARKS. 1976. Science **194:** 632–636.
10. KLINE, N. W. & H. E. LEHMANN. 1979. *In* Endorphins in Mental Health Research. E. Usdin, W. E. Bunney, Jr. & N. S. Kline, Eds.: 500–517. Macmillan. New York.
11. GERNER, R. H., D. H. CATLIN, D. A. GORELICK, K. K. HUI & C. H. LI. 1980. Arch. Gen. Psychiat. **37:** 642–647.
12. PICKAR, D., G. C. DAVIS, S. C. SCHULTZ, I. EXTEIN, R. WAGNER, D. NABER, P. W. GOLD, D. P. VAN KAMMEN, F. K. GOODWIN, R. J. WYATT, C. H. LI & W. E. BUNNEY. 1981. Am. J. Psychiat. **138**(2): 160–166.
13. WAHLSTRÖM, A., L. JOHANSSON & L. TERENIUS. 1976. *In* Opiates and Endogenous Opioid Peptides. H. W. Kosterlitz, Ed.: 49–56. Elsevier/North-Holland. Amsterdam.
14. TERENIUS, L., A. WAHLSTRÖM, L. LINDSTRÖM & E. WIDERLÖV. 1976. Neurosci. Lett. **3:** 157–162.
15. DOMSCHKE, W., A. DICKSCHAS & P. MITZNEGG. 1979. Lancet **1:** 1024.
16. WAGEMAKER, H. & R. CADE. 1977. Am. J. Psychiat. **134:** 684–685.
17. PALMOUR, R., R. ERVIN, H. WAGEMAKER & R. CADE. 1979. *In* Endorphins in Mental Health Research.[10] : 581–593.
18. LEWIS, R. V., L. D. GERBER, S. STEIN, R. L. STEPHEN, B. I. GROSSER, S. F. VELICK & S. UDENFRIEND. 1979. Arch. Gen. Psychiat. **36:** 237.
19. ROSS, M., P. A. BERGER & A. GOLDSTEIN. 1979. Science **200:** 974–981.
20. BLOOM, F., D. SEGAL, N. LING & R. GUILLEMIN. 1976. Science **194:** 630–632.
21. DAVIS, G. C., W. E. BUNNEY, JR., M. S. BUCHSBAUM, E. G. DE FRAITES, W. DUNCAN, J. C. GILLIN, D. P. VAN KAMMEN, J. KLEINMAN, D. L. MURPHY, R. M. POST, V. REUS & R. J. WYATT. 1979. *In* Endorphins in Mental Health Research.[10] : 393–406.
22. WATSON, S. J., P. A. BERGER, H. AKIL, M. J. MILLS & J. D. BARCHAS. 19, Science **201:** 73–75.

23. EMRICH, H. M., C. CORDING & S. PIREE. 1977. Pharmakopsychiatr. Neuro-Psychopharmakol. **10:** 265–270.
24. LEHMANN, H., N. P. VASAVAN NAIR & N. S. KLINE. 1979. Am. J. Psychiat. **136:** 762–766.
25. PICKAR, D. & W. E. BUNNEY, JR. 1981. In Biological Psychiatry, Proceedings of IIIrd World Conference, Stockholm.[7] C. Perris, G. Struwe & B. Jansson, Eds.: 394–397.
26. ANGST, J., V. AUTENRIETH, F. BREM, M. KOUKKOU, H. MEYER, H. STASSEN & U. STOREK. 1979. In Endorphins in Mental Health Research.[10] : 518–528.
27. KLINE, N. S., C. H. LI, H. E. LEHMANN, A. LAJTHA, E. LASKI & T. COOPER. 1977. Arch. Gen. Psychiat. **34:** 1111–1113.
28. CATLIN, D. H., D. GORELICK, R. H. GERNER, K. K. GUI & C. H. LI. 1980. In Advances in Biochemical Pharmacology: Regulation and Function of Neuropeptides. E. Costa & E. M. Trabucchi, Eds.: 465–472. Raven Press. New York.
29. JUDD, L. L., D. S. JANOWSKY, D. S. SEGAL & L. Y. HUEY. 1978. In Characteristics and Function of Opioids.[8] : 173–174.
30. DAVIS, G. C., W. E. BUNNEY, JR., E. G. DE FRAITES, I. EXTEIN, F. K. GOODWIN, W. HAMILTON, J. KLEINMAN, W. MENDELSON, R. POST, V. REUS, D. SHILING, D. VAN KAMMEN, D. WEINBERGER, R. J. WYATT & C. H. LI. 1978. Presented at the Seventeenth Annual Meeting of the American College of Neuropsychopharmacology, Maui, Hawaii.
31. JANOWSKY, D. S., M. K. KHALED & J. M. DAVIS. 1974. Psychosom. Med. **36:** 248–257.
32. JANOWSKY, D. S., K. EL-YOUSEF, J. M. DAVIS & H. I. SEKERKE. 1973. Arch. Gen. Psychiat. **28:** 542–547.
33. DAVIS, K., P. A. BERGER, L. E. HOLLISTER & E. G. DE FRAITES. 1978. Arch. Gen. Psychiat. **35:** 119–222.
34. RISCH, S. C., R. M. COHEN, D. S. JANOWSKY, N. H. KALIN & D. L. MURPHY. 1980. Science **209:** 1545–1546.
35. AKIL, H., P. A. BERGER, S. J. WATSON & J. D. BARCHAS. 1982. In preparation.
36. BERGER, P. A., S. J. WATSON, H. AKIL, J. D. BARCHAS & C. H. LI. 1980. In Enzymes and Neurotransmitters in Mental Disease.[4] : 45–64.
37. JANOWSKY, D. S., D. S. SEGAL & F. BLOOM. 1977. Am. J. Psychiat. **134:** 926–927.
38. VOLAVKA, J., A. MALLYA, S. BAIG & J. PEREZ-CRUET. 1977. Science **196:** 1227–1228.
39. KURLAND, A. A., O. MCCABE, T. E. HANLON & D. SULLIVAN. 1977. Am. J. Psychiat. **134:** 1408–1410.
40. SPITZER, R. L., J. ENDICOTT & E. ROBINS. 1978. Research Diagnostic Criteria (RDC) for a Selected Group of Functional Disorders, 3rd ed. Biometrics Research, New York State Psychiatric Institute. New York.
41. SPITZER, R. L., J. ENDICOTT & E. ROBINS. 1978. Arch. Gen. Psychiat. **35:** 773–782.
42. OVERALL, J. E. & D. R. GORHAM. 1962. Psychol. Rep. **10:** 799–812.
43. CLINICAL GLOBAL INVENTORY (CGI). 1967. The Clinical Global Impressions Scale. Psychopharmacology Research Branch and National Institute of Mental Health. Bethesda, MD.
44. SINHA, Y. N., F. W. SELBY, U. J. LEWIS & W. P. VANDERLAAN. 1973. J. Clin. Endocrinol. Metab. **36:** 509–516.
45. TOWER, B. B., B. R. CLARK & R. T. RUBIN. 1977. Life Sci. **21:** 959–966.
46. TOWER, B. B., M. B. SIGEL, R. T. RUBIN, R. E. POLAND & W. P. VANDERLAAN. 1978. Life Sci. **23:** 2183–2192.
47. AKIL, H., S. J. WATSON, J. D. BARCHAS & C. H. LI. 1979. Life Sci. **24:** 1659–1666.

48. SIEGEL, S. 1956. Nonparametric Statistics: For the Behavioral Sciences. McGraw-Hill. New York.
49. PFEFFERBAUM, A., P. A. BERGER, G. R. ELLIOTT, J. R. TINKLENBERG, B. S. KOPELL, J. D. BARCHAS & C. H. LI. 1979. Psychiat. Res. 1: 83–88.
50. RIVIER, C., W. VALE, N. LING, M. BROWN & R. GUILLEMIN. 1977. Endocrinology 100: 238–241.
51. CUSAN, L., A. DUPONT & G. S. KLEDZIK. 1977. Nature (London) 268: 544–547.
52. GUIDOTTI, A. & L. GRANDISON. 1979. In Endorphins in Mental Health Research.[10] : 416–422.
53. LABRIE, F., A. DUPONT & L. CUSAN. 1979. In Endorphins in Mental Health Research.[10] : 335–343.
54. TOLIS, G., J. HICKEY & H. GUYDA. 1975. J. Clin. Endocrinol. Metab. 41: 797–800.
55. GOLD, M. S., R. K. DONABEDIAN, M. DILLARD, JR., F. W. SLOBETZ, C. E. RIORDAN, & H. D. KLEBER. 1977. Lancet 2: 398–399.
56. OJEDA, S. R., P. G. HARMS & S. M. MCCANN. 1974. Endocrinology 95: 1694–1703.
57. FERLAND, L., P. KELLY, F. DENIZEAU & F. LABRIE. 1978. In Characteristics and Function of Opioids.[8] : 353–354.
58. WIKLER, A. 1954. J. Nerv. Ment. Dis. 120: 157–175.
59. FINK, M., A. ZAKS, J. VOLAVKA & J. ROUBICEK. 1971. In Narcotic Drugs: Biochemical Pharmacology. D. H. Clouet, Ed.: 452–467. Plenum Press. New York.
60. KREBS, E. & J. ROUBICEK. 1979. Pharmakopsychiatr. Neuro-Psychopharmakol. 12: 86–93.
61. PEZALLA, P. D., M. LIS, N. G. SEIDAH & M. CHRETIEN. 1978. Can. J. Neurol. Sci. 5: 183–188.
62. RAPOPORT, S. I., W. A. KLEE, K. D. PETTIGREW & K. OHNO. 1980. Science 207: 84–86.
63. GUNNE, L. M., L. LINDSTRÖM & L. TERENIUS. 1977. J. Neural. Transm. 40: 13–19.
64. BERGER, P. A., S. J. WATSON, H. AKIL & J. D. BARCHAS. 1981. Am. J. Psychiat. 138(7): 913–918.

DISCUSSION OF THE PAPER

J. V. VOLAVKA (*New York University School of Medicine, New York*): This was pointed out to me by Dr. Emrich when I discussed with him recent findings on some patients responding to naloxone. We injected schizophrenics with intravenous naloxone and found a significant increase in the circulating endorphin levels. Dr. Emrich points out that we are actually increasing their β-endorphin levels and while the naloxone is short-acting the endorphin may get to the receptor. Maybe this is why they improve.

P. A. BERGER: (*Stanford University School of Medicine, Stanford, CA*): I am pleased by those data. I think that is one of the numerous possible explanations that we considered. Of course, we also considered such things as rapid receptor modifications since the naloxone effect appears to occur after the normal duration of action of the naloxone, but, I think these results are exciting. Maybe Dr. Emrich could comment on them himself?

H. M. EMRICH (*Max Planck-Institut für Psychiatrie, Munich, FRG*): My comment to this is part of my presentation. At the moment I would like to comment on the hemodialysis investigations.

In our group in Munich we (Dr. Hokslark and Dr. Goland) were able to show, that hemodialysis in reality induces a strong increase of β-endorphin in plasma and possibly this is due to the stress of this method and possibly, although this was not investigated by us, the sham dialysis has less effect. So, some of the beneficial effects of hemodialysis and apparently of the sham hemodialysis in regard to schizophrenic symptoms (interestingly also shown now in depressive patients) could be due to this endorphin-activating stress effect by the procedure.

BERGER: That is an extremely interesting finding. Unfortunately, as you know, it is going to be very, very difficult to test because if you do not use sham dialysis as the control, it is extremely difficult to establish the efficacy. It would have to be a non-stressful procedure and it is hard to picture a control for dialysis that would be non-stressful.

A. J. MANDELL (*University of California at San Diego, La Jolla*): Dr. Berger, it occurs to me that you may have physiological action in your power spectrum in the sense that the power spectrum is a normalized variance and you have the alpha peak getting very much stronger, but, you do not show where that power came from. You only went up to thirty hertz and the dominant finding in EEGs now in schizophrenics, if you believe them from 1978, through 1980 and 1981, is forty hertz or above or sixty hertz activity. If you get increased stability, there is some nice second order work done with EEGs in which you follow the time-dependent power variations in the frequency band and morphine stabilizes that so that one might expect that if you extended your spectrum out, you would see a disappearance of power in the forty hertz or above and that being shunted into the alpha which, then, in second order variations would fit the morphine work. In other words, it stabilizes that frequency. You have the data for it if you would just extend the analysis.

BERGER: That is exactly what we should do and I think we will extend it out to sixty hertz in these patients. Thank you for the suggestion.

β-ENDORPHIN ADMINISTRATION TO ACUTE SCHIZOPHRENIC PATIENTS: A DOUBLE BLIND STUDY

Bertalan Pethö,* László Gráf,† István Karczag,* János Borvendég,†
István Bitter,* István Barna,† Ilona Hermann,† Judit Tolna,*
and Krisztina Baraczka *

* Semmelweis Medical University
Budapest, Hungary
† Institute for Drug Research
Budapest, Hungary

Apparently incompatible experimental findings and considerations support the hypothesis that the endogenous opioids participate, in some way, in maintaining the psychic equilibrium. Terenius et al.[1, 2] first drew attention to the possible connection between disorders in the metabolism of endogenous opioids and the different psychoses. According to their investigations, the measurable concentration of partially purified Fraction I, an opioid peptide different from enkephalins and β-endorphin, is considerably higher in the CSF of schizophrenics than in that of control patients. This tendency was more marked in acute cases and parallel with the improvement of the clinical condition. Neuroleptic therapy reduced Fraction I levels that were initially above the control value.[2] This recognition raised the possibility of treating schizophrenic patients with opiate antagonists (e.g., naloxone),[3] but most authors have reported on the failure of therapy.[4] Interpretation of the findings is greatly hampered by the fact that the opiate antagonists block the effect not only of Fraction I, but of all the other endogenous opioids, including those which other authors consider to play a psychopathological role antagonistic to that of Fraction I. This latter view is essentially based on two experimental observations. Jacquet and Marks [5] suggested a similarity between certain pharmacological properties of β-endorphin and the neuroleptics, while de Wied et al.[6] demonstrated neuroleptic activity for γ-endorphin, one of the fragments of β-endorphin also released under physiological conditions.[7]

After studying the complex psychiatric literature on alkaloid narcotics and endogenous opioids, Verebey et al.[8] have proposed that the endogenous opioids contribute to maintaining psychic equilibrium through their anxiolytic, tranquilizing, antidepressant, anger-, aggression-, and delusion-reducing effects, and their action in reducing insufficiency and suicidal tendencies. Consequently, reduction of the level of endogenous opioids would result in manifestations antagonistic to the above favorable effects (anxiety, hypersensitivity to average stress, reduced self-esteem, etc.).

With the successful chemical synthesis of human β-endorphin [9] it became possible to conduct clinical tests of the polypeptide. Kline and Lehmann [10] administered β-endorphin in intravenous doses of 1.5–9.0 mg to 15 psychiatric patients on 42 occasions. On the basis of the nature and duration of the effects, the authors distinguished four phases in the action: I. autonomous (30–120 sec); II. antidysphoric (1–6 hours); III. inhibitory (2–3 hours); IV. therapeutic (1–10 days). Vegetative reactions appeared in phase I and

460

0077–8923/82/0398–0460 $01.75/0 © 1982, NYAS

favorable therapeutic effects (improved mood, relief from anxieties, etc.) could be observed in phases II–IV.[10] The main technical shortcomings in these and in the investigations by Angst *et al.*[11] giving rise to the possibility of error, were as follows: (1) the investigations were not carried out in blind design; (2) the authors did not use a structured evaluation;[12] and (3) the medication given at the same time as the treatment or its interruption could influence the effect of the β-endorphin.

We report here studies on β-endorphin treatment of six acute schizophrenic patients in a double-blind design. These patients did not receive any other medication during the trial period. During the preparation of our preliminary report [13] on these studies, double-blind clinical studies with β-endorphin have also been reported by two other groups.[14, 15]

MATERIALS AND METHODS

Human β-endorphin was produced by solid-phase peptide synthesis [19] in Prof. C. H. Li's laboratory (University of California, San Francisco). We checked the homogeneity of this β-endorphin preparation with end-group and amino acid analyses and paper and gel electrophoreses (see ref. 16 for the methods). Following intracerebroventricular (i.c.v.) administration, the analgesic effect determined by the rat tail-flick test was the same as that of pig β-endorphin isolated from natural source.[17]

Synthetic human β-endorphin was dissolved in physiological saline solution, strained through a Millipore HA 0.22 μ filter, and filled in ampules under sterile conditions. Each ampule contained 4.0 mg of β-endorphin in 10 ml of physiological saline solution. The ampules were stored at −20°C.

Since β-endorphin has not yet been administered to patients suffering from manifest psychosis, we selected such patients for our investigation (TABLE 1). Six patients each received 4 mg of β-endorphin intravenously, while three patients were given the same volume of physiological saline solution. The injection lasted 5 minutes in all cases.

Our investigations were conducted in a double-blind design, with the psychopathological examination recorded according to the factor construct rating scale (FCRS) [18] in patients who had received no medication for at least 10 days and who were not receiving any other medication during the course of the study. The injection was administered at 10 A.M. The psychopathological and pain sensation tests were conducted at the following times: (1) at 8:30 A.M. on the day of treatment; (2) in 15 minutes immediately following the treatment; (3) hourly on the day of treatment up to 5 P.M.; and (4) at 9 A.M. and 1 P.M. on the days following treatment for one week unless it became necessary before the end of this period to give other (neuroleptic, anxiolytic) medication.

One hour before the β-endorphin injection and at the same time on the third day, we took 9–10 ml of CSF by lumbar puncture with the patient in a seated position. After removal the CSF was immediately frozen and was then lyophilized and dissolved again in 0.9–1.0 ml distilled water in order to determine the β-endorphin content by radioimmunoassay (RIA). For the details of the β-endorphin RIA method we refer to the description given by Borvendeg *et al.*[19] We used a pig β-endorphin antibody produced in rabbits in a dilution of 1:30,000; the lower limit of sensitivity, 20 pg β-endorphin, gave a 100% cross reaction with reference human β-endorphin.

TABLE 1

MAIN DATA ON PATIENTS

Patient	Sex	Age	Months Since Onset of Illness	Course of Illness	No. of Hospitalizations	Present Syndrome	Diagnosis
1. M.N.	female	31	22	Full remission after first psychosis; now recovered 4 months	2	Acute anxiety psychosis with delusions of reference	Cycloid psychosis
2. B.F.	male	19	¼	Hyperacute onset after six-day prodromal period; recovered in 3 months	1	Confusion, with religious and megalomaniac exaltation	Cycloid psychosis
3. R.L.	female	42	2	First psychosis disappeared after 3 weeks; acute onset of subsequent psychosis; second remission followed by another relapse 2 months later	2	Auditory, visual and olfactory hallucinations, anxiety, delusions of reference, incoherence	Affect-laden paraphrenia
4. C.B.	male	25	110	Chronic schizophrenia, chronically autistic and incapable of work. Deterioration every 2–3 years	5	Anxiety, bewilderment, auditory hallucinations, catatonic symptoms	Parakinetic catatonia
5. K.B.	male	25	96	Chronic schizophrenia; has been engaged in hospital work therapy for 5 years; deterioration approx. every six months	10	Somaesthesic hallucinations; auditory hallucinations; anxiety, depersonalization; mild schizophasia	Cataphasia

6. C.M.	female	24	82	Chronic schizophrenia; has been incapable of work for years; vagrant. Deterioration every 6–12 months	12	Emotional blunting; mannerisms; unreasonable euphoria and irritability; infantile joking; heteronomous abnormal physical sensations; incoherence	Shallow hebephrenia
Control patients who received only intravenous saline injection:							
7. J.I.	male	27	34	Has been unable to work since the first psychosis; lives with family. Chronic schizophrenia	4	Mannerisms, inactive, blunting, indifferent, hesitant, mild anxiety	Manneristic catatonia
8. T.M.	female	36	170	Chronic schizophrenia; lives with parents, reduced capacity for work and adjustment. Emotional blunting	11	Auditory hallucinations, delusions of reference, mild anxiety and incoherence	Autistic hebephrenia
9. E.L.	male	22	2	Subacute onset of illness	1	Inhibited, slightly tense, inactive, bewildered, mild delusions of reference	Cycloid psychosis

Note: The more precise diagnosis was based on Leonhard.[24] We classified the cycloid psychosis[25] into the schizophrenia spectrum disorder.

TABLE 2

TREND IN PSYCHOPATHOLOGICAL SYMPTOMS MEASURED BY FCRS IN PATIENTS TREATED WITH β-ENDORPHIN

Patient	Time of FCRS	Before β-endorphin	After	2	3	4	5	6	7	8
1. M.N.	Σ	46	(−)	(−)	(−)	(−)	(+)	+		
	1+2	9	(−)	(−)	(−)	(−)	(−)	(−)		
	5	5								
	6	1	(+)		(+)	(+)	(+)	+		
	9	6	(−)							
	10	1	(+)	++	(+)	(+)	+	++		Neurolepsis
	17	5	+							
	Σ	48		++						
	1+2	11								
	5	1								
2. B.F.	6	5	(−)	++	Neurolepsis					
	9	1								
	10	6								
	17	1								
	Σ	37	−	(−)	(+)	(+)	+	++	(+)	
	1+2	7	++	(+)			+	++	++	
	5	1		−						
3. R.L.	6	3	−	−	−	−	− +	(+)	++	
	9	4	−	+	−	−	+	+	++	
	10	1	+	+	(−) +	(+)	− +			
	17	5	−	−	+		+			
	Σ	48	−							Neurolepsis
	1+2	8	−						++	
	5	5	−					+	++	

	Score	Neurolepticum	Neurolepticum 20 days later
4. C.B.			
6	1		
9	3		−
10	1	(−)	(−)
17	5		−
Σ	41	++	(+)
1 + 2	6	(+)	(−)
5	3		

	Score	Neurolepticum
5. K.B.		
6	3	−
9	1	(−)
17	1	
17	3	(+)
Σ	60	(+)
1 + 2	11	+
5	1	

	Score	Neurolepticum	Neurolepticum 10 days later
6. C.M.			
6	1	(−)	−
9	1		
10	5		
17	17		

Legend: Σ = overall FCRS score; 1 + 2 = cognitive disorders of form and content; 5 = psychomotor retardation; 6 = agitation-excitement; 9 = depressive mood; 10 = elevated mood; 17 = anxiety-tension; (−), (+) = change in score ± 1 (in the case of Σ, less than 5% of total score); −, + = change in score ± 2 (in the case of Σ, 6–15% of total score); − −, + + = change in score ± 3 or more (in case of Σ, more than 16% of total score).

Results

Marked and lasting somnolence developed in two patients (3 and 6) on the day of the β-endorphin injection. A milder degree of somnolence could also be observed in the other four patients. We did not observe a reduction in the pain sensation in any of the patients when the skin was pricked with a needle. There was a change in the psychiatric symptoms in patients 1, 2, and 3 even within 30 minutes and one hour, particularly on the first day. The characteristic daily values for the FCRS scores are given in TABLE 2. Cognitive disorders showed a minimal improvement only in patient 6 and here too, only after days 6 and 7 following the treatment. With the exception of patient 4, psychomotor activity showed normalization in the first days. Where inhibition had been more marked before treatment with β-endorphin it declined, and where agitation and excitement were more prominent, these were reduced. There was a similar reciprocal change in mood in patient 3 compared to the initial value before administration of β-endorphin. Transient euphoria also occurred in two other patients (1 and 5). Patients 2 and 6 were in such a state of prolonged euphoria prior to treatment that any further increase in euphoria would have been difficult to detect. Anxiety was definitely reduced in four patients (1, 3, 4, and 5) but later—also in the case of patient 2—just because of the very marked increase in anxiety—neuroleptic-anxiolytic treatment had to be started. There was no substantial change in the other items of the FCRS. In four cases the intensity of the psychosis as reflected in the FCRS overall score first declined and then rose, in one case (5) it rose immediately and rapidly and in another one (6) it did not change.

Among the three control patients (whose FCRS scores are not shown), patient 7 improved suddenly and substantially after the psychological saline injection was given. For 3 days he was bright, active, and sociable, although his manneristic behavior remained unchanged. It was only in this case that the "blind" observer felt certain that the patient had received β-endorphin. His symptoms returned after 3 days and he had to be given anxiolyticums for his acute anxiety. The psychosis of control patient 8 grew gradually and steadily worse until we administered a neuroleptic drug on day 4. The behavior of control patient 9 was slightly improved, but he also had to be given neuroleptics on day 3.

In agreement with the data in the literature,[20] the β-endorphin immuno-reactivity in the CSF of the patients before the treatment gave a value in the range of 12-50 pg β-endorphin/ml. The CSF β-endorphin levels determined three days after treatment with β-endorphin in patients 4, 5, and 6 and in the two control patients examined (7 and 8), coincided with the initial values while in three patients (1, 2, and 3) we found a significant rise in the level (TABLE 3).

Discussion

All of our six patients given β-endorphin treatment showed a certain improvement for a shorter or longer period. This improvement was restricted to the area of mood and activity. The nature of the improvement depended on the initial symptoms; in all cases they indicated a tendency to restore the homeostasis. Contrary to the earlier data in the literature,[10, 11] the formal symptoms (e.g. mannerism) and cognitive disorders did not improve. For this reason, at least in the case of acute psychoses, β-endorphin treatment probably represents only "temperament therapy." There was no easing of the delusions and hallucinations and at most, the influence of the latter on experience and behavior declined as a result of the shift in mood.

It would appear that the more intensive the psychosis, the less the homeostatic influence of β-endorphin. In the six cases we studied it is questionable whether β-endorphin had any influence whatsoever in relieving the psychosis. We consider it probable that we are evaluating the so-called "own effect" of β-endorphin, that is, the effect by which it invariably induces transitory improvement in healthy people too. On the other hand, β-endorphin does not seem to have any real antipsychotic effect. The psychic disorders (retardation, confusion, bewilderment (see refs. 10, 21) produced by β-endorphin administered to persons free of psychopathological symptoms could indicate

TABLE 3

β-ENDORPHIN IMMUNOREACTIVITY (pg per ml) IN THE CSF OF THE PATIENTS BEFORE β ENDORPHIN TREATMENT AND ON THE THIRD DAY AFTER TREATMENT

Patient	β-Endorphin Immunoactivity	
	Before Treatment	After Treatment
1.	12 ± 1.4 *	24 ± 5.3
2.	17 ± 1.5	64 ± 12.2
3.	24 ± 8.4	85 ± 2.8
4.	13 ± 0.1	17 ± 1.6
5.	21 ± 0.2	23 ± 0.5
6.	15 ± 3.9	22 ± 1.8
7.	50 ± 0.8	48 ± 1.8
8.	27 ± 4.5	32 ± 5.3
9.	17 ± 0.5	— †

* Mean ± standard deviation of 4 parallel measurements.
† Measurement was not performed.

that the "own effect" of β-endorphin also acts to upset the psychic equilibrium. The result of the "own effect," which is bipolar from the viewpoint of homeostasis, almost certainly depends to a great extent on the initial condition of the organism which, in our cases, was seriously altered. We suggest that the widely differing duration of the "therapeutic phase" from patient to patient can be interpreted on the basis of these considerations: the "therapeutic phase" lasts only until the psychosis cancels out the "own effect"; the length of time this takes depends on the initial condition (in patient 2, for example, this was slightly less than one day).

This interpretation may help to resolve the apparent discrepancy between the two recent clinical studies showing either slight improvement [14] or significant worsening in the schizophrenic symptoms [15] after β-endorphin administration. Our results are more consistent with those of Berger *et al.*[14] who gave β-endorphin intravenously, whereas Gerner *et al.*[15] gave β-endorphin by infusion. The manner of administration may also affect the clinical results.

As regards the change in the β-endorphin level measured in the CSF (TABLE 3) it is striking that we observed a marked rise in level only in the three (1–3) schizophrenic syndromes accompanied by strong affective symptoms ("schizo-affective" psychosis). Since according to Foley et al.,[22] the half-life of human β-endorphin administered to humans intravenously and intracerebroventricularly is 37 and 93 minutes, respectively, it is improbable that the β-endorphin immunoactivity measured on the third day would be caused by the exogenous polypeptide. However, the possibility arises that β-endorphin introduced could stimulate the biosynthesis or release of cerebral (or hypophyseal?) β-endorphin through some, as yet unknown, mechanism. If confirmed, this observation could give a new angle to the investigation of the pathogenesis of the schizo-affective psychoses. The selective susceptibility of the schizophrenic subgroups is also an open question.[23]

In drawing our conclusions, not only the small number of patients but also the experience with the control patients point to the need for increased caution. As the example of patient 7 shows, the intravenous placebo injection can result in a transitory remission of the patient that misleadingly resembles the "temperament therapy" that can be expected from β-endorphin.

ACKNOWLEDGMENT

We are grateful to Professor C. H. Li (University of California, San Francisco) for supplying us with synthetic human β-endorphin.

REFERENCES

1. TERENIUS, L., A. WAHLSTRÖM, I. LINDSTRÖM & E. WIDERLÖV. 1976. Neurosci. Letters 3: 157–162.
2. TERENIUS, L., A. WAHLSTRÖM & L. JOHANSSON. 1979. In Endorphins in Mental Health Research. E. Usdin, W. E. Bunney & N. S. Kline, Eds.: 553–560. MacMillan Press. London.
3. GUNNE, L. M., I. LINDSTRÖM & L. TERENIUS. 1977. J. Neural. Transm. 40: 13–19.
4. DAVIS, G. C., W. E. BUNNEY, E. G. DE FRAITES, J. E. KLEINMAN, D. P. VAN KAMMEN, R. M. POST & R. J. WYATT. 1977. Science 197: 74–77.
5. JACQUET, Y. F. & N. MARKS. 1976. Science 194: 632–635.
6. DE WIED, D., G. L. KOVACS, B. BOHUS, J. M. VAN REE & H. M. GREVEN. 1978. Eur. J. Pharmacol. 49: 427–436.
7. BURBACH, J. P. H., J. G. LOEBER, J. VERHOEF, V. M. WIEGANT, E. R. KLOET & D. DE WIED. 1980. Nature 283: 96–97.
8. VEREBEY, K., J. VOLAVKA & D. CLOUET. 1978. Arch. Gen. Psychiatry 35: 877–888.
9. LI, C. H., D. YAMASHIRO, L.-F. TSENG & H. H. LOH. 1977. J. Med. Chem. 10: 325–328.
10. KLINE, N. S. & H. E. LEHMANN. 1979. In Endorphins in Mental Health Research. E. Usdin, W. E. Bunney & N. S. Kline, Eds.: 500–517. Macmillan Press. London.
11. ANGST, J., V. AUTENRIETH, F. BREM, M. KOUKKOU, H. MEYER, H. H. STASSEN & U. STOCK. 1979. In Endorphins in Mental Health Research. E. Usdin, W. E. Bunney & N. S. Kline, Eds.: 518–528. Macmillan Press. London.

12. WATSON, S. J., H. AKIL, P. A. BERGER & J. D. BARCHAS. 1979. Arch. Gen. Psychiatry **36:** 35–41.
13. PETHÖ, B., L. GRÁF, I. KARCZAG, I. BITTER, J. TOLNA, K. BARACZKA & C. H. LI. 1981. Lancet, January 24.: 212–213.
14. BERGER, P. A., S. J. WATSON, H. AKIL, G. R. ELLIOTT, R. T. RUBIN, A. PFEFFERBAUM, K. L. DAVIS, J. D. BARCHAS & C. H. LI. 1980. Arch. Gen. Psychiatry **37:** 635–640.
15. GERNER, R. H., D. H. CATLIN, D. A. GORELICK, K. S. HUI & C. H. LI. 1980. **37:** 642–647.
16. GRÁF, L., A. KENESSEY, A. PATTHY, A. GRYNBAUM, N. MARKS & A. LAJTHA. 1979. Arch. Biochem. Biophys. **193:** 101–109.
17. SZÉKELY, J. I., A. Z. RÓNAI, Z. DUNAI-KOVÁCS, E. MIGLECZ, I. BERZÉTEI, S. BAJUSZ & L. GRÁF. 1977. Eur. J. Pharmacol. **43:** 293–294.
18. OVERALL, J. E., B. W. HENRY & J. R. MARKETT. 1972. Psychiat. Res. **9:** 87–99.
19. BORVENDEG, J., L. GRÁF, I. HERMANN, M. PALKOVITS & K. MERETEY. 1978. *In* Endorphins '78. L. Gráf, M. Palkovits & A. Z. Ronai, Eds.: 177–186. Akademiai Kiado. Budapest.
20. EMRICH, H. W., C. CORDING & S. PIREE. 1977. Pharmakopsychiatr. Neuropsychopharmakol. **10:** 265–270.
21. OYAMA, T., T. FIN, R. YAMAYA, N. LING & R. GUILLEMIN. 1980. Lancet, January 19: 122.
22. FOLEY, K. M., I. A. KOURIDES, C. E. INTURRISI, R. F. KAIKO, C. G. ZAROULIS, J. B. POSNER, R. W. HOUDE & C. H. LI. 1979. Proc. Natl. Acad. Sci. USA **76:** 5377–5381.
23. VAN PRAAG, H. M. & W. M. A. VERHOEVEN. 1981. Comprehensive Psychiat. **22:** 125–146.
24. LEONHARD, K. 1979. The Classification of Endogenous Psychoses. Irvington. New York.
25. PERRIS, C. 1974. Cycloid Psychosis. Munksgaard. Copenhagen.

CLINICAL TRIAL OF DES-TYROSYL-γ-ENDORPHIN IN MENTAL ILLNESS

H. M. Emrich,* M. Zaudig, W. Kissling,† G. Dirlich,
D. v. Zerssen, and A. Herz

*Max-Planck-Institut für Psychiatrie
Munich, Federal Republic of Germany
† Klinikum rechts der Isar der Technischen Universität
Munich, Federal Republic of Germany*

INTRODUCTION

The therapeutic risks (namely, the development of an irreversible dyskinetic syndrome, i.e. tardive dyskinesia,[1, 2] severe leukopenic reactions,[3] and the neuroleptic malignant syndrome [4]) in a few patients in addition to the subjectively uncomfortable side effects (sedation, dyskinesia, etc.) associated with conventional neuroleptic therapy emphasize that one cannot be satisfied with the pharmacotherapeutic arsenal presently used in the treatment of schizophrenic psychoses. A challenging concept, introduced by de Wied,[5] suggests that schizophrenia results from a metabolic defect in the decomposition of γ-endorphin, insofar as the non-opioid derivatives of γ-endorphin (DTγE, DEγE [6]) are regarded as "endogenous neuroleptics." The idea of a deficiency of these in schizophrenics, based on animal experiments demonstrating neuroleptic-like effects of γ-endorphin (in particular, its des-tyrosyl derivative [7]) in several animal tests, prompted therapeutic trials as to a possible antipsychotic efficacy of DTγE in schizophrenic patients. The sensational reports of van Praag's and de Wied's groups,[8, 9] documented a strong antipsychotic effect of daily doses of 1 mg DTγE (i.m.), initially in an open trial in six schizophrenic patients, and subsequently in a double-blind placebo-controlled investigation in eight patients with schizophrenic psychoses. These findings demanded replication in view of the highly interesting practical and theoretical implications of the concept.

REVIEW

Reevaluative therapeutic investigations as to a possible antipsychotic action of DTγE have, so far, been performed by Bourgeois et al.,[10] Emrich et al.,[11, 12] Manchanda and Hirsch,[13] Casey et al.,[14] Busch et al.,[15] Metz et al.,[16] and Tamminga et al.[17] Unpublished data have been collected by the groups of P. Berger, M. Fink, and L. Sjöström. TABLE 1 provides an overview of the type of studies performed and the therapeutic results obtained in these investigations. The therapeutic trial performed by Bourgeois et al.[10] represents a multicenter collaborative investigation of the effects of 1.0-2.0 mg DTγE, i.m. (daily for 5–12 days) in 15 schizophrenic patients. The study was

* Supported by a grant (Heisenberg-Programm) of the Deutsche Forschungsgemeinschaft.

0077–8923/82/0398–0470 $01.75/0 © 1982, NYAS

TABLE 1

REPLICATION STUDIES ON THE EFFECT OF DTγE IN SCHIZOPHRENIA

Authors	Acute Cases	Chronic Cases	Type of Study	Results
Bourgeois *et al.*[10]	—	15	open/single-blind	2 slight improvements
Emrich *et al.*[11, 12]	6	7	double-blind, placebo-controlled	6 improvements (4 in acute, 2 in chronic cases)
Manchanda & Hirsch[13]	6	5	open	2 improvements in acute cases
(Casey *et al.*[14]	—	10	open	no change within 24 hrs) *
Busch *et al.*[15]	2	6	open	1 marked improvement in an acute case, 1 marked and 1 moderate improvement in 2 chronic cases
Tamminga *et al.*[17]	—	5	double-blind, placebo-controlled	very slight reduction in BPRS total scores
Fink *et al.* (personal communication)	7	—	double-blind, placebo-controlled	3 improvements
	21	38 (48)		6 improvements in 38 (48) chronic cases (15.8%) 10 improvements in 21 acute cases

* short-term application of DTγE

performed in a partially open, partially single-blind design. All patients suffered from chronic schizophrenia and neuroleptic treatment was continued during the trial. Two of the 15 patients (evaluated by use of the BPRS) showed a slight improvement.

The investigation of Manchanda and Hirsch,[13] represents an open study in schizophrenic patients (nuclear schizophrenia: n = 5; catatonic schizophrenia: n = 2; schizophrenia without first rank symptoms: n = 1; paranoid psychosis: n = 1; schizoaffective psychosis: n = 2). The patients were treated with daily doses of 1.0–2.0 mg DTγE for 12 days. Five of the 10 patients who com-

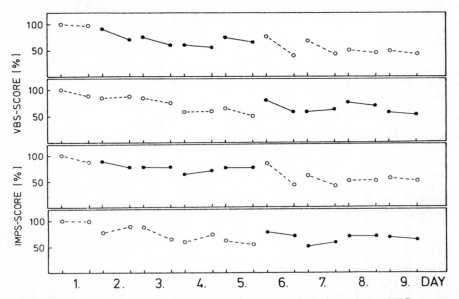

FIGURE 1. *Top*: Course of mean values of psychopathological scores (VBS course assessment scale [26] of the 13 schizophrenic patients treated with 2.0 mg DTγE for 4 days. *Open circles*: placebo, *dots*: DTγE. *Upper half*: 6 patients with DTγE phase prior to placebo phase; *lower half*: 7 patients with placebo phase prior to DTγE phase. Data normalized to initial values.

Bottom: Course of mean values of IMPS-subscales PCP, PAR, GRN, EXC, HOS. Symbols as in the upper part.

pleted the trial had an acute episode of their psychosis. All patients were evaluated by use of the Present State Examination (PSE [18, 19]), the Brief Psychiatric Rating Scale (BPRS [20]), the Manchester Scale,[21] and a nurses' rating scale. One patient showed an overall improvement of psychotic symptomatology, another patient lost hallucinations, delusions, and depressive symptoms and became hypomanic. Both patients who improved belonged to the subgroup of patients with an acute episode of their psychosis. Casey *et al.*,[14] similarly using an open type of design, administered 4.0–16.0 mg DTγE (i.m.) to 10 chronic schizophrenic patients. They observed no change in the psychotic status during a 24-hour post-injection assessment period employing the Comprehensive Psychiatric Rating Scale (CPRS [22]). In this trial, furthermore, no influence of DTγE upon the symptoms of tardive dyskinesia were observed. Tamminga *et al.*,[17] in a further study employing DTγE, investigated the effects of 0.5-2.0 mg DTγE daily over 8 days upon five patients with chronic schizophrenia by use of a placebo-controlled double-blind design. These patients, free of neuroleptic drugs for at least 8 days, had received, prior to the investigation, long-term neuroleptic treatment for a minimum of 5 years. Psychopathological evaluation, performed by use of the BPRS [20] and the Psychosis Change Scale,[23] revealed only a very slight reduction in the BPRS total score, not attributable to the psychotic symptomatology, since the BPRS psychosis subscale showed no difference at all during the course of the trial. The data are interpreted by the authors to reflect fluctuations in anxiety. In an open study using 1.0–5.0 mg DTγE i.m. (daily over 10 days), Busch *et al.*[15] observed in two of four patients exhibiting a recent exacerbation of their psychosis a clear clinical improvement, and a slight improvement in psychotic symptomatology and social functioning upon DTγE treatment in the others. Furthermore, Metz *et al.*,[16] belonging to the same group of investigators, observed a significant reduction of secondary facilitation of the H-reflex recovery curve upon DTγE treatment of eight schizophrenic patients (1.0–10.0 mg/d for 12 days). This result is similar to the effects observed after treatment with classical neuroleptic drugs; therefore, a similar pharmacological action of DTγE and of neuroleptics was suggested. Comparative *in vitro/in vivo* studies, recently performed on ³H-spiperone-binding in the corpus striatum and nucleus accumbens of the rat,[24] demonstrated evidence for an indirect DTγE-induced inhibition of central dopaminergic activity, whereas, on the contrary, a direct *in vitro* effect of DTγE upon dopamine receptors was lacking.

Employing a sequential design (daily doses of 1.0 mg DTγE over a period of 21 days) L. Sjöström treated three pairs of schizophrenic patients (DTγE vs. placebo) and observed a more pronounced improvement under DTγE. Fink *et al.* (personal communication), furthermore, applying daily doses of 1.0 mg DTγE for 6–15 days in seven patients with recurrent schizophrenia, by use of a placebo-controlled design, observed improvement in three cases.

The investigations as to the possible antipsychotic effects of DTγE, performed at the Max-Planck-Institute for Psychiatry, included, by use of a placebo-controlled cross-over design, 13 schizophrenic patients undergoing continuous neuroleptic therapy. All these patients exhibited productive psychotic symptomatology (e.g., hallucinations, acute delusions), seven of them in a chronic course and five in an acute course of frequently relapsing psychoses. In one further acute case the differential diagnosis of an exacerbation of chronic schizophrenia was obtained. A single-blind placebo period of 1 day (intramuscular injection at 1100 h) was followed by two double-blind treatment periods of 4 days each, with intramuscular injections of either 2.0 mg DTγE or placebo at 1100 h. Informed consent was obtained from the patients and/or close relatives. No adverse psychic or somatic effects were observed during the course of the trial. Psychopathological assessment was performed at 1100 h (before injection) and at 1500 h throughout the 9 days of the study by the Inpatient Multidimensional Psychiatric Scale (IMPS [25]) and the Verlaufs-Beurteilungs-Skala (VBS [26]), the latter an eight-point rating scale that can be adapted to reflect particular psychotic symptoms in individual patients.

Analysis of the results in all 13 patients, a selection of types similar to these of Verhoeven *et al.*,[8, 9] showed that placebo and DTγE reduced symptoms to approximately the same degree (FIG. 1). The majority of the curves showed a tendency towards an improvement and did not differ in steepness (in the average of all 13 patients of the study) during the DTγE as compared to placebo periods.

A comparative analysis of the data derived from chronic and acute cases, however, revealed a different pattern of results: if an improvement in the scores over 4 days of DTγE treatment of more than 20% (after correction

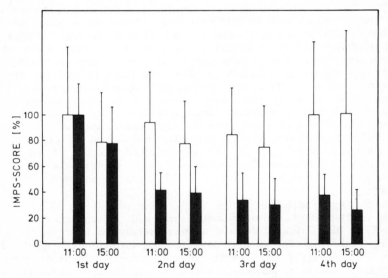

FIGURE 2. Course of mean IMPS-scores in 5 acute cases during DTγE/placebo treatment, normalized to initial values. *Open columns*: placebo; *shaded columns*: DTγE. *Bars*: S.E.M.

for individual placebo effect) is regarded as a positive DTγE response, only two patients in the group of seven chronic cases were DTγE responders, whereas in the group of six acute cases, four patients were classified as apparently responding to the drug. It may, thus, be hypothesized that the probability of a response is greater in acute cases than in cases of chronic schizophrenia. A quantitative comparative analysis of the results obtained from chronic and acute cases is possible only if the data of the DTγE treatment phases and of the placebo phases are pooled, irrespective of their sequence within the trial. Such a comparison is shown in FIGURE 2. The (normalized) mean IMPS-data (the sum scores of psychosis-specific subscales PCP + PAR + GRN + EXC + HOS) of the five acute cases show a pronounced tendency towards an improvement after DTγE treatment, whereas placebo apparently has no effect. The differences between treatment and placebo are statistically significant on days 2, 3, and 4 in both scales (VBS and IMPS; Wilcoxon-test: p < 0.05). However, the application of statistical tests to *post hoc* classification is not, perhaps, absolutely justified. The results can, therefore, only be regarded as an indication of the desirability for a replication of the study.

DISCUSSION

As shown in the present review, a corroboration of the provocative novel concept of de Wied's group concerning the antipsychotic efficacy of the proposed endogenous neuroleptic DTγE has not been achieved as concerns chronic schizophrenic patients. However, since chronic schizophrenia possibly represents a peculiar subgroup of psychoses, a reevaluation of possible antipsychotic effects of DTγE/DEγE in acute types of psychoses appears most necessary. The data, acquired in our own study, and those revealed in a review of literature, lead to the assumption that there may be some therapeutic efficacy of DTγE in acute cases and that it is much higher than in chronic schizophrenia where out of a total number of 38 cases, only 6 exhibited a slight DTγE response. This finding of the present evaluation suggests that it may be legitimate for a further effort to be made to explore the possible antipsychotic activity of DTγE/DEγE in acute schizophrenia, a strategy suggested theoretically as well as practically in view of the fascinating conundrum of the role of opioid and non-opioid peptides in the normal and abnormal functioning of the brain.

ACKNOWLEDGMENTS

For the supply of DTγE our thanks are due to Drs. R. M. Pigache and S. Krempl of Organon International, Holland and Germany.

REFERENCES

1. CHOUINARD, G., L. ANNABLE, A. ROSS-CHOUINARD & J. N. NESTOROS. 1979. Factors related to tardive dyskinesia. Am. J. Psychiatry **136:** 79–83.
2. DEGKWITZ, R. & O. LUXENBURGER. 1965. Das terminale extrapyramidale Insuffizienz- bzw. Defektsyndrom infolge chronischer Anwendung von Neuroleptics. Nervenarzt **36:** 173–175.
3. DUKES, M. N. G. 1981. Side Effects of Drugs. Annual 5. Excerpta Medica. Amsterdam.
4. CAROFF, S. N. 1980. The neuroleptic malignant syndrome. J. Clin. Psychiat. **41:** 79–83.
5. WIED, D. DE. 1979. Schizophrenia as an inborn error in the degradation of β-endorphin—a hypothesis. Trends Neurosci. **2:** 79–82.
6. REE, J. M. VAN, W. M. A. VERHOEVEN, H. M. VAN PRAAG & D. DE WIED. 1981. Neuroleptic-like and antipsychotic effect of γ-type endorphins. *In* The Role of Endorphins in Neuropsychiatry (Mod. Probl. Pharmacopsychiat.). H. M. Emrich, Ed. Vol. 17.: 266–278. Karger. Basel.

7. WIED, D. DE, G. L. KOVACS, B. BOHUS, J. M. VAN REE & H. M. GREVEN. 1978. Neuroleptic activity of the neuropeptide β-LPH$_{62-77}$ ([des-Tyr^1]-γ-endorphin; DTγE). Eur. J. Pharmacol. **49:** 427–436.

8. VERHOEVEN, W. M. A., H. M. VAN PRAAG, P. A. BOTTER, A. SUNIER, J. M. VAN REE & D. DE WIED. 1978. [Des-tyr^1]-γ-endorphin in schizophrenia. Lancet i: 1046–1047.

9. VERHOEVEN, W. M. A., H. M. VAN PRAAG, J. M. VAN REE & D. DE WIED. 1979. Improvement of schizophrenic patients treated with [des-Tyr^1]-γ-endorphin (DTγ-E). Arch. Gen. Psychiatry **36:** 294–298.

10. BOURGEOIS, M., E. LAFORGE, J. MUYARD, J. BLAYAC & J. LEMOINE. 1980. Endorphines et schizophrénies. II. Les essais de traitement des schizophrénies. Ann. Méd. Psych. **138:** 1112–1119.

11. EMRICH, H. M., M. ZAUDIG, D. V. ZERSSEN, A. HERZ & W. KISSLING. 1980. Des-tyr^1-γ-endorphin in schizophrenia. Lancet ii: 1364–1365.

12. EMRICH, H. M., M. ZAUDIG, W. KISSLING, G. DIRLICH, D. V. ZERSSEN & A. HERZ. 1980. Des-tyrosyl-γ-endorphin in schizophrenia: A double-blind trial in 13 patients. Pharmakopsychiatrie **13:** 290–298.

13. MANCHANDA, R. & S. R. HIRSCH. 1981. (Des-Tyr^1)-γ-endorphin in the treatment of schizophrenia. Psychol. Med. **11:** 401–404.

14. CASEY, D. E., S. KORSGAARD, J. GERLACH, A. JÖRGENSEN & H. SIMMELGAARD. 1981. Effect of des-tyrosine-γ-endorphin in tardive dyskinesia. Arch. Gen. Psychiatry **38:** 158–160.

15. BUSCH, D. A., B. J. TRICOU, A. ROBERTON & H. Y. MELTZER. 1982. Effect of (des-tyr)-γ-endorphin in schizophrenia. Psychiatry Res. In press.

16. METZ, J., D. A. BUSCH & H. Y. MELTZER. 1981. Des-tyrosine-γ-endorphin: H-reflex response similar to neuroleptics. Life Sci. **28:** 2003–2008.

17. TAMMINGA, C. A., P. J. TIGHE, T. N. CHASE, E. G. DEFREITES & M. H. SCHAFFER. 1981. Des-tyrosine-γ-endorphin administration in chronic schizophrenics. Arch. Gen. Psychiatry **38:** 167–168.

18. WING, J. K., J. E. COOPER & N. SARTORIUS. 1974. The Measurement and Classification of Psychiatric Symptoms. Cambridge University Press. London.

19. WING, J. K., J. M. NIXON, S. A. MANN & J. P. LEFF. 1977. Reliability of the PSE (9th ed.) used in a population study. Psychol. Med. **7:** 505–516.

20. OVERALL, J. E. & D. R. GORHAM. 1962. The brief psychiatric rating scale. Psychol. Rep. **10:** 799–812.

21. KRAWIECKA, M., D. GOLDBERG & M. VAUGHAN. 1977. A standardised psychiatric assessment scale for rating chronic psychotic patients. Acta Psychiat. Scand. **55:** 299–308.

22. ÅSBERG, M., S. A. MONTGOMERY, C. PERRIS, D. SCHALLING & G. SEDVALL. 1978. A comprehensive psychopathological rating scale. Acta Psychiat. Scand., Suppl. **271:** 5–27.

23. TAMMINGA, C. A., M. H. SCHAFFER, R. C. SMITH & J. M. DAVIS. 1978. Apomorphine improves schizophrenic symptoms. Science **200:** 567–568.

24. YAMADA, S., E. HAYASHI, N. W. PEDIGO, H. SCHOEMAKER & H. I. YAMAMURA. 1982. Neurochemical studies of des-tyrosine-γ-endorphin, a proposed endogenous neuroleptic. In Psychobiology of Schizophrenia. M. Namba and H. Kaiya, Eds.: 165–171. Pergamon Press. Oxford.

25. LORR, M., C. J. KLETT, D. M. NCNAIR & J. J. LASKY. 1962. Inpatient Multidimensional Psychiatric Scale. Consulting Psychologists Press. Palo Alto, CA.

26. EMRICH, H. M., C. CORDING, S. PIREE, A. KÖLLING, D. V. ZERSSEN & A. HERZ. 1977. Indication of an antipsychotic action of the opiate antagonist naloxone. Pharmakopsychiat. **10:** 265–270.

DISCUSSION OF THE PAPER

J. PLESS (*Sandoz Ltd., Basel, Switzerland*): If one administers peptides into the body, a large amount of compound is of course present in the peripheral system, giving rise to all kind of desired and undesired peripheral effects. On the other hand, owing to the poor penetration into the CNS the low concentration of peptides in this region will not cause significant CNS effects such as analgesia. Between these two extreme situations, namely, saturated periphery and unsufficient concentration in CNS of exogenously given peptide drug, there is the region of hypothalamus-pituitary. In this case the protection by the blood-brain barrier is not complete, in fact the existing fenestration permits a moderate penetration into the area even for peptides, causing a variety of endocrine effects. I think that great part of the episodical and unclear CNS activities by peptides found in literature are indirect and are rather consequences of peripheral or hypothalamic-pituitary effects. Peptides are not ideal substrates for CNS activities.

THE USE OF THE SYNTHETIC PEPTIDES γ-TYPE ENDORPHINS IN MENTALLY ILL PATIENTS

Jan M. van Ree,* Wim M. A. Verhoeven,† David de Wied,*
and Herman M. van Praag †

* Rudolf Magnus Institute for Pharmacology
† Department of Psychiatry
Medical Faculty, University of Utrecht
3521 GD Utrecht, the Netherlands

The discovery of peptides with opiate-like activity in pituitary and brain tissue initiated several hypotheses that implicated the endorphins in psychopathology such as schizophrenia. From these, three main hypotheses were formulated: endorphin excess, endorphin deficiency, and changes in β-endorphin fragmentation. The endorphin excess postulate stems from the findings showing an increased level of endorphins in cerebrospinal fluid (CSF) of schizophrenic patients [1] and a catatonia-like syndrome following injection of β-endorphin (β-LPH_{61-91}) into the CSF of rats.[2] This excess hypothesis was tested in schizophrenic patients using opiate antagonists and hemodialysis. It was found that about 25–30% of the patients responded to treatment with opiate antagonists, in that auditory hallucinations in particular diminished or disappeared for about 2–6 hours after injection.[3–5] In some schizophrenic patients a remission of symptomatology was observed following hemodialysis although others have questioned this finding.[6] The endorphin deficiency hypothesis originated from the observation that injection of β-endorphin into the periaqueductal gray of the rat brain stem caused a neuroleptic-like syndrome [7] and from some earlier reports about beneficial effects of opiates in schizophrenia. Clinical studies in which β-endorphin or the highly potent enkephalin analog FK 33–824 was administered to schizophrenic patients, indeed show some decrease of symptomatology following treatment with these endorphins [8–10] (for further references see ref. 11). However, the response to β-endorphin was not impressive and that to FK 33–824 was accompanied by morphine-like side effects.

The present paper deals with the third postulate, namely changes in β-endorphin fragmentation, particularly a deficiency in the generation of γ-type endorphins in schizophrenia.

To the γ-Type Endorphin Hypothesis

β-Endorphin induced typical morphine-like effects in animals (for ref. see 11) and additionally exhibits effects that are apparently not mediated by brain opiate receptors. Thus, extinction of pole jumping avoidance behavior was delayed by a single subcutaneous injection with β-endorphin and this effect persisted in the presence of naltrexone.[12] This action of β-endorphin was mimicked by the β-endorphin fragments α-endorphin (β-LPH_{61-76}), β-LPH_{61-69} and Met-enkephalin (β-LPH_{61-65}). α-Endorphin was found to be the most potent peptide in this respect.[12] γ-Endorphin (β-LPH_{61-77}) had

0077–8923/82/0398–0478 $01.75/0 © 1982, NYAS

an opposite effect on this behavior in that it facilitated extinction of pole jumping avoidance behavior of ras made resistant to extinction.[13] Also this effect could be differentiated from the opiate-like effects of γ-endorphin. The non-opiate-like γ-endorphin fragment, (des-Tyr[1])-γ-endorphin (DTγE, β-LPH$_{62-77}$) induced an effect similar to that of γ-endorphin and was even more potent.[13] Since impaired acquisition and facilitated extinction of conditioned avoidance behavior are characteristic for neuroleptic activity, the behavioral effects of DTγE were further explored and compared to those of the classical neuroleptic haloperidol. It was found that both DTγE and haloperidol attenuated passive avoidance behavior [13, 14] and were active in various grip tests.[13] Subcutaneous treatment with haloperidol caused in addition immobility, extension of the lower limbs, and ptosis. These effects of haloperidol were less pronounced following intracerebroventricular administration of this drug.[13] These observations led to the postulate that DTγE, or a closely related neuropeptide, is an endogenous neuroleptic with a profile more specific than that of currently used neuroleptic drugs and that an inborn error in the generation or metabolism of this peptide from β-endorphin might be an pathogenetic factor in psychopathological states for which neuroleptic drugs are beneficial.[15]

The first question that was raised was whether the neuroleptic-like activity of γ-type endorphins was limited to DTγE. Structure-activity relationship studies in which several γ-endorphin fragments were tested on extinction of pole jumping avoidance behavior and on activity in two grip tests, used as measures of neuroleptic-like activity, revealed that (des-enkephalin)-γ-endorphin (DEγE, β-LPH$_{66-77}$) is the shortest sequence with activity similar to DTγE.[16] β-LPH$_{67-77}$ was less active and β-LPH$_{66-76}$, which belongs to the α-type endorphin, was not active or induced even an opposite effect. That DEγE might be the active moiety mediating the neuroleptic-like activity of γ-type endorphins was confirmed by the finding that this but not shorter pepides antagonized certain behavioral effects of apomorphine (see below).

The second question concerned the presence and generation of these peptides in the body. Using high pressure liquid chromatography (HPLC) to separate the several related peptides and different radioimmunoassays to measure the amount of the peptides in the collected HPLC fractions, the β-endorphin fragments, γ-endorphin, DTγE, DEγE, α-endorphin and (des-Tyr[1])-α-endorphin (DTαE) were found in rat pituitary and brain,[17] in guinea pig ilea,[18] in human CSF,[19] and recently in human brain (Wiegant *et al.*, unpublished data). The levels are susceptible to change. For example, it was found that chronic exposure of guinea pigs or their ilea to morphine resulted in an increased level of the various β-endorphin fragments.[18] In addition, the fragmentation of β-endorphin *in vitro* was studied by incubating brain synaptosomal membrane (SPM) fractions with β-endorphin. The generation of γ-endorphin, DTγE, α-endorphin, and DTαE was established.[20] The fragmentation pattern appeared to be dependent on the pH of the incubation medium: when the pH was 6.7 accumulation of γ-endorphin and DTγE was found and when the pH was 5.9, especially α-endorphin, but also γ-endorphin and DTαE accumulated. This may suggest that the fragmentation pattern of β-endorphin depends on the activity of the different enzyme systems, involved in the conversion of β-endorphin to biologically active peptides. That the activity of these enzymes is susceptible to change can also be concluded from the finding that in membrane preparations of morphine-tolerant guinea pig ilea the accumulation of γ-endorphin, α-endorphin and DTαE was enhanced as compared to those of control ilea.[21] Incubation of brain SPM with DTγE, revealed that DEγE was one of the main accumulated peptides.[22] Thus, the brain and other tissues contain the γ-endorphin fragments DTγE and DEγE and have enzyme systems that can generate these fragments from β-endorphin and which activity can be influenced by various conditions (e.g., pH change, chronic morphine exposure).

The third question dealt with the characteristics of the neuroleptic-like action of γ-type endorphins, including their mode of action as compared to that of classical and atypical neuroleptics. These studies and their implications will be discussed later (see possible mode and site of action).

To test the hypothesis that γ-type endorphins possessed antipsychotic activity, clinical trials were performed in which DTγE and DEγE was administered to schizophrenic patients (see next section).

ANTIPSYCHOTIC EFFECTS OF γ-TYPE ENDORPHINS

Our first clinical trial with DTγE was a pilot experiment in which 1 mg of the peptide was given daily for 8–14 days to six schizophrenic patients, who had psychotic symptoms despite neuroleptic medication. This maintenance medication was withdrawn 1 week before DTγE treatment, resulting in an increase of psychotic symptoms in most of the patients. Symptoms of the patients were assessed using a Patient Specific Symptom Scale (PSSS, a three point rating scale comprising the main psychopathological symptoms). The patients could be divided into two groups of three patients on the basis of their response to treatment with DTγE.[23, 24] In the first group the psychotic symptoms (e.g. hallucinations and delusions) were diminished on day 3 and 4 of treatment, but thereafter the patients relapsed and became more or less aggressive and/or agitated. The other three patients improved from day 4 of treatment and their psychotic symptoms decreased for 2 weeks after the end of DTγE treatment. A second treatment for 4 days in two of these patients about 3 weeks after the end of the first treatment, when some symptoms, although at a moderate level, had returned, resulted again in a disappearance of the symptoms. The Brief Psychiatric Rating Scale (BPRS) assessed before and after the treatment revealed a response of less than 20% in three patients and a response of about 50% in one patient, while two patients responded more than 80%.

In a subsequent trial a double blind cross-over design was followed. Eight schizophrenic patients were treated for 8 days with placebo or DTγE (1 mg i.m. once daily) followed by 8 days with DTγE or placebo. This treatment was preceded and followed by 4 days of placebo injections. The neuroleptic medication of six patients (one patient was also involved in the first trial) was maintained during experimentation; the other two patients were and remained free of neuroleptic therapy. Scoring of the symptoms was performed in a similar way as outlined for the first study. The psychotic symptoms of the patients were hardly affected by placebo treatment, but diminished on active treatment.[24] In some patients the symptoms recurred some days after DTγE medication, whereas in others the effect of DTγE persisted longer. Although all patients more or less responded, according to the PSSS, the scoring on the BPRS revealed a more differential response pattern. The response of two patients was less than 20%, in two it was between 20 and 50%, in two between 50 and 80%, and in two patients it was more than 80%. The latter patients had had a short recent psychotic episode and were free of neuroleptic medication at admission.

In the third clinical trial with DTγE, which was also performed using a double blind, cross-over design, 10 patients were treated daily with 1 mg DTγE i.m. for 10 days.[25] The neuroleptic therapy of eight patients was discontinued at least 3 weeks before the start of the trial; two patients were not treated with neuroleptics. Symptoms were rated (once daily) during and after the experimental period using the BPRS. Little decrease of the symptoms (less than 15% of baseline score) was observed during placebo treatment. Treatment with DTγE did not affect the symptoms in three patients (<20% improvement), induced a slight effect in three patients (20–50% improvement), a moderate effect in one patient (50–80% improvement), and a marked effect in three patients (>80% improvement).[25] In general, the decrease of psychotic symptoms started on days 2 to 5 of active treatment. Interestingly, two of the three patients with a marked response were not treated with neuroleptics in the 6-month period before the trial. One of these patients remained free from psychotic symptoms for more than 12 months, while the other was treated again with DTγE (3 mg i.m. daily) for 10 days about 4 weeks after the first DTγE treatment, because psychotic symptoms recurred. After this second treatment period only mild psychotic symptoms (less than 10% of BPRS baseline score) persisted. This patient has been treated with DTγE (3 mg, s.c., twice weekly) for 6 months without relapsing.

Since animal experiments revealed that DEγE is the shortest fragment of γ-endorphin with neuroleptic-like action, this peptide was tested for antipsychotic activity. In a pilot experiment (single blind design) four schizophrenic patients were treated with DEγE (1 or 10 mg. i.m. daily) for 10 days. Thereafter, in a double-blind, placebo-controlled trial 13 patients were given 10 days of DEγE treatment (3 mg i.m. daily) and 6 patients received placebo treatment. Before and after the treatment the patients received placebo injections for 5 days. The neuroleptic therapy was maintained during the trial. Symptoms of the patients were scored using the BPRS. In none of the patients was a change in BPRS score of more than 20% noted during placebo treatment.[26] Two patients did not respond to DEγE treatment (<20% change), a slight response was found in five patients (20–50% improvement), a moderate response in six patients (50–80% improvement) and a marked response in six patients (>80% improvement). In 11 patients the reduction of symptoms was temporary in that they relapsed at the end or shortly after DEγE treatment, while in 6 patients the effect for DEγE was more long lasting, in that the decrease of symptoms persisted for at least 2 weeks. In three of the latter patients a second treatment with DEγE was given 2–4 weeks after the first treatment period. Also this treatment led to a decrease of symptomatology. In two of the six patients with a more long lasting response, psychotic symptoms recurred 2 months after the last treatment with DEγE, while the other four patients remained free of psychopathological symptoms for a period of at least 6 months.

The data collected so far indicate that the γ-endorphin fragments DTγE and DEγE have an antipsychotic effect in a number of schizophrenic patients. A marked response was observed in 11 of the 40 treated patients, a moderate or slight response in 9 and 11 patients respectively, while 9 patients did not respond. The BPRS data of the third DTγE and the DEγE study were further analyzed using the five BPRS subscales. In patients who moderately or markedly responded to peptide treatment, it was found that all five groups of symptoms decreased. No marked differences in the decrease of the groups of symptoms was present, neither in terms of degree of improvement nor in that of time course.[25, 26] Thus, both the positive and negative symptoms of the schizophrenic patients [27] may be affected by γ-type endorphin treatment. That the whole schizophrenic syndrome of the responding patients improved can also be inferred from the therapeutic effect of peptide treatment as assessed with the Clinical Global Impressions Scale, which was scored at the end of active treatment in the third DTγE and the DEγE trial (TABLE 1). A fairly good relationship was found between the decrease of symptomatology as assessed with the BPRS and the therapeutic effect of treatment. Of the 40 patients treated with DTγE or DEγE, 9 patients remained free of psychotic symptoms for at least 6 months. Eight of these patients had returned to society, 4 with maintenance of neuroleptic therapy and 4 without any drug treatment. The other patient was treated with DTγE during the 6 months follow-up period. The main psychopathological data of these 9 patients are presented in TABLE 2. Eight of these patients had one or more previous admissions. Comparing the period between the last and present admission and the period after peptide treatment, it appears that:

(1) Before peptide treatment seven out of eight patients were treated with neuroleptics and after peptide treatment four out of nine patients.

(2) Before peptide treatment four patients functioned inadequately (in-

TABLE 1

THERAPEUTIC EFFECT OF γ-TYPE ENDORPHINS IN SCHIZOPHRENIC PATIENTS AS ASSESSED WITH THE CLINICAL GLOBAL IMPRESSIONS SCALE AT THE END OF ACTIVE TREATMENT *, †

	Therapeutic Effect	BPRS Response (%)			
		< 20	20–50	50–80	> 80
DTγE	worse	—	—	—	—
(n = 10)	unchanged	3	1	—	—
	minimal	—	2	—	—
	moderate	—	—	1	—
	marked	—	—	—	3
DEγE	worse	—	—	—	—
(n = 17)	unchanged	2	—	—	—
	minimal	—	3	1	—
	moderate	—	2	4	1
	marked	—	—	1	3

* This effect is compared to the maximal decrease of symptoms as assessed with the BPRS scoring.

† Of the 6 patients treated with placebo only, 5 were scored unchanged and 1 as minimally improved, while the response to the BPRS of all these patients was less than 20%.

active, no job); three patients adequately but in a half-way house (job in a protected environment); and one patient functioned on a premorbid level (job in normal society). After treatment none of the patients functioned inadequately; five patients adequately, but in a half-way house; and three patients were on a premorbid level.

(3) The mean time interval between two psychotic episodes was just before peptide treatment 1.4 years and after treatment >1.9 years; however till now only three patients have relapsed after peptide treatment.

Summarizing, the mental status of the patients was unchanged in two patients and improved in six patients when comparing the period before and that after peptide treatment. These preliminary data suggest that treatment with γ-type endorphins might have some beneficial effects on he course of illness of some schizophrenic patients who are susceptible to γ-type endorphin treatment. One patient (TABLE 2, nr. 7) had no previous admission and was only very shortly treated with neuroleptics. The course of illness and their responsiveness to DEγE is presented in detail in FIGURE 1.

Apart from a slight euphoric reaction in few patients, which may not directly be related to γ-type endorphin treatment, no side-effects of treatment with these peptides were noted. It is of particular significance that the peptides did not cause motor side effects of an extrapyramidal nature. However, it must be kept in mind that most patients were treated for 10 days only. In some patients the antipsychotic effects of γ-type endorphin treatment was even more pronounced in the period just after discontinuation of peptide treatment (see TABLE 2).

RESPONDERS VERSUS NON-RESPONDERS

Our data indicate that some patients showed a marked reduction in symptoms while others hardly responded at all to γ-type endorphin treatment. Thus, we have looked in more detail at the symptoms, illness course, and drug history in order to investigate whether the degree of response to γ-type endorphins co-varies with certain characteristics of the individual patients. The maximal response to γ-type endorphin treatment was counted as response. This was assessed by calculating the difference between the total score on the BPRS of each patient before the experimental trial (baseline score) and that at the end or during 2 weeks after active treatment. This difference was expressed as percentage of the baseline score.

Diagnosis

The diagnosis of the patients was based on the criteria as indicated by Spitzer and coworkers,[28] the course of illness,[29] and on the data obtained from the Present State Examination interview.[30] The patients were divided into various subtypes of schizophrenia as indicated by the World Health Organization (ICD-9) classification.[31] There appears to be some relation between the diagnosis and the response to γ-type endorphins (TABLE 3). In fact, patients suffering from hebephrenic type of schizophrenia responded best, followed by those suffering from the paranoid type. Less response was found in patients with a catatonic type of schizophrenia. No marked differences in this respect were observed between DTγE and DEγE. Interestingly, patients with residual schizophrenia or suffering from a schizoaffective psychosis did not respond to DTγE.

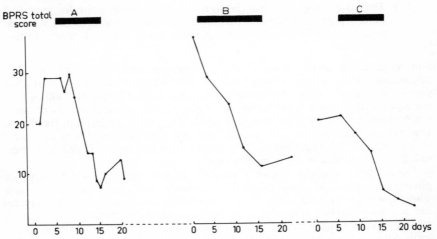

FIGURE 1. BPRS scoring of a patient treated with DEγE (no. 7, TABLE 2). The patient, a 57-year-old widow, was hospitalized for the first time because of a progressive psychotic disintegration that went on for 6 months. Since she had lost her husband 3 years ago she led a socially restricted life mostly together with her only son. At admission she described auditory and tactile hallucinations. Thinking was slightly incoherent, with thought reading, and she was preoccupied with paranoid ideas. There were delusions of grandiosity, reference, and of being influenced by radio-waves and X-rays. Her behavior was characterized by mannerisms and stereotypies. The diagnosis of schizophrenia of a paranoid type was made. She was treated with clopenthixol or haloperidol for a short period, but this treatment had to be discontinued because of severe extrapyramidal side effects. After a wash-out period of 6 weeks she was treated with DEγE (1 mg i.m. daily) for 10 days, following a single-blind design. During active treatment a progressive reduction of psychotic symptoms was observed (**A**). Emotional withdrawal and blunted affect persisted moderately. A slight relapse with mild psychotic symptoms was observed in the 2-week period after discontinuation of treatment. She was then treated with 10 mg DEγE s.c. for 10 days (single blind), during which period psychotic symptoms nearly completely disappeared in that only vague ideas of reference persisted (BPRS score: 3). Three months later she was discharged without any treatment. Control as an out-patient for 6 months did not reveal any psychotic symptoms, while social functioning was adequate. However, 2 months later she relapsed. Except for her delusions of grandiosity, the same psychotic symptoms as at the first admission were present. She was treated again with DEγE (3 mg i.m. daily, double-blind) for 15 days, after which period only a slight paranoid attitude persisted (**B**). Still in the psychiatric hospital, she relapsed 4 months later and was treated for the fourth time with DEγE (3 mg i.m. daily, single blind). Psychotic symptoms hardly changed during the initial 5-day period of placebo injections and completely disappeared during active treatment for 10 days (**C**). Two weeks later she was discharged and subsequently treated with 3 mg DEγE s.c. twice weekly. Out-patient control for 2 months did not reveal any change in her mental status.

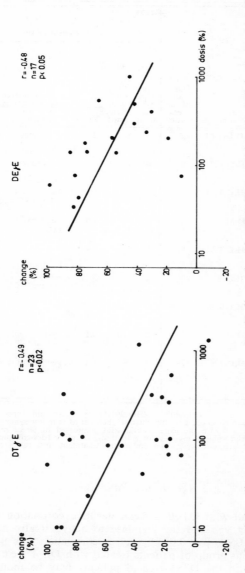

FIGURE 2. Correlation diagrams of the response to (des-Tyr¹)-γ-endorphin (DTγE) and (des-enkephalin)-γ-endorphin (DEγE) versus the dosage of neuroleptic medication. The response is given as the maximal decrease (in % of baseline score) of symptoms according to the BPRS score. The dose of neuroleptics is expressed as percentage of the mean normal dose (see TABLE 2).

TABLE 2

DATA OF PATIENTS WHO REMAINED FREE OF PSYCHOTIC SYMPTOMS FOR AT LEAST 6 MONTHS
AFTER TREATMENT WITH γ-TYPE ENDORPHINS

								Course of Illness		
No.	Sex	Age	Diagnosis*	Symptoms†	Duration of Illness (years)	Previous Admissions	Duration Last Admission (mo)	Years	Time between Last and Present Admission Medication	Functioning
1	f	19	H	H,D,T,M	2	1	5.5	1	3 dd 1 mg haloperidol (intermittent)	premorbid level
2	m	30	P	H,D,T	9	4	2	3	fluphenazine dec. 50 mg/2w	half-way house, adequate
3	m	22	H	H,D,T,M	0.5	1	2	0.25	haloperidol 2 mg/3 dd	inactive, social inadequate
4	m	36	P	D,M	7	3	3	1.5	fluphenazine dec. 75 mg/3w	inactive, social inadequate
5	m	23	P	H,D,T,M	8	5	2.5	1.4	—	inactive, social inadequate
6	f	40	P	H,D,T	7	4	6	3	perazine 100 mg/3 dd	half-way house adequate
7	f	57	P	H,D,T,M	0.75	0	—	—	—	—
8	f	20	H	H,D,T	1	2	1.5	0.1	clopenthizol 25 mg/3 dd	inactive
9	m	33	P	H,D,T	17	9	4	1.2	penfluridol 20 mg/w	private half-way house adequate

* H = hebephrenic type of schizophrenia (WHO:295.1); p = paranoid type of schizophrenia
† H = hallucinations; D = delusions; T = thought disturbances; M = motor symptoms.
‡ During the last 6 weeks before the experimental trial, expressed in % of mean normal dose
§ DTγE = (des-Tyr¹)-γ-endorphin 1 mg/day for 8-10 days; DEγE = (des-enkephalin)-γ-endorphin
¶ Time is indicated between end of γ-type endorphin treatment and relapse; > = at present

Age of the Patients

In patients treated with DTγE a weak negative correlation was observed between their present age and the response to active treatment (correlation coefficient (c.c.): -0.42, $p < 0.05$). Such a correlation was not present in the more homogeneous group of patients treated with DEγE (c.c.: 0.09). The correlation observed in the DTγE-treated patients may be induced by other factors than the age of the patients, since age was positively correlated with the duration of illness, the duration of recent psychotic episode, and the duration of previous neuroleptic therapy in the case of DTγE, but not in that of DEγE.

Previous Neuroleptic Medication		Present Admission					After Treatment		
			γ-Type Endorphin Treatment						
				Total BPRS Score					
Duration (years)	Dosage‡ (%)	Duration Psychotic Episode (mo.)	Peptide§	Baseline	End 1st Trial	14 Days After Final Treatment	Discharge Medication	Functioning	Relapse¶ (years)
1	311	4	DTγE	27	3	3	—	premorbid level	>3,6
9	114	12	DTγE (2×)	46	5	2	fluphenazine dec. 50 mg/2w	half-way house, adequate	2,2
0.4	52	0.5	DTγE	23	0	0	—	premorbid level	>3,4
4	—	0.7	DTγE	29	13	2	—	premorbid level	1,3
0.5	—	2	DTγE (2×)	42	18	4	DTγE for 6 months 3 mg/2xw	resocialization in hospital adequate	>1,6
7	133	5	DEγE (10 mg)	22	6	3	flupenthizol dec. 40 mg/3w	private/half-way house adequate	>1,6
0.25	174	7	DEγE (1&10 mg) (2×)	29	7	3	—	premorbid level	0,9
0.5	56	0.5	DEγE (2×) (3 mg)	18	4	0	haloperidol 5 mg/3dd	private/half-way house adequate	>0,8
10	40	3	DEγE (3 mg)	18	9	3	penfluridol 20 mg/w	private half-way house adequate	>1.2

(WHO:295.3).

recommended for this type psychosis.
1 or 3 or 10 mg/day for 10 days; Some patients were treated twice (:2×).
(1-11-81) no relapse.

Duration of Illness

The first symptoms of the patients were taken as starting point to determine the duration of illness. This duration was negatively correlated with the response to DTγE, but not with that to DEγE (c.c.: −0.56, p < 0.02, and −0.14, respectively). Since this item was also correlated with age, duration of recent psychotic episode, and the duration of previous neuroleptic therapy, in the case of DTγE, other factors may be involved. Moreover, the distribution of the data with DTγE indicated a deviation from the normal distribution.

TABLE 3

MAXIMAL DECREASE (IN %) OF SYMPTOMS ACCORDING TO BPRS-SCORE AT THE END OR DURING 2 WEEKS AFTER (DES-TYR^1)-γ-ENDORPHIN (DTγE) OR (DES-ENKEPHALIN)-γ-ENDORPHIN (DEγE) OR PLACEBO TREATMENT OF PATIENTS SUFFERING FROM DIFFERENT SCHIZOPHRENIC PSYCHOSES

Treatment	Diagnosis	WHO Classification	Number of Patients	Response (%)				Mean ± SEM
				<20	20–50	50–80	>80	
DTγE	hebephrenic type	295.1	2	—	—	—	2	94.5 ± 5.5
	catatonic type	295.2	3	—	3	—	—	39.2 ± 5.6
	paranoid type	295.3	11	—	3	3	5	66.4 ± 8.0
	residual schizophrenia *	295.6	3	3	—	—	—	8.6 ± 9.2
	schizoaffective type	295.7	4	4	—	—	—	16.0 ± 2.2
	all diagnoses		23	7	6	3	7	49.0 ± 7.0
DEγE	hebephrenic type	295.1	1	—	—	—	1	100.0
	catatonic type	295.2	5	1	3	1	—	40.8 ± 5.9
	paranoid type	295.3	11	1	2	5	3	62.2 ± 7.2
	all diagnoses		17	2	5	6	4	55.4 ± 6.1
Placebo			6	6	—	—	—	9.8 ± 3.0

* Patients had been in a psychiatric hospital for at least 5 years.

Duration of Recent Psychotic Episode

This duration was negatively correlated with the response to DTγE as well as to DEγE (c.c.: −0.50, p < 0.02 and −0.54, p < 0.05, respectively). Although this item was positively correlated with other analyzed variables and its distribution deviated from the normal one in the case of DTγE, these factors were not present in the patients treated with DEγE. Thus, a long duration of recent psychotic episode may lead to less responsiveness to γ-type endorphins.

Dosage and Duration of Previous Neuroleptic Medication

The dosage of neuroleptics during the last 6 weeks before the start of the trial was expressed as percentage of the mean dose, recommended for this type of psychosis.[32] In the case of DTγE, both the dosage and the duration of neuroleptic therapy was negatively correlated with the response to active treatment (c.c.: −0.49, p < 0.02 and −0.42, p < 0.05, respectively), while with DEγE only a negative correlation was observed with the dosage of neuroleptics (c.c.: −0.48, p < 0.05 and −0.36 respectively) (FIG. 1). Thus, especially a high dosage of neuroleptic therapy seems to make the patient less susceptible to γ-type endorphin treatment.

The outcome of these analyses suggests that a beneficial effect of γ-type endorphins can be expected in patients whose most recent psychotic episode is short and who are without medication or treated with a low dose of neuroleptic drugs. This accords well with findings of others that DTγE is more effective in acute schizophrenia than in chronic schizophrenia (see refs. 33–36, and Metz *et al.*, this volume). One might speculate about the special influence of the dosage of neuroleptic medication and the duration of last psychotic episode on the response to γ-type endorphins. It may be that these peptides are not effective in those patients who are rather insensitive to neuroleptic drugs and consequently had received high doses of these drugs and had a long duration of last psychotic episode. Another possibility is that high doses of neuroleptics and/or a long psychotic episode may disturb functional brain systems temporarily or perhaps even permanently and that as the result the interaction of γ-type endorphins with its substrate is less effective. Before more definite conclusions can be drawn in this respect, it seems necessary to have more knowledge about the mode of neuroleptic-like action of γ-type endorphins.

POSSIBLE MODE AND SITE OF ACTION

The neuroleptic-like action of γ-type endorphins was based on the similarities between the effects of these peptides and those of haloperidol on extinction of pole jumping avoidance behavior and on passive avoidance behavior and because both entities induce a grasping response.[13, 14] This latter response may be regarded as a physiological form of catalepsy.[37] Accordingly, bilateral lesions of the nucleus parafascicular of the thalamus induced a grasping response similar to that observed with γ-type endorphins.[38]

To further explore the neuroleptic-like actions of the peptides, experiments were performed that were focused on brain dopamine (DA). It has been suggested that a hyperactivity of brain DA systems plays a key role in the pathogenesis of schizophrenia.[39–42]

Most currently used neuroleptic drugs are potent blockers of DA activity.[43] Thus, in the first place the possible interaction of DTγE with DA binding sites was investigated. It was found that DTγE, in contrast to classical neuroleptics, did not interfere with the binding of DA-agonists and antagonists to brain homogenates *in vitro*.[44, 45] However, injections of DTγE led to a reduction of *in vivo* spiperone binding, suggesting that this peptide may indirectly affect DA receptor systems.[46]

Second, DTγE and DEγE, like neuroleptics, increased brain DA turnover.[47, 48] The action of the peptides was however less widespread in the brain and limited to some regions, particularly those innervated by the intradiencephalic DA systems. An increase in brain dopamine activity may be the underlying cause of the DTγE-induced decrease of plasma prolactin levels observed in patients [25] and under certain conditions in rats,[49] since the release of prolactin from the pituitary is under the inhibitory control of dopamine.[50]

Third, the intracranial electrical self-stimulation (ICSS) procedure was used. It was found that DTγE decreased the self-stimulation rate of animals with electrodes in the ventral tegmental-medial substantia nigra area, where the cell bodies of the mesolimbic DA pathways are located.[51] Similar effects were found for haloperidol. However, DTγE was effective especially when threshold currents were presented to the rats, while haloperidol was similarly effective at high current intensities. DTγE and haloperidol affected in the same way ICSS when the electrodes were implanted in the nucleus accumbens region [52] suggesting that the site of action of DTγE in this respect may be in the terminal region of the mesolimbic DA system.

Fourth, the interaction of γ-type endorphins with the effects of DA agonists was studied. Neuroleptic drugs attenuate the effects of the directly or indirectly acting DA-mimetics (e.g. apomorphine and amphetamine, respectively). Amphetamine and relatively high doses of apomorphine induce stereotypy and increase locomotion. In contrast, low doses of apomorphine result in hypoactivity and sedation. These differential effects of apomorphine have among others served to underline the concept of multiple DA receptor systems. Besides D1, D2, D3, and D4 dopamine receptors [53] and DAi versus DAe receptors,[54] pre- and postsynaptically located DA receptor systems have been proposed,[55] which have an opposite effect, namely, decreasing and increasing DA activity, and which may explain the opposite effects of low and high doses of apomorphine. Interestingly, systemic administration of γ-type endorphins (DTγE and DEγE) dose-dependently antagonized the hypoactivity induced by low doses of apomorphine, but had no effect on the stereotypy elicited by high doses of apomorphine or by amphetamine.[56] Thus, these peptides act directly or indirectly as antagonist on DA receptor systems, presumably located presynaptically and sensitive to low doses of apomorphine. Also others have suggested an action of DTγE on presynaptic DA receptor systems.[57, 58] Chronic treatment with DA antagonists leads to supersensitivity of post- as well as presynaptically located DA receptors.[59, 60] In rats treated subcutaneously with DEγE for 4 days the hypoactivity induced by apomorphine was enhanced, suggesting that repeated injection with this peptide leads to supersensitivity of γ-type endorphin–sensitive DA receptor systems.[56]

Fifth, the site of action of γ-type endorphins in the brain was investigated using a microinjection procedure. Most injections were done in the nucleus accumbens area, since DA systems in this area may be concerned in schizophrenia.[61] Moreover, ICSS from this area is affected by DTγE and DA systems in this area are implicated in the effects of apomorphine on locomotion (for ref. see 62). It was observed that microgram amounts of DTγE injected into the accumbal area attenuated the ACTH-induced excessive grooming. Similar effects were found following microinjection with DA-antagonists.[63] Also the phenylphenidate-induced hyperactivity was inhibited by high doses of DTγE when both entities were injected into the nucleus accumbens.[58] Intra-accumbal injection of picogram amounts of γ-type endorphins mimics the action of systemic administration of these peptides on passive avoidance behavior.[64] Low doses of apomorphine (1–100 ng) injected into the nucleus accumbens induced hypoactivity.[65] This action of apomorphine was dose-dependently antagonized by local injection with DEγE (10–100 pg). A similar antagonism was found following intra-accumbal injection with the classical neuroleptic haloperidol (10 pg) and the atypical neuroleptics sulpiride (10 pg) and clozapine (100 ng).[62] Thus, γ-type endorphins as well as classical and atypical neuroleptics induce the same effect in this respect, which may be of relevance for the antipsychotic action of these entities. As observed after systemic injection, subchronic treatment with DEγE into the nucleus accumbens for 4 days led to an enhanced response to low doses of apomorphine, suggesting that supersensitivity of the apomorphine sensitive receptor system had developed.[62] Since γ-type endorphins are present in the brain and in the nucleus accumbens,[17, 66] these peptides may physiologically interfere with the sensitivity of the DA receptor systems mediating apomorphine-induced hypoactivity. This hypothesis was tested by injecting DEγE or γ-endorphin antiserum into the nucleus accumbens for 10–12 days. Chronic treatment with DEγE resulted in hypoactivity and that with γ-endorphin antiserum in hyperactivity, which was present at least 3 days following discontinuation of treatment.[67] Assuming that the DA receptor systems mediating apomorphine-induced hypoactivity are located presynaptically on DA neurons involved in locomotion, the present data suggest that γ-type endorphins are involved in the setpoint regulation of these DA neurons. Chronically increased levels of γ-type endorphin may result in a decreased DA output and consequently in hypoactivity and chronic decreased levels—a chronic deficiency induced by γ-endorphin antiserum—in increased DA output and as a consequence hyperactivity. This accords well with the postulate that schizophrenic psychosis is related to a deficiency of γ-type endorphins and that distinct brain dopaminergic systems are hyperactive in this mental disorder. Interestingly, rats treated chronically with γ-endorphin antiserum into the nucleus accumbens have difficulties in habituation and/or adaptation and are impaired in cognitive capacities, disturbances that are not uncommon in schizophrenic patients.[67]

Although more studies are needed to substantiate at least some of the findings, it may be proposed that:

(1) γ-Type endorphins interfere selectively with certain DA systems,
(2) Chronic treatment with γ-type endorphins results in supersensitivity of these systems.

(3) γ-Type endorphins may be involved physiologically in the control of these DA systems.

(4) DA systems sensitive to γ-type endorphins are present in the nucleus accumbens.

(5) These DA systems are also sensitive to classical and atypical neuroleptics.

(6) These DA systems may be involved in the antipsychotic action of γ-type endorphins as well as in that of the classical and atypical neuroleptics.

However, it should be kept in mind that no direct evidence is available that the neuroleptic-like and antipsychotic action of γ-type endorphins is mediated by brain DA. Moreover, DA systems present in brain areas other than the nucleus accumbens may be involved in γ-type endorphin action as well.

CONCLUDING REMARKS

The similarities between certain behavioral effects of γ-type endorphins and haloperidol led to the postulate that these peptides are implicated in the pathogenesis of schizophrenic psychoses. Subsequently, an antipsychotic action of these peptides was observed in a number of schizophrenic patients. That not all treated patients responded to peptide treatment may be due to the heterogeneity of the schizophrenic syndrome, thus suggesting that a certain subgroup of schizophrenic patients is susceptible to γ-type endorphin treatment, or due to factors related to the course of illness and previous neuroleptic therapy of the patients. In fact, we found that a long psychotic episode and a high dose of previous neuroleptic medication diminished the responsiveness of the patient to γ-type endorphin treatment. Evidence has been obtained that γ-type endorphins interact with distinct DA systems in the brain and particularly in the nucleus accumbens. Since these peptides did not interfere with apomorphine- or amphetamine-induced stereotypy, effects presumably mediated by the nucleus caudatus DA systems, the γ-type endorphins may be devoid of extrapyramidal side effects. So far, such effects were not observed in patients treated with these peptides. Thus, in comparison to the classical neuroleptics with extrapyramidal side effects and the atypical neuroleptics with a lower incidence of these effects, the γ-type endorphins may be considered as prototypes of antipsychotic substances without extrapyramidal side effects.

REFERENCES

1. TERENIUS, L., A. WAHLSTRÖM, L. LINDSTRÖM AND E. WIDERLÖV. 1976. Neurosci. Lett. 3: 157–162.
2. BLOOM, F., D. SEGAL, N. LING & R. GUILLEMIN. 1976. Science 194: 630–632.
3. TERENIUS, L. 1978. The implications of endorphins in pathological states. In Characteristics and Function of Opioids. J. M. Van Ree & L. Terenius, Eds.: 143–158. Elsevier/North-Holland. Amsterdam.
4. DAVIS, G. C., M. S. BUCHSBAUM & W. E. BUNNEY, JR. 1979. Schizophr. Bull. 5: 244–250.

5. VERHOEVEN, W. M. A., H. M. VAN PRAAG & J. T. V. M. DE JONG. 1981.
   Neuropsychobiology **7:** 159–168.
6. FOGELSON, D. L., S. R. MARDER & T. VAN PUTTEN. 1980. Am. J. Psychiatry
   137: 605–607.
7. JACQUET, Y. F. & N. MARKS. 1976. Science **194:** 632–635.
8. KLINE, N. S., C. H. LI, H. E. LEHMANN, A. LAJTHA, E. LASKI & T. COOPER. 1977.
   Arch. Gen. Psychiatry **34:** 1111–1113.
9. BERGER, PH. A., S. J. WATSON, H. AKIL, G. R. ELLIOT, R. T. RUBIN, A.
   PFEFFERBAUM, K. L. DAVIS, J. D. BARCHAS & C. H. LI. 1980. Arch. Gen.
   Psychiatry **37:** 635–640.
10. JØRGENSEN, A., R. FOG & B. VEILIS. 1979. Lancet **i:** 935.
11. VAN REE, J. M. & D. DE WIED. 1981. Neuropharmacology **20:** 1271–1277.
12. DE WIED, D., B. BOHUS, J. M. VAN REE & I. URBAN. 1978. J. Pharmacol.
    Exp. Ther. **204:** 570–580.
13. DE WIED, D., G. L. KOVÁCS, B. BOHUS, J. M. VAN REE & H. M. GREVEN.
    1978. Eur. J. Pharmacol. **49:** 427–436.
14. KOVÁCS, G. L. & D. DE WIED. 1978. Eur. J. Pharmacol. **53:** 103–107.
15. DE WIED, D. 1978. Psychopathology as a neuropeptide dysfunction. *In*
    Characteristics and Function of Opioids. J. M. Van Ree & L. Terenius, Eds.:
    113–122. Elsevier/North-Holland. Amsterdam.
16. DE WIED, D., J. M. VAN REE & H. M. GREVEN. 1980. Life Sci. **26:** 1275–
    1279.
17. VERHOEF, J., J. G. LOEBER, J. P. H. BURBACH, W. H. GISPEN, A. WITTER & D.
    DE WIED. 1980. Life Sci. **26:** 851–859.
18. OPMEER, F. A., J. G. LOEBER & J. M. VAN REE. 1980. Life Sci. **27:** 2393–
    2400.
19. LOEBER, J., J. VERHOEF, J. P. H. BURBACH & J. M. VAN REE. 1979. Acta
    Endocrinol. **91:** 74.
20. BURBACH, J. P. H., J. G. LOEBER, J. VERHOEF, V. M. WIEGANT, E. R. DE KLOET
    & D. DE WIED. 1980. Nature **283:** 96–97.
21. OPMEER, F. A., J. P. H. BURBACH, V. M. WIEGANT & J. M. VAN REE. 1982.
    Life Sci. **31:** 323–328.
22. BURBACH, J. P. H., P. SCHOTMAN, J. VERHOEF, E. R. DE KLOET & D. DE WIED.
    Biochem. Biophys. Res. Commun. **97:** 995–1004.
23. VERHOEVEN, W. M. A., H. M. VAN PRAAG, P. A. BOTTER, A. SUNIER, J. M. VAN
    REE & D. DE WIED. 1978. Lancet **i:** 1046–1047.
24. VERHOEVEN, W. M. A., H. M. VAN PRAAG, J. M. VAN REE & D. DE WIED.
    1979. Arch. Gen. Psychiatry **36:** 294–298.
25. VERHOEVEN, W. M. A., H. G. M. WESTENBERG, A. W. GERRITSEN, H. M. VAN
    PRAAG, J. H. H. THIJSSEN, F. SCHWARZ, J. M. VAN REE & D. DE WIED. 1981.
    Psychiatry Res. **5:** 293–310.
26. VERHOEVEN, W. M. A., J. M. VAN REE, A. HEEZIUS-VAN BENTUM, D. DE WIED
    & H. M. VAN PRAAG. 1982. Arch. Gen. Psychiat. **39:** 648–657.
27. MACKAY, A. V. P. & T. J. CROW. 1980. Br. J. Psychiat. **137:** 379–386.
28. SPITZER, R. L., J. ENDICOTT & E. ROBINS. 1978. Arch. Gen. Psychiat. 35:
    773–782.
29. VAN PRAAG, H. M. 1976. Compr. Psychiat. **17:** 481–497.
30. WING, J. K., J. E. COOPER & N. SARTORIUS. 1975. The Measurement and
    Classification of Psychiatric Symptoms. Cambridge University Press.
31. WORLD HEALTH ORGANIZATION. 1977. Manual of the International Statistical
    Classification of Diseases, Injuries and Causes of Death. Geneva.
32. VAN PRAAG, H. M. 1978. Psychotropic Drugs: A Guide for the Practitioner.
    Brunner/Mazel. New York.

33. EMRICH, H. M., M. ZAUDIG, W. KISSLING, G. DIRLICH, D. VON ZERSSEN & A. HERZ. 1980. Pharmakopsychiatrie **13:** 290–298.
34. MANCHANDA, R. & S. R. HIRSCH. 1981. Psychol. Med. **11:** 401–404.
35. TAMMINGA, C. A., P. J. TIGHE, TH. N. CHASE, E. G. DEFRAITES & M. H. SCHAFFER. 1981. Arch. Gen. Psychiatry **38:** 167–168.
36. BOURGEOIS, M., E. LAFORGE, J. MUYARD, J. BLAYAC & J. LEMOINE. 1980. Ann. Med. Psychol. **138:** 1112–1119.
37. VAN REE, J. M. & D. DE WIED. 1982. Trends Pharmacol. Sci. **3:** 358–361.
38. VAN REE, J. M., B. BOHUS & D. DE WIED. 1980. Similarity between behavioral effects of des-tyrosine-γ-endorphin and haloperidol and of α-endorphin and amphetamine. *In* Endogenous and Exogenous Opiate Agonists and Antagonists. E. Leong Way, Ed.: 459–462. Pergamon Press.
39. MATTHYSSE, S. 1974. Schizophrenia: Relationships to dopamine transmission, motor control and feature extraction. *In* The Neurosciences, F. O. Schmitt & F. G. Worden, Eds. 733–737. MIT Press. Cambridge, MA.
40. MELTZER, H. Y. & S. M. STAHL. 1976. Schizophrenia Bull. **2:** 19–76.
41. VAN PRAAG, H. M. & J. KORF. 1976. Am. J. Psychiatry **133:** 1171–1177.
42. VAN KAMMEN, D. P. 1979. Psychoneuroendocrinology **4:** 37–46.
43. NIEMEGEERS, C. J. E. & P. A. J. JANSSEN. 1979. Life Sci. **24:** 2201–2216.
44. VAN REE, J. M., A. WITTER & J. E. LEYSEN. 1978. Eur. J. Pharmacol. **52:** 411–413.
45. PEDIGO, N. W., N. C. LING, T. D. REISINE & H. I. YAMAMURA. 1979. Life Sci. **24:** 1645–1650.
46. PEDIGO, N. W., T. SCHALLERT, D. H. OVERSTREET, N. C. LING, P. RAGAN, T. D. REISINE & H. I. YAMAMURA. 1979. Eur. J. Pharmacol. **60:** 359–364.
47. VERSTEEG, D. H. G., E. R. DE KLOET & D. DE WIED. 1979. Brain Res. **179:** 85–93.
48. VERSTEEG, D. H. G., G. L. KOVÁCS, B. BOHUS, E. R. DE KLOET & D. DE WIED. 1982. Brain Res. **231:** 343–351.
49. LAMBERTS, S. W. J., M. DE QUIJDA, J. M. VAN REE & D. DE WIED. Neuropharmacology. In press.
50. CLEMENS, J. A. & C. J. SHAAR. 1980. Fed. Proc. **39:** 2588–2592.
51. DORSA, D. M., J. M. VAN REE & D. DE WIED. 1979. Pharmacol. Biochem. Behav. **10:** 899–905.
52. VAN REE, J. M. & A. P. OTTE. 1980. Neuropharmacology **19:** 429–434.
53. SEEMAN, PH. 1980. Pharmacol. Rev. **32:** 229–313.
54. COOLS, A. R. & J. M. VAN ROSSUM. 1980. Life Sci. **27:** 1237–1253.
55. CARLSSON, A. 1975. Receptor-mediated control of dopamine metabolism. *In* Pre- and Postsynaptic Receptors. E. Usdin & W. E. Bunney, Eds.: 49–66. Marcel Dekker. New York.
56. VAN REE, J. M., H. INNEMEE, J. W. LOUWERENS, R. S. KAHN & D. DE WIED. Neuropharmacology. In press.
57. NICKOLSON, V. J. & H. H. G. BERENDSEN. 1980. Life Sci. **27:** 1377–1385.
58. DAVIS, K. L., A. SAMUEL, A. A. MATHE & R. C. MOHS. 1981. Life Sci. **28:** 2421–2424.
59. MULLER, P. & PH. SEEMAN. 1978. Psychopharmacology **60:** 1–11.
60. VERIMER, T., D. B. GOODALE, J. P. LONG & J. R. FLYNN. 1980. J. Pharm. Pharmacol. **32:** 665–666.
61. CROW, T. J. 1979. Dopaminergic mechanisms in schizophrenia: Site and mechanisms of antipsychotic effect and postmortem studies. *In* Neuroleptics and Schizophrenia. J. M. Simister, Ed.: 29–40. Lundbeck. Luton, England.
62. VAN REE, J. M., A. M. CAFFEE & G. WOLTERINK. Neuropharmacology. In press.
63. GISPEN, W. H., D. ORMOND, J. TEN HAAF & D. DE WIED. 1980. Eur. J. Pharmacol. **63:** 203–207.

64. KOVÁCS, G. L., G. TELEGDY & D. DE WIED. 1982. Neuropharmacology.
    21: 451–457.
65. VAN REE, J. M. & G. WOLTERINK. 1981. Eur. J. Pharmacol. **72:** 107–111.
66. DORSA, D. M., L. A. MAJUMDAR & M. B. CHAPMAN. 1981. Peptides. **2** (Suppl.
    1): 71–77.
67. VAN REE, J. M., G. WOLTERINK, M. FEKETE & D. DE WIED. Neuropharmacology.
    In press.

DISCUSSION OF THE PAPER

UNIDENTIFIED SPEAKER: I am not familiar with the background of the des-compounds. What is their binding to the various types of opiate receptors?

J. M. VAN REE (*Medical Faculty, University of Utrecht, the Netherlands*): They do not bind to opiate receptors.

CLINICAL, ELECTROPHYSIOLOGICAL, AND BIOCHEMICAL EFFECTS OF DES-TYROSINE-γ-ENDORPHIN IN PSYCHIATRIC PATIENTS *

John Metz, Daniel A. Busch, and Herbert Y. Meltzer

The Pritzker School of Medicine
University of Chicago
Chicago, Illinois 60637
Illinois State Psychiatric Institute
Chicago, Illinois 60612

Des-tyrosine-γ-endorphin (DTγE), a derivative of γ-endorphin, has been found to have some behavioral effects in rats consistent with a post-synaptic dopamine receptor blocking action *in vivo*.[1-3] There is also electrophysiological evidence [4,5] and biochemical evidence consistent with a direct or indirect neuroleptic-like action in rats.[6] However, several types of biochemical evidence are inconsistent with a dopamine receptor antagonist action.[7-9] DTγE may also influence pre-synaptic DA synthesis and release.[10-12]

Because of the reports of possible neuroleptic-like action, DTγE has been administered to psychotic patients. Several studies demonstrated that DTγE was effective in treating some psychotic patients,[13-15] whereas others have shown equivocal responses [16,17] or that DTγE was entirely ineffective in treating chronic schizophrenics.[18,19]

We report here the results of an open pilot study using DTγE in the treatment of patients with schizophrenia. The compound used in our study was supplied by Organon, Inc. An open design, dose-finding study was carried out because of uncertainty as to the potency of each batch of the new material.

METHODS

Subjects

The study included eight patients hospitalized on the research wards of the Laboratory of Biological Psychiatry of the Illinois State Psychiatric Institute. Entrance to the study was dependent upon diagnosis of schizophrenia made by consensus of two psychiatrists and a psychologist following completion of the Present State Examination (PSE) (20), Eighth Edition. All patients met Research Diagnostic Criteria (RDC) [21] for the diagnosis of schizophrenia or schizoaffective illness, mainly schizophrenic type. Six met diagnostic criteria for chronic schizophrenia, one for subacute schizophrenia, and one for acute schizoaffective illness, mainly schizophrenic. Demographic data for each patient, as well as data on previous course and response to previous neuroleptic treatment are presented in TABLE 1a. There were five males and three females. The mean age was 24.8 years (range 20 to 42). The mean num-

* Supported in part by United States Public Health Service Grants MH 29206 and MH 30938 and by the State of Illinois Department of Mental Health. H.Y.M. is recipient of United States Public Health Service Grant MH 47808.

0077–8923/82/0398–0496 $01.75/0 © 1982, NYAS

ber of previous hospitalizations was 2.3 (range 1 to 6). The mean duration of the current episode was 4.1 years (range 1 month to 23 years) and the mean duration of illness was 8 years (range 2 to 23). All patients gave informed consent for participation in this study. Of the eight patients, two (subjects 2 and 3) had received high doses of neuroleptics immediately prior to admission. No other patients had received neuroleptics within 3 months prior to admission.

Following admission, the patients were kept off active medication for a period of 9 to 25 days. During this time, they were observed for stability of symptomatology and baseline biological studies were carried out. At the end of this period, treatment with DTγE was begun, with an initial dose of 1 mg i.m. daily for at least 3 days. FIGURE 1 indicates the dose of DTγE for each patient on each treatment day. The dose varied from 3–10 mg/day for the rest of the 10–12 day period. The maximum dose, which was randomly assigned, was 3 mg/day in four patients; 5 mg/day in two; and 10 mg/day in two.

Following treatment with DTγE, patients were not given active medication for at least a week. At the end of this post-DTγE period five patients received conventional neuroleptic treatment and two refused further treatment; in one case, no further neuroleptic treatment was felt to be clinically indicated.

Assessment of Clinical Changes

The instruments used to exaluate patients were the Global Assessment Scale (GAS),[22] at the beginning and end of placebo period and at end of the study, and an expanded version of the Schedule for Affective Disorders and Schizophrenia-Change Scale (SADS-C),[23] which included additional items taken from the PSE concerned with rating of psychotic phenomena. Nurse ratings were done using the Nurses Observation Scale for Inpatient Evaluation (NOSIE).[24]

Data from the SADS-C has been divided into 26 scales. Because of the small number of subjects, we examined only the scales most relevant to psychotic symptomatology: auditory hallucinations (sum of scores for five items), first rank symptoms (eight items), delusions of reference and persecution (two items), incomprehensibility (three items), impact of hallucinations (one item), and impact of delusions (one item). We also developed four NOSIE scales: sociability (10 items, maximum score 40); neatness (4 items, maximum score 16); calmness (5 items, maximum score 20); cooperativeness (3 items; maximum score 12). Copies of the modified SADS-C and NOSIE scales are available on request.

Clinical assessment of change was made in weekly ward research meetings through discussion with the ward psychiatrists, psychologists and psychiatric residents. These changes were assessed on a scale consisting of Marked Improvement, Moderate Improvement, Minimal Improvement, No Change, or Deterioration. Clinicians were also asked to describe areas in which clinical improvement or deterioration occurred.

TABLE 1

A. DESCRIPTIVE DATA ON PATIENTS

Subject No.	Age	Sex	RDC Diagnosis	Age at Onset	Duration of Current Episode	Previous Course	Number of Previous Hospitalizations	Previous Neuroleptic Response
1	22	M	Schizophrenia chronic undifferentiated	19	2 months	Recurrent illness, good but incomplete remission	3	Uncertain probably minimal
2	42	M	Schizophrenia, chronic undifferentiated	19	23 years	Chronic illness, continuous impairment	6	Minimal improvement—less angry
3	21	M	Schizophrenia, chronic undifferentiated	19	2 years	Chronic illness, continuous impairment	1	Minimal improvement
4	35	F	Schizoaffective, acute, manic mainly schizophrenic	27	6 months	Acute illness, complete remission	1	Excellent
5	20	M	Schizophrenia, chronic disorganized	16	3 years	Chronic illness, continuous severe impairment	1	Minimal improvement—less angry
6	31	M	Schizophrenia chronic undifferentiated	uncertain	uncertain	Chronic illness, partial remission	1	Uncertain
7	20	F	Schizophrenia, subacute undifferentiated	18	1 month	Recurrent illness, good but incomplete remissions	1	Excellent

| 8 | 27 | F | Schizophrenia, chronic undifferentiated | 24 | 4 months | Chronic illness, partial remissions | 4 | Good |

B. Descriptive Data on Patients

Subject No.	Presenting Symptomatology	Change during Placebo Period
1	Withdrawn with occasional laughter. Nightmares. Delusions of influence, control, reference and persecution. Thought insertion, thought withdrawal.	Stable
2	Anxious, irritable. Thought disorder. Recent increased attention to chronic fantastic grandiose and persecutory delusions and auditory hallucinations.	Marked deterioration. Increased irritability and hostility
3	Anxious with blunted affect. Concern with peculiar ideas. Thought disorder. Passivity experiences. Referential delusions. Continuous auditory hallucinations, some first rank. Visual, tactile, gustatory hallucinations.	Auditory hallucinations stopped. But, more preoccupied with peculiar ideas.
4	Florid psychosis; tense, restless, with elevated, anxious mood. Incoherent. Persecutory delusions. Delusions of control. Thought insertion, thought withdrawal. Auditory, olfactory, visual gustatory hallucinations.	Stable
5	Withdrawn with occasional angry outbursts. Thought disorder.	Initial improvement followed by marked deterioration with angry outbursts, visual hallucinations, delusions
6	Withdrawn. Thought disorder. Persecutory delusions; thought insertion, thought withdrawal, thought broadcasting. Auditory hallucinations.	Stable
7	Very withdrawn. Nearly mute with occasional laughter. Bizarre somatic delusions. Auditory hallucinations.	Slight improvement, especially in bizarre somatic delusions
8	Withdrawn and haughty. Bizarre somatic and persecutory delusions. Delusions of control. Thought insertion, thought withdrawal. Auditory hallucinations.	Stable

C. DESCRIPTIVE DATA ON PATIENTS' CLINICAL RESPONSE TO DTγE

Subject No.	Presenting Symptomatology	Degree of Change
1	Improvement by third day of treatment; full remission of psychotic symptoms by ninth day. More sociable, but still exhibited some irritating, inappropriate laughter, and tendency to be withdrawn.	Marked improvement
2	Initially showed continuation of the deterioration that began during placebo period; then became less hostile and more sociable. No change in delusions or hallucinations.	Minimal improvement
3	Much more socially active; no longer preoccupied with peculiar ideas. No change in delusions or hallucinations.	Marked improvement
4	Little behavioral change. Less pressure of speech and incoherence. No change in delusions or hallucinations.	No change
5	Initially showed continuation of deterioration that began during placebo period; then became more sociable and realistic with disappearance of some delusions.	Moderate improvement
6	More sociable and cooperative; however, felt more angry. No change in delusions, hallucinations, thought disorder.	No change
7	Minimally more talkative, though displayed more inappropriate laughter. Improvement in bizarre somatic delusions.	Minimal improvement
8	Slight improvement during first week: more sociable, improvement in paranoid delusions. During second week, thinking became better organized, but patient again became more withdrawn.	Minimal improvement

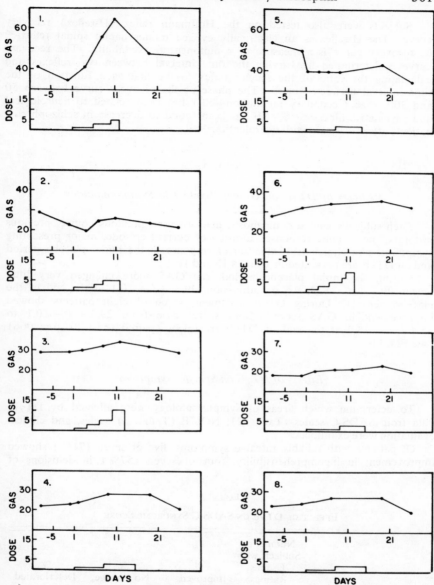

FIGURE 1. Global Assessment Scale (GAS) score ratings in eight patients before, during, and after treatment with DTγE.

Biological Measurements

Regular blood samples were taken during the placebo periods and during the DTγE and neuroleptic treatment periods for the assessment of prolactin and platelet monoamine oxidase (MAO) levels.

Subjects were also tested on the Hoffmann reflex (H-reflex) recovery curve. The H-reflex is an electrically evoked monosynaptic spinal reflex;[25] its recovery curve is a measure of α-motoneuron excitability. The recovery curve is determined by varying the time interval between two reflexes and calculating the ratio of the second reflex to the first as a function of the time interval between stimuli. The phase of the recovery curve between 50 and 300 msec (secondary facilitation—SF) has been related to neurological and psychiatric illnesses.[26-30] SF has been found to decrease in schizophrenic patients after treatment with neuroleptics.[31]

RESULTS

Effects of DTγE on Global Psychiatric Symptomatology

Each subject's age, sex, diagnosis, age of onset, previous course, previous history of neuroleptic response, duration of current episode, major presenting symptoms, and clinicians' evaluation of response in the initial placebo period and on DTγE are presented in TABLES 1b and 1c.

During the initial placebo period, the GAS score changed very little (mean 29.3 + / − S.D. 9.5 on admission, 29.3 + / − 10.1 at the end of the placebo period). During DTγE treatment, seven of eight patients showed improvement in GAS scores. GAS scores rose from 29.3 + / − 10.1 to 35.4 + / − 13.7 at the end of DTγE treatment (paired t = 1.70, p = .066) (see FIG. 1).

Effects of DTγE on Specific Symptoms

To determine which areas of symptomatology were affected by DTγE, data from SADS-C scales (TABLE 2), NOSIE (TABLE 3) scales, and clinical evaluation were examined.

Of patients with reliably rateable symptoms, five of seven (71%) showed improvement in incomprehensibility, four of seven (57%) in delusions of

TABLE 2

EFFECT OF DTγE ON SADS-C SYNDROME SCORE

	Number of Subjects with Usable Ratings	% Improved	% No Change	% Deteriorated
Auditory hallucinations	5/8	1(20)	4(80)	0(0)
First rank symptoms	5/8	2(40)	3(60)	0(0)
Delusions of reference and persecution	7/8	4(57)	1(14)	2(29)
Severity of hallucinations	7/8	2(29)	4(57)	1(14)
Severity of delusions	6/8	0(0)	2(35)	4(67)
Incomprehensibility	7/8	5(71)	1(14)	1(14)

TABLE 3

EFFECT OF DTγE ON GAS AND NOSIE RATINGS

	% Improved	% No Change	% Deteriorated
GAS	7(87.5)	0(0)	1(12.5)
NOSIE scales	5(62.5)	0(0)	3(37.5)
1. Sociability	6(75)	0(0)	2(25)
2. Neatness	2(25)	2(25)	4(50)
3. Calmness	2(25)	4(50)	2(25)
4. Cooperativeness	4(50)	1(12.5)	3(37.5)

reference and persecution, and two of five (40%) in first rank symptoms. The ability to give answers which could be evaluated was improved in six of seven patients (86%). On the other hand, SADS-C items relating to the degree to which the patient claimed to be influenced by delusions and hallucinations did not indicate any beneficial effect of DTγE.

Of the NOSIE items (see TABLE 3), the most impressive change was in social withdrawal (Sociability Scale) which improved in 6 of 8 (75%) of the patients. There was little overall change in the degree to which patients were cooperative (Cooperativeness Scale) in the ward routine and the extent to which they were easily upset (Calmness Scale). On the negative side, four of eight (50%) of the patients showed a tendency to take less care of their physical appearance (Neatness Scale).

Clinicians' assessments indicated that two patients showed marked overall improvement, one showed moderate improvement, three showed minimal improvement, and two showed no change. The assessment by clinicians suggests that treatment with DTγE was associated with improved functioning in several areas; patients were less withdrawn, more sociable, cooperative, and realistic. However, clinicians observed little change in delusions and hallucinations on DTγE except in patient 3.

Relationship of Demographic Variables and Treatment History to DTγE Response

There were no significant relationships between changes in GAS scores from before to after DTγE treatment and any of the following variables: age, duration of illness, duration of current episode, or presence of neuroleptic treatment in the three months prior to admission. Of the four patients who had a good or excellent previous response to neuroleptics, one had a doubtful response to DTγE, two a minimal response, and one a marked response. Of the three patients who had a minimal response to neuroleptics, one had a minimal response to DTγE, one a moderate, and the third a marked response. One patient had a doubtful response to both neuroleptic and DTγE. Thus, there was no correlation between previous neuroleptic response and clinical response to DTγE.

Time Course and Dose Effects on Clinical Change during DTγE Treatment

FIGURE 1 indicates GAS scores for all subjects during DTγE treatment as well as shortly before starting and discontinuing DTγE. The dose of DTγE is also shown for each day of the treatment. The data suggest that in most subjects clinical change associated with DTγE began within the first week of treatment on DTγE (1 mg/day), and that increasing the dose of DTγE above 3 mg/day did not result in an increase in the rate of improvement. Two patients (subjects 2 and 5) showed deterioration on the 1 mg/day dose followed by modest improvement after several more days of DTγE treatment. By way of contrast, one patient (subject 8) after some improvement on the 1 mg/day dose did not improve further when the dose was increased to 3 mg/day.

Clinical Response to Discontinuation of DTγE

Responses after discontinuation of DTγE were highly variable, but by the end of the post-DTγE washout period, six of eight patients showed evidence of deterioration on GAS (FIG. 1). The GAS scores (mean $+/-$ S.D.) fell from $35.4 +/- 13.7$ to $30.5 +/- 10.9$ (paired $t = 2.16$, $p = .034$).

Clinical Response to Post-DTγE Neuroleptic Treatment

Following a post-DTγE washout period, five of eight patients received neuroleptics for more than a week. The five patients all showed substantial clinical improvement as indicated by GAS scores (FIG. 1) on neuroleptics. Time of onset of improvement on neuroleptics was variable, ranging from several days in the case of subject 7 to 3 weeks in the case of subject 4.

Untoward Effects of DTγE

There was initial deterioration on DTγE followed by improvement in two of eight patients (FIG. 1). In the case of subject 2, this appears to have been a continuation of progressive deterioration which began after he was placed on placebo medication early in hospitalization rather than a result of DTγE; furthermore, during the course of DTγE treatment, he became slightly less withdrawn and hostile. Subject 5 acutely decompensated during the first day of DTγE, which coincided with several intense stresses in his life. After 3 days on DTγE, he began to improve, particularly in sociability and in a more realistic approach to problem-solving. We consider it highly unlikely that pharmacological effects of DTγE contributed to his sudden decompensation.

Through the course of DTγE no physical side effects or extrapyramidal symptoms were noted.

Effect of DTγE on Biological Variables

Six of the eight patients had slight decreases in MAO at the end of DTγE treatment compared to placebo (average decrease of about 6% from 11.4 to 10.7). This change was not statistically significant, but was in the same direction and about the same magnitude as would be expected from a comparable period of neuroleptic treatment. On the other hand, prolactin values showed no systematic change through the course of the study.

H-reflex secondary facilitation in the DTγE condition was significantly lower than in the baseline condition (52 +/− 17 vs. 64 +/− 19). Direct muscle responses and unconditioned H-reflexes were unaffected by DTγE. Of the eight patients, only subject 4 failed to show a decrease in SF following DTγE.

For comparison purposes, FIGURE 2 shows the values obtained before and after DTγE in this study and the values we obtained in a similar study of standard neuroleptics and other antipsychotic agents.[31] In that study, we found that psychiatric patients treated with placebo, lithium carbonate, tricyclic antidepressants, or monoamine oxidase inhibitors all failed to show any change in the H-reflex recovery curve when tested under conditions similar to those of this study. On the other hand, each of the three groups of patients which received neuroleptic treatment for at least 2 weeks all had SF values significantly lower than baseline. Thus, the present results with DTγE are very similar to the results previously observed following neuroleptic treatment.

Five of the patients were retested during the second placebo period. For three, SF values returned to the baseline levels; for the other two, SF remained at the level at the end of the DTγE period.

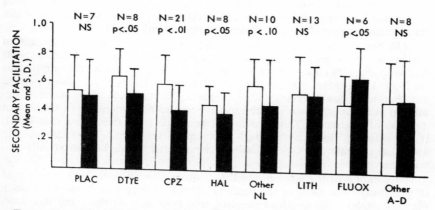

FIGURE 2. Effects of different chronic medications on H-reflex secondary facilitation. Different groups of patients were studied before □ and after ■ receiving placebo (PLAC), des-tyrosine-γ-endorphin (DTγE), chlorpromazine (CPZ), haloperidol (HAL), other neuroleptics, including trifluoperazine, fluphenazine, thioridazine, and loxapine (Other NL), lithium carbonate (LITH), fluoxetine (FLUOX), and other anti-depressants, including imipramine, amitriptyline, nortryptyline, and phenelzine (Other A-D). In each case, statistical significance was determined by two-tailed, repeated measures, t-tests.

We have recently completed H-reflex testing on two additional subjects, not part of the original group, using DTγE from a different batch. As with the first group, both subjects had lower SF after DTγE than in placebo conditions (decreases of 5% and 19% relative to placebo). When the subjects were later treated with reserpine and prolixin-d, they showed even greater decreases in SF (20% and 28% less than placebo condition). These subjects were tested once or twice a week throughout the 3 weeks of DTγE treatment and for up to 3 weeks of treatment with reserpine or prolixin. The SF responses of DTγE were about as rapid as to reserpine and prolixin (clear decreases were seen within a week), but for both subjects there was more variability in the measurement of SF during DTγE treatment than during the period of treatment with reserpine or prolixin. Clinical and biochemical data have not yet been analyzed on these two subjects, but it appears that neither showed more than minimal improvement while receiving DTγE.

DISCUSSION

We conducted an open trial of DTγE in eight schizophrenic patients. Patients received DTγE in doses ranging from 1 to 10 mg/day for 12 days.

Our data indicated marked improvement in two subjects; four other subjects showed minimal improvement in delusions, hallucinations, or thought disorder. Six of the eight subjects showed evidence of increased sociability during the trial of DTγE. No subject showed continuing deterioration throughout the trial of DTγE.

The question of whether DTγE has significant antipsychotic properties cannot be definitively answered by this study. The trials were brief; both patients and staff were aware that the patients were receiving a new drug which had been reported to be highly effective in previous studies and which represented a new class of potential antipsychotic agents.

The magnitude of the changes in GAS scores (a mean improvement of 5.4 points) was greater than that in a comparison group of 21 patients receiving single-blind treatment with low to moderate doses of chlorpromazine for 2 weeks (a mean improvement of 2.5 points). Cotes et al.[32] have pointed out that in a double-blind study comparing flupenthixol with placebo, significant neuroleptic versus placebo differences did not emerge until the end of 3 weeks of treatment. Thus, we cannot conclude from these data that DTγE is less effective than conventional neuroleptic treatment. However, we can state that the rate and type of improvement noted by Verhoeven et al.[14] was not observed.

Exploration of the appropriate DTγE dosage on an open basis was a goal of this study. For most of the patients, clinical change was gradual and took place throughout the length of the drug trial beginning on the 1 mg/day dose. However, subjects 2 and 5 did not follow this pattern. Both showed continued deterioration while on the 1 mg/day dose but then began to improve on 3 mg/day dose. Whether this was related to the dose increase, the number of days on DTγE, or other factors cannot be determined. There was no evidence that further dosage increases enhanced the rate of recovery. By way of contrast, subject 8 showed improvement on the 1 mg/day dose but showed a plateau in improvement on the 3 mg/day dose, raising the possibility that there is a therapeutic dose range above which clinical deterioration may occur. On the basis of these findings, a dose of 1–3 mg/day appears to be most beneficial. Whether it will be necessary to characterize the dose for each batch of DTγE will require further study.

It is quite unclear what group of patients are most likely to respond to DTγE. The type of patients studied may be an important variable in accounting for the differences in DTγE effectiveness reported by different groups. In our study, we were unable to establish a relationship between response to DTγE and such variables as diagnostic subtype, age, duration of illness or episode, or previous response to neuroleptic treatment.

The response of H-reflex recovery curves to DTγE treatment, decreased SF, suggests a pharmacological action similar to neuroleptics, independent of behavioral effects. However, decreased SF is not necessarily an effect unique to antipsychotic or neuroleptic drugs. At this time we do not know the precise biochemical and anatomical systems which regulate the H-reflex recovery curve, nor have we studied a diverse group of pharmacological agents which might affect it. Therefore, the fact that DTγE and neuroleptics are the only two types of agent which consistently reduce SF in psychotic patients must be viewed as suggestive, but not conclusive, evidence that the drugs have some common pharmacological action.

In conclusion, the efficacy of DTγE in the treatment of schizophrenia is uncertain at this time, and further double-blind studies comparing DTγE with placebo must be performed before concluding that DTγE is or is not an effective treatment of schizophrenia. The diverse basic research studies demonstrating an antidopaminergic effect of DTγE in rats and the effect on the H-reflex recovery function in man provide a sufficient rationale in our mind for continuing the clinical studies. There may be only a few RDC schizophrenics who improve with DTγE and this may be intermittent, but it would be of great importance to identify these individuals because of the profound impetus it would provide to peptodergic-dopaminergic studies.

REFERENCES

1. DE WIED, D., B. BOHUS, J. M. VAN REE, G. L. KOVACS & H. M. GREVEN. 1978. Lancet **1:** 1046.
2. DE WIED, D., G. L. KOVACS, B. BOHUS, J. M. VAN REE & H. M. GREVEN. 1978. Eur. J. Pharmacol. **49:** 427.
3. GISPEN, W. H., D. ORMOND, J. TEN HAAF & D. DE WIED. 1980. Eur. J. Pharmacol. **63:** 203.
4. DORSA, D. M., J. M. VAN REE & D. DE WIED. 1979. Pharmacol. Biochem. Behav. **10:** 899.
5. VAN REE, J. M., D. DE WIED, W. M. A. VERHOEVEN & H. M. VAN PRAAG. 1980. Lancet **1:** 363.
6. PEDIGO, N. W., T. SCHALLERT, D. H. OVERSTREET, N. C. LING, P. RAGAN, T. D. REISINE & H. I. YAMAMURA. 1979. Eur. J. Pharmacol. **60:** 359.
7. WEINBERGER, S. B., A. ARNSTEN & D. S. SEGAL. 1979. Life Sci. **24:** 1637.
8. VAN REE, J. M., A. WITTER & J. E. LEYSEN. 1978. Eur. J. Psychiatry **52:** 411.
9. PEDIGO, N. W., N. C. LING, T. D. REISINE & H. I. YAMAMURA. 1979. Life Sci. **24:** 1645.
10. SCHOEMAKER, H. & V. J. NICKOLSON. 1980. Life Sci. **27:** 1371.
11. NICKOLSON, V. J. & H. H. G. BERENDSEN. 1980. Life Sci. **27:** 1377.

12. DAVIS, K. L., A. SAMUEL, A. A. MATHE & R. C. MOHS. 1981. Life Sci. 28: 2421.
13. VERHOEVEN, W. M. A., H. M. VAN PRAAG, P. A. BOTTER, A. SUNIER, J. M. VAN REE & D. DE WIED. 1978. Lancet 1: 1046.
14. VERHOEVEN, W. M. A., H. M. VAN PRAAG, J. M. VAN REE & D. DE WIED. 1979. Arch. Gen. Psychiatry 36: 294.
15. VAN REE, J. M. & A. P. OTTE. 1980. Neuropharmacology 19: 429.
16. EMRICH, H. M., M. ZAUDIG, D. V. ZERSSEN, A. HERZ & W. KISSLING. 1980. Lancet 1: 1364.
17. MANCHANDA, R. & S. R. HIRSCH. 1981. Psychol. Med. 11: 401.
18. CASEY, D. E., S. KORSGAARD, J. GERLACH, A. JORGENSEN & H. SIMMELSGAARD. 1981. Arch. Gen. Psychiatry 38: 158.
19. TAMMINGA, C. A., P. J. TIGHE, T. N. CHASE, E. G. DEFRAITES & M. H. SCHAFFER. 1981. Arch. Gen. Psychiatry 78: 167.
20. WING, J. K., J. E. COOPER & N. SARTORIUS. 1974. The Measurement and Classification of Psychiatric Symptoms. Cambridge University Press. Cambridge, England.
21. SPITZER, R. L., J. ENDICOTT & E. ROBINS. 1977. Research Diagnostic Criteria, Third Edition. New York State Psychiatric Institute. New York.
22. ENDICOTT, J., R. L. SPITZER, J. L. FLEISS & J. COHEN. 1976. Arch. Gen. Psychiatry 33: 766.
23. SPITZER, R. L. & J. ENDICOTT. 1977. Schedule for Affective Disorders and Schizophrenia (SADS-C), Third Edition. New York State Psychiatric Institute. New York.
24. HONIGFELD, G., R. D. GILLIS & C. J. KLETT. 1966. NOSIE-30: A Treatment Sensitive Ward Behavior Scale, Report No. 66. Central Neuropsychiatric Research Laboratory, Perry Point, MD.
25. MAGLADERY, J. W. 1955. Pflugers Arch. 261: 301.
26. OLSEN, P. Z. & E. DIAMANTOPOULOS. 1967. J. Neurol. Neurosurg. Psychiatry 30: 325.
27. CRAYTON, J. W., H. Y. MELTZER & D. J. GOODE. 1977. Biol. Psychiatry 12: 545.
28. GOODE, D. J., H. Y. MELTZER, J. W. CRAYTON & T. A. MAZURA. 1977. Schizophr. Bull. 3: 121.
29. YAP, C.-B. 1967. Brain 90: 887.
30. MASLAND, W. S. 1972. Arch. Neurol. 26: 313.
31. METZ, J., D. J. GOODE & H. Y. MELTZER. 1980. Psychol. Med. 10: 541.
32. COTES, P. M., T. J. CROW, E. C. JOHNSTONE, W. BARTLETT & R. C. BOURNES. 1978. Psychol. Med. 8: 657.

CLOSING REMARKS

Karl Verebey

New York State Division of Substance Abuse Services
Testing and Research Laboratory
Brooklyn, New York 11217
and
State University of New York
Downstate Medical Center
Brooklyn, New York 11203

Up until about the time this conference received approval by the New York Academy of Sciences the subject of the opioids' influence and possible therapeutic value in mental illness was somewhat suspect and apt to come under heavy criticism. "There aren't enough well-controlled studies," the critics said. While this is true, we must note that the reason for such lack is that prior to the discovery of opiate receptors and the endorphin system in the brain, there were only historical accounts and clinical observations suggesting that opioids were potentially antipsychotic drugs. These accounts did not provide sufficient scientific bases for clinical trials. Also, opiates were so closely perceived with addiction by professionals and the public that their stigma even prevented their use for relief of pain in terminally ill cancer patients. Because of this stigma most institutional review boards would decline permission for studies of opiates in mental illness. In this emotional and political environment, trials of opiates in a nonopiate-related disorder were nearly impossible.

My purpose for organizing this conference was to bring together evidence and knowledge; to bring together clinicians from all over the country and the world who have made similar observations on the effectiveness of opiates in various forms of psychopathology. Basic scientists were also invited to help construct a scientific basis that may explain the historical accounts of the therapeutic use of opiates and the more recent clinical observations. The basic scientist's input has been badly needed in the total effort to legitimize the "opiate-behavioral" field, and this input has finally emerged in this conference. Thus, future clinical experiments can be firmly built on the information reported in this volume.

Several basic research studies indicate that one of the physiological roles of opiates is the inhibitory modulation of certain sympathetic neurons. This mechanism may explain the tranquilizing, fear-alleviating, and antiaggressive effects of opiates described in the psychiatric literature. In schizophrenia and other mental disorders a major symptom is the loss of stress tolerance. Normal individuals may utilize their endogenous opioids as brain "shock absorbers" during stress. Thus, the sympathetic discharge is dampened by the inhibitory modulation of endorphins. This system appears to be deficient in schizophrenics. Thus, theoretically in some individuals whose deficit is not related to opiate receptor dysfunction, external opioid supplementation may be therapeutic. This view may help to rationalize the use of exogenous opioids to supplement the deficient endogenous opiate system just as insulin is used in diabetes.

The appearance of tardive dyskinesia after chronic neuroleptic treatment is only one reason—and a serious one at that—for finding new antipsychotic agents without such side effects. Chronic opiate use does not result in tardive dyskinesia, and overall it is safer than the chronic use of phenothiazine-like drugs. The antiaggressive effect of opiates makes them desirable for the treatment of violent patients. Presently, no effective antiaggression medication is available. Another group of patients who may benefit from opiate therapy are the psychotic depressives who are considered for electroconvulsive therapy but who cannot receive it for medical reasons. Acute psychosis has been treated by opiates successfully by the "street pharmacologists" after "bad trips" caused by hallucinogenic drugs like LSD and phencyclidine (PCP). Similar success was reported for the use of meperidine and morphine for the treatment of PCP-induced psychosis during the first clinical trial of PCP in 1959. It behooves us to test opioids in well-controlled clinical trials for the treatment of acute psychosis, especially in patients who are difficult to manage.

Future research also faces other than social and political obstacles, and these are related to the extremely complex pharmacology of the opiates. It is not unusual to find in the old "opiate-behavioral" literature nearly identical experimental conditions reporting diametrically opposing results. This occurs not because the observations were wrong, but because they were not correlated with the time–action of the particular drug studied. Thus, the drug action that is described in a report may have represented the effects of the drug's *absence* rather than presence, and obviously the two situations are radically different. To further complicate the situation, the following pharmacologic characteristics of opioids make these drugs difficult to study: tolerance, physical dependence, different route of drug administration, different affinity of opiates to the various types of opiate receptors, and, of importance, the individual differences among subjects with respect to both receptors and metabolic characteristics. Thus, in order to produce reliable data, clinical studies must be well planned and monitored by experienced pharmacologists and psychiatrists. Treatment successes should not be statistically eliminated even if only one or two of ten subjects responds. Individual responders to opiate therapy should be thoroughly studied, searching for unique characteristics that may identify such patients objectively in an untreated group.

Although there is a great deal of information present in this volume, it is only the beginning. High-quality research is needed now to develop opiate therapy for the future benefit of the mentally ill. I am certain that the participants in this conference and researchers in this field will meet again, and that the ideas that were present as seeds planted at this conference will grow into a healthy tree of knowledge elucidating the role of opiates in mental illness.

Index of Contributors

(Italicized page numbers refer to comments made in discussion.)

511